T0188139

OXFORD MEDICAL PUBLICATIONS

# Oxford Handbook of
# Rheumatology

## Published and forthcoming Oxford Handbooks

Oxford Handbook for the Foundation Programme 3e
Oxford Handbook of Acute Medicine 3e
Oxford Handbook of Anaesthesia 2e
Oxford Handbook of Applied Dental Sciences
Oxford Handbook of Cardiology
Oxford Handbook of Clinical and Laboratory Investigation 3e
Oxford Handbook of Clinical Dentistry 4e
Oxford Handbook of Clinical Diagnosis 2e
Oxford Handbook of Clinical Examination and Practical Skills
Oxford Handbook of Clinical Haematology 3e
Oxford Handbook of Clinical Immunology and Allergy 2e
Oxford Handbook of Clinical Medicine—Mini Edition 8e
Oxford Handbook of Clinical Medicine 8e
Oxford Handbook of Clinical Pharmacy
Oxford Handbook of Clinical Rehabilitation 2e
Oxford Handbook of Clinical Specialties 8e
Oxford Handbook of Clinical Surgery 3e
Oxford Handbook of Complementary Medicine
Oxford Handbook of Critical Care 3e
Oxford Handbook of Dental Patient Care 2e
Oxford Handbook of Dialysis 3e
Oxford Handbook of Emergency Medicine 4e
Oxford Handbook of Endocrinology and Diabetes 2e
Oxford Handbook of ENT and Head and Neck Surgery
Oxford Handbook of Expedition and Wilderness Medicine
Oxford Handbook of Gastroenterology and Hepatology
Oxford Handbook of General Practice 3e
Oxford Handbook of Genitourinary Medicine, HIV, and Sexual Health 2e
Oxford Handbook of Geriatric Medicine
Oxford Handbook of Infectious Diseases and Microbiology
Oxford Handbook of Key Clinical Evidence
Oxford Handbook of Medical Sciences
Oxford Handbook of Nephrology and Hypertension
Oxford Handbook of Neurology
Oxford Handbook of Nutrition and Dietetics
Oxford Handbook of Obstetrics and Gynaecology 2e
Oxford Handbook of Occupational Health
Oxford Handbook of Oncology 3e
Oxford Handbook of Ophthalmology
Oxford Handbook of Paediatrics
Oxford Handbook of Palliative Care 2e
Oxford Handbook of Practical Drug Therapy 2e
Oxford Handbook of Pre-Hospital Care
Oxford Handbook of Psychiatry 2e
Oxford Handbook of Public Health Practice 2e
Oxford Handbook of Reproductive Medicine and Family Planning
Oxford Handbook of Respiratory Medicine 2e
Oxford Handbook of Rheumatology 3e
Oxford Handbook of Sport and Exercise Medicine
Oxford Handbook of Tropical Medicine 3e
Oxford Handbook of Urology 2e

# Oxford Handbook of
# Rheumatology

**Fourth Edition**

## Gavin Clunie
Consultant Rheumatologist and Metabolic Bone Physician,
Addenbrooke's Hospital, Cambridge, UK

## Nick Wilkinson
Consultant Paediatric and Adolescent Rheumatologist,
Evelina London Children's Hospital, London, UK

## Elena Nikiphorou
Consultant Rheumatologist, Whittington Hospital;
Clinical Researcher, Academic Rheumatology Department,
King's College London, UK

## Deepak Jadon
Consultant Rheumatologist and Director of the
Rheumatology Research Unit,
Addenbrooke's Hospital, Cambridge, UK

OXFORD
UNIVERSITY PRESS

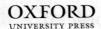

# OXFORD
UNIVERSITY PRESS

Great Clarendon Street, Oxford, OX2 6DP,
United Kingdom

Oxford University Press is a department of the University of Oxford.
It furthers the University's objective of excellence in research, scholarship,
and education by publishing worldwide. Oxford is a registered trade mark of
Oxford University Press in the UK and in certain other countries

© Oxford University Press 2018

The moral rights of the authors have been asserted

First Edition published in 2002
Second Edition published in 2006
Third Edition published in 2011
Fourth Edition published in 2018

Published in the United States of America by Oxford University Press
198 Madison Avenue, New York, NY 10016, United States of America

British Library Cataloguing in Publication Data

Data available

Library of Congress Control Number: 2017960672

ISBN 978–0–19–872825–2

Printed and bound in Turkey by Promat

# Foreword

I am pleased to introduce you to the 4th edition of the *Oxford Handbook of Rheumatology*. This edition has increased in size, but continues to be just as accessible. It presents the reader with a pragmatic approach to making a differential diagnosis. The approach to thinking about how to make sense of the history and clinical findings is clear. The common rheumatological conditions are covered well, and the new edition incorporates relevant sections on paediatric and adolescent rheumatology.

From the days of Sir William Osler, the art of listening to and observing the patient has been a key focus of what defines a good doctor. Medicine has advanced considerably since his day, but the core values of a physician have not changed.

The focus on good clinical history taking and examination technique is a reminder of the core skill set that we use as physicians. When all else fails, go back to the basic principles, and back to the patient. This book shows us how important that skill set is.

Professor Jane Dacre MD, PRCP
President
Royal College of Physicians
London, UK

# Preface

Rheumatic musculoskeletal conditions are common both in general and hospital practice. Musculoskeletal symptoms are a primary feature of many multisystem illnesses, not only in the autoimmune joint and connective tissue diseases, but also metabolic, endocrine, neoplastic, and infectious conditions. Symptoms are also common in the context of injury, age-related change, and psychological distress. Many conditions in rheumatology are a major source of morbidity and mortality.

We have kept the format of the previous edition for this version but importantly have updated the text to include paediatric and adolescent rheumatology.

*Part I* remains as a guide to evaluation of rheumatic and musculoskeletal disease from the point of referral and reflects the way clinical problems/ symptoms present to the clinician in real life. We have considered how this happens for adults, and new in this version, for children and adolescents, affected by rheumatological and musculoskeletal disease. The reader will find detail on musculoskeletal anatomy and functional anatomy in this part of the book.

*Part II* remains as the section of the book where the reader can find disease-specific information (e.g. spondyloarthritis, vasculitis, back pain, and so on). We have included paediatric sections in each chapter where there is relevance for disease occurring in children and adolescents, noting the difference in disease and its management in children and adolescents compared with adults.

*Part III* remains as medicine management and contains chapters on drugs used in rheumatology practice, glucocorticoid injection therapy, and rheumatological emergencies.

We have tried to avoid duplication but cross reference between chapters. We hope this book is helpful and informative for all doctors, physiotherapists, and specialist nursing practitioners who are faced with managing people and patients with undiagnosed musculoskeletal symptoms or established rheumatic musculoskeletal diseases.

# Acknowledgements

The authors would like to acknowledge the work of the co-founder author-editor of the textbook Dr Alan Hakim for his contribution, whom together with Dr Clunie, devised and wrote the book from the first edition and co-author-editor Dr Inam Haq (who joined for the 2nd and 3rd editions), in helping to establish the *Oxford Handbook of Rheumatology* as the market leader small textbook for rheumatology.

# Contents

# Contributors

**Dr Emma Davies**
Specialist Registrar in
Rheumatology, Royal National
Hospital for Rheumatic Diseases,
Bath, UK

**Dr Catherine Fairris**
Specialist Registrar in
Rheumatology, Royal National
Hospital for Rheumatic Diseases,
Bath, UK

**Dr Shabina Habibi**
Senior Clinical Research Fellow,
Royal National Hospital for
Rheumatic Diseases, Bath, UK

**Dr Philip Hamann**
PhD Research Fellow &
Specialist Registrar in
Rheumatology, Royal National
Hospital for Rheumatic Diseases,
Bath, UK

**Dr Dobrina Hull**
Specialist Registrar in
Rheumatology, Guys and
St Thomas' Hospital NHS
Foundation Trust, London, UK

**Dr Eiphyu Htut**
Specialist Registrar in
Rheumatology, Addenbrooke's
Hospital, Cambridge University
Hospitals NHS Foundation Trust,
Cambridge, UK

**Dr Anthony Isaacs**
Specialist Registrar in
Rheumatology, The Whittington
Hospital NHS Trust,
London, UK

**Dr Ritu Malayia**
Specialist Registrar in
Rheumatology, Guys and
St Thomas' Hospital NHS
Foundation Trust, London, UK

**Dr Seraina Palmer**
Fellow in Paediatric
Rheumatology, Kinderspital,
Zürich, Switzerland

**Dr Elizabeth Reilly**
Specialist Registrar in
Rheumatology, Royal National
Hospital for Rheumatic Diseases,
Bath, UK

**Dr Maliha Sheikh**
Specialist Registrar in
Rheumatology, Addenbrooke's
Hospital, Cambridge University
Hospitals NHS Foundation Trust,
Cambridge, UK

**Dr Giulia Varnier**
Fellow in Paediatric
Rheumatology, Evelina London
Children's Hospital, Guys and
St Thomas' Hospital NHS
Foundation Trust, London, UK

**Dr Natasha Weisz**
Specialist Registrar in
Rheumatology, The Whittington
Hospital NHS Trust, London, UK

**Dr Cee Yi Yong**
Specialist Registrar in
Rheumatology, Norfolk and
Norwich University Hospitals
NHS Foundation Trust,
Norwich, UK

# Symbols and abbreviations

| | |
|---|---|
| $\rightarrow$ | cross-reference |
| α | alpha |
| β | beta |
| ↑ | increased |
| ↓ | decreased |
| ↔ | normal |
| > | greater than |
| < | less than |
| ~ | approximately |
| ∴ | therefore |
| AAV | ANCA-associated vasculitis |
| ABA | abatacept |
| AC | adhesive capsulitis |
| ACA | anticentromere antibody |
| ACE | angiotensin-converting enzyme |
| AChA | acrodermatitis chronicum atrophicans |
| AC(J) | acromioclavicular (joint) |
| ACL | anticardiolipin |
| ACPA | anticitrullinated peptide antibody(-ies) |
| ACR | American College of Rheumatology |
| AD | autosomal dominant |
| ADM | abductor digiti minimi |
| AFF | atypical femoral fracture |
| AICTD | autoimmune connective tissue disease |
| AIS | autoinflammatory syndrome |
| AKI | acute kidney injury |
| ALNT | anterolateral neospinothalamic tract |
| ALP | alkaline phosphatase |
| ALT | alanine transaminase |
| AMA | amyloid A |
| AML | amyloid L |
| ANA | antinuclear antibody |
| ANCA | antineutrophil cytoplasmic antibody |
| Anti-β2GP1 | anti-β2 glycoprotein-1 |
| AOSD | adult-onset Still's disease |
| AP | anteroposterior |

| APB | abductor pollicis brevis |
| APL | abductor pollicis longus |
| APL | antiphospholipid |
| APRIL | a proliferation inducing-ligand |
| APS | antiphospholipid (antibody) syndrome |
| APTT | activated partial thromboplastin time |
| AR | autosomal recessive |
| ARA | American Rheumatism Association |
| ARB | angiotensin II receptor blocker |
| ARDS | adult respiratory distress syndrome |
| ARTEMIS | Abatacept Treatment in Polymyositis and Dermatomyositis trial |
| AS | ankylosing spondylitis |
| ASAS | Assessment of Spondyloarthritis International Society |
| AST | aspartate transaminase |
| ASOT | antistreptolysin O titre |
| ASU | avocado/soybean unsaponifiable |
| ATN | acute tubular necrosis |
| axSpA | axial spondyloarthritis |
| AZA | azathioprine |
| β2GP1 | β2 glycoprotein-1 |
| BAFF | B-cell activating factor (see also BLyS) |
| BAL | bronchoalveolar lavage |
| BCP | basic calcium phosphate (crystals) |
| BD | Behçet's disease |
| bDMARD | biologic disease-modifying antirheumatic drug |
| BILAG | British Isles Lupus Assessment Group |
| BLyS | B-lymphocyte stimulator (see also BAFF) |
| BMC | bone mineral content |
| BMD | bone mineral density |
| BMI | body mass index |
| BSR | British Society of Rheumatology |
| BVAS | Birmingham Vasculitis Activity Score |
| C | cervical (e.g. C6 is the sixth cervical vertebra) |
| CA | coracoacromial |
| CADM | clinically amyopathic dermatomyositis |
| CAMPS | CARD14-mediated psoriasis |
| CANDLE | chronic atypical neutrophilic dermatosis with lipodystrophy and elevated temperature |
| cAPS | catastrophic antiphospholipid syndrome |
| CAPS | cryopyrin-associated periodic fever syndromes |

| CARD | caspase activation and recruitment domain |
| CBT | cognitive and behavioural therapy |
| CCP | cyclic citrullinated peptide |
| CDAI | Clinical Disease Activity Index |
| CHB | congenital heart block |
| CHCC | Chapel Hill Consensus Conference |
| CINCA | chronic, infantile, neurological, cutaneous, and articular syndrome |
| CK | creatine kinase |
| CKD | chronic kidney disease |
| CMC(J) | carpometacarpal (joint) |
| CMP | comprehensive metabolic panel |
| CMV | cytomegalovirus |
| CNO | chronic non-bacterial osteomyelitis |
| CNS | central nervous system |
| COMP | cartilage oligomeric matrix protein |
| COX | cyclooxygenase |
| CPP | calcium pyrophosphate |
| CPPD | calcium pyrophosphate deposition |
| CREST | calcinosis, Raynaud's, (o)esophageal dysmotility, sclerodactyly, telangiectasia (syndrome) |
| CRMO | chronic recurrent multifocal osteomyelitis |
| CRP | C-reactive protein |
| CRPS | complex regional pain syndrome |
| CS | congenital scoliosis |
| CSF | cerebrospinal fluid |
| CT | computed tomography |
| CTX | collagen X-link |
| cTnC | cardiac troponin C |
| cTnT | cardiac troponin T |
| CTS | carpal tunnel syndrome |
| CWP | chronic widespread pain |
| CXR | chest radiograph |
| CYC | cyclophosphamide |
| DAS | Disease Activity Score |
| dcSScl | diffuse cutaneous systemic sclerosis |
| DIC | diffuse intravascular coagulation |
| DILE | drug-induced lupus erythematosus |
| DIP(J) | distal interphalangeal (joint) |
| DIRA | deficiency of IL-1 receptor agonist |
| DISH | diffuse idiopathic skeletal hyperostosis |

| DITRA | deficiency of interleukin 36 receptor antagonist |
| DLCO | diffusion capacity for carbon monoxide |
| DOMS | delayed-onset muscular strain |
| DM | dermatomyositis |
| DMARD | disease-modifying antirheumatic drug |
| DVT | deep vein thrombosis |
| DXA | dual-energy X-ray absorptiometry |
| EA | enteropathic arthritis |
| EANM | European Association of Nuclear Medicine |
| EBV | Epstein–Barr virus |
| ECG | electrocardiogram |
| ECM | erythema chronicum migrans |
| ECRB | extensor carpi radialis brevis |
| ECRL | extensor carpi radialis longus |
| ECU | extensor carpi ulnaris |
| ED | extensor digitorum |
| EDL | extensor digitorum longus |
| EDM | extensor digiti minimi |
| EDS | Ehlers–Danlos syndrome |
| EED | erythema elevatum dictinum |
| EHL | extensor hallucis longus |
| EI | extensor indicis |
| EGPA | eosinophilic granulomatosis and polyangiitis |
| ELISA | enzyme-linked immunosorbent assay |
| ELMS | Eaton–Lambert myasthenic syndrome |
| EM | erythema migrans |
| EMG | electromyography |
| EN | erythema nodosum |
| ENA | extractable nuclear antigen |
| ENT | ear, nose, and throat |
| EPB | extensor pollicis brevis |
| EPL | extensor pollicis longus |
| ERA | enthesitis-related arthritis |
| ESR | erythrocyte sedimentation rate |
| ESSG | European Spondyloarthropathy Study Group |
| EULAR | European League Against Rheumatism |
| F | female |
| FBC | full blood count |
| FCAS | familial cold autoinflammatory syndrome |
| FCR | flexor carpi radialis |

| FCU | flexor carpi ulnaris |
| FD | fibrous dysplasia |
| FDA | Food and Drug Administration |
| $^{18}$F-FDG | fluorine-18 fluorodeoxyglucose |
| FDL | flexor digitorum longus |
| FDP | flexor digitorum profundus |
| FDS | flexor digitorum superficialis |
| FENa | fractional excretion of sodium |
| FFS | Five-Factor Score |
| FGF | fibroblast growth factor |
| FHB | flexor hallucis brevis |
| FHH | familial hypocalciuric hypercalcaemia |
| FJ | facet joint |
| FLS | Fracture Liaison Service |
| FM | fibromyalgia |
| FMF | familial Mediterranean fever |
| FPL | flexor pollicis longus |
| FR | flexor retinaculum |
| FVSG | French Vasculitis Study Group |
| GALS | gait, arms, legs, spine (examination) |
| GARA | gut-associated reactive arthritis |
| GBS | Guillain–Barré syndrome |
| GC | glucocorticoid |
| GCA | giant cell arteritis |
| GFR | glomerular filtration rate |
| GH(J) | glenohumeral (joint) |
| GI | gastrointestinal |
| GIO | glucocorticoid-induced osteoporosis |
| GLA | gamma linoleic acid |
| GOA | generalized osteoarthritis |
| GORD | gastro-oesophageal reflux disease |
| HA | hydroxyapatite |
| HAQ | Health Assessment Questionnaire |
| HCQ | hydroxychloroquine |
| HDCT | hereditary disorder of connective tissue |
| h-EDS | hypermobility (type) Ehlers–Danlos syndrome |
| HELLP | haemolysis, elevated liver enzymes, and low platelets |
| HIDS | hyper IgD syndrome |
| HIV | human immunodeficiency virus |
| HLA | human leucocyte antigen |

| HMG-COA | 3-hydroxy-3-methyl-glutaryl-coenzyme A |
| --- | --- |
| HPOA | hypertrophic pulmonary osteoarthropathy |
| HPT | hyperparathyroidism |
| HRT | hormone replacement therapy |
| HSCT | haematopoietic stem cell transplantation |
| HSP | Henoch–Schönlein purpura |
| HUS | haemolytic uraemic syndrome |
| HTLV | human T-cell leukaemia virus |
| IA | intra-articular |
| IBD | inflammatory bowel disease |
| IBM | inclusion-body myositis |
| ICD | implantable cardioverter defibrillator |
| IFN | interferon |
| IgG4-RD | immunoglobulin G4-related disease |
| IGRA | interferon gamma release assay |
| IIM | idiopathic inflammatory myopathy |
| IL | interleukin |
| ILAR | International League of Associations for Rheumatology |
| ILD | interstitial lung disease |
| IM | intramuscular(ly) |
| IMM | idiopathic inflammatory myopathy |
| INR | international normalized ratio |
| IP | interphalangeal |
| ISCD | International Society of Clinical Densitometry |
| ISG | International Study Group |
| ISN | International Society for Nephrology |
| ITB | iliotibial band |
| IV | intravenous(ly) |
| IVDU | intravenous drug user |
| IVIg | intravenous immunoglobulin |
| JAK | Janus kinase |
| JAS | juvenile ankylosing spondylitis |
| JCA | juvenile chronic arthritis |
| JDM | juvenile dermatomyositis |
| JIA | juvenile idiopathic arthritis |
| JIIM | juvenile idiopathic inflammatory arthritis |
| JIO | juvenile idiopathic osteoporosis |
| JPM | juvenile polymyositis |
| JPsA | juvenile psoriatic arthritis |
| JRA | juvenile rheumatoid arthritis |

| JSLE | juvenile systemic lupus erythematosus |
| JSpA | juvenile spondyloarthritis |
| KD | Kawasaki disease |
| KUB | kidney ureter bladder |
| L | lumbar (e.g. L5 is the fifth lumbar vertebra) |
| LA | lupus anticoagulant |
| LCL | lateral collateral ligament |
| lcSScl | limited cutaneous systemic sclerosis |
| LDA | low-dose aspirin (75–150 mg/day) |
| LDH | lactate dehydrogenase |
| LE | lupus erythematosus |
| LEF | leflunomide |
| LFTs | liver function tests |
| LGL | large granular lymphocyte |
| LH | luteinizing hormone |
| LHE | lateral humeral epicondylitis |
| LIP | lymphocytic interstitial pneumonitis |
| LLLT | low-level laser therapy |
| LMWH | low-molecular-weight heparin |
| M | male |
| MAA | myositis-associated autoantibodies |
| MAGIC | mouth and genital ulcers with inflamed cartilage |
| MAS | macrophage activation syndrome |
| MCL | medial collateral ligament |
| MCP(J) | metacarpophalangeal (joint) |
| MCTD | mixed connective tissue disease |
| MDI | Myositis Disease Index |
| MDP | methylene diphosphonate |
| MDT | multidisciplinary team |
| MEN | mycophenolate mofetil |
| MEVK | mevalonate kinase |
| MFS | Marfan syndrome |
| MG | myasthenia gravis |
| MHC | major histocompatibility complex |
| MKD | mevalonate kinase deficiency |
| MMF | mycophenolate mofetil |
| MMPI | Minnesota Multiphasic Personality Inventory |
| MMT | manual muscle test |
| mNY | modified New York |
| MPA | microscopic polyangiitis |

| MPO | myeloperoxidase |
| MR | magnetic resonance |
| MRA | magnetic resonance angiography |
| MRI | magnetic resonance imaging |
| MSA | myositis-specific autoantibodies |
| MSK | musculoskeletal |
| MSU | monosodium urate |
| MTP(J) | metatarsophalangeal (joint) |
| MTX | methotrexate |
| MUA | manipulation under anaesthesia |
| MVA | mevalonic aciduria |
| MVK | mevalonate kinase |
| MWS | Muckle–Wells syndrome |
| MYOACT | myositis disease activity index |
| MYODAM | myositis damage index |
| NAI | non-accidental injury |
| NCS | nerve conduction study |
| NICE | National Institute for Health and Care Excellence (UK) |
| NLE | neonatal lupus erythematosus |
| NLRs | NOD-like receptors |
| NMS | neuromuscular scoliosis |
| NO | nitrous oxide |
| NOAC | novel oral anticoagulant |
| NOD | nucleotide-binding oligomerization domain |
| NOMID | neonatal-onset multisystem inflammatory disease |
| NSAID | non-steroidal anti-inflammatory drug |
| NSF | nephrogenic systemic fibrosis |
| OA | osteoarthritis |
| OI | osteogenesis imperfecta |
| OMIN | Online Mendelian Inheritance in Man |
| ONFH | osteonecrosis of the femoral head |
| OO | osteoid osteoma |
| OT | occupational therapist |
| PAH | pulmonary artery hypertension |
| PAMPS | pathogen-associated molecular patterns |
| PAN | polyarteritis nodosum |
| PAPA | pyogenic arthritis, pyoderma gangrenosum, and acne |
| PBC | primary biliary cirrhosis |
| PCR | polymerase chain reaction |
| PDB | Paget's disease of bone |

| PDE5 | phosphodiesterase type 5 |
| PE | pulmonary embolism |
| PET | positron emission tomography |
| PFAPA | periodic fever, aphthous stomatitis, pharyngitis, adenitis syndrome |
| PHP | pseudohypoparathyroidism |
| PIN | posterior interosseous nerve |
| PIP(J) | proximal interphalangeal (joint) |
| PL | palmaris longus |
| PM | polymyositis |
| PML | progressive multifocal leucoencephalopathy |
| PMN | polymorphonuclear neutrophil |
| PMR | polymyalgia rheumatica |
| PoTS | postural orthostatic tachycardia syndrome |
| PRR | pattern-recognition receptor |
| Ps | psoriasis |
| PsA | psoriatic arthritis |
| PSA | prostatic-specific antigen |
| PTH | parathyroid hormone |
| PUO | pyrexia of unknown origin |
| PV | plasma viscosity |
| PVNS | pigmented villonodular synovitis |
| RA | rheumatoid arthritis |
| RAID | rare autoinflammatory disease |
| RAPS | rivaroxaban for antiphospholipid antibody syndrome |
| RCT | randomized controlled trial |
| RD | Raynaud's disease |
| ReA | reactive arthritis |
| RF | rheumatoid factor |
| RhF | rheumatic fever |
| RNA | ribonucleic acid |
| RNP | ribonuclear protein |
| ROD | renal osteodystrophy |
| RP | relapsing polychondritis |
| RPS | Renal Pathology Society |
| RSD | reflex sympathetic dystrophy (algo/osteodystrophy) |
| RSI | repetitive strain injury |
| RS$_3$PE | remitting seronegative symmetrical synovitis with pitting oedema |
| RTA | renal tubular acidosis |

| RTX | rituximab |
| --- | --- |
| sACE | serum angiotensin converting enzyme |
| SAI | subacromial impingement |
| SAA | serum amyloid A |
| SADAI | Simplified Disease Activity Index |
| SAPHO | synovitis, acne, palmoplantar pustulosis, hyperostosis, aseptic osteomyelitis (syndrome) |
| SARA | sexually acquired reactive arthritis |
| SC | subcutaneous |
| SC(J) | sternoclavicular (joint) |
| Scl | systemic scleroderma |
| SCS | spinal cord stimulation |
| SD | standard deviation |
| sDMARD | synthetic disease-modifying antirheumatic drug |
| SERM | selective oestrogen receptor modulator |
| SHPT | secondary hyperparathyroidism |
| SI(J) | sacroiliac (joint) |
| SIP | Sickness Impact Profile |
| SLE | systemic lupus erythematosus |
| SLEDAI | Systemic Lupus Erythematosus Disease Activity Index |
| SLICC | Systemic Lupus International Collaborating criteria |
| SNRI | serotonin-norepinephrine re-uptake inhibitors |
| SoJIA | systemic-onset juvenile idiopathic arthritis |
| SpA | spondyloarthritis |
| SRC | scleroderma renal crisis |
| SRP | signal recognition peptide |
| SS | Sjögren's syndrome |
| SScl | systemic sclerosis |
| SSRI | selective serotonin reuptake inhibitor |
| SSZ | sulfasalazine |
| STIR | short tau inversion recovery |
| SUA | serum uric acid |
| SUFE | slipped upper femoral epiphysis |
| T | thoracic (e.g. T5 is the fifth thoracic vertebra) |
| TA | Takayasu arteritis |
| TB | tuberculosis |
| TCZ | tocilizumab |
| TENS | transcutaneous electrical nerve stimulation |
| TFT | thyroid function test |
| TGF | transferring growth factor |

| | |
|---|---|
| TIA | transient ischaemic attack |
| TLRs | Toll-like receptors |
| TM(J) | temporomandibular (joint) |
| TNFα | tumour necrosis factor (alpha) |
| tPA | tissue plasminogen activator |
| TPMT | thiopurine S-methyltransferase |
| TRAPS | tumour necrosis factor-associated periodic syndrome |
| TSH | thyroid-stimulating hormone |
| TTP | thrombotic thrombocytopenic purpura |
| U&E | urea and electrolytes (in UK test includes creatinine) |
| UC | ulcerative colitis |
| uPCR | urine protein:creatinine ratio |
| US | ultrasound |
| UV | ultraviolet |
| VAS | visual analogue scale |
| VDI | Vasculitis Damage Index |
| vs | versus |
| WBC | white blood cell |
| WHO | World Health Organization |
| WRD | work-related disorder |
| XLHR | X-linked hypophosphataemic rickets |

# Part I

# The presentation of rheumatic disease

# Evaluating rheumatological and musculoskeletal symptoms

# Introduction

Adults and children can present with musculoskeletal (MSK), inflammatory, and autoimmune diseases in varied ways. Symptoms can be simple and focal, such as regional pain, or general and non-specific, often in the context of a generalized process such as fever or fatigue. The following are important points in assessing the time, type, and nature of presentation:

- Why someone has presented at a particular time.
- What is the impact of symptoms, emotionally and functionally.
- The individual's perceptions, fears, or cultural references that might modify (amplify or suppress) expression of the symptoms.
- What fears, beliefs, and factors might present a barrier to effective medical engagement.
- The same pathological processes might present variably at different ages: broadly speaking, the young, adults, and the elderly.

In this chapter, the assessment of symptoms has been separated into two parts. First, the assessment of symptoms in adults and second, the patterns of disease presentation in children and adolescents.

# Musculoskeletal pain in adults

## Introduction

The most common presenting symptom to the rheumatologist is unexplained or ineffectively treated MSK pain.

- Pain is defined by its subjective description, which may vary depending on its physical (or biological) cause, the patient's understanding of it, its impact on function, and the emotional and behavioural response it invokes.
- Pain is particularly prone to be 'coloured' by cultural, linguistic, and religious differences. Therefore, pain is not merely an unpleasant sensation to many; it is, in effect, an 'emotional change'.
- Pain experience is different for every individual.

## Localization of pain

Adults usually localize pain accurately, although there are some situations worth noting in rheumatic disease where pain can be poorly localized (Table 1.1):

- Adults may not clearly differentiate between periarticular and articular pain, referring to bursitis, tendonitis, and other forms of soft tissue injury as 'joint pain'. Therefore, it is important to confirm the precise location of the pain on physical examination.
- Pain may be well localized but caused by a distant lesion, e.g. interscapular pain caused by mechanical problems in the cervical spine, or right shoulder pain caused by acute cholecystitis.
- Pain caused by neurological abnormalities, ischaemic pain, and pain referred from viscera is harder for the patient to visualize or express, and the history may be given with varied interpretations.
- Bone pain is generally constant despite movement or change in posture—unlike muscular, synovial, ligament, or tendon pain—and often disturbs sleep. Fracture, tumour, and metabolic bone disease are all possible causes. Such constant, local, sleep-disturbing pain should always be investigated.

**Table 1.1** Clinical pointers in conditions in adults where pain is poorly localized

| Diagnosis | Clinical pointer |
| --- | --- |
| Periarticular shoulder pain | Referred to deltoid insertion—not specific for lesion but typical in rotator cuff lesions |
| Carpal tunnel syndrome | Nocturnal paraesthesias and/or pain, often diffuse—patients often report symptoms in all fingers but detailed assessment then is needed to disclose 5th finger sparing |
| Insertional gluteus medius tendonitis/enthesitis | Nocturnal pain lying on affected side |
| Hip synovitis | Groin/outer thigh pain radiating to the knee |

- Patterns of pain distribution are associated with certain MSK conditions. For example, polymyalgia rheumatica (PMR) typically affects the shoulder girdle and hips, whereas rheumatoid arthritis (RA) affects the joints symmetrically, with a predilection for the hands and feet.
- Patterns of pain distribution may overlap, especially in the elderly, who may have several conditions simultaneously, e.g. hip and/or knee osteoarthritis (OA), peripheral vascular disease, and degenerative lumbar spine all may cause lower extremity discomfort.

## The quality of pain

Some individuals find it hard to describe pain or use descriptors of severity. A description of the quality of pain can often help to discriminate the cause. Certain pain descriptors in adults are associated with non-organic pain syndromes (Table 1.2):

- Burning pain, hyperpathia (i.e. an exaggerated response to painful stimuli), and allodynia (i.e. pain from stimuli that are normally not painful) suggest a neurological or central 'pain sensitization' cause.
- A change in the description of pain in a patient with a long-standing condition is worth noting, since it may denote the presence of a second condition, e.g. a fracture or septic arthritis in a patient with established RA.
- Repeated, embellished, or elaborate descriptions ('catastrophizing') may suggest non-organic pain, but be aware that such a presentation may be cultural. Such descriptions may associate with illness behaviour in the consultation or during the examination.

**Table 1.2** Terms from the McGill pain scale that help distinguish between organic and non-organic pain syndromes (adults)

| Organic | Non-organic |
| --- | --- |
| Pounding | Flickering |
| Jumping | Shooting |
| Pricking | Lancinating ('shooting') |
| Sharp | Lacerating |
| Pinching | Crushing |
| Hot | Searing |
| Tender | Splitting |
| Nagging | Torturing |
| Spreading | Piercing |
| Annoying | Unbearable |
| Tiring | Exhausting |
| Fearful | Terrifying |
| Tight | Tearing |

## Pain from trauma/damage to tissues ('mechanical') in adults

In general, mechanical disorders are worsened by activity and relieved by rest. This does not mean pain is not present at rest; in severe mechanical/ degenerative disorders, pain disturbs sleep.

- A good knowledge of anatomy and functional anatomy should allow localization of affected structures though localization of pains in young children can be difficult.
- An appreciation of secondary muscle spasm is important as such pain can mask, to a degree, localization of a mechanical pain, particularly in the back.

## Inflammatory musculoskeletal pain in adults

Inflammatory lesions causing pain typically do so with or after immobility, such as when getting out of bed or after a long car journey.

- Inflammatory MSK pain is often described with 'stiffness'.
- Inflammatory joint pains from RA, inflammatory OA and peripheral joint disease in psoriatic arthropathy (PsA) or axial spondyloarthritis (axSpA) can be present on waking and ease with joint movement.
- An assessment of inflammatory back pain is a key assessment in a young adult with back pain (pain at night, pain/stiffness in the early morning easing with movement; resolution or significant improvement with non-steroidal anti-inflammatory drugs (NSAIDs); associated posterior pelvic/buttock pains of similar quality and description); axSpA needs to be ruled out.

# Elicited pain on examination in adults

In adults, eliciting pain or discomfort by the use of different examination techniques may be used to provide clues to the diagnosis:

- Palpation and comparison of active and passive range of motion can be used to reproduce pain and localize pathology. This requires practice and a good knowledge of anatomy.
- Many of the classic physical exam signs and manoeuvres have a high degree of inter-observer variability. Interpretation should take into account the context in which the examination is done and the effects of suggestibility.
- Palpation and passive range of motion exercises are performed while the patient is relaxed.
- The concept of 'passive' movement is the assumption that when the patient is completely relaxed, the muscles and tendons around the joint are removed as potential sources of pain; in theory, passive range of motion is limited only by pain at the true joint. This assumption has its own limitations, however, since passive movements of the joint will still cause some movement of the soft tissues. In some cases (e.g. shoulder rotator cuff disease), the joint may be painful to move passively because of subluxation or impingement due to a musculotendinous lesion.
- The clinician should be aware of myofascial pain when palpating musculotendinous structures, especially around the neck and shoulder regions. Myofascial pain is said to occur when there is activation of a trigger point that elicits pain in a zone stereotypical for the individual muscle. It is often aching in nature.
- Trigger points are associated with palpable tender bands. It is not clear whether trigger points are the same as the tender points characteristic of fibromyalgia.
- Some lesions may cause pain primarily on movement and may not be amenable to disclosure from static palpation (e.g. enthesitis). Do not dismiss the report of focal pain (or think of it as referred only) if there is no tenderness at the site on static examination. Pain may only occur with tissue function/movement.
- Local anaesthetic infiltration at the site of a painful structure is sometimes used to help localize pathology, e.g. injection under the acromion may provide substantial relief from a 'shoulder impingement syndrome'. However, the technique is reliable only if localization of the injected anaesthetic can be guaranteed. Few, if any, rigorously controlled trials have shown it to give specific results for any condition.
- Always complete a regional MSK examination by examining the adjacent more proximal structures/joint. Typically, patterns of pain referral extend distally so problems at one joint can cause symptoms in the area of the adjacent distal joint.

# Other presenting symptoms in adults

## Stiffness

Stiffness is a common presenting symptom of MSK rheumatological disease. It may be a manifestation of inflammation or reduced movement due to mechanical pathology including swelling, or be used by an individual to describe reduced movement due to pain

- Stiffness is often worse after a period of rest. Short periods (<30 min) of stiffness that persist after mobilizing is not a meaningful observation. Stiffness lasting >30 min and often several hours after mobilizing is a typical symptom of inflammatory arthritis.
- Stiffness can occur in normal joints. Individuals typically click or crack their joints to stretch the tissues and gain relief.
- Stiffness may be a manifestation of tissue fibrosis; in tendons, for example, fibrosis may cause nodules to form that in their most extreme lead to locking or triggering.
- Swelling may arise as a result of synovitis in a joint or tendon, oedema, cellulitis, haematoma or varicosities, ganglia (common around the wrist), tophi (fingers, toes), cysts, or nodules (e.g. RA nodules over elbows, or nodules in fascia as in Dupuytren's in the hand).

## Swelling

- The report of swelling has shown to be unreliable in many instances. Regard 'swelling' as a sign on examination unless the description of it as a symptom is convincing and the story has been elicited very carefully.
- Nerve compression or irritation can often be perceived as swelling (think of how your lip feels—but isn't—after a dental anaesthetic i.e. swollen!) and can colour the reporting of carpal tunnel syndrome symptom.

## Clunks, snaps, and clicks

- 'Clicks' are often the focus of symptom reports and can cause some anxiety. However, 'clicks' from many different structures are not specific for 'pathology'.
- Induced snaps like cracking knuckles are usually noises created from the quick expansion of gas/air within a confined space.
- 'Clunks', however, may denote structural loss of integrity (e.g. femoroacetabular impingement, multidirectional instability of shoulder in hypermobile Ehlers–Danlos syndrome (EDS)) and are arguably then more likely to be associated with 'pathology' compared with 'clicks'.

## Constitutional symptoms

Fatigue, fevers, sweats, and excessive sweating sometimes occur with many different rheumatological diseases.

- It is key to ascertain what is meant by fatigue, differentiating it from lack of sleep, deconditioning, or specific muscle weakness.
- Fatigue is experienced by many patients in association with systemic illness, anaemia, endocrinopathy, or metabolic pathology but also from more insidious (psychosocial influenced) processes such as frustration, stress, and anxiety or as a consequence of disturbed sleep.

- Fatigue often has to be interrogated as sometimes patients won't report it, thinking it is part of ageing, or because of their stage in life (e.g. menopause), or because of their work pattern.
- Fevers and sweats can, on the face of it, suggest systemic infection, but these symptoms can be associated with autoimmune connective tissue diseases particularly systemic lupus erythematosus (SLE), and in systemic vasculitis and severe cases of crystal-induced inflammatory disease (e.g. gout).
- Flushes are often drug induced but are often used to describe generalized vascular reactivity or a response to tachycardia or other symptoms (secondary effects).
- Excessive sweating is associated with glucocorticoid (GC) use, generalized inflammatory diseases such as giant cell arteritis (GCA) and autoimmune conditions such as SLE. True hyperhidrosis is associated with acne and SAPHO (synovitis, acne, palmoplantar pustulosis, hyperostosis, aseptic osteomyelitis) syndrome.

## Rashes

There are many rheumatological conditions that are manifest in part by rashes. The association may be temporally related or separate in time so a broad view of the history of the rash needs to be taken. The latter is exceptionally important for the diagnosis of psoriasis disease.

- Erythematous rashes occur with viral arthritis, with SLE (as urticarias) and adult-onset Still's disease (AOSD) typically.
- Acne or acneiform rashes can occur in SAPHO syndrome, Behçet's disease, and psoriasis disease.
- Pustules occur in a form of psoriasis disease, can denote gonococcal disease in the right clinical context, and are a hallmark lesion of vasculitides (with palpable purpura).
- Livedo reticularis is a key feature of SLE but most notably antiphospholipid syndrome (APS). It can be severe enough to cause a localized vasculitis.
- A brawny, violaceous, slightly raised, confluent, skin eruption is typical of dermatomyositis (upper trunk, periorbital, and backs of hands typically).
- Psoriasis is notoriously varied and differs particularly in relation to where it is. An atlas of typical psoriasis appearances is a very useful tool in the rheumatology clinic.

# The adult gait, arms, legs, spine (GALS) screening examination

As an introduction to a general MSK examination it is helpful to be familiar with the GALS screen,[1] designed to quickly identify the regions of the body functionally affected. Table 1.3 and Fig. 1.1, and Table 1.4 and Fig. 1.2 demonstrate this process in text and visual format.[2]

- The numbering in Table 1.3 corresponds with that in Fig. 1.1.
- Table 1.4 documents the verbal commands required in Fig 1.2.

The adult GALS and paediatric GALS (pGALS) examination screens are valuable, quick assessment tools for identifying sites of major MSK abnormalities and function before entering into a more detailed physical examination.

The adult GALS screen is summarized in Table 1.4. The pGALS screen (video format) is detailed at: ✍ http://www.arthritisresearchuk.org/health-professionals-and-students/video-resources/pgals.aspx

**Table 1.3** Examination in adults—general inspection

| Position | Observation |
|---|---|
| *Observe from the front:* | |
| 1 Neck | Abnormal flexion (torticollis, effect of kyphosis) |
| 2 Shoulder | Muscle bulk across the chest, shoulder swelling, acromioclavicular joint OA, chest deformities |
| 3 Elbow | Full (or hyper) extension, joint swelling, nodules |
| 4 Pelvis | Level—tilted lower on one side may be leg length difference or spinal curvature (scoliosis) |
| 5 Quadriceps | Muscle bulk |
| 6 Knee | Alignment—bow-legged (varus deformity) or knock-kneed (valgus deformity); swelling above patella (synovitis) |
| 7 Midfoot | Swelling, operation scars |
| | Loss of midfoot arch—flat feet |
| *Observe from the back:* | |
| 8 Shoulder | Muscle bulk across deltoid, trapezius, and scapular muscles |
| 9 Spine alignment | Scoliosis/kyphosis |
| 10 Gluteal | Muscle bulk/pelvic asymmetry |
| 11 Knee | Swelling |
| 12 Calf | Muscle bulk, swelling |
| 13 Hindfoot | Out-turning (eversion) of the heel associated with flat-foot |
| | Achilles tendon swelling |
| *Observe from the side:* | |
| 14 Spine alignment | Cervical—normal lordosis; dorsal/thoracic—normal kyphosis; lumbar—normal lordosis |
| 15 Knee | Excessive extension—hypermobility |

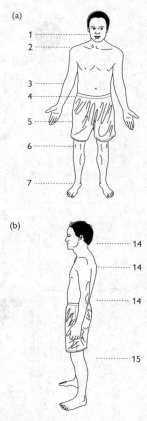

**Fig. 1.1** Physical examination—general inspection. Measure lumbar flexion using the Schöber test. With the patient standing upright, make a horizontal mark across the sacral dimples and a second mark over the spine 10 cm above. The patient then bends forward as far as possible. Re-measure the distance between the marks. It should increase from 10 to >15 cm; less suggests restriction. Adapted from Houghton AR, Gray D. (2010) *Chamberlain's Symptoms and Signs in Clinical Medicine: An Introduction to Medical Diagnosis*, 13th edition. Hodder Arnold, London.

(c)

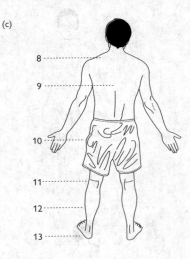

8
9
10
11
12
13

(d)

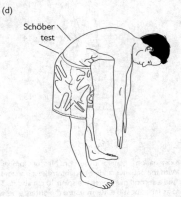

Schöber test

**Fig. 1.1** (Continued).

**Table 1.4** Physical examination screening tool—gait, arms, legs, and spine (GALS) in adults

| Position | Observation/action | Cue to patient for active movements |
|---|---|---|
| **Gait and spine** Patient standing Active (patient-initiated) movements | **Gait:** smooth movement, arm swing, pelvic tilt, normal stride length, ability to turn quickly | 'Walk to the end of the room, turn, and walk back to me' |
| | **Lumbar spine:** | |
| | Lumbar forward flexion | 'Bend forward and touch your knees/ankles/toes' |
| | Lumbar lateral flexion | 'Place your hands by your side; bend to the side running your hand down the outside of your leg toward your knee' |
| | Trendelenburg test. If opposite side of the pelvis drops below the horizontal, suggests weakness of the hip abductors on the weight-bearing leg | 'Stand on one leg . . . now the other' |
| **Neck and thoracic spine** Patient sitting facing you Active (patient-initiated) movements | **Neck:** smooth movement, no pain/stiffness | |
| | Forward flexion | 'Put your chin to your chest' |
| | Side flexion | 'Tip your ear onto your shoulder' |
| | Extension | 'Tilt your head back' |
| | Rotation | 'Turn your head onto your shoulder' |
| | **Thoracic spine:** smooth movement, no pain/stiffness | |
| | 1) Lateral chest expansion | |
| | 2) Rotation | 'Fold your arms, turn body to the . . .' |
| **Hands, wrists, elbows, and shoulders** Patient sitting facing you Active (patient-initiated) movements and palpation | **Hand, wrist, finger:** swelling deformity | 'Place both hands out in front, palms down and fingers straight' |
| | **Hand pronation:** observe palms and grip function | 'Turn the hands over, palms up'—'make a fist' |
| | Gently squeeze the MCP joints by compressing the row of joints together. Assess for pain. Feel for warmth. Look for operation scars | 'Place palms of hands together as if to pray, with elbows out to the side' |
| | Wrist extension and flexion | 'With the elbows in the same position place the hands back to back with the fingers pointing down' |
| | **Elbows:** look for nodules, rash | 'Bend your elbows bringing your hands up to your shoulders' |
| | **Shoulders:** Abduction to 180° | 'Raise arms sideways, up to point at the ceiling' |
| | Rotation | 'Touch the small of your back' |

*(Continued)*

**Table 1.4** (*Contd.*)

| Position | Observation/action | Cue to patient for active movements |
|---|---|---|
| Hips, knees, and ankles | **Hips:** lift leg (bended knee) and position upper leg vertical. Rotate lower leg | |
| Patient supine on couch | **Knees:** | |
| Passive examination of hips and knees | Flex and extend knee feeling the patella with palm of hand for 'crepitus' and with back of hand for warmth | |
| Some active movements | Feel back of the knee, calf, and Achilles tendon for pain and swelling | |
| | **Ankles and feet:** gently squeeze the MTP joints by compressing the forefoot. Assess for pain. | 'Turn your ankles in a circular motion' 'Now up and down' 'Wiggle your toes' |

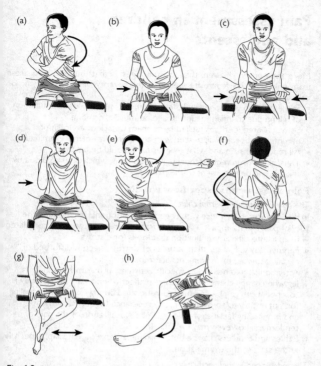

**Fig. 1.2** Physical examination screening manoeuvres. Adapted from Houghton AR, Gray D. (2010) *Chamberlain's Symptoms and Signs in Clinical Medicine: An Introduction to Medical Diagnosis*, 13th edition. Hodder Arnold, London.

## References

1. Doherty M, Dacre P, Dieppe P, Snaith M. The 'GALS' locomotor screen. *Ann Rheum Dis* 1992;51:1165–9.
2. Hakim AJ. The musculoskeletal system. In: Houghton AR, Gray D (eds), *Chamberlain's Symptoms and Signs in Clinical Medicine*, 13 ed. London: Hodder Arnold, 2010.

# Pain assessment in children and adolescents

## Introduction

More apparent in children, than at other ages, is that the level of distress from pain does not correlate well with the severity of the underlying or causative pathology.

- Some children will complain little of pain, but 'silently' lose the function of a limb due to inflammation of a joint, muscle, or bone.
- Some children, perhaps fuelled by concern or lack of concern of a parent, may become distressed with an essentially normal examination.
- All reports of pain and what relieves pain should be believed.
- Thus, all children require thorough assessment, which here is guided by the age and development of the patient.

## Pain assessment in specific scenarios

### The non- or minimally verbal child

In the very young, or those with cognitive or emotional impairment, the history of pain and its impact is sought from the parent or carer and correlated with an astute clinical examination that looks for distress.

- Parents may volunteer that, at times of distress, sleep is disturbed or certain activities or movements are impaired.
- Attention should be paid to specific activities such as movement of a leg when nappy changing or change in affect when a part of the body is touched. Both can be carefully corroborated during examination feeling for, but not trying to overcome, any resistance to joint movement and monitoring facial expressions. Precise localization of the pain or tenderness, however, may be difficult.
- Babies and toddlers may be better examined on a parent's lap, especially at the start of the examination.

### The toddler and school-aged child

- Children from <3 years old can volunteer helpful information and attempts to engage them in friendly discussion will provide reassurance before examination.
- Engagement of the young child is also optimized with an appropriate environment that includes freely accessible toys, a play specialist, and relaxed parents who feel they have been heard.
- Young children might not understand the word pain and parents may help in the choice of language. Use of a picture or cuddly toy may help to localize the site of pain and the use of the Faces Pain Scale is a standard tool to indicate pain intensity, see: ℘ http://www.iasp-pain. org/Education/Content.aspx?ItemNumber=1519.
- A lot of information can be gained from watching a child at play while history taking and thereafter all children and toddlers are best approached with confidence and ease.
- Beginning with the pGALS as a playful exercise of copying often facilitates cooperation with the more formal regional exam (see ➜ 'The paediatric GALS screen' and also at ℘ http://www.arthritisresearchuk. org/health-professionals-and-students/video-resources/pgals.aspx).

- Look, feel, and move limbs and joints with careful facial observation and appropriate reassurance. Swelling may arise from subcutaneous tissues, tendons, or joints, and may include oedema, lymphoedema, cellulitis, and haematoma.
- Clicking is common and normal unless associated with a jarring or locking movement.
- Pain at end of range of joint movement typically indicates intra-articular pathology.

*Teenagers*
- By speaking directly to the young person, a more accurate clinical picture will be acquired than from speaking to parents alone.
- Direct, friendly questioning will also help engage and optimize examination and any future appointment.
- Supplemental information from parents may be helpful as may any discordance between histories.
- Where possible, teenagers should be offered to be seen on their own, with parents included fully in the consultation thereafter. This is now considered best practice.
- Explain confidentiality, and respect for privacy and modesty will also promote trust and optimize clinical assessment.
- Avoid non-verbal signals that appear to judge the individual.
- Identify problems with sleep. Early morning wakening with pain may be associated with inflammatory or malignant conditions, whereas difficulty with sleep initiation or maintenance may be associated with chronic pain.
- In particular, insufficient sleep is associated with pain amplification and reduced resilience.
- In a study of chest pain, only 1 in 300 patients had associated cardiac pathology which was clearly apparent on examination.
- Over 90% of back pain is benign or biomechanical in nature.
- Frequent associations with chronic pain include bowel, bladder, and psychological disturbances.

# Limp and gait concerns in children and adolescents

Most cases of limp (an asymmetric gait pattern) present acutely and so are commonly seen in A&E/emergency room by an orthopaedic surgeon to rule out infection and malignancy if there are systemic features, or Perthes disease and slipped upper femoral epiphysis (SUFE) if there are no systemic features. Most cases of acute limp, however, have a preceding illness and are diagnosed as irritable hip or transient tenosynovitis. Subacute or long-standing limp or concerns about gait may present to rheumatologists.

## Age-specific assessment

### Toddlers and pre-school children

- Review the child with reference to normal development and spend time observing the gait, first noting normal variants (see ➔ pp. 37–9).
- Enquire about age of onset (when onset is at the time of first walking, consider developmental hip dysplasia).
- Note any preceding illness or trauma.
- Take care not to simply ascribe limp to trauma in the presence of other features and if the history is incongruent, consider non-accidental injury (NAI) history.
- Immunosuppression may mask sepsis.
- Morning stiffness is typical of juvenile idiopathic arthritis (JIA).
- Carefully observe foot position when the child is walking for foot and ankle involvement in JIA.
- Consider that referred pain from the abdomen or groin may be present and avoid a simple focus on the hip.
- Weakness predominates in neuromuscular conditions and there may have been slow or even loss of gross motor milestones.
- Localizing pain or tenderness may be difficult for young children and the young child should be assessed as previously described for pain.
- The soles of the feet should be examined.

### School-aged children and adolescents

- An insidious onset of limp is typical of Perthes disease and JIA, the latter having associated stiffness after prolonged rest.
- Other osteochondroses should also be considered (see ➔ Table 16.11).
- Association with exercise and evening predominance is typical of biomechanical conditions.
- New-onset limp in adolescents raises concerns for chronic SUFE or bone tumour.
- Hip restriction or pain at the limits of internal or external rotation requires further investigation.

# Pyrexia, fatigue, and unexplained acute-phase response in children and adolescents

## Fever and pyrexia of unknown origin (PUO)

- Persistent or intermittent low-grade fever especially when associated with failure to gain or loss of weight will raise suspicion of malignancy and multisystem disease, such as SLE.
- Documenting the periodicity of fever may be helpful.
- A subacute fever or PUO (intermittent or persistent fever >38°C for >3 weeks) may indicate contact with infectious diseases, travel, tick bite exposure, medication use ('drug fever'), and sexually acquired infection (in an adolescent).
- A full systems enquiry should be backed up by a detailed examination including nailfold capillaries, lymph node assessment, fundoscopy, and cardiac auscultation.
- 'Phone photos (taken by the child, adolescent, or parent) of rashes can help in the assessment of relapsing–remitting rashes and ultimately as a record to share with other professionals, such as a dermatologist.

## Unexplained acute-phase response

- An unexplained erythrocyte sedimentation rate (ESR) >15 mm/min has a differential diagnosis similar to that of fever/PUO and a complete history and examination is required.
- Persistent increase (over 6–12 weeks) in platelet count and C-reactive protein (CRP) increases the likelihood of an inflammatory disease being found.
- Biopsy of any suspected lesion can be helpful and whole-body magnetic resonance imaging (MRI) can be a helpful screen for malignancy or to locate sources of localized inflammation.
- Other causes include renal disease especially when there is azotaemia, multiple myeloma, and anaemia of chronic disease associated with iron deficiency.

## Fatigue

- It is unclear from what age children report negative experiences of generalized exhaustion, which as in adults may accompany any illness, but it may be reported by parents as a presenting symptom.
- It is key to ascertain what is meant by fatigue, differentiating it from lack of sleep, deconditioning, or specific muscle weakness.
- It is important to understand specific concerns of the parent (e.g. a sense of not being listened to).
- Other enquiries should include details about the onset of fatigue, medication, and appetite.
- A full systems enquiry may raise suspicion of active inflammation; malignancy; endocrine disorder; distress from pain, bowel, or bladder dysfunction; skin sensitivities; and other functional disorders.
- Investigations are usually directed by suspicion of any underlying disorder, but, as in pain assessment, care should be taken to avoid unnecessary or endless investigations that prevent effective engagement in a management plan. Simple screening tests include inflammatory markers, full blood count (FBC), thyroid function, and antinuclear antibody (ANA).

# The paediatric GALS screen

The adult GALS MSK disease screening examination has been modified to a paediatric form (pGALS) to facilitate engagement of patients as young as 2 years and to account for subtleties in joint restriction of joints typically involved in JIA.

- Limbs should be adequately exposed to permit full examination and the pGALS is demonstrated by the doctor facing the patient and encouraging them to copy. In this way, a full screening joint examination can be played out as a game without touching the patient initially, thereby building rapport and patient confidence.
- Gait examination is discussed in detail in ➔ pp. 37–9.
- Supplemental to neck examination is range of motion and asymmetry of jaw opening. Temporomandibular joint movement should allow three fingers of the patient's hand to be held vertically in their open mouth.
- Joint movement restriction is a sign of disease activity in JIA conditions. As a result, where JIA is suspected, increased attention should be paid to flexion at all finger joints, extension of the elbow, and inversion and eversion of the foot, checking subtalar and midfoot joints.
- A full demonstration of pGALS can be found at ℛ http://www. arthritisresearchuk.org/health-professionals-and-students/video-resources/pgals.aspx

# Musculoskeletal assessment and patterns of disease: making a working diagnosis

# Introduction

- When evaluating a person—child or adult—with focal or widespread pain, it is important to consider that the pain may be derived from joints. Sometimes it won't be obvious. MSK pain may arise from joints (disease of synovium, cartilage, or bone) but also entheses, tendons, muscles, or a combination of structures, or can be referred from site to site (usually from proximal to distal), or can be associated with/ secondary to neurogenic lesions. *Patterns* of presentation of pain can be useful pointers to diagnosis.
- More than one in five general practitioner (GP) consultations are for patients with MSK problems, with osteoarthritis (OA) the most common cause of chronic pain and restricted activity in the over 50s.
- MSK pain is the presenting symptom in 6–13% of consultations in paediatric primary care with additional consultations for concerns about gait, swelling, and weakness.
- MSK pain in the paediatric population is common and its prevalence increases with age. Chronic severe pain, lasting >3 months and affecting quality of life, is common too, with a prevalence of up to 16% in secondary school-aged girls.
- The majority of causes (>80%) of MSK pains are self-limiting and have minimal impact on quality of life. In this respect, pain is not a sensitive marker of disease yet it is still important to provide reassurance to avoid symptom amplification and prolonged disability.
- But also, MSK pain can be a presenting feature of conditions not to be missed and other long-term conditions that may result in tissue damage or significantly affect participation and quality of life.
- The challenge is to understand pain in the context of other symptoms and signs. Many diagnoses can be made without investigations.
- To categorize the approach to assessment, we have subclassified the patterns of pain/disease into:
  - features/conditions not to be missed.
  - normal variants.
  - inflammatory arthritis.
  - non-inflammatory MSK pain.
- To help in the assessment of inflammatory arthritis, we have categorized by age, number of joints, and by joint number. Although not the convention in paediatrics, we have taken a threshold of 3 joints to define multi-articular involvement:
  - mono/oligoarticular arthritis in children (1–2 joints).
  - monoarthritis in adults.
  - oligoarthritis in adults.
  - poly-articular arthritis in children (≥3 joints).
  - poly-articular arthritis in adults.
  - arthritis and systemic features (children and adolescents).
- Widespread pains are also the presenting feature of chronic pain syndromes.

# Musculoskeletal (MSK) features not to be missed (that may be indicative of serious disease)

## General considerations

Among the many MSK, inflammatory, and autoimmune diseases that present to rheumatologists, some require prompt intervention including life-threatening conditions: cancer, infection, and non-accidental injury (NAI) in children and vulnerable adults (Box 2.1). Complex regional pain syndrome (CRPS) is included here due to the level of associated incapacitation and early intervention being essential.

---

**Box 2.1 Conditions 'not to be missed' in children and adolescents**

Key features that may indicate these conditions include systemic symptoms, a history of trauma that does not adequately explain examination findings, focal unexplained bone pain and tenderness lasting more than a few weeks, and in children marked disability or loss of developmental milestones.
- Septic arthritis, osteomyelitis
- Acute lymphoblastic leukaemia, lymphoma
- Bone tumours (e.g. sarcoma)
- Neuroblastoma in children
- NAI
- CRPS.

---

- Unexplained and persistent focal pain and bony tenderness in children is a 'red flag'. Such pain lasting more than 2 weeks raises the suspicion of bone cancers.
- 'Focal' means able to clearly point to the site of bone pain or tenderness and is often associated with a limp or disability, and where the pain cannot be explained by osteochondroses, trauma, or infection.
- In children, bone cancers are typically associated with weight loss and fatigue. Early metastasization is associated with increased mortality necessitating early recognition.

## Key features which should trigger referral for further assessment in children and adolescents

- Limp (see also ➔ 'Assessment of the limping child' pp. 37–9).
- Persistent localized (unilateral) pain through the night.
- Joint restriction or persistent joint swelling.
- Impaired functional ability.
- School absence or teacher concern.
- Morning symptoms unexplained by the previous day activities and tiredness after disturbed sleep.
- Widespread pain.

- Worrying thoughts or anxiety of the patient or parent.
- Systemic features such as fever, malaise, anorexia, weight loss, rash, raised acute-phase response and abnormal growth or development. For example, these features might lead to disclosure of:
  - septic arthritis or osteomyelitis (high fever, hot and tender joint, or limb pain).
  - leukaemia, lymphoma neuroblastoma, lupus, or vasculitis (persistent >2 weeks of low-grade fever typically associated with a rash).
  - Kawasaki disease (high spiking fever in under 6s with limb pains).
  - multisystem inflammatory disorders.
  - reactive arthritis.
  - chronic infections including tuberculosis (TB) (travel history and contact tracing is important).
  - other reactive illnesses with or without clear infection (e.g. Lyme disease, *Streptococcus*, Henoch–Schönlein purpura (HSP)); in all of these, the presence of rash may be indicative of diagnosis.
- A history of trauma incongruent with exam findings could be consistent with NAI or CRPS. In NAI, the mechanism of injury may not explain its extent or severity, and should be discussed with a paediatrician or lead clinician. In CRPS, there is frequently a history of minor trauma.
- Reported loss of milestones.
- Loss of peer or social contact or significant reduction in physical activity. These changes should not be dismissed as behavioural or anxiety induced (whether parent or child) without plans for a timely review of resolution or progression.
- Suspicion of neuromuscular disease. The onset of muscular dystrophies, congenital and metabolic myopathies, and neuropathies are often insidious in onset. Muscle weakness, muscle fatigue, numbness, and delayed development predominate but may be associated with widespread or focal pain that is the presenting feature.
- Suspected problems with pain processing. Notably CRPS, juvenile fibromyalgia, and sensory integration-autistic spectrum and anxiety disorders can be associated with very high levels of disability due to altered pain processing. There can be complete school absence and grossly abnormal sleep routines attributed to pain.
- Hypermobility with widespread pain. Hypermobility does not indicate the cause of the pain. Care must be taken when using the term 'hypermobility' as it can be perceived as disabling with a poor outcome. The cause of pain is often complex, but with effective communication and a range of integrated strategies that includes a focus on self-management and resilience, the outcome will be excellent with full participation in a normal quality of life.
- In considering the above-listed features, which should prompt further referral, there are other key points which may be helpful in the assessment:
  - Attributing pain to non-specific trauma or sprain or internal disruption of the joint can be reassessed after 2–3 weeks to see if it has resolved.

- Arthritis is commonly associated with persistent and prolonged morning stiffness and joint restriction. Pain is not a major feature and any report of joint swelling unreliable.
- Bone lesions are indicated by pain and focal tenderness often with consistent symptoms at night. Pain is often intense (e.g. osteoid osteoma or leukaemia with marrow involvement).
- Pain from muscle lesions localize well to the affected muscle. Functional weakness, not attributable to fear of movement from pain, may be indicated by walking on tiptoes and difficulties climbing stairs, and putting on T-shirts or jumpers.
- Lesions from ligaments, tendons, and entheses may be difficult to establish due to the symptoms they cause coexisting with symptoms from associated muscle and bone lesions.
- Focal tenderness may be revealing, particularly at entheses including the heel, patella, anterior superior iliac spine, and plantar fascia.
- Entheseal and ligamentous pain can be intense and often seemingly disproportionate to examination findings.
- Weight falling across centiles or unexplained weight loss >5% in an adolescent needs detailed assessment.

## Key features to identify prompting further urgent rheumatological assessment—adults

For non-rheumatologists, generally the more systemic features present associated with MSK symptoms, the more the need to obtain urgent assessment:

- Fevers and sweats can indicate sinister disease but can denote infection and both autoinflammatory and autoimmune disease.
- Fever and sweats can accompany severe gout or vasculitis, including GCA in the elderly.
- Arthralgias and myalgias can be part of a paraneoplastic syndrome— however, features are not specific and the condition is rare.
- Most rheumatologists would consider obtaining an extensive panel of lab investigations and chest X-ray (CXR) in patients with severe MSK symptoms and systemic features.
- Systemic features in the context of a positive ANA require that a thorough examination is done and urinalysis obtained to rule out renal disease associated with SLE.
- Severe pain and swelling in a joint with or without systemic features requires prompt assessment, and aspiration of fluid from the joint for Gram stain, culture, and polarized light microscopy (?crystals).
- Incipient cord compression can present with progressive stiffness and limb weakness without pain. Such 'neurological' stiffness reported as a symptom, is a mimic of stiffness from symptoms associated with peripheral MSK lesions.

## Key features necessitating timely rheumatological referral—adults

Many healthcare systems do operate a basic MSK service in primary care setting to support primary care doctors in managing the extensive amount benign/self-limiting of MSK disease seen. However, all systems sensibly require triage processes to promptly identify patients that require prompt onward referral to a rheumatologist:

- Key symptoms to identify and why:
  - Multiple small joint pain/stiffness—might be RA which requires early treatment to reduce permanent joint damage and disability.
  - Inflammatory back pain (see ⊃ Chapter 8)—which can predict the presence of axSpA/AS.
  - Systemic symptoms plus positive ANA might be an autoimmune connective tissue disease (e.g. SLE) which can in some patients cause serious organ disease.
  - Severe unexplained temporal head pain and/or scalp sensitivity and/or amaurosis fugax with high CRP or ESR—might be GCA and require prompt steroid treatment.
- A pragmatic way of screening for inflammatory small joint arthritis has been adopted as an educational initiative by The UK Royal College of General Practitioners. The 3 'Ss': Stiffness, Swelling, and a positive Squeeze test (pain elicited by squeezing the knuckles).
- Insidious cord compression can present with progressive stiffness and limb weakness without pain. Such 'neurological' stiffness is a mimic of 'MSK' stiffness.
- Gout and septic arthritis can look exactly the same—so aspirate!
- Polymyalgia rheumatica (PMR)-type symptoms can be the predominant type of MSK symptomology in a number of conditions including pyrophosphate arthritis, psoriasis-related MSK disease, axSpA, and autoimmune connective tissue diseases. A wise GP considers the condition a symptom-complex which may have an underlying disease explanation.

# Assessment of children and adolescents

## Normal variants

Effective reassurance that a child has a normal variant avoids unnecessary referral, investigation, and intervention. See Table 2.1.

**Table 2.1** Normal MSK variation in children and adolescents

| Normal variant | Prevalence | Notes |
|---|---|---|
| Genu varum (bow legs) | Very common <2 yrs old | If progressive consider Blount's disease, rickets, skeletal dysplasia |
| Genu valgum (knock knees) | Physiological 4–7 yrs; and as a mild condition is common thereafter | Refer if intermalleolar distance >8 cm, unilateral, gait is modified, deteriorating, or new onset in adulthood |
| In-toeing/ out-toeing | Common in under 5s | Usually resolves by 9 yrs. Causes include metatarsus adductus, femoral anteversion, and tibial torsion. Refer >9 yrs if gait affected |
| Toe walking | 7–24% of children (especially in autistic spectrum disorder) | Usually resolves by 3 yrs. If obligate, new onset, progressive, or unilateral consider neuromuscular and orthopaedic disorders |
| Femoral anteversion | Common 4–7 yrs | Presents as in-toeing and occasionally limb pain. Rarely requires surgical intervention |
| Hypermobile hands | Very common <5 yrs. At 13 yrs is present in 30% boys, 46% girls | No clear association with pain. May be associated with development and coordination delay needing writing support |
| Hypermobile knees | Common <5 yrs. Affects 8–11% at age 13 yrs | May be associated with patellofemoral pain and associated biomechanical imbalance |
| Flat feet (pes planus) | Universal initially. Affects >40% at ages 3–6 yrs and 1 in 7 adults. Longitudinal arch develops at 3–5 yrs | Shoe inserts stabilize but do not correct the foot. Exercises will address biomechanical pain. Rigid flat foot indicates bone or neural problem |
| High arch (pes cavus) | Affects 10% of the population | Assess biomechanics and for neuromuscular disorder if progressive or concern. Consider spinal tumour if unilateral |
| Benign nocturnal limb pain of childhood | Common in children 3–12 yrs. Peaks at age 6 yrs. Occurs in up to 40% under 5s | Further assessment if associated with disability, focal tenderness, systemic features, significant morning stiffness, swelling, erythema, weakness |

## Inflammatory arthritis in children and adolescents

The key features of recognizing inflammatory arthritis are:
- Consistent morning stiffness lasting >30 min.
- Swelling with joint restriction.
- Associated muscle atrophy
- Involvement of >1–2 joints (see Table 2.2).

### Infectious features

- The features of a reactive arthritis may include preceding symptoms of a viral infection such as coryza or non-specific rash.
- Other viral features include 'slapped cheek' of parvovirus, a widespread and facial macular rash of rubella, and sore throat of mumps, although these are rarely seen due to vaccination. In this respect, a *vaccination history* is required.
- Vaccinations may be associated with arthralgia and myalgia but are not associated with the development of JIA.

**Table 2.2** Typical patterns of joint involvement in the various inflammatory juvenile conditions

|  | 1–2 joints | ≥3 joints |
|---|---|---|
| Septic arthritis including TB | xx | |
| JIA | xx | xx |
| Reactive/viral arthritis | xx | x |
| Post-streptococcal arthritis | xx | x |
| Rheumatic fever | | x |
| Inflammatory bowel disease (IBD)-related arthritis | x | x |
| Henoch–Schönlein purpura (HSP) | x | x |
| Haemophilia | x | |
| Lyme disease | x | |
| Foreign body synovitis | x | |
| Malignancy | x | x |
| Autoinflammatory disease (e.g. familial Mediterranean fever (FMF)) | x | x |
| Multisystem autoimmune disease | | x |
| Pigmented villonodular synovitis (PVNS) | x | |
| Chronic recurrent multifocal osteomyelitis (CRMO) | x | x |
| Sarcoid | x | x |
| Non-inflammatory conditions | x | |

- A non-SpA reactive arthritis is usually short lived, typically 3–6 weeks in duration although may be up to 8 weeks. However, a uniphasic reactive arthritis in a child who is human leucocyte antigen (HLA)-B27 positive (with related features such as conjunctivitis, urethritis, psoriasiform rash) may be considerably longer. In this situation, there is typically a history of diarrhoea in children.
- Associated diarrhoea, especially bloody diarrhoea and a fever, should alert to enteric organisms such as *Shigella*, *Yersinia*, *Campylobacter*, and *Salmonella*, which may be cultured from the stool.
- *Escherichia coli* and *Clostridium difficile* are also known to trigger a reactive arthritis.
- Post-streptococcal arthritis is typically associated with a sore throat *without* cough and a very painful, marginally swollen, often flitting polyarthritis. Mucocutaneous features may include rash of scarlet fever and strawberry tongue.
- Acute rheumatic fever (RhF) should also be considered with the above-listed features (see ➋ Chapter 17) and additional clinical features may include erythema marginatum, skin nodules, a pericardial rub or new-onset murmur (and prolonged ECG PR interval), and chorea.
- In moderate- to high-risk incidence populations there are newly revised international guidelines for the diagnosis of RhF (2015 Statement of American Heart Association). Low risk is an incidence of RhF <2 per 100,000 school-aged children or all-age prevalence of rheumatic heart disease <1 per 1000. New criteria include echocardiographic and Doppler findings and monoarthritis and polyarthralgia as major criteria.

### History of trauma

- Trauma is common and often the event that draws attention to an already swollen joint.
- Haemarthrosis from internal joint disruption or periarticular swelling from quadriceps contusion or tear occurs within 2 hours of trauma.
- Trauma may include a penetrating injury with a punctum from a blackthorn or similar foreign body.
- A mechanism of injury incongruous with examination findings may raise suspicion of NAI or CRPS (see ➋ Chapter 22).

### Systems enquiry and past medical history

- May indicate features of coeliac or IBD or raise suspicion of multisystem inflammatory disorders such as SLE or vasculitis.
- Other conditions associated with an increased risk of arthritis include cystic fibrosis, coeliac disease, Down's syndrome, and other genetic conditions.

### Family history

- Enquire about arthritides including axSpA/AS and related conditions such as IBD, psoriasis, and previous iritis.
- Patients may volunteer haemophilia, FMF, SLE, and other autoimmune diseases.
- The family history is also very helpful in raising parental or patient worries about cancer or perceptions about arthritis or joint pains as witnessed in an older family member who may have RA, osteoarthritis, or fibromyalgia or other conditions.

*Travel history and infectious contacts*

- Previous travel history may raise suspicion of TB, *Salmonella*, and other enteric organisms.
- Travel history should incorporate enquiry about unusual infections such as brucellosis and leishmaniosis from endemic areas. Enquiry about consumption of unpasteurized milk products may be helpful.
- Insect bites and contact with tics including travel to endemic rural areas may lead to consideration of Lyme disease (see ➔ Chapter 17) and other conditions.
- Scratches from a cat and associated lymphadenitis or lymphangina is suggestive of *Bartonella* infection.

*Response to medication*

- The outcome of medication use can be viewed as a 'test' in itself. Results of the 'test' will help guide future management.
- Failure to respond to intra-articular steroids can raise the suspicion of undiagnosed TB and PVNS.

*Examination*

- Routine examination should include height and weight and a well-practised paediatric pGALS (see ➔ Chapter 1).
- Observe the child at play first and respect the privacy of adolescents.
- Be attentive of and reassuring about painful movements.
- pGALS is a quick, excellent screening tool for joint restriction, often key to finding multiple joint involvement when just 1 or 2 joints were initially suspected. It is also a valuable and playful way of engaging a younger child in examination without touching the child and avoiding distress.
- Even subtle differences in range of motion may signify synovial thickening.
- Any doubt about the presence of synovitis can be addressed with ultrasound (or MRI, as directed later in this section).

*Regional MSK examination*

- Subsequent assessment should include comparison of both sides, assessment for muscle wasting, scars, deformity, tenosynovitis, enthesitis, and spinal and hip disease.
- Muscle wasting, a clear sign of chronicity, typically affects vastus medialis with knee involvement and calf with ankle involvement. Upper limb muscle wasting is usually less prominent than in adults.
- Tenosynovitis is more commonly seen around the ankle, but may be mechanical in origin rather than inflammatory. It is not associated with any specific subtype of JIA.
- Involvement of the tendons of the hand may result in trigger finger.
- Enthesitis discriminates enthesitis-related arthritis from other forms of JIA; areas of tenderness include Achilles' insertion, patellar tendon, attachment of quads and hamstrings to pelvis, and plantar fascia.
- Examination of the spine should include the Schöber test of spinal drift in enthesitis-related arthritis (ERA; see ➔ Chapter 9) and distraction of the sacroiliac joints (with four quadrant test) to illicit any discomfort of these joints.

*Characteristic rashes*
- Psoriasis and associated nail pits (see ➔ Chapter 8).
- Palmar pustulosis and acne of SAPHO (see ➔ Chapter 8).
- Henoch–Schönlein purpura (HSP; see ➔ Chapter 18).
- Erythema chronicum migrans of Lyme disease (see ➔ Chapter 17).
- Erythema marginatum.
- Erythema nodosum of vasculitis and sarcoid (see ➔ Chapters 15 and 18, respectively).
- Lipodystrophy and/or skin thickening with pink halo in scleroderma.
- Other vasculitic rashes especially involving the palm or finger tips.
- Nail bed capillary changes of systemic sclerosis (SScl), SLE, and autoimmune overlap conditions.

*Investigations: imaging*
It is recommended that imaging should be discussed with a radiologist whenever possible:
- Ultrasound (US) can be helpful when exam findings are equivocal.
- But US is associated with a high false-negative rate in routine clinical situations especially for feet, ankles, and small joints of the hand.
- US can pick up early erosions that may guide changes in medication.
- MRI may be less available or immediate but is better for demonstrating chondral changes and bone and entheseal oedema. It has a very low false-negative rate for synovitis and low false-positive rate when using gadolinium enhancement.
- MRI is the investigation of choice for pelvic and spinal assessment and has characteristic findings for PVNS.
- Radiographs can be helpful when suspicious of skeletal dysplasia or metabolic bone disease (including rickets and scurvy) and for assessing bone mineralization.
- Radiographs may also demonstrate periarticular osteopenia, erosions, and loose bodies of osteochondritis although US is the preferred investigation in this circumstance.
- DXA scanning grades bone mass (BMD) against average expected but data needs adjustment for bone growth and pubertal changes (bone mineral apparent density (BMAD)). A number of approaches to data correction exist, but should be interpreted with caution.
- When malignancy or infection is suspected, a whole-body MRI (+fat suppression sequences) may be helpful, and has replaced bone scintigraphy and fluorine-18 fluorodeoxyglucose ([18]FDG) positron emission tomography–computed tomography (PET-CT) scans, which impart high radiation.
- Whole-body MRI is also used when non-bacterial osteomyelitis (including CRMO and SAPHO (see ➔ Chapter 18 and Chapter 8, respectively) is suspected.

*Laboratory tests*
- Autoimmune serology is helpful in multisystem inflammatory disorders but not typically in JIA, for which there are no diagnostic tests.
- ANA is not diagnostic. It is now considered a risk factor for uveitis although eye inflammation still occurs in those who are ANA negative. Further research into the value of testing ANA is ongoing.

- ESR and FBC may be normal in active JIA.
- Thrombocytosis is common in most inflammatory conditions and can be very high in systemic-onset JIA, along with neutrophilia.
- Platelet and lymphocyte counts are commonly low in juvenile SLE and antiphospholipid syndrome.
- A low platelet and neutrophil count in the presence of raised inflammatory markers and arthritis may indicate malignancy.
- A high neutrophil count—especially with 'bands' on film inspection—may indicate infection.
- Interpretation of antistreptolysin O titre (ASOT) can be difficult. The most reliable clinical feature for streptococcal infection is sore throat without cough. Serial ASOT are required and combined measurement of anti-streptococcal DNAseB and streptozyme may be helpful.
- Rheumatoid factor (RF)-positive polyarticular JIA occurs in <5% of JIA and has a characteristic symmetrical appearance. RF should not be considered a routine test and is more likely to be misinterpreted when falsely positive.
- Lyme serology should only be requested in keeping with Lyme disease diagnostic guidelines (see ➔ Chapter 17).
- For suspected TB, interferon-γ assays (IGRA), CXR, and Mantoux tests are important if synovial aspiration for culture is not done.

### Joint aspiration and synovial biopsy

Care should be taken to avoid psychological trauma when undertaking this procedure as it may lead to loss of trust and future problems with venesection, routine examination, as well as repeat steroid injection.

- Joint injections may be done under general anaesthesia or with the aid of inhaled agents such as Entonox®.
- Joint aspiration for Gram stain and culture is the investigation of choice for septic arthritis and when considering TB synovitis.
- In some centres, synovial fluid cell differentials can be determined which may be helpful in differentiating between low-grade sepsis and autoimmunity.
- Bloody taps are common but if the blood runs through the whole of the sample, haemarthrosis should be considered and may be attributable to trauma, bleeding diathesis, PVNS, or haemangioma.
- Crystal arthropathy is very rare in children and adolescents and is not a common presentation of hyperuricaemia.
- Synovial biopsy is helpful when considering PVNS, sarcoid, chronic infections, and malignancy. Arthroscopic biopsy has a higher yield than needle biopsy.

## Assessment of gait and the limping child

The normal gait is a complex automatic process that in a child requires development of muscles, bones, joints, and ligaments effectively controlled and coordinated by the neurological system. Imbalances in any of this process will lead to problems but in general, a delayed gait is usually attributable to slower cephalocaudal myelinization of normal development. It is inappropriate to ascribe hypermobility or hypotonia to this delay or related problems with balance and coordination. Slower development may be perceived as a problem, but is not a medical disorder. Catch up with peers takes time and the finer adjustments to the gait pattern may not occur until the child is 8–10 years of age.

A simple view of normal gait includes a:

- *Stance phase* starting with the heel strike, progressing through plantar-flexion to toe-off. Assessment also looks at base width and single-limb support time.
- *Swing phase* from toe-off to heel strike with forward rotation and tilting of the pelvis and a stable lumbar spine and abdomen. Assessment also includes cadence and stride length.

*Assessment of a limp*

A limp is an asymmetric gait, but many people interpret other abnormalities of gait as a limp. Some abnormalities of gait are listed as follows. Examples of causes of limp in children attending A&E are shown in Table 2.3.

- *Antalgic gait* results from pain or stiffness leading to a shorter stance phase.
- *Trendelenburg limp or gait* is attributable to weak hip abduction causing a body sway in stance phase and a droop of the hip in the swing phase.
- *Waddling gait* is attributable to neuromuscular or articular stiffness around the pelvis.
- *Stiff-legged (peg-leg) gait* results from loss of knee flexion and circumduction with pelvic elevation on the affected side.

**Table 2.3** Causes of a limp in children seen in A&E; median age 4.4 years (interquartile range 2.9–7.5 years)

| Final diagnosis | No. (%) | Median days to presentation |
|---|---|---|
| 'Irritable hip' | 96 (40%) | 1 |
| No final diagnosis | 72 (30%) | 1 |
| Muscle strain/overuse | 42 (17%) | 3 |
| Perthes disease | 5 (2%) | 30 |
| Osteomyelitis | 4 (2%) | 0.5 |
| Local infection | 5 (2%) | N/A |
| JIA | 2 (1%) | N/A |
| Trauma/fracture/toddler fracture | 4 (1%) | 2 |
| Osteochondrosis | 2 (1%) | N/A |
| Neoplasia | 2 (1%) | N/A |
| Back/abdominal | 3 (1%) | N/A |
| Slipped Upper Femoral Epiphysis (SUFE) | 1 (0.5%) | 30 |
| Other | 5 (1.5%) | |
| Total | 243 (100%) | |

- *Toe walking* may be habitual, typically resolving at 3 years or may be due to muscle contractures or spasticity. Check whether the child can heel strike when concentrating. Unilateral toe walking may indicate a lower-extremity length inequality or be from a wound to the heel.
- *High stepping gait* may result from difficulties with dorsiflexion of the foot, usually associated with peroneal neuropathies lower motor neuron neurological disease (e.g. spina bifida, polio) and peripheral neuropathies (e.g. hereditary motor sensory neuropathy I/II).
- *Stooped gait* might indicate abdominal pathology.
- *Clumsy gait* is often described but rarely seen in formal assessment. It is in part the result of inattention and may also be from subtle physiological developmental delay (often associated with handwriting difficulties and learning delay or disability). May include more frank neurodevelopmental or metabolic disorders.
- *Ataxic gait.*

*Further gait assessment*

Should follow general MSK assessment plus:
- Localize site of pathology (and include back and abdomen; see
  ➜ Chapter 3)—20% of limps are not associated with pain.
- Look for biomechanical imbalances.
- Trivial injury or trauma may be unwitnessed and toddler fractures missed on conventional radiographs.
- Incongruence or inconsistency in history raises suspicion of NAI.
- Consider sports-related injuries and overuse syndromes.
- Neurovascular status, including strength, sensation, and reflexes, can also be assessed while the child is sitting or supine.
- Measure and compare lower-extremity lengths.
- Walk, run, and hop allow assessment of coordination, strength, and bring out subtle abnormality and provide developmental assessment.
- Also assess skin, sole of feet, nails, and shoes.

## Assessment of muscle pain and weakness in children and adolescents

Changes in gait, and difficulty climbing stairs and putting on jumpers or T-shirts may be attributable to muscle pain or weakness.
- In the history of acute muscle pain there should be enquiry about trauma, previous biomechanical muscle pains, preceding viral infection, and fever and site.
- Benign myositis of childhood is a transient illness that typically presents with calf pain in the 4–10-year-old age range 3 days after onset of fever and is associated with a high creatine kinase (CK). Guillain–Barré syndrome also affects distal muscles and follows certain viral or bacterial infections but will be associated with gradual progression, marked weakness, sensory symptoms, and normal CK.
- Chronic myositis may also be associated with a low-grade fever, muscle tenderness and high CK.
- Juvenile dermatomyositis, SLE, pyomyositis, and some periodic fevers with myalgia will have characteristic rashes.

- Non-inflammatory causes of muscle weakness include neuromuscular conditions, such as muscular dystrophies, that are progressive with loss of motor milestones; upper motor neuron lesions including spinal compression with increased reflexes; or anterior horn cell conditions, neuropathies, and metabolic muscle disease with absent reflexes. These conditions rarely cause muscle tenderness.
- Muscle weakness and Trendelenburg gait are also seen in gross deconditioning from sedentary behaviour and chronic pain conditions. Tenderness is common along with symptomatic deterioration towards the end of the day.
- Widespread myalgias of juvenile fibromyalgia and enthesitis may be confused with each other.

### Joint pains with systemic features in children and adolescents

Where there is fever, rash, and arthritis, diagnoses *other than* systemic-onset JIA (SoJIA; previously known as Still's disease) ought to be considered first and before a trial of steroids which will mask infections, malignancy, and Kawasaki disease.

- Travel, infection contact, social, and family histories are vital in terms of disclosing a history suggestive of infection.
- There should be a full enquiry about symptoms referable to each organ system, which may point to a diagnosis of multisystem inflammatory disease.
- Characterizing the fever, including fluctuation throughout the day, periodicity, and duration may be diagnostic of SoJIA, Kawasaki disease, and specific periodic fevers (see ➔ Chapter 18).
- A 'quotidian' fever occurring once or twice a day with return to baseline is characteristic of SoJIA, Kawasaki disease has a high spiking fever for at least 5 days. For periodic fevers see ➔ Chapter 18.
- Look for and characterize any rash. This may facilitate diagnoses of SoJIA for which there are multiple typical rashes, lupus, dermatomyositis, periodic fevers and vasculitis. Other important rashes are those of pyoderma and neutrophilic dermatoses, scleroderma, and Behçet's disease; all may need distinguishing from viral exanthems and fungal infection.
- Ocular features may include red eye, pain, double vision, photophobia, and blurring.
- Ear, nose, and throat (ENT) features may include sinusitis, crusting, bloody discharge, tinnitus, hearing loss, facial weakness, oral ulceration, sore throat, parotitis, and dry mouth.

### Non-inflammatory MSK conditions in children and adolescents
(See also Box 2.2.)

*Principles of diagnosis*
- Biomechanical and non-inflammatory pain is very common in healthy children and adolescents and is by far the commonest cause of MSK pain.

## Box 2.2 Typical non-inflammatory MSK disorders in children and adolescents

*Painful conditions from focal lesions*
- Patellofemoral syndrome
- Other biomechanical imbalances
- Tendinopathy and enthesitis (including ERA)
- Perthes disease (groin, thigh)
- Slipped Upper Femoral Epiphysis (SUFE) (groin, thigh)
- Osteochondroses
- Neuroblastoma
- Osteoid osteoma
- CRPS
- Osteosarcoma
- Stress fracture
- PVNS (usually large joint).

*Conditions that may be associated with widespread MSK pain*
- Haemophilia
- Juvenile fibromyalgia
- NAI
- Skeletal dysplasias
- Marfan syndrome
- Ehlers–Danlos syndrome
- Osteogenesis imperfecta (focal or multiple fractures)
- Muscular dystrophies and other neuromuscular conditions
- Rickets
- Vitamin C deficiency-scurvy
- Hyperparathyroidism
- X-linked hypophosphataemic rickets (fractures/bone pain).

- Hypermobility in the normal population is common and care should be taken before ascribing focal or widespread MSK pain to the hypermobility syndrome/Ehlers–Danlos syndrome (EDS) type 3. Inappropriate/over-zealous use of the diagnostic label can reflect a misunderstanding of the multifactorial nature of MSK pain and project a 'disabling' rather than 'enabling' formulation onto patients. In turn, this can lead to parental confusion, a lack of flexibility over treatment strategies, and excess disability.
- Biomechanical pain typically increases with activity and occurs in the evening or following morning or two after increased physical activity. It may be associated with stiffness at these times.
- Biomechanical pain may be associated with minor swelling and tenderness and may occur with inflammatory or other conditions. It commonly occurs with chronic arthritis due to muscle and joint inhibition from active inflammation and subsequent MSK imbalance.
- Focal bone pain occurs with osteochondroses and osteoid osteoma and although very rare, osteosarcomas should be considered in the absence of typical features of an osteochondrosis.
- Neuromuscular conditions manifest by weakness may present with (often initially focal) pain.

*Contributory factors to chronic non-inflammatory MSK pains and their impact*

- MSK imbalance—from tight and/or weak musculature or ligaments (patellofemoral syndrome is an example).
- General deconditioning—whether through overall lack of background effective physical activity, excess sedentary behaviour, or avoidance of activity due to pain.
- Repetitive physical activity in the presence of suboptimal muscular control.
- Subchondral or other bony stress.
- Features of gross motor development (including proprioception) which are slower than global development or development of peers and siblings—development requires nerve myelination and neuromuscular imprinting, so practice will not improve rate of change (as occurs with nocturnal enuresis).
- The pace of proprioceptive movement programming, which continues to develop until puberty.
- Suboptimal strength for range of joint movement (as with some hypermobile joints).
- Adverse gait or other patterns of movement including tracking of patella. For example, gait maturation and improvements in gait efficiency continue until after skeletal maturity.
- A 'boom and bust' approach to physical activity.
- Loss of confidence in specific movements.
- Difficulties in pain self-appraisal.
- Central and peripheral pain pathway (or neuromatrix) sensitization.
- Difficulties with background sensory processing as occurs in patients with autistic spectrum disorders.
- Ruminating or attentive behaviours.
- Reinforcing parental or other family member responses.
- Social and environmental factors including those at school.

*Notable features in the history ('pearls')*

- Osteochondroses develop gradually and are associated with pain and tenderness at typical tendon insertion or joint sites.
- Locking or gelling of a joint may indicate an osteochondritis dissecans lesion (typically elbow, knee, ankle).
- Weakness may be indicated by difficulty climbing stairs, or getting up from the floor (e.g. at school assembly).
- Non-participation in physical education lessons, extracurricular sport, and other physical activity may indicate either a significant impact of a condition or general deconditioning and reflect cycles of behaviour in response to pain.
- Disruption at the hip may present as insidious onset of knee pain or limp. This includes Perthes disease in children aged 4–10 years and subacute SUFE in peripubertal adolescents with an increased incidence in those overweight.

- With respect to knee joint pain/lesions:
  - Meniscal tears are associated with an acute event.
  - Cruciate ligament tears are also associated with acute trauma and there may be a history of popping within the knee and immediate swelling.
- Skeletal dysplasias may present with limb pain and deformity but usually present with a family history and disproportionate short stature or in the case of osteogenesis imperfecta, fractures. Occasionally, suspicion arises when polyarthropathy fails to respond to conventional treatments for arthritis and bilateral hip dysplasia or Perthes disease.

*Other aspects of the history*
- Typical features which might suggest a functional disorder include irritable bowel syndrome, dizziness, paraesthesiae, headaches, and bladder dysfunction.
- Family history may indicate other painful conditions but these are very unlikely to be genetically related other than through body type and patterns of movement and behaviour.
- Response to medication will help to guide future management.
- Engagement with, and response to, other treatments including physiotherapy, osteopathy, and complementary therapies will also help guide future management.
- Assessment of 'engagement' includes an understanding of the patient's cooperation with home exercise programmes and this can be correlated with exam findings (e.g. persistence of tight musculature or specific areas of deconditioning).

*Examination: general*
- Routine examination should include measuring height and weight and a pGALS (see ➔ Chapter 1).
- There should be a general assessment of conditioning and posture, which includes the presence of spinal contour noting any hyperlordosis or loss of lordosis.
- Gait has predictive patterns (see also ➔ 'Gait assessment', pp. 37–9):
  - Note any antalgic gait from trauma or inflammation.
  - A Trendelenburg or waddling gait can occur from hip abductor weakness from neuromuscular disorders or hip joint disorders.
  - Circumduction gait from hemiplegia or leg length discrepancy attributable to chronic knee synovitis (see ➔ Plate 1).
  - Ataxia due to neurological involvement.
  - Toe walking—if unilateral or not correctable with advice, upper motor neuron or lysosomal disorders should be considered.
- Weakness can be assessed though the Gower sign in a younger child, rising out of a chair without use of upper limbs, sustained neck flexor strength, and winging of scapulae when pushing against a wall.
- Regional MSK assessment is described in ➔ Chapter 3 and is usually key to diagnosis and management of non-inflammatory conditions.
- Regional examination should include assessment of adjacent regions given the functional connection between regions.

*Investigations: imaging*

The principles of imaging in young children are to minimize procedure time and radiation exposure wherever possible and to request imaging judiciously following discussion with a paediatric radiologist.

- Radiographs are often normal in early joint inflammation, but they are the investigation of choice if considering periosteal lesions, traumatic or stress fractures, mineralization defects (e.g. rickets), or major structural conditions such as skeletal dysplasia.
- Consider US if there is likelihood of joint/tendon synovitis, an osteochondral lesion, or a ligament, enthesis, or tendon lesion.
- MRI and further radiological investigation may include assessment of any organ, especially for feet and ankles, hips, and spine.
- Where there is a pyrexia of unknown origin or similar broad differential diagnosis, whole-body MRI (with fat suppressed *sequences*) may be helpful.

*Investigations: laboratory tests*

- All investigations should be performed with a clear understanding of how to interpret the results and specific tests (such as serology for multisystem disorders, *Streptococcus*, *Borrelia*, etc.) should be interpreted according to the pre-test probability.
- Weak positive results for lupus anticoagulant, RF, ANA, ENA, and ASOT may need repeating.
- Serological tests should also be interpreted with caution after immunoglobulin infusions or serious infections and HIV.

## Chronic pain without identifiable MSK abnormalities in children and adolescents

*Key considerations*

Chronic pain is defined (for research purposes) as the presence of pain or discomfort for >3 months. This may be continuous in the same location or intermittent. This may be a useful definition for clinical purposes and to help raise chronic pain syndromes or disorders in the differential diagnosis.

- In most circumstances, there is a characteristic history and examination findings and a positive diagnosis should be made. This does not require investigation.
- Treating these conditions as diagnoses of exclusion tends to undermine the diagnosis and raise suspicion in the patient or parent that sufficient investigation has not been done to rule out alternative causes of pain.
- If investigations are ordered, the exact purpose of this investigation should be explained and should be framed in the context of a positive diagnosis.
- In children and adolescents, both local, or regional, and widespread chronic pain occurs. This includes the current terminology of complex regional pain syndrome (CRPS) and juvenile fibromyalgia (FM), both pain processing or neuromatrix problems. There should be guarded use of these terminologies as there is a far better prognosis in children and adolescents than in adults and use of such terms may lead to unintended interpretations.

- The commonest cause of regional and widespread pain, however, remains biomechanical problems typically associated with growth and development. This includes benign nocturnal limb pains of childhood.
- It is likely that patients will have seen other professionals and at the beginning the patient or parent should be asked what they hope from the consultation.
- Localized pain such as CRPS is typically associated with an episode of minor trauma (major trauma is usually associated with high levels of appraisal and adjustment) in circumstances that may be challenging or alarming (e.g. unanticipated summersault on a trampoline, unexpected fall, excessively boisterous play, road traffic accident, or the presence of exhaustion from lack of sleep or heat stroke).
- The pain often builds up over time and the source of pain is considered mysterious and unexplained to patient and/or parent. This is frequently compounded by inconsistent assessment and explanation by health professionals and by agitating family members or friends.
- Widespread idiopathic pain including juvenile FM is usually insidious in onset with gradual imposition on quality of life over time.
- The levels of disability and distress for both localized and widespread chronic pain are usually well in excess of the clinical findings from history and examination, but should not be dismissed.
- The needs of patients with chronic pain should be clearly identified to help direct an effective treatment strategy that often requires a multidisciplinary approach (input from experienced physiotherapist, occupational therapist (OT), and psychologist).
- The role of medication is unclear and if used, medicine use should be closely monitored for benefit and side effects. Medication tends to be most effective when used to support engagement with other physical and psychological therapeutic strategies.

# Assessment of patterns of MSK features in adults

When evaluating an adult with joint, tendon, and muscle problems, it helps to initially consider what is normal variation and what is abnormal and, in the case of joint pains, the likely number of joints involved. Whether monoarticular (1 joint), oligoarticular (2–3 joints), or polyarticular (>3 joints) will influence the initial differential diagnosis and working diagnosis.

- For example, RA can present with monoarthritis but it would be a very unusual presentation whereas gout in men typically presents as a single site of inflammation.
- The differential diagnosis generates a working diagnosis which in turns dictates to a degree what tests are done and in what order.

## Normal variants

Normal variant features of MSK origin in children are usually developmental in origin (see ➔ Table 2.1, p. 32). In adults, varied skeletal morphological appearances are not usually associated with disease directly, though their mechanical effects may lead to secondary MSK problems, notably early degeneration.

- In adults, asymmetric MSK appearances, however, are more likely to represent relevant pathology.
- Adults can come to clinical attention, reporting noticeable change in MSK appearance though invariably, such changes, if indeed present at all, but without pain and other features, are not sinister and rarely indicate serious disease.
- Adult MSK appearances do vary notably. Typical sites of high variation are neck length, kyphotic/hyperlordotic lumbar thoracolumbar spine contour, degree of shoulder protraction, sloping shoulders, degree of elbow valgus, pelvis width and tilt, degree of femoral anteversion angle, Q-angle at the knee, degree of tibial torsion, in-toeing/out-turn, and reducible plano-valgus in the feet.
- Subtle appearances of some MSK structures, however, can indicate an underlying condition and occasionally are not identified through childhood and adolescence and lead to (a late) diagnosis of the condition in adulthood (e.g. trichorhinophalangeal syndrome, hypermobility syndrome/EDS3, and Scheuermann's disease).

## Monoarticular pain in adults

- Acute pain and swelling of a joint follows intra-articular trauma such as cruciate or meniscus tears in the knee. History will be key indiscriminating trauma or spontaneous inflammation; MRI is essential to identify the cause of trauma.
- Acute inflammatory monoarthritis is commonly due to crystal arthropathies in the older patient (see ➔ Chapter 7), infection (particularly gonococcal in the younger adult; ➔ Chapter 17) or haemarthrosis, the causes of which include trauma, bleeding disorder, vitamin C deficiency, synovial haemangioma, and PVNS.

- Aspiration of fluid for Gram stain, culture, and polarized light microscopy is an early priority of management.
- A fracture across the joint line may also cause an acute monoarthritis. Stress fractures occur as the result of repetitive loading of bone, and can be found with occupational, recreational, or athletic activities. Stress fractures may be small and therefore can be missed on plain radiographs; MRI may be more sensitive and should be considered if the patient is at risk.
- Non-gonococcal septic arthritis is particularly important to consider in the elderly, who may not present with the signs and symptoms expected with infection. Non-gonococcal septic arthritis is a rheumatological emergency (see ➔ Chapters 17 and 25), and should be treated with intravenous antibiotics immediately on suspicion.
- In the UK, although *Staphylococcus aureus* is the most common organism causing septic arthritis in the elderly, it is prudent to consider atypical infections (e.g. Gram negative).
- Septic arthritis preferentially occurs in patients with RA, in patients with renal disease, and immunocompromised patients.
- The presence of crystals in monoarticular joint fluid aspirates does not exclude infection.
- Distinguishing a swollen digital joint from a swollen digit is important in discriminating dactylitis—usually associated with PsA and other spondyloarthritides.
- Not all great toe pain/swelling is gout. The great toe is very commonly affected in PsA—check if digit is dactylitic and there is nail disease—see ➔ Chapter 8.
- Boxing glove-type swelling of a hand is a typical manifestation of calcium-containing crystal-induced inflammation, particularly calcium pyrophosphate deposition (CPPD)-pseudogout—on hand radiographs look for the joint space loss and marked sclerosis of articular surfaces of bones in CPPD of the carpal joints and chondrocalcinosis in the wrist triangular fibrocartilage complex.

## Oligoarticular pain in adults

(See also Table 2.4.)

### The assessment of an inflamed joint

The clinical features of inflammation and pain at any given synovial joint and the differential diagnosis in the context of other possible regional MSK diagnoses are discussed in ➔ Chapter 3.

Synovitis is the term given to inflammation of the synovial lining. This inflammation may be a consequence of a range of cellular processes, and is not specific for any one diagnosis. Joint effusions often accompany synovitis.

Inflammation of periarticular tissues may accompany synovitis. Enthesitis (inflammation at a tendon or ligament insertion into bone) or tenosynovitis (inflammation of the tendon itself) may be the most prominent feature.

**Table 2.4** Common causes of monoarticular/oligoarticular joint inflammation and typical patterns of presentation (adults)

| Disease | Typical pattern |
|---------|-----------------|
| Gout (see ➲ Chapter 7) | Age >40 yrs. Initially presents as an acute monoarthritis. Strong association with hyperuricaemia, renal impairment, and diuretics. Possible general symptoms mimicking sepsis. Possible family history. Acute-phase reactants and serum white blood cells often high. Joint fluid urate crystals seen by polarized light microscopy. Joint erosions and tophi occur in chronic disease |
| Spondyloarthritis (see ➲ Chapter 8) | Age <40 yrs, men more than women. Mostly oligoarticular lower limb joint enthesitis/synovitis. May occur with sacroiliitis, urethritis or cervicitis, uveitis, gut inflammation, psoriasis (scaly or pustular). Possible family history. ESR/CRP may be normal. More severe course if HLA-B27 positive |
| CPPD arthritis (see ➲ Chapter 7) | Mean age 72 yrs. Oligoarticular, acute monoarticular (25%), and occasionally polyarticular patterns of synovitis |
| Haemarthrosis | Obvious trauma does not always occur. Swelling usually considerable. Causes include trauma (e.g. cruciate rupture or intra-articular fracture), PVNS, bleeding diatheses, and chondrocalcinosis |
| Osteoarthritis (see ➲ Chapter 6) | Soft tissue swelling is usually not as obvious as bony hypertrophy (osteophytes). Typical distribution (e.g. first carpometacarpal and knee joints) |
| Rheumatoid arthritis (see ➲ Chapter 5) | Can initially present with an oligoarthritis that evolves into a symmetrical polyarthritis. Can rarely present as an acute monoarthritis |
| Septic arthritis (excluding *Neisseria gonorrhoeae*) (see ➲ Chapter 17) | Most common cause *Staphylococcus aureus*. Associated with chronic arthritis, joint prostheses, and reduced host immunity. Peak incidence in elderly. Systemic symptoms common and sometimes overt. Synovial fluid is Gram +ve in 50% of cases and culture +ve in 90% of cases |
| Gonococcal arthritis (see ➲ Chapter 17) | Age 15–30 yrs in urban populations and with inherited deficiency of complements C5 to C9. One form presents as an acute septic monoarthritis. Organism detected by Gram stain of joint fluid in 25% and by culture in 50% in the second group |

*History: general points*
- Pain and stiffness are typical features of synovitis and enthesitis. Both are often worse in the morning, or after periods of immobility. The presence or absence of stiffness does not discriminate between different causes of synovitis.
- Pain is often severe in acute joint inflammation. In chronic situations, pain may be less severe (due to mechanisms that increase physical and psychological tolerance). There are no specific descriptors that discriminate pain from synovitis or enthesitis.

- Swelling, either due to synovial thickening or effusion, often accompanies synovitis.
- A patient's report of swelling is not always reliable. Patients with carpal tunnel syndrome, for example, will frequently report that their hands are swollen, even when no swelling is visible.
- Reduced mobility in a joint affected by enthesitis/synovitis is almost universal regardless of its cause.

*Examination: general points*

- Swelling may be observed or detected by palpation. Its absence does not rule out synovitis or enthesitis. Synovial swelling needs to be discriminated from bony swelling, fat, and other connective tissue swellings (e.g. ganglia, nodules, etc.). Without imaging or attempting to aspirate joint fluid, it may be difficult to discriminate synovial thickening from effusion.
- Skin erythema (implying periarticular inflammation) and warmth do not always accompany joint inflammation, but they are common with crystalline and septic arthritis. Erythema can also occur in reactive arthritis, rheumatic fever, and with nascent Heberden's or Bouchard's nodes in osteoarthritis (OA; see ➲ Chapter 6).
- Tenderness of thickened synovium is common, but is not always present. Severely tender swelling suggests joint infection, haemarthrosis, or an acute inflammatory reaction to crystals.
- Inflammation of entheses results in 'bony' tenderness at joint margins, and sites of tendon or ligament insertion.
- Decreased range of motion is almost always demonstrable in a joint affected by synovitis or enthesitis. The degree to which passive and active range of motion is reduced depends on a number of often interdependent factors (e.g. pain, size of effusion, periarticular muscle weakness, or pain).
- Movement of a joint affected by synovitis or enthesitis will induce pain and stiffness, although neither is specific. Affected joints will demonstrate reduced range on active or passive range of motion exercises; moving the joint beyond that point will elicit pain.
- The age, sex, and occupation of the patient give non-specific, but important clues:
  - Oligoarthritis is uncommon in young adults. SpA, especially reactive arthritis, is likely to be the main cause; 75% of patients who develop reactive arthritis are <40 years old.
  - Gout typically occurs in those >40 years old, and is the most common cause of inflammatory arthritis in men (self-reported in 1 in 74 men and 1 in 156 women).
  - The mean age of patients with CPPD arthritis is about 72 years (range 63–93 years).
  - Areas endemic for tick infection (forestation) with *Borrelia* are at risk of Lyme arthritis.

*History: which joints are affected?*

Some processes are more common in certain joints than others:

- Shoulder synovitis is typical in hydroxyapatite arthritis (Milwaukee shoulder/knee syndrome) and AL amyloidosis (see ➔ Chapter 18).
- Involvement of a shoulder or hip is extremely unusual in gout.
- CPPD arthritis (as pseudogout) occurs rarely in the small finger joints (see ➔ Chapter 7).
- The knee is the commonly involved in acute crystalline arthropathy and septic arthritis (both gonococcal and non-gonococcal).
- Large knee effusions are common with Lyme arthritis, but this is a non-specific finding. Large effusions can also be seen with septic and psoriatic arthritis (see ➔ Chapter 8).
- In theory, there are many causes of synovitis in a single first metatarsophalangeal (MTP) joint, but the majority of cases will be due to gout; 50–70% of first attacks occur in this joint. Care is needed in not mistaking dactylitis due to PsA for gout.

*History: preceding factors*

Factors preceding swelling of a single joint or oligoarthritis may be highly relevant. These include trauma and infection:

- Acute non-traumatic monoarticular synovitis is most commonly due to crystal-induced synovitis or synovitis associated with SpA.
- A preceding history of trauma typically suggests intra-articular fracture (with/without haemarthrosis), a meniscus tear (knee), or an intra-articular loose body, such as an osteochondral fragment (which may cause the patient to complain about a 'locking' knee).
- Twinges of joint pain often precede an acute attack of gout. Acute arthritis ('pseudogout') occurs in 25% of patients with CPPD arthritis.
- In hydroxyapatite arthritis, synovitis is usually mild to moderate, gradual in onset, and typically worse at night.
- An acute monoarthritis with fever in FMF (see ➔ Chapter 18) is a mimic of septic arthritis. Such joint manifestations are present in up to 75% of cases.
- Septic arthritis should always be considered (and promptly ruled out) as a cause of acute joint swelling (see ➔ Chapter 25).

*History: family and social history*

There may be important clues from the family and social history:

- Both gout and SpA have a familial component. Between 6% and 18% of patients with gout also have a family history of gout. There may be a family history of SpA or uveitis in patients who have reactive, psoriatic, or enteropathic arthritis or ankylosing spondylitis (AS).
- Gout in young adults suggests an inherited abnormality (usually increased urate production from 5-phosphoribosyl-1-pyrophosphate synthetase 'super'-activity, since the other enzyme deficiencies present in childhood).
- Excessive alcohol consumption is associated with gout. Alcohol can also contribute to lactic acidosis that inhibits urate breakdown.
- Consider Lyme disease if patients live, work, or visit endemic areas; outside of the United States, this includes Europe, Russia, China, and Japan. Peak incidence occurs during the summer.

- Brucella arthritis is generally monoarticular and occurs primarily in areas where domesticated animals are infected and poor methods of animal husbandry, feeding habits, and hygiene standards coexist.

*History: ask about other associated features*

Associated extra-articular features include previous eye, gastrointestinal, cardiac, and genitourinary symptoms:

- Low-grade fever, malaise, and anorexia occur commonly in both septic arthritis and gout. Marked fever can occur in gout and only occurs in about a third of patients with septic arthritis.
- Ask about any current or previous features which might suggest SpA:
  - back or buttock pain (enthesis or sacroiliitis).
  - swelling of a digit (dactylitis).
  - plantar heel pain (plantar fasciitis).
  - red eye with irritation (anterior uveitis).
  - urethritis, balanitis, cervicitis, recurrent or acute diarrhoea (reactive arthritis)—be suspicious of previous diagnosis of IBD—ask about getting up at night to open bowels and passing slime/mucus—both suggestive symptoms for IBD.
  - psoriasis.
  - symptoms of inflammatory bowel disease.
- Behçet's disease (see ➲ Chapter 18) can cause an oligoarthritis. Other features include painful oral and genital ulcers, and uveitis.
- The involvement of more than one joint does not rule out septic arthritis. In up to 20% of cases, multiple joints can become infected.

*Examination: general*

- Always compare sides, to establish if the changes are symmetric or asymmetric.
- It is important to establish from the examination whether there is true synovial swelling. A history of swelling is not always reliable and other, non-synovial, pathology can present with single or oligoarticular joint pain.

*Examination of affected joints*

Examine the affected joints for tenderness. Check passive range of motion for evidence of locking or instability:

- Acute processes such as crystal arthritis, infection, and post-traumatic effusion often lead to painful swelling, marked tenderness of swollen soft tissues, and painfully restricted active and passive movement of the joint. These features are usually less overt with chronic arthritis.
- Instability of an acutely inflamed joint or tests for cartilage damage in the knee may be difficult to demonstrate. Further examination will be necessary after drainage of joint fluid.
- Detection of enthesis tenderness around the affected joints or at other sites is a useful clue to the diagnosis of SpA.

*Examination of other musculoskeletal structures*

- Examine the low back and typical sites of bony tenderness—sacroiliitis and enthesitis are common features of SpA.
- Tendonitis is not specific and can occur in gout, CPPD arthritis, SpA, and gonococcal infection.

*Examination: look for skin rashes and any inflammation*

Oligoarthritis may be part of a systemic inflammatory or infectious condition:

- Temperature and tachycardia can occur with some non-infectious causes of acute arthritis (e.g. crystal arthritis), although their presence in the context of oligoarticular joint swelling requires exclusion of joint infection.
- Gouty tophi may be seen in the pinnae and in other peripheral locations. They can be difficult to discriminate clinically from rheumatoid nodules. Polarized light microscopy of material obtained by needle aspiration will be diagnostic for tophi.
- The hallmark of relapsing polychondritis (see ➔ Chapter 18) is lobe-sparing, full-thickness inflammation of the pinna.
- Mouth ulcers are common; however, crops or large painful tongue and buccal lesions associated with oligoarticular arthritis suggest Behçet's disease.
- A typical site for the osteitis (tender swelling of bone) of SAPHO syndrome (see ➔ Chapter 16) is around the sternum and clavicles.
- Skin erythema over a joint suggests crystal arthritis or infection.
- Associated skin rashes may include erythema nodosum (associated with ankle/knee synovitis in acute sarcoid), purpuric pustular rashes (Behçet's, gonococcal infection, and SAPHO syndrome), erythema marginatum (rheumatic fever), or keratoderma blennorrhagica (aggressive-looking rash of the sole of the foot in sexually acquired reactive arthritis).
- Psoriasis may be associated with both synovitis and enthesitis.

*Investigations*

The presence of synovitis can be confirmed by obtaining US or MRI of the joints in question. At larger joints, both are sensitive for the detection of effusion and synovial thickening. Inflammation at periarticular or capsular entheses can also be seen.

*Laboratory tests: joint fluid*

The most important investigation of a patient with monoarticular synovitis is joint aspiration and prompt examination of fluid. Fluid should be sent in sterile bottles for microscopy and culture:

- The appearance of synovial fluid is not specific; however, blood or bloodstaining suggests haemarthrosis from trauma (including the aspiration attempt), a haemorrhagic diathesis, haemangioma, PVNS, and synovioma.
- Turbidity (decreased clarity) of fluid relates to cellular, crystal, lipid, and fibrinous content. Synovial fluid in septic arthritis and acute crystal arthritis is frequently turbid due to the effects of a high number of neutrophils.
- Cell counts give some diagnostic guidance but are non-specific (Table 2.5). There is a high probability of infection or gout if the neutrophil differential is >90%.
- Joint fluid eosinophilia is not specific.

**Table 2.5** Characteristics of joint fluid

| Characteristic | Normal | Group I (non-inflammatory) | Group II (inflammatory) | Group III (septic) |
|---|---|---|---|---|
| Viscosity | Very high | High | Low | Variable |
| Colour | None | Straw | Straw or opalescent | Variable with organisms |
| Clarity | Clear | Clear | Translucent or opaque | Opaque |
| Leucocytes (cells/mm³) | 200 | 200–2000 | 2000–50,000 | >50,000 |
| Polymorphonuclear neutrophils (%) | <25 | 25 | Often >50 | >75 |

- Polarized light microscopy of fluid can discriminate urate (3–20 μm in length, needle-shaped, and negatively birefringent—blue and then yellow as the red plate compensator is rotated through 90°) and calcium-containing crystals such as calcium pyrophosphate (positively birefringent crystals, typically small and rectangular or rhomboid in shape).
- Lipid and cholesterol crystals are not uncommon in joint fluid samples, but their significance is unknown.
- Crystals appearing in synovium less commonly, but in typical settings include hydroxyapatite associated with Milwaukee shoulder (and knee) syndrome (alizarin red-S stain positive), calcium oxalate in end-stage renal failure on dialysis (may need scanning electron microscopy to confirm), cystine in cystinosis, and xanthine in xanthinosis.
- The presence of crystals in joint fluid does not exclude infection.
- The most common causes of non-gonococcal septic arthritis in Europe and North America are *Staphylococcus aureus* (40–50%), *Staphylococcus epidermidis* (10–15%), *Streptococcal* species (20%), and Gram-negative bacteria (15%).

*Investigations: radiographs*

Radiographs can confirm an effusion, show characteristic patterns of chondral and bone destruction (e.g. in infection or erosive gout), and can reveal intra-articular calcification associated with CPPD or hydroxyapatite arthritis.

- Septic arthritis causes patchy osteopenia and loss of bone cortex.
- 'Punched-out' erosions (within joints or around metaphyses; 'Lulworth Cove erosions'), soft tissue swellings (tophi), and patchy calcification are hallmarks of chronic gout.
- Intra-articular calcification may commonly be either chondrocalcinosis (fine linear or punctate fibrocartilage calcification) or larger loose bodies (often with prolific osteophytes)—both are associated with CPPD arthritis.
- Numerous regularly shaped calcific masses in a joint may be due to synovial chondromatosis (most common in middle-aged men; 50% of cases affect the knee).

- The presence of erosions does not implicate RA. The arthritis may be due to an enthesitis associated with SpA or erosive OA. Discrimination of erosive enthesitis, RA erosions, OA-associated subchondral cysts, and gout erosions is often poorly done by non-MSK radiologists and the unwary/unlearned rheumatologist!

### Investigations: further imaging

Further imaging should be discussed with your radiologists:
- MRI confirmation of traumatized structures such as meniscus damage in the knee and labral damage in the shoulder should be sought if suspected.
- US of knee or shoulder might be first-line imaging depending on the experience of the radiologist when considering periarticular lesions (e.g. anterior knee structure lesions around the patellar ligament or the rotator cuff of the shoulder).
- MRI can confirm synovitis, although appearances are usually non-specific. Characteristic MRI appearances of enthesitis and associated osteitis and PVNS are recognized.

### Other laboratory investigations to consider

- FBC, acute-phase response (ESR, CRP). Neutrophilia is not specific for infection and can occur in crystal arthritis.
- Blood urea, electrolytes, creatinine, and urate (e.g. hyperuricaemia and renal impairment associated with gout).
- Blood calcium, phosphate, albumin, alkaline phosphatase (±PTH), thyroid function tests, and ferritin to screen for hyperparathyroidism, thyroid disease, and haemochromatosis, all of which can be associated with CPPD arthritis.
- Autoantibodies: RF and anticitrullinated peptide antibody (ACPA) may help identify early RA. RF is not specific for RA and is less specific than ACPA. Be aware of the association of RF with primary Sjögren's syndrome.
- Immunoglobulin M (IgM) *Borrelia burgdorferi* serology may help diagnose Lyme disease in patients at risk (e.g. acute arthropathy or migratory arthritis).
- Antibodies to the streptococcal antigens streptolysin O (ASOT) DNAase B, hyaluronidase, and streptozyme may be useful in patients who have had sore throat, migratory arthritis, or features of rheumatic fever (see ➲ Chapter 18).

### Investigations: synovial biopsy

- If there is a haemarthrosis or suspicion of PVNS, MRI of the joint is wise before biopsy to characterize the vascularity of a lesion.
- Consider a biopsy to evaluate a monoarthritis of unclear aetiology. Biopsy may be helpful to diagnose sarcoid arthropathy (see ➲ Chapter 18), infectious arthritis, or crystal arthropathy when the usual diagnostic tests are negative.
- Formalin fixation of samples is sufficient in most cases. Samples for polarized light microscopy are best fixed in alcohol (urate is dissolved by formalin). Snap freezing in nitrogen is essential if immuno-histochemistry is required.

- Arthroscopic biopsy will yield more tissue than needle biopsy and will allow joint irrigation.
- Congo red staining of synovium, ideally with polarized light microscopy, should be requested if AA, AL, or $\beta_2$-microglobulin amyloid is a possibility (see ➔ Chapter 18). This should be considered in patients with myeloma (AL) and long-term dialysis patients ($\beta_2$-microglobulin). AA amyloid is an uncommon, but recognized complication of RA, AS, FMF, and Crohn's disease.

## Widespread MSK pains in adults

Widespread MSK pain is a common reason for adults to seek medical advice (Table 2.6). Although some patients will have a polyarticular arthritis, many conditions are characterized by MSK symptoms which may be diffuse or multicentric. In addition, the interpretation and reporting of symptoms varies considerably and can be a source of confusion. This section reviews important aspects of the history, examination, and investigations in the initial evaluation of patients who present with non-localized, multicentric pains.

### Initial impressions

- Think broadly about the possible diagnoses.
- Use what you know about the epidemiology of likely conditions. For example, a 35-year-old man with peripheral joint pains is more likely to have psoriatic arthritis (see ➔ Chapter 8) than RA or generalized OA (see ➔ Chapter 6), SLE (see ➔ Chapter 10), or PMR.

**Table 2.6** Broad categories of conditions that may present with widespread MSK pain

| | |
|---|---|
| Common | Inflammatory polyarthritis (e.g. RA or psoriatic arthritis) |
| | Generalized (nodal) OA (see ➔ Chapter 6) |
| | Fibromyalgia/chronic pain syndromes (see ➔ Chapter 22) |
| | Non-specific myalgias and arthralgias* associated with infection (e.g. viruses) (see ➔ Chapter 17) |
| Less common | Myoarthralgias* in autoimmune connective tissue diseases |
| | Myalgias/muscle inflammation (e.g. polymyositis) (see ➔ Chapter 14) |
| | Myoarthralgias* with neoplasia and/or skeletal metastases |
| | Polyostotic Paget's disease (see ➔ Chapter 16) |
| Rare | Metabolic bone diseases (e.g. osteomalacia, see ➔ Chapter 8) |
| | Metabolic myopathies (e.g. hypokalaemia; see ➔ Chapter 14) |
| | Neurological disease (Parkinson's disease) |

* In certain situations/conditions patients may complain of both muscle and joint pains. This is easily appreciated if you've ever had influenza!

*Age, gender, and racial background*
- What clues can be drawn from the age, sex, and racial background?
- The degree to which these factors influence the likelihood of disease varies according to the prevalence of the disease in the local population. Review what you know about epidemiology of diseases.

*Previous diagnoses*
Presenting features may be put in context early if you have knowledge of MSK associations of diagnoses that have already been made. For example:
- Synovitis in patients with (radiological) chondrocalcinosis (CPPD disease/arthritis).
- Arthropathy in patients with hyperparathyroidism and hypercalcaemia (see ➋ Chapter 16, CPPD arthritis/pseudogout).
- Enthesitis/synovitis in patients with Crohn's disease or ulcerative colitis (see ➋ Chapter 8, Spondyloarthritis).
- Polyarticular synovitis and myalgia in patients with lymphoma.
- Crystal-induced or β₂-microglobulin deposition arthritis and osteodystrophy in chronic renal disease (see ➋ Chapter 16).

*Taking a history*
First, establish whether pains arise from joints or tendons/entheses, muscles, bone, or are neurologic.
- Although the patient may report 'joint pains', take time to establish whether the pains are truly from the joint or periarticular tissues.
- Listen carefully to the description of the pains; try to determine if the patient has a single condition or a number of overlapping causes of pain.

*Obtain a detailed history of the pain at different sites*
- A good history should help narrow the differential diagnosis considerably. For example, a 70-year-old man referred with 'widespread joint pains mostly in his legs' could have multiple weight-bearing joint OA or lumbosacral nerve root claudication symptoms (see ➋ Chapters 3 and 6 and ➋ Chapter 21, respectively). A middle-aged woman with 'hand and neck pain' could have an arthropathy or radicular pain associated with cervical spondylosis.
- Widespread pain due to bone pathology could be due to skeletal metastasis. Bony pain is often unremitting, and changes little with changes in posture and movement.
- One pitfall is to assume that all pains arise from a single pathological process. For example, in an older patient, multiple pathologies frequently exist and can be complicated to unravel. The following are all common in the elderly:
  - osteoarthritis (any/multiple joints).
  - CPPD arthritis.
  - rotator cuff arthropathy.
  - sarcopenia/falls risk.
  - PMR.
  - spinal stenosis of lumbar canal with leg symptoms.
  - primary hyperparathyroidism.
  - CKD-related MSK symptoms.
  - hypovitaminosis D/osteomalacia.

*Joint pain at rest, after rest, or with joint use?*

Establish whether pain arises from joints or tendons/entheses.

- Pain occurring with inflammation is conventionally regarded as being associated with morning stiffness or stiffness after periods of rest. It tends to be prominent in conditions such as RA, SpA, PMR, and myositis. Inflammatory joint pain often improves in the day.
- Mild degrees of immobility-associated pain and stiffness occur in some other conditions, such as OA and fibromyalgia, although such forms of stiffness generally last for <1 h. Stiffness may also be a feature of muscle spasm and soft-tissue oedema.
- Mechanical joint damage such as OA is also painful. Unlike inflammatory joint pain, mechanical joint pain is worsened by use, and improves with rest.

*Ask, and document in detail, which joints are affected*

- A symmetric polyarthritis affecting the small joints is typical for RA. RA can also present with carpal tunnel syndrome, tenosynovitis, tennis elbow, or an asymmetric pattern of joint involvement, and can be preceded by a palindromic pattern of joint pain (see ➜ 'Ask about the pattern of joint symptoms over time', pp. 57–8).
- Arthritis from parvovirus B19 infection may also be polyarticular and symmetric but also may cause myopathy and general symptoms.
- Small joint pain in the hands occurs in nodal generalized OA. Distal interphalangeal joints (DIPJs), proximal interphalangeal joints (PIPJs), and thumb joints are usually affected. OA is also associated with pain in the spine, hips, and knees.
- The combination of sacroiliac (low back and buttock), pelvic, and lower limb joint/enthesis pain, typically in an asymmetric oligoarticular pattern, is suggestive of SpA. Typical sites of involvement include anterior knee, posterior and inferior heel (plantar fascia).
- Enthesitis can affect the wrists and small joints of the hand and feet (e.g. plantar fascia origin and insertion at metatarsal heads) and may be difficult to distinguish from RA on clinical grounds alone.
- CPPD typically favours the large and medium-sized joints, but a picture of multiple joint involvement similar to that in RA is possible (including tenosynovitis).
- Widespread arthralgias/arthritis occurs in patients with leukaemia, lymphoma, myeloma, and certain infections.

*Ask about the pattern of joint symptoms over time*

- A short, striking history of marked, acute polyarticular symptoms often occurs with systemic infection (Table 2.7). Prominent malaise and fever should raise suspicion of infection.
- There may be a longer history than is first volunteered. Autoimmune rheumatic and connective tissue diseases may evolve over a period of time and often naturally relapse and remit; the first symptoms of disease may be dismissed by the patient as irrelevant.
- Conventionally, persistent inflammatory joint symptoms should be present for at least 6 weeks before RA is diagnosed.

**Table 2.7** Common infections that can present with acute polyarthritis and a raised acute-phase response

| Infection | Common extra-articular clinical features | Key laboratory diagnostic tests in acute infection |
|---|---|---|
| Rheumatic fever (group A haemolytic streptococci) | Acute infection 1–2 weeks earlier, fever, rash, carditis | Positive throat swab culture. High ASOT (in 80%) |
| Post-streptococcal | Acute infection 3–4 weeks earlier, tenosynovitis | As above |
| Parvovirus B19 (adults*) | Severe flu-like illness at onset, various rashes | Anti-B19 IgM |
| Rubella (also post-vaccine) | Fever, coryza, malaise, brief rash | Culture. Anti-rubella IgM |
| Hepatitis B | Fever, myalgia, malaise, urticaria, abnormal liver function | Bilirubin+, ALT+, AST+, anti-HBsAg, anti-HBcAg |
| Lyme disease (*Borrelia burgdorferi*) | Tick bites, fever, headache, myalgias, fatigue, nerve palsies | Anti-Bb IgM (ELISA + immunofluorescence) |
| *Toxoplasma gondii* | Myositis, paraesthesias | Anti-Toxo IgM |

Even if serological tests have high sensitivity and specificity, the positive predictive value of the test is low if the clinical likelihood of the infection is low. Therefore, do not use serological tests indiscriminately.

\* The presentation of parvovirus B19 illness may be quite different in children.

- Migratory arthralgias occur in 10% of RA patients initially: a single joint becomes inflamed for a few days then improves and a different joint becomes affected for a few days and so on. A similar pattern can occur in post-streptococcal arthritis, granulomatosis with polyangiitis (previously known as Wegener's granulomatosis), sarcoidosis, Lyme disease, and Whipple's disease.
- Recurrent pains from various MSK lesions, which have occurred from injury or have developed insidiously, are typical in patients with underlying hypermobility (e.g. EDS including hypermobility-EDS, OI, Marfan Syndrome etc) (see ➔ Chapter 19).
- The onset of enthesopathy may be insidious or acute.

### Is there widespread muscle pain?

If you think there is widespread muscle pain, consider that:
- The myalgias may be fibromyalgia or enthesitis.
- Pain locating to muscle group areas may be ischaemic or neurologic in origin, and not necessarily due to intrinsic muscle disease.
- The differential diagnosis of polymyositis (PM) and dermatomyositis (DM) is broad, but many of these conditions are rare (Table 2.8 and see ➔ Chapter 14).

**Table 2.8** The major causes of myopathies and conditions associated with diffuse myalgia

| | |
|---|---|
| Infectious myositis | Viruses (e.g. influenza, hepatitis B or C, Coxsackie, HIV, HTLV-I) |
| | Bacteria (e.g. *Borrelia burgdorferi* (Lyme disease)) |
| | Other (e.g. malaria toxoplasmosis) |
| Endocrine and metabolic | Hypo/hyperthyroidism |
| | Hypercortisolism |
| | Hyperparathyroidism |
| | Hypocalcaemic, hypokalaemic |
| Autoimmune diseases | Polymyositis |
| | Dermatomyositis |
| | SLE |
| | Systemic sclerosis (SScl) |
| | Sjögren's syndrome |
| | RA, Vasculitis (e.g. PAN, AAV, rheumatoid vasculitis) |
| | Myasthenia gravis |
| | Eosinophilic fasciitis |
| Carcinomatous myopathy | |
| Idiopathic | Fibromyalgia (muscles should not be weak) |
| | Inclusion body myositis |
| | Sarcoid myositis |
| Drugs | Lipid-lowering drugs (e.g. fibrates, gemfibrozil, niacin) |
| | Anti-immune (e.g. colchicine, ciclosporin, penicillamine*) |
| | Rhabdomyolysis (e.g. alcohol, opiates) |
| | TNFα inhibitors |
| | Others (e.g. azathioprine, chloroquine*) |
| Muscular dystrophies | Limb girdle |
| | Facioscapulohumeral |
| Congenital myopathies† | Mitochondrial myopathy |
| | Myophosphorylase deficiency |
| | Lipid storage diseases |

* Drugs most likely to cause painful myopathy.

† Because of variable severity, some conditions may not present until adulthood.

Note: Guillain–Barré syndrome and motor neuron disease may be considered in the differential diagnosis of non-painful muscle weakness

*Ask about the distribution and description of myalgias and weakness*

- True weakness may denote either myopathy or a neurological condition. However, patients may report a feeling of weakness if muscles are painful, therefore, rely more on your examination before deciding muscles are weak.
- PMR (rare in patients <55 years old), myositis, and endocrine or metabolic myopathies typically present with proximal weakness.
- PMR does not lead to objective weakness; instead, patients experience proximal muscle pain and stiffness that is worse in the morning, and is frequently described by the patient as 'weakness'.
- Although rare, truncal muscle pain, and stiffness can be a presenting feature of Parkinson's disease.
- Cramp-like pains may be a presenting feature of any myopathy (e.g. hypokalaemic) or even motor neuron disease. However, some patients may interpret radicular (nerve root) pains as 'cramp-like'.
- Inflammatory, endocrine, and metabolic myopathies are often not painful.
- Occasionally, some genetic muscle diseases (e.g. myophosphorylase, acid maltase deficiency), can present atypically late (in adults) with progressive weakness that may be mistaken for PM.

*Ask about the pattern of muscle pains over time*

- Severe, acute muscle pain occurs in a variety of conditions. The most common causes are viral, neoplastic, and drugs. Some toxic causes may result in rhabdomyolysis, myoglobinuria, and acute kidney injury (AKI).
- Usually PM/DM is characterized by slowly evolving but progressive muscle pain and weakness (e.g. weeks to months).
- Low-grade episodic muscle pains may denote a previously undisclosed hereditary metabolic myopathy.
- Fibromyalgia (see ➲ Chapter 22) is a chronic pain syndrome and symptoms may have been present for a considerable time at presentation.

*Are the pains ischaemic?*

- Ischaemic muscle pain often occurs predictably in association with repeated activity and eases or resolves on rest ('claudication'). Consider this especially if pains are confined to a single limb or both legs.
- The distribution of pains may give clues as to sites of underlying pathology, e.g. upper extremities are affected by subclavian artery stenosis and thoracic outlet syndrome; lower extremities are affected by atherosclerotic vascular disease or lumbar nerve root stenosis.
- Ischaemic pains in the context of a highly inflammatory state may suggest systemic vasculitis, such as polyarteritis nodosa.

*Widespread pain may be due to bone pathology*

- Bone pains are unremitting and disturb sleep. They could denote serious pathology—radiographic and laboratory investigations are important.
- The major diagnoses to consider include disseminated malignancy, multiple myeloma, metabolic bone disease (e.g. renal osteodystrophy, hyperparathyroidism, osteomalacia), and polyostotic Paget's disease.

Specific questions are often required because previous problems may not be regarded as relevant by the patient. For example:
- For those with joint pains a history of the following may be of help:
  - other autoimmune diseases (increased risk of RA, SLE, etc.).
  - Raynaud's phenomenon (association with SScl, RA, and SLE).
  - dry eyes (possible Sjögren's syndrome).
  - uveitis or acute 'red eye' (association with SpA).
  - recurrent injuries/joint dislocations (association with joint hypermobility syndrome.
  - genital, urine, or severe gut infection (link with SpA).
  - psoriasis (association with SpA).
  - diabetes (cheiroarthropathy).
- For those in whom myalgias/myositis seems likely:
  - preceding viral illness (possible viral myositis).
  - foreign travel (tropical myositis).
  - other autoimmune disease (associated with PM/DM).
  - previous erythema nodosum (sarcoid).
  - drugs and substance abuse.
- For all patients:
  - weight loss or anorexia (association with malignancy).
  - fevers or night sweats (association with infection).
  - sore throat (possible post-streptococcal condition).
  - persistent spinal pain (association with fibromyalgia).
  - rashes (association with Lyme disease, SLE, DM, vasculitis).
- For those with widespread bony pain:
  - history of rickets (association with osteomalacia).
  - chronic renal disease (will precede renal osteodystrophy and may predispose to crystalline arthritis and osteoarticular deposition of $\beta_2$-microglobulin).

## Psychosocial and sexual history
- Preceding sexual activity and genital infection is important primarily because of an association of *Chlamydia trachomatis* infection with reactive arthritis and enthesitis/SpA (see ➲ Chapter 8).
- Reactive arthritis has an association with HIV. HIV is also associated with PM, and is a risk factor for pyomyositis.
- There is an association of anxiety and depression with FM (see ➲ Chapter 22).

## Ask about travel
- Residence in, or travel to, rural areas populated by deer might be important in indicating a risk of exposure to *Borrelia burgdorferi* and contracting Lyme disease (the spirochete is carried by ticks that colonize deer, boar, and other animals and bite other mammals).
- *Plasmodium falciparum* (intertropical areas), *Trypanosoma* (mainly South America), *Trichinella*, and cysticerci (tapeworm larval cysts) infections are associated with myalgias/myositis.

*Family history*

Ask about family with arthritis or autoimmune diseases:

- There is a hereditary component to psoriatic arthritis, SpA, large joint and generalized nodal OA, and hyperuricaemia/gout.
- The risk of developing any autoimmune condition is higher in families of patients with autoimmune diseases than generally.
- Hypermobility per se (not necessarily joint hypermobility syndrome) and FM show a strong heritability in twin studies.

*Drug history*

- The following drugs have been reported to cause a myopathy (those marked* are more likely to be painful): lithium, fibrates, statins, penicillin, colchicine, penicillamine*, sulphonamides, hydralazine, ciclosporin, phenytoin, cimetidine* (muscle cramps), zidovudine, carbimazole, TNFα inhibitors, and tamoxifen.
- The myositis that occurs with penicillamine is not dose dependent or cumulative dose dependent. It can be life-threatening.
- Drug-induced SLE, which is characterized commonly by arthralgias, aching, and malaise, and less commonly by polyarthritis, can occur with a number of drugs including hydralazine, procainamide, isoniazid, minocycline, TNFα inhibition therapy. Quinidine, labetalol, captopril, phenytoin, methyldopa, and sulfasalazine *may* also cause similar symptoms.
- Mild myalgias and arthralgias may be caused by a number of commonly used drugs, e.g. proton pump inhibitors and quinolone antibiotics.
- Alcohol in excess and some illegal drugs are associated with toxic myopathy occasionally resulting in rhabdomyolysis.

*Ask about chest pain, dyspnoea, palpitations, cough, and haemoptysis*

- Cardiac abnormalities are features of autoimmune rheumatic and connective tissue diseases, but are infrequent at initial presentation. Cardiac infection is associated with widespread aches and pains (e.g. rheumatic fever/post-streptococcal myalgias/arthralgias, infective endocarditis).
- Chronic effort-related dyspnoea due to interstitial lung disease occurs in many patients with autoimmune connective tissue and rheumatic diseases. Up to 40% of RA patients may have CT evidence of lung disease. In many sedentary patients, however, symptoms are not prominent. Dyspnoea may be present at presentation.
- Respiratory failure and aspiration pneumonia can occur as a result of a combination of truncal striated, diaphragmatic, and smooth muscle weakness in PM.
- There is an association between bronchiectasis and RA.
- The most common neoplasm in patients diagnosed with malignancy-associated myositis, is of the lung.

*Ask specifically about dysphagia, abdominal pain, and diarrhoea*
- Patients may not mention gastrointestinal symptoms if they
  have resolved. There are many links between bowel disease and
  inflammatory arthritis (SpA linked to IBD is probably the commonest).
  - Ask specifically about previous severe diarrhoeal or dysenteric ery-
    thema migrans in Lyme disease.
  - Erythema marginatum in rheumatic fever.
  - UV sensitive rash on face/arms in SLE.
  - Violaceous rash on knuckles/around eyes/base of neck in DM.
  - Livedo reticularis in SLE and APS.
  - Purpuric rash in vasculitis (e.g. HSP).
  - Erythema nodosum in sarcoidosis.
- Illnesses such as those caused by *Campylobacter, Yersinia, Shigella*, or
  *Salmonella*, will be relevant to diagnosing reactive arthritis/SpA.
- Gut smooth muscle may be affected in polymyositis and give rise to
  dysphagia and abdominal pain.

## Examination

In patients with widespread pain, a full medical examination is always
necessary.

*Skin and nails*
In all patients look carefully at the skin and nails:
- Nails may show prominent ridges or pits in psoriatic arthropathy,
  splinter haemorrhages in infective endocarditis, systemic vasculitis or
  APS, or periungual erythema in scleroderma and the inflammatory
  myopathies.
- Look for skin rashes in conditions characterized by widespread pain.
  For example, lymphadenopathy may be present with either infection or
  inflammation and is non-specific. However, if prominent it may denote
  lymphoma.
- Signs of anaemia are a non-specific finding in many chronic systemic
  autoimmune diseases.
- Clubbing of the digits may be present in Crohn's disease and ulcerative
  colitis (associated with SpA) and bronchiectasis (associated with RA).
- Oedema can occur in both upper and lower extremities in a subset of
  patients presenting with inflammatory polyarthritis/tenosynovitis. The
  condition has been termed RS$_3$PE (remitting seronegative symmetric
  synovitis with pitting oedema). This condition is striking in that it occurs
  suddenly, often in patients 60–80 years old and is very disabling. It
  may be associated with other conditions. It may be a manifestation of
  pseudogout in CPPD disease.

*Examination of the joints*
Important points to note when examining joints:
- Each joint should be compared to the joint on the opposite extremity,
  first by observation, then palpation, then by its active and passive range
  of motion exercises.
- Useful examination tools include a tape measure to record swelling
  (circumferential) and a goniometer (protractor with arms) to measure
  the range of joint movement.

*Patterns of abnormality*

Note the specific cause of joint swelling and site of tenderness, distribution of affected sites, and hypermobility:

- In nodal generalized OA, osteophytes (bony swelling—may be tender) can be noted at DIPJs (Heberden's nodes) and PIPJs (Bouchard's nodes). Periosteal new bone at sites of chronic enthesitis may be palpable and tender.
- Nodules may occur in nodal OA, RA, polyarticular gout, ANCA-associated vasculitis, multicentric reticulohistiocytosis, or hyperlipidaemia (xanthomata).
- Soft tissue swelling with tenderness and painful restriction of the joint on movement suggests an inflammatory arthritis. There is often adjacent muscle wasting. This is most easily appreciated in the interosseous muscles in patients with hand arthritis, or the quadriceps in patients with knee arthritis.
- The 'painful joints' may be inflamed tendons or entheses. Tender tendon insertions and periarticular bone tenderness, often without any joint swelling, may denote enthesis inflammation associated with SpA.
- Tendonitis may be part of many autoimmune rheumatic or connective tissue diseases. Look specifically for thickening of the digital flexors and swelling of the dorsal extensor tendon sheath in the hand, and tenderness/swelling of both peroneal and posterior tibial tendons in the foot.
- Gross swelling with painful restriction of small joints is unusual in SLE. Often there is little to find on examination of joints.
- General joint hypermobility may lead to joint and other soft tissue lesions. An examination screen for hypermobility may be helpful (Table 2.9; also see ➲ Chapter 19). Check also for associated features.

**Table 2.9** Features of hypermobility. These are the 'Brighton' criteria

| Examination screen (scored out of 9) | Ability to extend fifth finger >90°at MCPJ (score 1 + 1 for R + L) |
|---|---|
| | Ability to abduct thumb (with wrist flexion) to touch forearm (score 1 + 1) |
| | Extension of elbows >10° (1 + 1) |
| | Extension of knees >10° (1 + 1) |
| | Ability to place hands flat on floor when standing with knees extended (1) |
| Associated features | Prolonged arthralgias |
| | Skin striae, hyperextensibility, and abnormal scarring |
| | Recurrent joint dislocations |
| | Varicose veins |
| | Uterine/rectal prolapse |
| | Recurrent soft-tissue lesions |
| | Marfanoid habitus |
| | Eye signs: drooping eyelids, myopia, down-slanting eyes |

*Examination of patients with widespread myalgia*

- Check for muscle tenderness and weakness. Document the distribution. Is there evidence of neurologic or vascular disease?
- The characteristic sites of tenderness in fibromyalgia should be confidently recognized (Fig. 2.1; see also ➜ Chapter 22). Despite discomfort, the muscles should be strong.
- Examine the strength of both truncal and limb muscle groups (Fig. 2.2). In the presence of pain, it may be difficult to demonstrate subtle degrees of muscle weakness.
- Patterns of muscle weakness are not disease specific; however, there are some characteristic patterns: symmetric proximal extremities in PM and DM; quadriceps and forearm/finger flexors in inclusion body myositis; limb muscles in mitochondrial myopathy. (Note: using specific apparatus physical therapists can help document isometric muscle strength in certain muscle groups.)
- Muscles in PMR are not intrinsically weak.
- Muscle wasting is not specific. If wasting is profound and rapid, consider neoplasia. Wasting will occur in most long-standing myopathies.
- Check for increased limb tone and rigidity—most evident by passive movement at a joint—consistent with extrapyramidal disease. There may be resting tremor in the hand, facial impassivity, and 'stiff' gait. Muscular tone in the limbs may also be increased in motor neuron disease; however, if presenting with muscle pains, the patient with motor neuron disease is more likely to have a lower motor neuron pattern of neuronal loss (progressive muscular atrophy) with muscular weakness/wasting, flaccidity, and fasciculations.
- The fatiguability of myasthenia gravis can be identified by determining the length of time the patient can keep their arms extended in front of them, or maintain an upward gaze.
- Muscle pains or cramps due to large-vessel ischaemia are likely to be non-tender at rest and strong. Demonstrate absent pulses and bruits and substantiate findings with US Doppler examination.

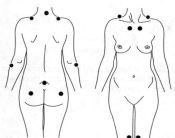

- Tenderness of skin overlaying trapezius
- Low cervical spine
- Midpoint of trapezius
- Supraspinatus
- Pectoralis, maximal lateral to the second costochondral junction
- Lateral epicondyle of the elbow
- Upper gluteal area
- Low lumbar spine
- Medial fat pad of the knee

Fig. 2.1 Typical sites of tenderness in fibromyalgia.

(a) Functional

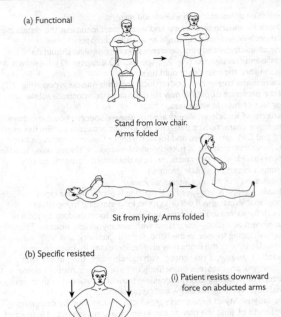

Stand from low chair.
Arms folded

Sit from lying. Arms folded

(b) Specific resisted

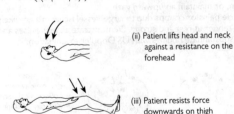

(i) Patient resists downward
force on abducted arms

(ii) Patient lifts head and neck
against a resistance on the
forehead

(iii) Patient resists force
downwards on thigh

**Fig. 2.2** Screening examination for proximal myopathy. (a) Functional movements requiring truncal and proximal lower limb muscle strength. (b) Resisted movement testing of deltoid (i), longitudinal flexors of the neck (ii), and iliopsoas/quadriceps (iii) strength.

- In suspected cases of PM and DM, examine for cardiopulmonary abnormalities. Other associated signs in DM include periungual erythema/telangiectasia, erythematous violaceous rash and skin calcinosis. Dysphonia and swallowing abnormalities occur in both PM and DM.
- Because of its associations, patients with myositis should be carefully examined for the following signs: dry eyes/mouth (Sjögren's syndrome; see ● Chapter 12), skin thickening/tenderness or discoloration (scleroderma; see ● Chapter 13), skin rashes (SLE; see ● Chapter 10), thyroid tenderness or enlargement (endocrine myopathy; see ● Chapter 4).

*Investigations: general points*
- ESR and CRP may be higher than normal in the setting of infection, malignancy, or active rheumatic disease. A slightly elevated ESR is a common finding in healthy elderly people.
- A positive ANA may occur in association with many autoimmune conditions, in other diseases (Table 2.10), and in some healthy people. It is, therefore, not diagnostic for SLE or any single condition; however, high-titre ANA may be significant and conversely, ANA-negative SLE is rare.
- ACPA is more specific for RA than RF (see ● Chapter 5), which can be positive in a number of inflammatory conditions.
- Controversy exists about the diagnosis of FM. It is prudent to only make a diagnosis of FM when other disorders can be confidently excluded. Consider: psoriasis-related MSK disease, SAPHO, sarcoid, autoimmune connective tissue diseases including APS, vasculitides.

**Table 2.10.** Examples of the prevalence of antinuclear antibodies (ANAs) in some diseases using ELISA, or Hep2 cells as substrate

| Population group | | Prevalence of ANAs ('up to') (%) |
|---|---|---|
| Normal population | | 8 |
| SLE | | 100 |
| Other autoimmune joint, vasculitis, or CTDs | Systemic sclerosis | 95 |
| | Sjögren's syndrome | 70–80 |
| | Psoriatic arthritis | 50 |
| | Polymyositis | 40 |
| | Polyarteritis nodosa | 18 |
| Examples from other diseases | Chronic active hepatitis | 100 |
| | Drug-induced lupus | 100 |
| | Myasthenia gravis | 50 |
| | Sarcoidosis | 30 |
| | Diabetes | 25 |

*Basic tests in patients with polyarthropathy*

- Urinalysis (dipstick) may show proteinuria or haematuria. Both glomerular and tubular damage are possible. Glomerulonephritis (in SLE, vasculitis, or endocarditis, for example) is usually associated with significant proteinuria and haematuria simultaneously. These patients will need urgent evaluation by a nephrologist.
- ESR and CRP are non-specific and may be normal in the early stages of these conditions. If very high, then consider infection or malignancy. There is often no evidence of an acute-phase response in patients with enthesitis (even though pain and bony tenderness may be widespread). A mild anaemia and thrombocytosis may accompany inflammation.
- Throat swab, ASOT, anti-DNAaseB antibodies may be useful to identify a recent post-streptococcal condition, but levels may remain mildly elevated long-term and indicate previous infection (IgG).
- Other tests which can be considered in the appropriate setting:
  - random blood sugar (diabetes).
  - TFTs/thyroid antibodies (hyper/hypothyroidism).
  - prostatic-specific antigen (malignancy).
  - fecal calprotectin (screening for inflammatory bowel disease in SpA).
- Joint fluid aspiration and culture is mandatory for patients in whom sepsis is a possibility. Fluid should be examined by polarized light microscopy in suspected cases of crystal-induced synovitis.
- In patients who are ANA-positive, test for extractable nuclear antigens (ENAs) to help characterize the type of autoimmune process.
- In many patients presenting with a short history of widespread joint pains, radiographs will be normal. An early sign of joint inflammation is periarticular osteopenia, but this is not specific. Recognized types of erosions, and bone reaction lesions and their distribution can be noted by experienced radiologists in specific conditions (e.g. RA, psoriatic arthritis, gout, CPPD arthritis).
- Referral to a sexual health clinic for further detailed investigations if there is a suggestion of recent or recurrent genital infection may help to strengthen the evidence for a diagnosis of sexually acquired reactive arthritis.

*Laboratory tests in patients with widespread muscle pain/weakness*

- Dipstick urinalysis: to screen for haematuria or myoglobinuria.
- FBC, ESR.
- Initial screening tests to consider: urea/electrolytes (U&E), creatinine, TFTs/TSH, bone profile, and 25-hydroxyvitamin D, liver function tests (LFTs), angiotensin-converting enzyme (ACE), CK, parathyroid hormone (PTH), ANA/ENAs, RF, myositis specific antibody panel and consider random cortisol and 24-hour urinary cortisol.
- Elevated CK or aldolase occurs in most cases of PM. ALT, AST, and lactate dehydrogenase (LDH) are non-specific markers of muscle damage. Note that specific muscle isoenzymes of CK and LDH exist and the normal range of all enzymes may vary in different populations. Muscle enzymes may be elevated after non-inflammatory causes of muscle damage, e.g. exercise/trauma.

- Check for ANA and, if positive, screen for ENAs. Antibodies to certain (cytoplasmic) tRNA synthetases (e.g. Jo-1, SRP) are myositis-specific.
- Think of checking for urinary myoglobin in cases where acute widespread muscle pain may be associated with myolysis—causes include excessive alcohol or ingestion of certain drugs (cocaine, amphetamines, ecstasy, heroin), exercise, or trauma. Such patients may be at risk of renal failure.
- PM can be a presenting feature of HIV. In HIV-positive patients, infections causing muscle disease include TB and microsporidia.
- Viral myositis may be clinically indistinguishable from PM. Serology may yield diagnostic clues.

*Electrophysiology and imaging in patients with muscle conditions*

- Electromyography (EMG) abnormalities occur in two-thirds of patients with muscle inflammation. More information is likely if studied in the acute rather than the chronic phase of the illness. In the acute phase, denervation and muscle degeneration give fibrillation potentials in 74% of PM and 33% of DM patients (see ➲ Chapter 14). Other features include low-amplitude short-duration motor unit and polyphasic potentials.
- EMG is poor at discriminating ongoing muscle inflammation in myositis from steroid-induced myopathy.
- There are characteristic MRI patterns of abnormality in PM and DM. MRI can be used to identify potential muscle biopsy sites to avoid false-negative results associated with patchy muscle inflammation.

*Muscle biopsy*

- Muscle biopsy should be considered in all patients evaluated for PM or DM.
- In PM, inflammatory infiltrates predominate in the endomysial area around muscle fibres without perifascicular atrophy. In DM, inflammation is more prominent in the perimysial area and around small blood vessels and there is typically perifascicular atrophy.
- Routine tests do not reliably distinguish PM from cases of viral myositis. Some of the glycogen storage diseases will become apparent from light microscopy of biopsy material.
- An autoimmune myositis is unlikely in the absence of positive HLA immunohistochemistry on biopsy material.

*Investigations for malignancy*

Investigations in adults with widespread bony pain should aim to rule out malignancy, particularly myeloma, gonadal tumours, and malignancies from breast, renal, and prostate cancers:

- Investigations should include mammography, urine cytology, PSA, renal US, serum and urinary protein electrophoresis.
- Hypercalcaemia may accompany these conditions; check blood calcium, phosphate, 25-hydroxyvitamin-D, PTH, PTH-related protein. PTH should also be checked in suspected cases of osteomalacia (raised due to calcium/vitamin D deficiency) together with 25-hydroxyvitamin D levels (low or low/normal), alkaline phosphatase (high/normal), 24-hour urinary calcium will be low.

- Radiographs of affected sites are important. Include a CXR.
- Bone scintigraphy can identify sites of neoplasia, Paget's disease, osteoporotic fractures, severe PTH bone disease, or osteomalacia. Characteristic patterns of abnormality exist.
- Whole-body CT scan is often the best single investigation to rule out deep tissue masses in abdomen and pelvis.
- Bone biopsy (maintained undecalcified by placing sample in 70% alcohol) of affected sites will be diagnostic in some, but not all, cases of osteomalacia, osteoporosis, and renal osteodystrophy. The best samples are obtained from a transiliac biopsy. Bone marrow can be aspirated for examination at the same time.
- PET-CT is now used to screen for suspected small tumours where other tests are negative, for locating lymphoma tissue for biopsy and in identifying deep tissue inflammation or sepsis where diagnosis is otherwise unclear.

# Regional musculoskeletal symptoms: making a working diagnosis

# Introduction

This chapter aims to provide a guide to constructing a differential diagnosis in the patient who presents with regional musculoskeletal (MSK) symptoms. It does not make reference to all possible diagnoses, only the most common.

## General considerations (adults)

- Findings from conventional clinical examination and imaging of the MSK system usually occur when the patient is at rest, and therefore only minimally symptomatic.
- Examination in the context of function (i.e. carrying, lifting, walking, bending, etc.) is not easy, although it is arguably more appropriate. Therefore, a thorough history utilizing a good depth of knowledge of functional anatomy is the best alternative and an invaluable way of obtaining good information about abnormal function and its causes.
- Time spent obtaining a detailed account of onset of symptoms is helpful whether or not the symptoms are of recent onset, or chronic, or associated with trauma. Patients usually have a clearer concept of injury-induced disease and may try to rationalize the appearance of non-trauma-related symptoms by association with an event or injury.
- Lay terms may reflect lay understanding. For example, the term 'repetitive strain injury' is commonly used by the layperson to denote a diagnosis. It is not a diagnosis, merely a description of a (unlikely!) mechanism by which injury has occurred. It is important to identify anatomically where the problem lies and to then enquire as to activities that may have induced or perpetuated the problem.
- Consider the possibility that the problem is a 'work-related disorder' (WRD). A WRD may not just be MSK; consider the possibility of associated respiratory (asthma, fibrosis), dermatological (dermatoses), neurological (neuropathy, behavioural), psychosocial (anxiety, depression), and infective (sewage, carcasses, needlestick) pathologies. Examples of MSK WRDs are given in this chapter.
- With children, it is important to obtain a history from both the child and a care provider. Second-hand information, even if provided by a parent, may be less reliable than direct information from someone who has the opportunity to observe the child during the day.
- Regional MSK lesions may be a presenting feature of a systemic disorder, such as an autoimmune rheumatic disease, malignancy, or infection. Clinical suspicion should guide the evaluation.
- Screening for disseminated malignancy, lymphoma, myeloma, and infection should at least include a FBC, metabolic screen, serum and urine protein electrophoresis with immunofixation, ESR, and CRP.
- Weakness (as a symptom) may be due to a neuropathic or myopathic condition or it may be perceived according to the impact of other symptoms such as pain.

## General considerations (children and adolescents)

Regional MSK assessment in children and adolescents differs from adult assessment, in the need to account for developmental variation, and motor 'competence'.

- Though MSK problems from congenital deformities can present for the first time in adults—to adult rheumatologists—it is more likely that congenital anomalies are disclosed initially in children. Regional MSK assessment in a child requires consideration of this.
- Although MSK pain is an ubiquitous experience in childhood, response to pain by an individual child depends on various states of anxiety, stress, and past experiences and can be influenced by the role of parents or other family members.

# Neck pain in adults

## Background epidemiology

- About 10% of the adult population has neck pain at any one time, although many people do not seek medical help.
- About 1% of adult patients with neck pain develop neurological deficits, but overall levels of disability are lower than for patients with low back pain.
- A continuum of radiological appearances exists in relation to age: intervertebral disc narrowing, marginal end-plate osteophytes, and facet joint changes. Appearances are often termed 'degenerative'; however, the correlation with presence and severity of pain is poor; Table 3.1 lists the major causes of neck pain in adults.

## Functional anatomy

- The neck is the most mobile (37 separate articulations), but least stable part of the spine. There are seven vertebrae (C1–C7) and five intervertebral discs (C2/3–C6/7). The C5/6 disc is most often associated with radicular symptoms. If it occurs, cord compression is most likely in this region, although atlantoaxial (C1–C2) subluxation may produce the same picture, especially among patients with RA.
- Minor congenital abnormalities are not infrequent and increase the risk of degenerative changes.
- Nerve roots C2 and C3 cover sensation over the back of the head, the lower jaw line, and the neck.
- Nerve roots (C4–T1) leave the spine in dural root sleeves, traverse the intervertebral foramina, and form the brachial plexus.
- Cervical nerves have a dermatomal representation (Fig. 3.1) and supply upper limb musculature in a predictable way.

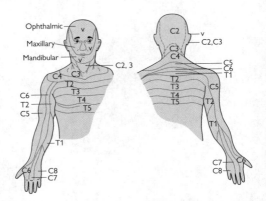

**Fig. 3.1** Dermatomal distribution of the cervical and upper thoracic nerves reflecting the radicular pattern of nerve root lesions.

**Table 3.1** The major causes of neck pain in adults

| | |
|---|---|
| Soft tissue lesions (posture, psychogenic, and overuse as modifiers) | Neck strain |
| | Torticollis |
| | Myofascial pain |
| | Trauma (e.g. acute flexion-extension injury ('whiplash')) |
| | Cervicothoracic interspinous bursitis |
| Degenerative and mechanical lesions | Spondylosis |
| | Disc prolapse |
| | Thoracic outlet syndrome |
| | Diffuse idiopathic skeletal hyperostosis (DISH) |
| Inflammatory conditions | Rheumatoid arthritis (see ➲ Chapter 5) |
| | Spondyloarthropathy (±fracture ±inflammatory discitis) |
| | Juvenile idiopathic arthritis (see ➲ Chapter 9) |
| | Polymyalgia rheumatica (PMR) |
| | Myelitis |
| Bone lesions | Traumatic fracture |
| | Osteomyelitis (e.g. TB) |
| | Osteoporosis (fracture) (see ➲ Chapter 16) |
| | Osteomalacia (bone disease or muscle pain) |
| | Paget's disease |
| Non-osseous infections | General systemic infection (general/cervical myalgias) |
| | Meningitis |
| | Discitis |
| Malignancy | Primary (rare) or secondary tumours (±pathological fracture) |
| | Myeloma, lymphoma, leukaemia |
| Brachial plexus lesions | Trauma |
| | Thoracic outlet syndrome (e.g. cervical rib) |
| Referred pain | Acromioclavicular or temporomandibular joint |
| | Heart and major arteries (e.g. angina, aorta dissection) |
| | Pharynx (e.g. infection, tumours) |
| | Lung and diaphragm (e.g. tumour, subphrenic abscess) |
| | Abdomen (e.g. gallbladder, stomach, oesophageal, or pancreatic disease) |
| | Shoulder (e.g. adhesive capsulitis) |

### Taking a history of neck pain in adults

*The site, radiation, and description of pain*

- Nerve root (radicular) pain is usually sharp and reasonably well localized in the arms. It is often 'burning' and associated with paraesthesia and numbness.
- Nerve root irritation and compression by an intervertebral disc are common causes of radicular pain. However, in older adults and those who suffer recurrent bouts of pain it is usually due to encroachment of vertebral end-plate or facet joint osteophytes, or thickened soft tissue or fibrosis on the nerve leading to stenosis of the exit foramen.
- Pain from deep cervical structures is common. It often localizes poorly across the upper back. It can be referred to the upper arms, is typically described as 'heavy' or 'aching' and is more diffuse than nerve root pain.
- Muscle spasm can accompany any lesion. It can be very painful.
- Pain from the upper cervical spine (C1–C3) can be referred to the temporomandibular joint (TMJ) or retro-orbital regions. Conversely, pain from both TMJ disorders and as a result of dental malocclusion can be referred to the neck.
- Pain from the lower neck may be referred to the interscapular and anterior thoracic wall regions. The latter may mimic cardiac ischaemic pain.
- Florid descriptions of the pain and of its extent and severity ('catastrophizing') are associated with prominent psychological modulators of pain.
- Evaluation of the shoulder joint is often necessary as pathology there often coexists and symptoms around the shoulder often complicate neck evaluation.
- Occipital headache is a common manifestation.

*Acute neck pain with trauma*

Acute neck pain with trauma requires urgent assessment, even if there are no obvious neurological symptoms:

- Acute trauma requires urgent evaluation for fracture, spinal cord damage, and vertebral instability. About 80% of serious injuries occur from an accelerating head hitting a stationary object.
- An abrupt flexion injury may fracture the odontoid (less common with extension); however, <1 in 5 injuries at C1/C2 produce neurological deficit because of the wide canal at this level.
- If not traumatic or osteoporotic (the latter being relatively rare in the cervical spine), fractures may occur in bone invaded by malignancy.

*New and/or associated symptoms*

Ask about associated leg weakness, and new bladder or bowel symptoms. New-onset acute neck pain with neurological features needs urgent evaluation. Neurological symptoms may also accompany chronic neck pain:

- Spinal osteomyelitis, meningitis, discitis (infection or inflammation), myelitis, and fracture may all present with acute or subacute neck pain. All may cause cord compression. Myelopathy due to spondylosis typically presents with a slowly progressive disability over weeks to months, although it can be acute, particularly if associated with central disc prolapse.

- Subacute pain, flaccid paralysis, and profound distal neurological signs may suggest myelitis, a condition caused mainly by infections and autoimmune diseases.
- Tinnitus, gait disturbance, blurring of vision, and diplopia associated with neck pain are all ascribed to irritation of the cervical sympathetic nerves.
- The vertebral arteries pass close to the facet joints just anterior to emerging nerve roots. Disruption of vertebral blood flow may cause dizziness in severe cases of neck spondylosis.

*Previous trauma*

Ask about previous trauma. It can precede and influence chronic pain:
- Acute and occupational (chronic overuse) trauma is a common antecedent of chronic neck pain.
- Cervical dystonia (torticollis) can occur 1–4 days after acute trauma, it responds poorly to treatment, and can be long-standing. It may also complicate arthropathy, such as in RA or Parkinson's disease.
- Whiplash injury is associated with chronic myofascial pain.
- In some patients with chronic pain following (sometimes trivial) trauma, there may be dissatisfaction with the quality of care received at the time of the injury.
- Unresolved litigation associated with trauma correlates with the persistence of neck pain and reported disability.

*Occupational and leisure activities*

Some occupations, sports and activities are associated with recurrent neck pain:
- Neck pain (and early spondylosis) is prevalent in people whose occupations require persistent awkward head and neck postures, e.g. professional dancers.
- Although biomechanical factors may be an important influence in initiating and aggravating neck pain, there may also be an underlying genetic predisposition to OA and/or hypermobility.

*Other points*

Establish whether the pain started or varies with non-MSK symptoms:
- Cardiac ischaemia, dyspepsia, or abdominal pain can result in referred pain to the neck (Table 3.1).

## Examination of the neck: adults

The neck is part of the functional upper limb and symptoms in the arms and legs may be relevant. Neurological examination of the arms is important:
- An adequate examination cannot be performed in a clothed patient. Despite the inconvenience, it is important to have the patient change into an examination gown to avoid missing relevant clues.
- Inspection from front and back may reveal specific muscle wasting or spasm and poor posture.
- Observing active movements reveals little if the patient has severe pain or muscle spasm. Inability to move the neck even small distances is characteristic in axial spondyloarthritis (axSpA; see ➲ Chapter 8).

- Tenderness often localizes poorly in degenerative disease. Exquisite tenderness raises the possibility of a disc lesion, osteomyelitis, or malignancy (the latter two are rare).
- There may be 'trigger points' in neck stabilizer and extensor muscles. Activation of a trigger point elicits myofascial pain in a zone that is stereotypical for the individual muscle.
- Tender points (localized, non-radiating pain elicited by pushing with the thumb), notably at the occipital origin of the trapezius, the medial scapular border, and the mid-belly of the trapezius, are features of fibromyalgia (FM; see → Chapter 22). It is not clear whether tender and trigger points are the same.
- Examination of passive mobility may be helpful primarily if it reveals gross asymmetry. The normal range of movement varies depending on age, sex, and ethnicity. Generally, at least 45° of lateral flexion and 70° of rotation should be achieved in a middle-aged adult. Global loss of passive mobility is non-specific and occurs with increasing age. The range of movement that might indicate hypermobility has not been established.
- Care should be taken if neck instability is a possibility (e.g. fracture, RA). Vigorous passive examination of forward flexion may exacerbate disc lesions.
- Examination of the shoulder is important to evaluate any referred pain or associated articular lesion (e.g. adhesive capsulitis).
- Neurological examination of upper and lower limbs is important in all cases where pain is referred to the arms and/or the legs if cord compression is a possibility: look for increased tone, clonus, pyramidal weakness, and extensor plantar response. Check for a cervicothoracic sensory level.

### Investigation of neck conditions in adults

#### Radiographs

Radiographs should be requested with specific objectives in mind:
- A lateral neck film may demonstrate soft tissue thickening in infection or synovium in RA (see → Chapter 5), will document spondylitis (syndesmophytes, discitis, and periosteal apposition in posterior elements associated with psoriasis), and the severity of spondylosis.
- Oblique views centred on the suspected level may show nerve root foramen stenosis from bony encroachment in patients with radiculopathy. There may be underlying OA (see → Chapter 6).
- High cervical flexion and extension views and a 'through-the-mouth' (odontoid) view are useful to see odontoid pathology.
- In an adult with RA, if the distance between the anterior arch of the atlas and odontoid process is >3 mm on a lateral (flexion) image there is likely to be C1/C2 subluxation in the sagittal plane.
- On a lateral image, superior odontoid subluxation in RA can be judged from a reduced distance from the antero-inferior surface of C2 to a line drawn between the hard palate and base of the occiput (McGregor's line). The distance should be >34 mm in men and >29 mm in women. Lateral odontoid subluxation is best demonstrated with magnetic resonance imaging (MRI).

- Stepwise vertebral subluxation throughout the cervical spine demonstrated on a lateral image is characteristic of advanced RA.
- There may be only a few, but important signs of spinal infection, such as a soft tissue mass or isolated loss of joint space.

*Magnetic resonance imaging and computed tomography (CT)*
- MRI has largely superseded CT, arthrography, and CT arthrography in assessing cervical spine/nerve, dural, vertebral, disc, and other soft tissue lesions in the neck.
- In many cases the relevance of some MRI findings is still being established—patterns of signal abnormality do occur in asymptomatic people. The frequency of these effects increases with age.
- MRI is the technique of choice for imaging disc prolapse, myelopathy (see ➐ Plate 2), myelitis and for excluding infection or tumours. MRI is used to help evaluate the need for, and plan, neurosurgical intervention in high cervical instability in RA patients.
- MRI may show soft tissue swelling around the odontoid in calcium pyrophosphate deposition (CPPD) disease (see ➐ Chapter 7), but the diagnosis is best made with CT, which shows calcification around the odontoid and of adjacent ligaments ('crowned dens syndrome').
- In patients with the combination of unexplained radiographic signs and generalized symptoms MRI is an important investigation. Cases of spinal infection such as tuberculosis (TB) or brucellosis and lymphoma and can be picked up (see ➐ Chapter 17).

*Bone scintigraphy*
- Despite improved image quality and tomographic images, the neck is poorly imaged using bone scintigraphy.

## Treatment of neck pain in adults
Fig. 3.2 shows the principles of treating mechanical cervical syndromes in adults and the timing of MRI scanning:
- Remember to review the diagnosis if pain persists despite treatment and symptoms seem disproportionate to the results of imaging.
- In our experience, inflammatory spondyloarthritis (SpA)-related neck pains can be mistaken as a result of 'cervical spondylosis'. This may be because the clinician too readily assumes the latter diagnosis and/or radiologists report degenerative changes only on radiographs.

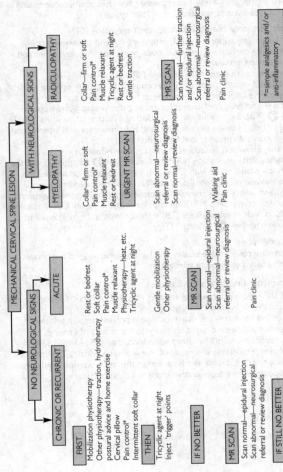

**Fig. 3.2** The principles of treating mechanical neck syndromes in adults and the timing of MRI scanning.

# Neck pain in children and adolescents

## General considerations

Neck pain in children is common. See Table 3.2. Though there are conditions specific to childhood below, this section should be read in association with neck pain assessment in adults p. 74 including functional anatomy and examination (for adolescents).

- The prevalence of neck pain in secondary school-aged children is ~11%.
- In one study, 60% of children experienced at least one episode of neck pain over a 2-year period and 9% experienced neck pain 'often'.
- Of those children with neck pain who present to A&E, 62% have had trauma, 19% presented following infection, in 18% neck pain is related to adverse posture, and just 1.2% had neck pain associated with other conditions. Neck pain resolves in 96% within 2 weeks.

## Clinical features

- In younger children, neck problems are most commonly manifest as torticollis or stiffness.
- Subacute or chronic infectious aetiology includes lymphadenitis, including tuberculous retropharyngeal abscess, and discitis.
- Bone pathology is very rare but causes include eosinophilic granuloma, non-bacterial osteomyelitis, and osteoid osteoma. Malignancy is usually associated with characteristic MRI findings.
- Systemic onset and other forms of JIA are associated with neck stiffness more than with pain.
- Studies in adulthood have indicated cervical spine involvement in up to 80% cases of polyarticular JIA.
- In JIA, neck involvement is often associated with TMJ involvement.

## Examination of the neck: children and adolescents

- General guidelines for the assessment of pain should be followed as outlined in ➔ Chapter 1.
- There should be full exposure of the spine for the examination and a neurological examination undertaken in all cases.
- A full examination includes assessment of posture and biomechanics of the shoulders and lower spine and pelvis.
- Examination of lymph nodes, pharynx, eyes, and joints is important.
- Imaging of choice is MRI.

**Table 3.2** The causes of neck pain in children

| | |
|---|---|
| Soft tissue injury | Neck strain, congenital torticollis, trauma including whiplash, and sporting injury |
| Inflammatory conditions | JIA, juvenile SpA, non-bacterial osteomyelitis, myelitis |
| Skeletal conditions | Osteomyelitis (including TB), osteoid osteoma, histiocytosis, malignancy, insufficiency fracture (e.g. idiopathic juvenile osteoporosis) |
| Non-skeletal infection | Lymphadenitis, meningitis, discitis, retropharyngeal abscess |
| Neurological conditions | Posterior fossa tumour, benign paroxysmal torticollis, syrinx |
| Other | Ocular torticollis (Duane syndrome, refractive error, nystagmus, visual field defect), chronic pain syndrome, thoracic outlet syndrome |

# Shoulder pain in adults

## Anatomy of the shoulder

(See Fig. 3.3.)
- The glenohumeral joint is a ball and socket joint. The shallow glenoid cavity permits a wide range of movement. The circular fibrocartilaginous labrum sits on the glenoid, increases the articular surface area, and acts as a static joint stabilizer.
- Normal glenohumeral movements include depression, then glide and rotation of the humeral head under the coraco-acromial (CA) arch to enable elevation of the arm. As the arm elevates, there is smooth rotation and elevation of the scapula on the thoracic wall.
- Shoulder movements are a synthesis of four joints: glenohumeral, acromioclavicular (AC), sternoclavicular (SC), and scapulothoracic.
- Movements at AC and SC joints enable slight clavicular rotation, shoulder elevation/depression, and protraction/retraction.
- The rigid CA arch protects the glenohumeral joint from trauma and it, and the overlying deltoid, are separated from the capsule by the subacromial (subdeltoid) bursa.
- A cuff of muscles surrounds the glenohumeral joint capsule. These 'rotator cuff 'muscles are the supraspinatus, infraspinatus, teres minor, and subscapularis.
- The supraspinatus initiates abduction by depressing the humeral head, then elevating the arm alone for the first 10° of movement. The more powerful deltoid then takes over abduction. Infraspinatus/teres minor and the subscapularis externally and internally rotate the arm in the anatomical position respectively (Fig. 3.4).
- Production of powerful shoulder movements requires some degree of arm elevation as the larger muscles, such as deltoid, latissimus dorsi (extensor), and teres major (adductor), work inefficiently with the arm in the anatomical position. Rotator cuff muscles act synchronously as joint stabilizers through the range of shoulder movement.
- The long head of the biceps tendon originates above the glenoid usually attached to the labrum and runs within the glenohumeral joint capsule anteromedially in a bony groove.

## Pain and shoulder lesions in adults

(See also ➲ Chapter 20.)
- Shoulder pain is common and may have its origin in articular or periarticular structures or may be referred from the neck or thoracic spine, thoracic outlet, or sub-diaphragmatic structures (Table 3.3).
- Shoulder lesions often produce pain referred to the humeral deltoid insertion (patient points to upper arm).
- Periarticular disorders, mainly shoulder subacromial impingement (SAI) disorders, are the most common cause of shoulder pain in adults (>90% of cases).
- Traumatic or inflammatory lesions of many different shoulder structures and conditions that result in neuromuscular weakness of the rotator cuff or scapular stabilizers may result in impingement pain.

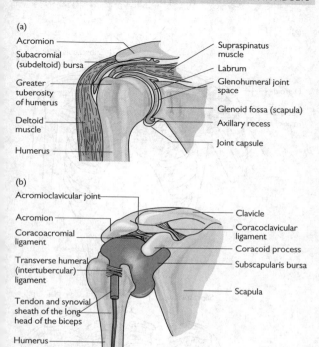

(a)
Acromion
Subacromial (subdeltoid) bursa
Greater tuberosity of humerus
Deltoid muscle
Humerus

Supraspinatus muscle
Labrum
Glenohumeral joint space
Glenoid fossa (scapula)
Axillary recess
Joint capsule

(b)
Acromioclavicular joint
Acromion
Coracoacromial ligament
Transverse humeral (intertubercular) ligament
Tendon and synovial sheath of the long head of the biceps
Humerus

Clavicle
Coracoclavicular ligament
Coracoid process
Subscapularis bursa
Scapula

**Fig. 3.3** (a) Major shoulder structures. (b) The relationship of the joint capsule to its bony surround and the coracoacromial arch.

- Pain from subacromial impingement syndrome is thought to be generated by the 'squashing' of subacromial structures between the greater tuberosity of the humeral head and the CA arch during rotation/elevation of the humeral head.

## Taking a history about shoulder pain in adults

### When did the pain start?

Shoulder injuries are common, and may be acute or chronic (overuse).
- Rotator cuff lesions (inflammation, degenerative weakness, or tear) are often associated with activities and occupations that involve straining the arm in abduction or forward flexion. A history of an acute injury, however, is not always obtained. Subsequent calcification in the tendon following a supraspinatus injury can be asymptomatic or present with acute pain.

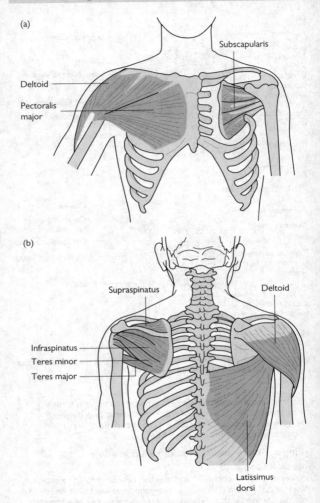

**Fig. 3.4** The muscles of the shoulder: (a) anterior view; (b) posterior view.

**Table 3.3** The most common causes of shoulder pain in adults

| | |
|---|---|
| Periarticular lesions (often manifest as subacromial impingement pain) | Rotator cuff tendonitis/tears (common >40 years) |
| | Calcific tendonitis |
| | Bicipital tendonitis |
| | Subacromial bursitis |
| | Enthesopathy associated with SpA, e.g. PsA |
| | Periarticular muscle weakness |
| Articular lesions | Synovitis (glenohumeral or AC joints) |
| | OA (glenohumeral or AC joints) |
| | Glenohumeral instability (e.g. labral tears) |
| | Adhesive capsulitis ('frozen shoulder') |
| Neurologic | Cervical nerve root and radicular referred pain |
| | Neurological amyotrophy |
| | Spinal cord lesions: tumours, syringomyelia |
| | Brachial neuromyopathy |
| Thoracic lesions (referred pain) | Mediastinal tumours |
| | Angina |
| Systemic and diffuse conditions | Polymyalgia rheumatica |
| | Myositis (see ⊃ Chapter 14) |
| | Chronic pain syndromes (see ⊃ Chapter 22) |
| | Polyarticular inflammatory arthritis |
| Bone disorders (see ⊃ Chapter 16) | Tumours |
| | Osteonecrosis |
| | Paget's disease |

- Manual labour is a risk factor for rotator cuff lesions. There is typically no acute injury, but a history of repetitive movements over years that lead to injury.
- Athletes who take part in throwing and racket sports are at risk of rotator cuff tendinopathy and labral tears. Rugby and American Football players and cyclists are at risk of clavicle fracture, shoulder dislocation and disruption of the AC joint.
- Pain from degenerative glenohumeral or AC joint arthritis might be a long-term sequela of a bone or joint injury.
- Myofascial pain of the shoulder girdle is common and may mimic the symptoms of cervical radiculopathy and even reflux oesophagitis or ischaemic heart disease.
- Severe, persistent, sleep-disturbing pain of recent onset may be indicative of avascular necrosis, osteomyelitis, or bony tumours.

*Where is the pain?*
- Pain from the shoulder may be referred to the deltoid insertion.
- Well-localized pain may occur with AC joint arthritis (e.g. patient places a finger on the affected joint), but remember that referred C4 nerve root pain and pain from bone lesions of the distal clavicle is maximal in the same area.
- Glenohumeral articular and capsulitis pain is not well localized (e.g. the patient covers their shoulder with their hand).
- Pericapsular pain may be associated with SAI, but may also be myofascial (typically) or referred from the cervicothoracic spine.
- Bilateral shoulder pain should increase suspicion of the presence of an inflammatory polyarthritis such as RA (see ➜ Chapter 5), psoriatic arthritis (see ➜ Chapter 8) or CPPD arthritis (see ➜ Chapter 7)—but these would be rare without other joint symptoms.
- Diffuse pain across the shoulder girdle muscles in those >55 years old raises the possibility of PMR. Pain is often associated with immobility and stiffness, particularly early in the day.
- A deep aching pain associated with stiffness is characteristic of adhesive capsulitis (frozen shoulder). The use of the term frozen shoulder is popular, but often incorrectly applied. It is a condition that is rare in patients <40 years of age. The condition occurs in three phase: a painful phase, an adhesive ('frozen') phase, and a resolution phase. Phases often overlap and the duration varies but long-term limitation of shoulder movement remains in up to 15% of patients. It is associated with diabetes.

*Does the pain vary?*
Movement- or posture-related pain may be a clue to its cause:
- Rotator cuff lesions often present to rheumatologists with a subacromial impingement pattern of pain—that is, pain reproducibly aggravated by specific movements during each day such as reaching up (overhead) with the arm. Articular, bone, and adhesive capsulitis pain is more likely to be persistent.
- A history of recurrent bouts of shoulder pain in young adults may suggest glenohumeral instability due to hypermobility or previous trauma, e.g. a labral tear.
- In an unstable shoulder, pain may result from synovitis, subchondral bone damage, or an SAI disorder. The frequency of recurrent anterior subluxation is inversely proportional to the age at which the initial dislocation occurs.

*Are there spinal symptoms?*
There is an association between neck conditions and shoulder pain. C4 nerve root pain is referred to the shoulder, adhesive capsulitis is associated with cervical nerve root symptoms (the nature of the link is unknown), and inflammatory conditions, such as CPPD and psoriatic spondylitis forms can be associated with bilateral shoulder pain referral and can mimic PMR.

## Examination of the shoulder in adults

### Visual inspection

Inspect the neck, shoulders, and arms from the front, side, and back with the patient standing.

- Abnormality of the contour of the cervicothoracic spine could indicate muscle imbalance/spasm or might be associated with a nerve root origin of pain.
- Scapular asymmetry at rest is especially relevant when examining children and may indicate a congenital bony deformity. Subtle degrees of asymmetry are common and are not usually due to specific pathology, nor are they of consequence.
- Diffuse swelling of the whole shoulder may suggest a shoulder effusion/ haemarthrosis or subacromial bursitis. In the elderly, Milwaukee shoulder should be considered. Swelling of the AC joint occurs with joint diastasis, arthritis, and distal clavicular bone lesions.
- Arm swelling and skin changes distally could indicate a complex regional pain syndrome.

### Elicit any tenderness

Eliciting tenderness of shoulder structures is often unrewarding:

- Tenderness of the AC joint, humeral insertion of the supraspinatus tendon, and the long head of biceps tendon may be clues to pathology, but palpation will not be specific for diagnosis.
- The deltoid origin is a typical enthesis involved in active PsA.
- An appreciation of trigger points associated with myofascial pain and tender points in fibromyalgia (see ➋ Chapter 22) is important in the interpretation of regional soft tissue tenderness.

### Document bilateral (active) shoulder movements

This aids diagnosis but also gives an indication of the level of functional impairment and can help in monitoring changes over time. The movements are first tested actively (the patient does the movement) and then passively (the clinician supports the limb). Muscle strength can also be assessed while testing active movement.

- Observe active arm elevation in the scapular plane from behind, noting symmetry of scapular movement, the pattern of pain during elevation, and the range of elevation. Hunching of the shoulder at the outset of arm elevation often occurs with an impingement problem. A painful arc may suggest a rotator cuff lesion. Inability to lift the arm suggests a rotator cuff tear or weakness, capsulitis, or severe pain, e.g. acute calcific supraspinatus tendonitis.
- Observe and compare active internal rotation of shoulders, which can be judged by how far up the back the hand can reach. Poor performance may be due to rotator cuff weakness, weakness of the scapular stabilizing muscles, or pain (generally from impingement syndrome). This manoeuvre assumes normal elbow function.

- Observe the active range of external rotation of the humerus from the front. Ask the patient to flex their elbows as if they were holding a tray and then rotate the arms outwards. Minor degrees of restriction caused by pain are not specific, but severe restriction is characteristic of adhesive capsulitis.
- Passive range of motion should be tested with two hands: one hand guides the movement, while the second rests on the shoulder. Many patients will subconsciously flex the spine to compensate for restricted range of motion at the shoulder; using both hands can help detect this and other abnormalities in movement at the joint.

### Test for subacromial impingement
- Always compare the affected with the non-symptomatic side and make conservative judgements about muscle weakness if there is pain impeding voluntary effort.
- Most tests rely on their ability to narrow the distance between the humeral head and the CA arch, by driving the greater tuberosity under the CA arch as the humerus rotates (Fig. 3.5).
- Whether the tests are specific for lesions of the subacromial structures or for the site of impingement is unknown.

### Movement of the glenohumeral joint
Move the glenohumeral joint passively in all directions by moving the upper arm with one hand and placing the other over the shoulder to feel for 'clunks', crepitus, and resistance to movement:
- If the humeral head can be slid anteriorly (often with a 'clunk') clearly without rotation in the glenoid it suggests instability.
- Grossly reduced passive shoulder movement (notably external rotation, with or without pain) is the hallmark of adhesive capsulitis.
- Pull down on both (hanging) arms. If the humeral head moves inferiorly (sulcus sign) there may be glenohumeral instability.

### Stress the acromioclavicular joint
Stressing the AC joint may reproduce the pain. This is conventionally done by compression or shear tests:
- These tests should not normally be painful. Although painful tests have not proved to be specific for AC pathology (pain from SAI may also be present), a positive test may provide a clue that the AC joint is arthritic, dynamically unstable, or that impingement of structures in the subacromial space under the AC joint is occurring.
- Hold the patient's arm in forward flexion (90°) and draw it across the top of the patient's chest. The resulting compression of the AC joint may produce pain. AC joint pain can also be elicited by passively elevating the arm through 180°, bringing the hand to the ceiling. Pain is experienced in the upper 10° or so of movement.

(a)

**Painful arc**
(active)

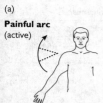

**Action:** Patient standing.
Slow arm abduction
(scapular plane).

**Positive** Pain onset (maximal)
**test:** at (variable) angular
range.

(b)

**Neer test**
(passive)

**Action:** Patient sitting/standing.
Passive forward flexion.
Scapula fixed.

**Positive** Pain at (variable) angle
**test:** of flexion.

(c)

**Empty can**
(active)

**Action:** Patient sitting/standing.
Active forward flexion
to 90° then internal
rotation—'can empties'.

**Positive** Pain with flexion or
**test:** rotation of arm.

(d)

**Kennedy–Hawkins**
(passive)

FIX

**Action:** Patient sitting/standing.
Passive forward flexion (90°).
Fix elbow with hand.
Passive internal rotation.

**Positive** Pain at some stage of
**test:** elevation or rotation.

**Fig. 3.5** Tests useful for eliciting subacromial impingement.

*Gauge strength in rotator and other shoulder muscles*
Once the potential active range of movement has been ascertained in the context of pain and you know which movements hurt (by testing actively and passively) then you can judge the validity of the examination of isolated muscle resistance testing (Table 3.4):
- Rotator cuff muscles need to be tested sub-maximally in regard of strength for strength against resistance—explain to the patient not to push too hard—see Table 3.4.
- Knowledge of nerve supply is important to know whether there might be a neuromyopathic cause for weakness and where a lesion might be (post-infective brachial neuritis can cause focal rotator cuff neuromyopathy and is not uncommon).

**Table 3.4** Isolated muscle testing of shoulder girdle muscles

| Muscle: nerve root, peripheral nerve, supply and muscle action | Muscle position | Isolated muscle test | Pathology affecting muscle strength/bulk |
|---|---|---|---|
| **Supraspinatus:** C5/C6. Suprascapular nerve. Initial humeral abduction and stability of raised upper arm | From behind, seen and felt above the scapular spine at rest and when activated | Abduct arm from neutral against resistance | Tear or disuse following damage, e.g. after a fall, chronic overuse stress, or in athletes (throwing arm) |
| **Infraspinatus:** C5/C6. Suprascapular nerve. External rotation and stability of humeral head | From behind, seen and felt arising from medial scapular border passing laterally (below the scapular spine) | External rotation of arm in neutral, elbow supported and flexed at 90° | Tear or disuse following chronic damage |
| **Serratus anterior:** C5–C7. Long-thoracic nerve. Pulls the scapula forward on the thoracic wall (extends forward reach of arm) | Appreciated from behind when patient is pushing against a wall with arms outstretched in front, in that scapula remains fixed | Test by pushing wall with an outstretched arm or push-up. If paralysed there will be lifting and lateral excursion of the scapula | Damage to long-thoracic nerve from trauma. Patient may also have SAI |
| **Deltoid:** C5/C6. Axillary nerve. Flexion, extension but mainly abduction of humerus | Arises from the scapular spine and acromion, then swathes the shoulder inserting into the humerus laterally | Wasting may be obvious. Weakness in isometric strength of an arm abducted to 90° | Lesions of axillary nerve damaged by anterior shoulder dislocation (external rotation may also be weak from denervation of teres minor) |

*Shoulder examination with the patient supine*

Examine the shoulders with the patient supine to test whether there is anterior cuff deficiency, glenohumeral joint laxity, or a labral tear: this is especially important in young adults and adolescents to identify an 'unstable shoulder'. Hold and support the upper arm held in slight abduction and external rotation (the elbow is flexed). Move the arm gently (cranially in the coronal plane) and apply gradual degrees of external rotation.

• Deficiency of anterior structures is suggested by patient apprehension that pain is imminent or that the shoulder will slip forward. With a labral tear, there may be an audible or palpable 'clunk'.

- Pressure down on the upper arm (taking the pressure off anterior shoulder structures by an anteriorly translocated humeral head) may relieve apprehension or pain associated with it (+ve relocation test).
- An unstable shoulder identified with the above tests may denote previous traumatic injury (e.g. shoulder dislocation) or a hypermobility disorder.

## Investigations of shoulder disorders in adults

Optimum initial imaging for investigating undiagnosed shoulder pain is disputed. Management of shoulder problems based on history and examination alone is a practical approach to a common problem, since many problems get better in the short term. The long-term sequelae of such management strategies, however, are unknown. Studies of shoulder pain primarily suggest that chronic shoulder problems are common, often despite initial improvement.

### Radiographs

- The standard projection for screening purposes is anteroposterior (AP), although the AP axial–lateral view taken with the arm abducted may add information about the relationship of the glenoid and humeral head. Look for calcific deposits in soft tissue basic calcium phosphate crystals: Milwaukee shoulder (see ➔ Chapter 7).
- Supraspinatus outlet views are often used to assess acromial configuration and identify inferior acromial osteophytes in patients with SAI.
- If recurrent dislocation is suspected, associated humeral head defects may be identified by an AP film with internal humeral rotation or a Stryker view. Bilateral films distinguish anomaly (invariably bilateral) from abnormality.
- Bilateral AP AC joint views with the patient holding weights may identify, and grade degrees of, AC joint diastasis (separation). Distal clavicular erosion may be due to RA, hyperparathyroidism, myeloma, metastases, or post-traumatic osteolysis.
- Although characteristic patterns of abnormality are associated with SAI (see ➔ Plate 3), minor age-related radiographic abnormalities are normal.

### Other imaging: ultrasound, arthrography, CT arthrography, MRI, isotope bone scan

- Ultrasound (US) scoring systems for locating and grading rotator cuff tears now exist. US permits examination of the rotator cuff with the shoulder in different positions, but is highly operator dependent.
- Patterns of rotator cuff abnormality and subacromial impingement are well recognized with both arthrography and MRI. However, there is no consensus about which of ultrasound, MRI, or arthrography is most accurate for detecting rotator cuff tears.
- Children, adolescents, and young adults suspected of having unstable shoulders should have an MRI examination, since detailed views of the humeral head, glenoid labrum, periarticular glenohumeral soft tissues, and subacromial area are important.

- MRI is the modality of choice in young adults when instability is diagnosed. Rotator cuff lesions and labral abnormalities are best assessed with MRI. Enhancement with IV contrast may increase the chance of detecting a labral tear.
- No specific patterns of bone scan abnormality have been consistently recognized for isolated shoulder lesions, although a phase study may be diagnostic for complex regional pain syndrome in the arm.

*Other investigations*

- Local anaesthetic injection may help disclose the site of shoulder pain, although it is possible that by the time anaesthesia occurs, the injected anaesthetic has spread to areas not intended as a target.
- Joint aspiration is essential if infection is possible. Fluid is usually aspirated easily from a distended shoulder capsule. Haemarthroses can occur in degenerate shoulders, with haemophilia, trauma, and pigmented villonodular synovitis (PVNS).
- Electrophysiological tests (electromyography (EMG)/nerve conduction study (NCS)) may confirm muscle weakness and help establish the presence of neuromuscular disease, e.g. myositis or neurological amyotrophy.
- Blood tests are required if considering infection or inflammation.
- A normal creatine kinase (CK) and aldolase will rule out myositis in the majority of cases.
- Blood urea, electrolytes, creatinine, alkaline phosphatase, calcium, phosphate, thyroid function tests, and myeloma screen should be considered if metabolic bone or myopathic disease is considered.

## Treatment of shoulder disorders in adults

- Physical therapy should play a focal part in encouraging mobilization of the joint, and early assessment is prudent.
- Know whether there is an additional neck/spinal generated pain component (physical therapists are independent diagnosticians and some may erroneously aim therapy at cervicothoracic segments for individual shoulder lesions).
- Do not refer to physiotherapy without knowledge of who will see the patient, and the approach that will be taken for instability and rotator cuff weakness.
- Simple analgesics are often necessary.
- Steroid injections can be considered in the following situations (see also ➔ Chapter 24):
  - Tendonitis of the rotator cuff.
  - Adhesive capsulitis (see ➔ Plate 4).
  - AC joint pain.
  - Subacromial bursitis (see ➔ Plate 5).
- The principles of steroid injection and rehabilitation are dealt with in ➔ Chapter 24.

- There are several situations where local steroids should be avoided:
  - Bicipital tendonitis (rest, analgesia, physical therapy).
  - The first 6 weeks of an acute rotator cuff tear.
  - When symptoms have become chronic and conservative therapy has not helped for a presumptive clinical diagnosis (this requires reassessment, imaging as surgery may be required).
- Surgical intervention may be: subacromial decompression arthroscopy, synovectomy of the SC joint and AC joint, or excision of the distal end of the clavicle:
  - Subacromial decompression may be necessary for chronic rotator cuff tendonitis especially when imaging has shown inferior acromial osteophytes.
  - Other interventions include repair of a rotator cuff or biceps tendon rupture and joint replacement (for pain relief rather than improvement in function mainly).
- Lithotripsy does not offer advantages over steroid injection and physical therapy for calcific supraspinatus tendonitis.

# Shoulder pain in children and adolescents

## General considerations

The prevalence of chronic shoulder pain in adolescents is 7–11%.

- The principal cause of shoulder pain is biomechanical imbalance either from deconditioning, sporting injury (e.g. labral tear or rotator cuff lesions), overuse, or secondary to direct trauma.
- The shoulder can be involved in JIA.
- Examination follows the principles of adult examination already described and paediatric guidelines on examination—see ➲ Chapter 1.

**Table 3.5** Causes of shoulder pain in children and adolescents

| | |
|---|---|
| Soft tissue injury | Biomechanical imbalance and deconditioning: adverse neuromuscular patterning/glenohumeral or scapular instability; subacromial impingement; biceps tendinopathy; rotator cuff tendinopathy; trauma; myositis |
| Joint pathology | AC joint injury; juvenile idiopathic arthritis; labral tear |
| Skeletal lesions | Proximal humeral stress injury to physis (including little leaguer's shoulder); osteomyelitis and non-bacterial osteomyelitis (especially of clavicle); osteoid osteoma; osteosarcoma (especially in adolescent); fracture; distal clavicular osteolysis |
| Other | Brachial plexus injury; chronic pain syndrome; referred pain (from the neck); thoracic outlet syndrome; periphrenic inflammation |

# Pain around the elbow in adults

### Functional anatomy

- The humero-ulnar articulation is the prime (hinge) joint at the elbow. The radius also articulates with the humerus and allows forearm and hand supination/pronation, with the ulna at the elbow (Fig. 3.6).
- Normal extension results in a straight arm, but some muscular people lack the last 5–10° of extension and some (especially women) have up to an extra 10° of extension (hyperextension).
- Normal flexion is to 150–160° and forearm supination/pronation range is around 180°.
- Due to obliquity of the trochlea, extension is associated with a slight valgus that can be accentuated in women (up to 15°).
- Unilateral acute traumatic or chronic overuse lesions of the elbow are common. Bilateral symptoms may occur in these situations, but also consider the possibility of an inflammatory arthritis affecting the elbows or referred pain from the neck.

### Taking a history of elbow pain in adults

*Is pain exclusively located in the elbow or referred from elsewhere?*

Establish whether the pain is associated with neck pain and whether it has neurogenic qualities or is associated with paraesthesias or numbness. Pain may be referred from proximal neurologic lesions (e.g. C6, C7) or from distal lesions such as carpal tunnel syndrome (CTS).

*Is there a history of acute or chronic (overuse) trauma?*

- Pain at the lateral epicondyle 1–2 weeks after a weekend of 'home maintenance' might suggest lateral epicondylitis (tennis elbow) following excessive use of a screwdriver, for example.
- Other common sites of pain, where characteristic conditions related to overuse are recognized, include the medial humeral epicondyle ('golfer's elbow') and the olecranon bursa (repetitive pressure/friction). Although typically acute in onset, these conditions may develop insidiously.

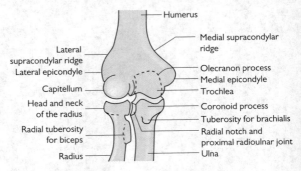

**Fig. 3.6** Bony configuration at the (right) elbow (anterior view).

- Fractures around the elbow and fractures/dislocations in the forearm are common.
- Dislocation of the radial head alone is rare and is usually associated with concurrent fracture of the ulna (radiographs may not identify the fracture). If not associated with fracture (and especially if recurrent), dislocation may be associated with generalized hypermobility (see ➔ Chapter 19) or shortening of the ulna due to bone dysplasia.

### Does the pain radiate distally?

- Forearm pain may be an additional clue to C6 or C7 radicular pain, but may also be due to the spread of MSK pain along the extensor group of muscles from lateral epicondylitis or from entrapment of the median nerve in the elbow region.
- Peritendonitis crepitans is pain, tenderness, and swelling in the forearm associated with occupational overuse. It is thought to be due to damage of the long wrist/hand flexors and extensors at the muscle–tendon junction.
- Diffuse pain in the forearm can occur as a result of overuse injury, particularly in musicians and typists, although there is overlap with regional pain syndromes.
- Pain around the forearm may also arise from inflammation at the wrist (see ➔ 'Wrist pain in adults', pp. 106–9) particularly in De Quervain's tenosynovitis.

### Is there prominent stiffness with the pain?

- Stiffness is often non-specific but may denote inflammation such as synovitis of the joint or olecranon bursa. It raises the possibility of an autoimmune rheumatic or crystal deposition disease.
- In the middle aged and elderly, gout (see ➔ Chapter 7) of the olecranon bursa and surrounding soft tissues, particularly overlying the border of the ulna, is common and is often misdiagnosed as a cellulitis.

### Ask about locking

Locking of the elbow either in flexion or supination/pronation may be due to loose intra-articular bodies. A single loose body is most commonly due to osteochondritis dissecans of the capitellum and multiple loose bodies are associated with OA or synovial chondromatosis.

### Is the pain unremitting and severe?

This type of pain suggests bony pathology:
- Although non-fracture bone pathology is rare in the elbow region, local bony pain might suggest osteochondritis or avascular necrosis or, if part of a wider pattern of bony pain, metabolic bone disease.
- In the elderly and others at high risk for osteoporosis, supracondylar, and other fractures may occur with surprisingly little trauma.

### Are there symptoms in other joints?

Ask about other joints, low back (sacroiliac) pains and risks for gout:
- Elbow synovitis is an uncommon presenting feature of adult RA.
- Periarticular enthesitis is a recognized feature of spondyloarthritis (SpA) (see ➔ Chapter 8) and may mimic tennis elbow.
- The periarticular tissue around the elbow is a common site for gout.

## Examination of the elbow in adults

Look for abnormality then palpate with the thumb. Observe the active, passive, and resisted active range of joint and related tendon movements, and consider examining for local nerve lesions. A complete assessment should include examination of neck, shoulder, and wrist.

### Visual inspection

Look for obvious deformity or asymmetry in the anatomical position:

- Up to 10° of extension from a straight arm is normal. More extension might suggest a hypermobility disorder.
- A child with an elbow lesion typically holds the extended arm close to the body, often in pronation.
- Swelling due to joint synovitis is difficult to see in the antecubital fossa unless it is florid: it is most easily seen (and more easily felt) adjacent to the triceps tendon insertion.
- The olecranon bursa, which may be inflamed, overlies the olecranon and does not as a rule communicate with the joint. Overlying erythema, though non-specific, may be a sign of infection or gout.
- Nodules over the extensor surface or ulna border may be associated with RA (see ➔ Chapter 5).
- Psoriatic plaques are commonly found at the elbow extensor surface.

### Observe active flexion and supination/pronation with the elbows held in 90° of flexion

- Although the range of movement may be affected by extra-articular pain, loss of range usually implies an intra-articular disorder.

### Palpate the lateral epicondyle of the humerus

- In lateral epicondylitis (tennis elbow), there is tenderness, which may extend distally. Resisted wrist and finger extension with the elbow in extension or passively stretching the tendons (make fist, flex wrist, pronate forearm, then extend elbow) may reproduce the pain.
- Lateral epicondyle tenderness may be due to inflammation of the radiohumeral bursa that lies under the extensor tendon aponeurosis.
- Note that tenderness of lateral and sometimes medial epicondyles can occur in chronic pain syndromes. In these cases, the relevant extensor or flexor tendon provocation tests are likely to be negative.

### Palpate the medial humeral epicondyle

- Tenderness suggests traumatic medial epicondylitis ('golfer's elbow'), a regional or chronic pain syndrome, or enthesitis. Confirm the site of the pain by stretching the wrist flexors—supinate the forearm then passively extend both the wrist and elbow simultaneously. Resisted palmar flexion of the wrist or forearm pronation with elbow extension may also cause pain. Tasks that rely on this repetitive movement are often the provoking cause.
- Consider osteochondritis of the medial humeral epicondyle as a cause of persistent pain following an injury.

*Passively flex and extend the elbow joint*

Passively flex and extend the joint and note the range of movement and 'end-feel' (the feel of resistance at the end of the range of passive joint movement):

- 'End-feel' may tell you whether there is a block to full flexion or extension from a bony spur or osteophyte (solid end-feel) or from soft tissue thickening/fibrosis (springy, often painful).
- Note any crepitus (often associated with intra-articular pathology) and locking (may have loose bodies in the joint).

*Supinate and pronate the forearm*

Passively supinate and pronate the forearm supporting the elbow in 90° of flexion with your thumb over the radioulnar articulation:

- There may be crepitus or instability/subluxation associated with pain. Instability might suggest a tear/damage to the annular ligament (due to trauma or chronic/aggressive intra-articular inflammation).

*Test peripheral nerve function if there are distal arm symptoms*

- Given its course around the lateral epicondyle, the integrity of the radial nerve should always be tested when a lateral elbow lesion is suspected.
- The median nerve runs in the antecubital fossa and may be affected in traumatic elbow lesions. It is particularly susceptible where it runs between the two heads of pronator teres (from medial epicondyle and the coronoid process of the ulna) and separates into anterior interosseous and terminal median nerve branches.
- The ulnar nerve lies in the groove behind the medial epicondyle. Bony or soft tissue abnormality in this area may affect nerve function and lead to reduced sensation in the little finger and weakness in the small muscles of the hand, the flexor carpi ulnaris (FCU), the extensor carpi ulnaris (ECU), or the abductor digiti minimi (ADM). The median and ulnar nerves are dealt with in more detail in the later sections on wrist and hand disorders.

## Investigation of elbow conditions in adults

*Radiographs and other imaging*

- Standard AP and lateral radiographs are the most straightforward way of imaging the elbow initially. CT or MRI may then be needed if the diagnosis is still obscure and referred pain can be ruled out.
- Look for periosteal lesions and enthesophytes (new bone spurs at clear entheses like the triceps insertion). Periosteal new bone and enthesophytes are typical in psoriatic arthritis (see ◗ Chapter 8).
- A lateral radiograph may identify displacement of the anterior fat pad associated with a joint effusion (sail sign).
- Dislocations of the radial head and associated ulna fractures in children are easily missed. To make this diagnosis a high degree of suspicion and further imaging are often needed.

*Needle arthrocentesis/olecranon bursocentesis*
- Arthrocentesis/bursocentesis with fluid sent for microscopy and culture should always be done in suspected cases of sepsis.
- Fluid should be sent for polarized light microscopy in cases of bursitis that may be due to gout. Serum urate is worth requesting but may not be raised in acute gout.
- Examination of fluid for crystals should always be considered in cases of monoarthritis in the elderly or patients on dialysis.

*Electrophysiology*
If nerve entrapment is suspected and there is some uncertainty after clinical examination, then electrophysiological tests may provide useful information. Testing can help identify the degree and likely site of nerve damage and can help to discriminate between a peripheral and nerve root lesion (if EMG of selected muscles requested also).

## Treatment of elbow conditions in adults
- The management of fractures is beyond the scope of this text.
- Epicondylitis is best managed early on with rest, splinting, analgesia, and local steroid injections. The efficacy of physical manipulation has not been proven, although there are theoretical reasons why ultrasound therapy could be of value (e.g. it passes through the myofascial planes and concentrates near bone). Resistant cases may benefit from surgery—a 'lateral release'.
- Steroid injections (see **⊋** Chapter 24) may be of value in the following situations:
  - lateral or medial epicondylitis (hydrocortisone). See **⊋** Plate 6.
  - inflammatory arthritis (usually long acting steroid).
  - olecranon bursitis.
  - ulnar nerve entrapment.
- Surgical procedures include excision of nodules and bursae, transposition of the ulnar nerve, synovectomy, excision of the head of the radius, and arthroplasty.
- Arthroplasty in inflammatory arthritis is best reserved for severe pain and should be undertaken by an experienced surgeon. Lesser procedures such as proximal radial head excision can be effective to improve pain and function if forearm pronation/supination are poor.
- Radiation synovectomy of the elbow (Re-186) for inflammatory arthritis, PVNS, or synovial chondromatosis requires ultrasound guidance (see guidelines available at ℘ http://www.eanm.org).

# Elbow pain in children and adolescents

## General considerations

The elbow is a common site of injury in children and adolescents; the growth plate and entheseal attachments are vulnerable to overuse injury before skeletal maturity.

- Characteristic injurious lesions are associated with specific activities (e.g. baseball pitching or throwing sports, gymnasts).
- The two main entheses at the elbow—origin of long tendons to the fingers at medial and lateral humeral epicondyles—can become inflamed or painful in people with juvenile PsA or SpA.
- Examination of the elbow in young people is as for adults see ➔ p. 100. See also functional anatomy see ➔ p. 98.

Table 3.6 Causes of elbow pain in children and adolescents

| | |
|---|---|
| Lateral elbow | Lateral humeral epicondylitis/enthesitis (caused by trauma or JSpA or JPsA); osteochondritis and osteochondritis dissecans (adolescent gymnasts); Panner's disease (osteonecrosis of capitellum seen in children aged 5–10 years and may be related to throwing injuries) |
| Medial elbow | Medial humeral epicondylitis/enthesitis caused by trauma— seen in children 9–12 yrs from throwing sports including pitching in baseball—and enthesitis in JSpA and JPsA; medial collateral ligament (MCL) injury; ulnar neuritis; pronator strain |
| Posterior elbow | Olecranon enthesitis; olecranon osteochondritis; olecranon impingement (overhead arm use in racket sports, swimming, boxing, etc.); triceps avulsion |
| Other | JIA; fracture; loose cartilaginous body; skeletal dysplasia |

# Wrist pain in adults

## Functional anatomy of the wrist

- The wrist includes radiocarpal (scaphoid and lunate) and intercarpal articulations. The ulna does not truly articulate with the lunate, but is joined to it, the triquetrum, and the radius (ulnar side of distal aspect), by the triangular fibrocartilage complex.
- The intercarpal joints are joined by intercarpal ligaments and are most stable when the wrist is in full extension. Anterior carpal ligaments are stronger than posterior ones and are reinforced by the flexor retinaculum. Wrist and finger flexor tendons, the radial artery, and the median nerve enter the hand in a tunnel formed by the carpal bones and the flexor retinaculum (carpal tunnel).
- Flexion (70°), extension (70°), radial and ulnar deviation (about 20° and 30° from midline, respectively) occur at the wrist but supination/pronation of the wrist and hand is due to radiohumeral movement at the elbow.
- Flexor carpi radialis (FCR) and ulnaris (FCU) are the main flexors of the wrist, although palmaris longus (PL) also helps (Fig. 3.7). They all arise from the medial humeral epicondyle.
- All carpal extensors arise from the lateral humeral epicondyle (Fig. 3.7).
- Radial deviation (abduction) occurs primarily when radial flexors and extensors act together. Ulnar deviation (adduction) occurs primarily when ulnar flexors and extensors act together.

## Taking a history of wrist pain in adults

Table 3.7 details the major diagnoses for painful conditions of the wrist and hand.

### Determine the exact location of the pain

- Pain localizing only to the wrist most likely comes from local tissue pathology. Cervical nerve root pain as a result of a C6, C7, or C8 lesion and pain from peripheral nerve lesions is likely to be located chiefly in the hand.
- Pain at the base of the thumb, aggravated by thumb movements, in middle and old age is typical of OA (see ➋ Chapter 6) of the trapezium-first metacarpal joint. Pain in this area might also be due to tenosynovitis of thumb tendons.

### Trauma history

Injury/post-injury conditions are common. Taking a history of trauma is important.

- Common fractures in adults are scaphoid and base of the first metacarpal (Bennett's), and head of the radius (Colles').
- Post-traumatic chronic wrist pain following injuries may be due to ligamentous injury and chronic carpal instability or osteonecrosis (lunate).
- Unusual or florid pain descriptors suggest a regional pain syndrome (e.g. CRPS; see ➋ Chapter 22).

(a)

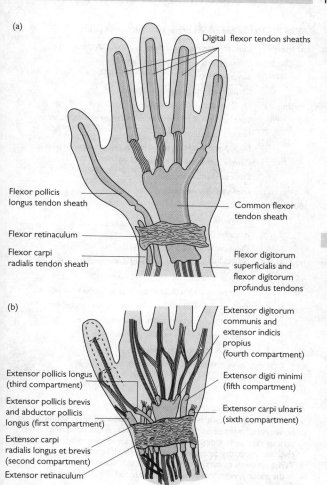

Digital flexor tendon sheaths

Flexor pollicis longus tendon sheath

Common flexor tendon sheath

Flexor retinaculum

Flexor carpi radialis tendon sheath

Flexor digitorum superficialis and flexor digitorum profundus tendons

(b)

Extensor digitorum communis and extensor indicis propius (fourth compartment)

Extensor pollicis longus (third compartment)

Extensor digiti minimi (fifth compartment)

Extensor pollicis brevis and abductor pollicis longus (first compartment)

Extensor carpi ulnaris (sixth compartment)

Extensor carpi radialis longus et brevis (second compartment)

Extensor retinaculum

**Fig. 3.7** Flexor (a) and extensor (b) tendon sheaths crossing the wrist. Flexor carpi radialis (FCR) inserts into the second and third metacarpals. Flexor carpi ulnaris (FCU) inserts into the pisiform, hamate, and fifth metacarpal. Extensor carpi radialis longus (ECRL) inserts into the base of the second, extensor carpi radialis brevis (ECRB) into the third, and extensor carpi ulnaris (ECU) into the fifth metacarpal, respectively.

**Table 3.7** Painful conditions of the wrist and hand (adults)

| | |
|---|---|
| Articular | Chronic inflammatory arthritis (e.g. PsA, RA, JIA, CPPD) |
| | Osteoarthritis |
| | Septic arthritis |
| | Carpal instability (e.g. lunate dislocation) |
| Periarticular | De Quervain's tenosynovitis |
| | Tenosynovitis of common flexor/extensor tendon sheath |
| | Flexor pollicis tenosynovitis |
| | Distal flexor stenosing tenosynovitis (trigger finger or thumb) |
| | Ganglia, subcutaneous nodules, tophi |
| | Diabetic cheiroarthropathy |
| | Dupuytren's contracture |
| Bone | Fracture |
| | Neoplasia |
| | Infection |
| | Osteochondritis (➜ Chapter 16) |
| Neurologic | Median nerve entrapment (carpal tunnel or at pronator teres) |
| | Anterior interosseous nerve syndrome |
| | Ulnar nerve lesions (cubital tunnel or in Guyon's canal in wrist) |
| | Posterior interosseous nerve or radial nerve entrapment |
| | Brachial plexopathy or thoracic outlet syndrome |
| | Cervical nerve root irritation or entrapment |
| | Complex regional pain syndrome |
| | Spinal cord lesions, e.g. syringomyelia |

### Are there features to suggest synovitis?

- Pain due to wrist joint synovitis may be associated with 'stiffness' and be worse at night or early morning. Stiffness 'in the hand' may have various causes including multiple tendon/small joint synovitis, diabetic cheiroarthropathy or systemic sclerosis (SScl; see ➜ Chapter 13).
- Wrist synovitis occurs commonly in adult RA and PsA.
- In the elderly, wrist synovitis may be due to CPPD arthritis (see ➜ Chapter 7).

### The quality of the pain

- Although primary bone pathology is rare, local bony pain (unremitting, severe, sleep disturbing) might suggest osteonecrosis or, if part of a wider pattern of bony pain, metabolic bone disease.
- Radicular pain may be burning in quality and is typically associated with numbness and paraesthesia. Such neurogenic pain is commonly due to nerve root irritation or compression.

*Other joint/MSK symptoms*

- Wrist and extensor tendon sheath synovitis is a common presenting feature of adult RA. Other joints may be affected.
- CPPD arthritis commonly involves the wrist, and can mimic RA in its joint distribution and presentation in the elderly.
- Wrist synovitis and enthesitis occurs in SpA. Pain may be considerable, although swelling is minimal. There may be inflammatory-type symptoms of spinal pain and enthesitis elsewhere.

*Ask specifically about job/leisure activities*

- Repetitive lateral and medial wrist movements with thumb adducted can cause tenosynovitis of the abductor pollicis longus (APL) or the extensor pollicis brevis (EPB), commonly called De Quervain's tenosynovitis.
- If there is no obvious history of trauma, tendonitis may be a presenting feature of a systemic autoimmune rheumatic disease or even gonococcal infection in adolescents and young adults.
- Overuse pain syndromes may occur as a result of repetitive activity. The term 'repetitive strain injury' is controversial. Objective assessment of pain, location of swelling, etc., from the outset is invaluable in assessing the response to treatment. Lack of objective findings (if imaging is normal) suggests a regional pain disorder.

## Examination of the wrist in adults

*Visual inspection*

Inspect the dorsal surface of both wrists looking for swelling, deformity, or loss of muscle bulk (see ➡ Plate 7a):

- Diffuse swelling may be due to wrist joint or extensor tendon sheath synovitis or both.
- A prominent ulna styloid may result from subluxation at the distal radioulnar joint owing to synovitis or radioulnar ligament damage.
- Prominence ('squaring') of the trapezoid–first metacarpal joint commonly occurs in OA of this joint.
- Loss of muscle bulk in the forearm may be due to a chronic T1 nerve root lesion or disuse atrophy.

*Flexion/extension range tests for major wrist lesions*

- The normal range of both flexion and extension in adults is about 70°. Synovitis invariably reduces this range.
- Substantial common flexor or extensor tendon swelling will probably block the full range of wrist movements.
- There is normally an additional 20° of flexion and extension to the active range with passive movement.
- Pain and crepitus are unlikely to be specific for any type of lesion.

*Examine the dorsum of the wrist in detail*

- Note any abnormal excursion of the ulnar styloid associated with pain and/or crepitus suggesting synovitis.
- Post-traumatic carpal instability, particularly scapulolunate dissociation, is relatively common. The latter is demonstrated by eliciting dorsal subluxation of the proximal scaphoid pole by firm pressure on its distal pole as the wrist is deviated radially from a starting position with the forearm pronated and the wrist in ulnar deviation. Note any gap between scaphoid and lunate, and any associated tenderness.
- Note any tenderness or thickening of the common extensor tendon sheath and tendon sheath of APL and EPB.
- Tenderness at the base of the thumb may be due to wrist synovitis, carpal or carpometacarpal OA, tenosynovitis, a ganglion, or a ligament lesion.
- Finkelstein's test for De Quervain's tenosynovitis may be used to elicit APL/EPB tendon pain. With the thumb adducted and opposed, the fingers are curled to form a fist. Passive ulnar deviation at the wrist stretches the abnormal tendons and elicits pain. Although it is a sensitive test, it is not specific for tendon pain.
- Protrusion of the thumb out of the fist on the ulnar side of the hand during the first part of this test is unusual and suggests thumb, and perhaps general, hypermobility.

*Test the integrity of the tendons*

Many muscles/tendons that move both the wrist and digits originate at the elbow; therefore, the quality of information gained from isolated tendon resistance tests (either for pain or strength) may be affected by pain elsewhere around the wrist, wrist deformity, or elbow lesions.

- Interpret findings cautiously.
- Useful information might be obtained by passive movement of a tendon, rather than by resisted active movement, and also by feeling for thickening or crepitus of the tendons.

## Investigation and treatment of wrist conditions in adults

The investigation and treatment of wrist conditions is covered in ➔ 'Symptoms in the hand in adults', pp. 112–21.

# Symptoms in the hand in adults

Symptoms in the hand are a common presenting feature of some systemic conditions, and localized neurological and MSK lesions are common, especially in adults. Detailed knowledge of anatomy is beyond the scope of this text. Functional anatomy is important and the more common abnormalities are summarized here.

## Functional anatomy of the hand

### The long tendons

- Digital power is provided primarily by flexor and extensor muscles arising in the forearm. Their action is supplemented and modified by small muscles in the hand. Precise movements of the hand are mainly due to small muscles.
- Powerful flexors (Fig. 3.7): flexor digitorum superficialis (FDS), flexor digitorum profundus (FDP), and flexor pollicis longus (FPL).
- FDS flexes proximal interphalangeal joints (PIPJs) and, more weakly, metacarpophalangeal joints (MCPJs)/wrist.
- FDP flexes distal interphalangeal joints (DIPJs) and, increasingly weakly, PIPJs, MCPJs/wrist.
- FPL flexes (at 90° to other digits) mainly the PIPJ, but also the whole thumb in a power grip (see later).

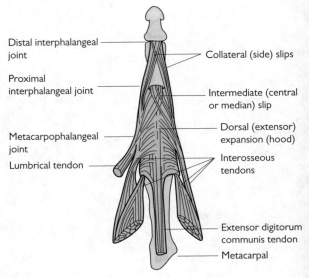

Distal interphalangeal joint

Proximal interphalangeal joint

Metacarpophalangeal joint

Lumbrical tendon

Collateral (side) slips

Intermediate (central or median) slip

Dorsal (extensor) expansion (hood)

Interosseous tendons

Extensor digitorum communis tendon

Metacarpal

**Fig. 3.8** Extensor expansion of a finger.

**Table 3.8** Muscles of the thenar eminence

| Muscle | Origin | Insertion |
| --- | --- | --- |
| Abductor pollicis brevis | Flexor retinaculum, scaphoid, and trapezium | Thumb proximal phalanx and dorsal expansion |
| Flexor pollicis brevis | Flexor retinaculum, trapezium, trapezoid, and capitate | Thumb proximal phalanx (base of radial side) |
| Opponens pollicis | Flexor retinaculum and tubercle of the trapezium | First metacarpal (lateral border) |
| Adductor pollicis | Capitate, bases of second/third metacarpals and distal third metacarpal | Thumb proximal phalanx (medial side) |

- Powerful digital extensors (Fig. 3.7 and Fig. 3.8): extensor digitorum (ED) arises from the lateral epicondyle splitting at the wrist to insert into each digital dorsal expansion (digits two to five) that attaches to all three phalanges. The fifth digit has an additional tendon, extensor digiti minimi (EDM) that also arises at the lateral epicondyle.
- APL abducts the thumb at the MCPJ, provided the wrist is stable.
- EPB and EPL extend the thumb.
- Extensor indicis (EI) arises from the ulna posterior border distal to EPL and joins the index finger ED tendon.
- The muscles of the thenar eminence (Table 3.8) act synchronously. All except adductor pollicis (ulnar nerve, C8/T1) are supplied by the median nerve from C8/T1 nerve roots. All three muscles are supplied by the ulnar nerve (C8/T1).

*The intrinsic muscles*

- The longitudinal muscles of the palm (four dorsal and four palmar interossei and four lumbricals) all insert into digits.
- Palmar interossei from metacarpals 1, 2, 4, 5, insert into dorsal tendons.
- Each dorsal interosseous arises from origins on two adjacent metacarpals. The muscles abduct the second and fourth fingers and move the middle finger either medially or laterally.
- The four lumbricals (Fig. 3.9 and Table 3.9) arise from tendons of FDP in the palm passing to the lateral side of each MCPJ inserting into the dorsal expansions.
- The interossei combine with lumbricals to facilitate fine control of flexion and extension of MCPJs and PIPJs.

*Grip*

- For power, the wrist extends and adducts slightly, and the long digital flexors contract.
- A modified power grip, the hook grip, is used to carry heavy objects like a suitcase. The thumb is extended out of the way and extension at MCPJs accompanies flexion at PIPJs/DIPJs.
- More precision in the grip can be obtained using varying degrees of thumb adduction, abduction, and flexion. The thumb can be opposed with any of the four other digits depending on the shape of the object to be held and the type of manipulation required.

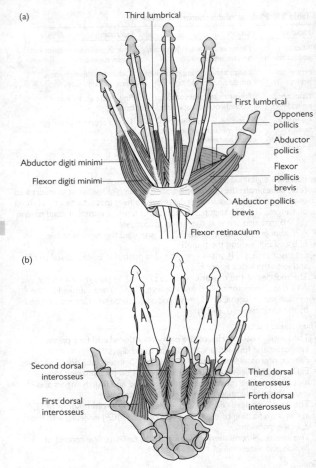

**Fig. 3.9** (a) Lumbrical muscles and muscles of the thenar and hypothenar eminences. (b) Dorsal interossei.

**Table 3.9** Muscles of the hypothenar eminence

| Muscle | Origin | Insertion |
|--------|--------|-----------|
| Abductor digiti minimi | Flexor retinaculum (FR), pisiform, and pisohamate ligament | Base of the fifth proximal phalanx and dorsal expansion |
| Flexor digiti minimi brevis | Flexor retinaculum and Hook of hamate | Base of the fifth proximal phalanx |
| Opponens digiti minimi | Flexor retinaculum and Hook of hamate | Medial side of the fifth metacarpal |

## Taking a history of hand symptoms in adults

A history of acute or overuse trauma with subsequent localized symptoms requires a straightforward application of anatomical knowledge, precise examination, and judicious choice of imaging techniques for diagnosis. However, there are subtler or less easily delineated patterns of symptoms in the hand, particularly when pain is diffuse or poorly localized.

*Is the pain associated with immobility or stiffness?*
- Stiffness may be associated with joint or tendon synovitis but is not specific. Prompting may provide more accurate localization of symptoms.
- If unilateral, especially on the dominant hand, be suspicious that diffuse hand pain may be due to a regional pain syndrome.

*Is stiffness local or diffuse?*
- Patterns of joint involvement in autoimmune rheumatic disease and polyarticular arthritis are summarized in ➲ Chapter 2.
- If localized in the palm, there may be Dupuytren's contracture (associated with diabetes). If diffuse, there may be thickening of soft tissue from a systemic process, e.g. hypothyroidism, SScl, diabetic cheiroarthropathy, or disorders of mucopolysaccharide metabolism (the latter especially in infants, although Fabry's disease can present in adulthood with acroparaesthesias and palmar telangiectasia).
- Stiffness due to an upper motor neuron lesion (an interpretation of increased tone) is unlikely to be confined to the hand and is likely to be associated with weakness. The pattern of symptoms over time should give a clue to its aetiology.

*Are there neurologic qualities to the pain or characteristics typical of a common nerve lesion?*
- 'Burning' or 'deep' episodic pain varying with head, neck, and upper spinal position is typical of cervical nerve root pain. Ask about occupation and other activities that are associated with neck problems, the relationship with sleep posture, and frequent headaches.
- Pain on the radial side of the hand waking the patient at night and often relieved, at least partially, by shaking the hand is typical of median nerve entrapment in the wrist. However, pain in this condition is often poorly localized at initial presentation. Remember: other lesions that produce pain in the area around the thumb base: trapezoid–first metacarpal joint OA, tenosynovitis of APL/EPB (De Quervain's) or EPL, referred pain from a C6 nerve root lesion, and ligament lesions (e.g. ulnar collateral ligament of first MCP—'skier's thumb').

*Tingling/pins and needles/numbness*

Make sure both you and the patient understand what you each mean by these terms:

- Symptoms usually denote cervical nerve root or peripheral nerve compression, although they can reflect underlying ischaemia.
- Tingling in the fingertips of both hands, however, is recognized to occur commonly in patients diagnosed with fibromyalgia.
- Symptoms associated primarily with specific positions of the whole arm may be due to thoracic outlet compression of neurovascular structures.

*Pain arising from bone*

Pain in the hands arising from bones may be difficult to discriminate. Radiographs will often lead to confirmation of the diagnosis:

- The most common tumour in the hand is an enchondroma. It is usually painless. If they are painful, then one should suspect infarction or malignant change.
- Secondary metastases and malignant bone tumours in the hand are rare, but must be ruled out in children, adolescents, and young adults with persistent localized bone pain.
- Paget's disease of hand bones can occur, but is relatively rare.
- Digital bone pain from osteomalacia/rickets occurs, but is unusual at presentation.
- Digital pain may rarely be due to sarcoidosis, hyperparathyroid bone disease, thyroid acropachy, hypertrophic (pulmonary) osteoarthropathy (HO), or pachydermoperiostitis. Look for clubbing.

*Ischaemic pain?*

A history suggestive of ischaemic pain in the hands is rare in rheumatologic practice. Persistent ischaemic digital pain can complicate systemic sclerosis and severe Raynaud's (see ➲ Chapter 13):

- Digital vasomotor instability (e.g. Raynaud's disease (RD); see ➲ Chapter 13) is episodic, triggered by cold and emotion, and characterized by digital colour changes: white/blue then red.
- Pain from vasculitis is likely to be persistent and associated with a purpuric rash, nailfold infarcts, or splinter haemorrhages.
- Ischaemic pain associated with cervicothoracic posture or prolonged arm elevation may be due to a lesion of the thoracic outlet.
- Pain may be due to thromboembolism (e.g. antiphospholipid syndrome) infective endocarditis, or thromboarteritis obliterans (Buerger's disease)

*'Swelling'*

Examination is more reliable than a history:

- Apart from isolated lesions, such as ganglia, patients' description of soft tissue or joint swelling may be unreliable and should be substantiated by examination.
- Nerve lesions can give the impression that swelling is present (think what a dentist's local anaesthetic does for your lip!). Patients with carpal tunnel syndrome, for example, can complain of the hand swelling at night.

### 'Weakness'

Ask about trauma, neck, and median nerve entrapment symptoms:

- Acute tendon injuries are common industrial accidents. Chronic occupational overuse may also lead to rupture.
- If weakness is profound and there has been no obvious trauma, the cause is likely to be neuromuscular.
- If not associated with pain, weakness is more likely to be neurological than MSK in origin.
- Weakness associated with pain may be due to a neurologic or MSK lesion, the latter situation often due to an inability to use the hand (or part of it) because of pain or an alteration in biomechanical function as a result of deformity, which may only be slight.
- True weakness associated with stiffness is associated with myelopathy or even motor neuron disease.
- A detailed history of the progression of symptoms is important and neurologic examination should be thorough.

### Trigger finger

This may denote tenosynovitis of a digital flexor tendon. Damage to the tendon and its sheath can result in a fibrous nodule attached to the tendon that moves and catches under the proximal annular ligament just distal to the MCPJ. It may not be painful. This most commonly affects the middle and ring fingers, and is prevalent among professional drivers, cyclists, and those in occupations requiring repeated use of hand-held heavy machinery.

## Examination of the hand: adults

The following sequence is comprehensive, but should be considered if a general condition is suspected. Often an examination only needs to be more specifically directed.

### Inspection of the nails and fingers

- Pits/ridges and dactylitis are associated with psoriatic arthritis (see → Plate 8 and → Chapter 8).
- Splinter haemorrhages may be traumatic, but are associated with infective endocarditis or vasculitis (see → Chapter 13).
- Obvious cuticle damage and punctate cuticle erythema (dilated capillary loops) are features of secondary RD or SScl (see → Plate 9).
- Periungual erythema is associated with a number of autoimmune rheumatic and connective tissue diseases.
- Multiple telangiectasias are associated with lcSScl (see → Chapter 13).
- Diffuse finger thickening (dactylitis) may be due to gross tendon thickening (e.g. SpA or sarcoid), or connective tissue fibrosis/thickening (SScl, cheiroarthropathy). Bony or soft tissue DIPJ or PIPJ swelling should be discriminated.
- A shiny/waxy skin appearance may indicate scleroderma/morphoea.
- Scattered, tiny, non-blanching dark red punctate lesions are typical of cutaneous skin vasculitis.
- Erythematous or violaceous scaly papules/plaques over MCPJs or PIPJs may suggest dermatomyositis (see → Chapter 14).

*Note any diffuse swelling of the hand*
- Diffuse soft tissue/skin swelling, may occur in association with RA, CPPD-pseudogout, CRPS, and SScl.
- RS$_3$PE (remitting seronegative symmetric synovitis with pitting oedema), which presents mainly in adults in their 70s, may be a distinct type of non-erosive polyarticular/tendon synovitis, but may be associated with other, often haematological, conditions.
- Swelling associated with CRPS may be localized or diffuse (see ⊃ Plate 10). Skin may be shiny and later there is often a dark red or blue mottled appearance.
- Typical skin appearances are critical to making a clinical diagnosis of scleroderma. The skin may be initially puffy, but later shiny and tight and, with progression, atrophic with contractures.

*Note any muscle wasting*
Wasting may be due to a degree of chronic denervation (e.g. the thenar eminence in CTS), disuse atrophy (e.g. painful polyarthropathy, joint hypomobility), or catabolism of muscle (e.g. polymyositis, RA). In the elderly, there may be age-related muscle loss ('sarcopenia').

*Note any deformity of digits*
- Deformities tend to occur with long-standing polyarticular joint disease, e.g. OA, severe RA, and psoriatic arthritis.
- Isolated deformities may be due to previous bone or tendon trauma, severe neurological lesions and Dupuytren's contracture. A mallet finger (loss of active DIPJ extension) is due to rupture of the distal extensor tendon expansion usually due to direct trauma.

*Inspect the palm and dorsum of the hand*
- Palmar erythema is not specific, but is associated with autoimmune disorders of connective tissue and joints.
- Check for Dupuytren's disease (fascial thickening on ulnar side).
- On the dorsum of the hand, ganglia and swelling of the common extensor tendon sheath are usually easily noted. Swelling of the extensor tendon sheath is commonly associated with RA in adults.

*Palpation of joints and nodules*
Palpation of joints and nodules is best done using thumb pads with the patient's wrist supported:
- Swelling should be noted for site, consistency, tenderness, and mobility. Osteophytes and exostosis are periarticular or at sites of pressure, may be tender, but are always fixed (see ⊃ Plate 7d).
- Ganglia are hard and usually quite mobile (can occur anywhere).
- Rheumatoid nodules (occur anywhere, but typically on the dorsum of the hand and the extensor surface of the elbow) and tophi (usually distal) are rubbery, hard, relatively fixed, but may be moved (see ⊃ Plate 7a).
- Synovitis is often represented by soft ('boggy'), often springy, swelling around a joint. It may be tender and warm but this is not invariable.
- Synovitis in a single joint may be due to autoimmune rheumatic disease, OA, infection, or foreign-body synovitis (e.g. rose thorn synovitis).

*Palpate tendons in the palm or on the volar aspect of the phalanges*
- Thickening, tenderness, and crepitus suggest tenosynovitis, but tenosynovitis can be hard to spot if it is mild.
- Tethering and thickening of tendons in the palm associated with excessive digital flexion when the hand is at rest and a block to passive finger extension suggests chronic flexor tenosynovitis (take care to note any contributory joint damage).
- Passive tendon movement by gently flexing/extending a proximal phalanx may disclose palpable tendon nodules, crepitus and tenderness.

*Discriminate Dupuytren's disease from flexor tendinopathy*
Dupuytren's disease (a fascia contracture) typically involves the fourth and fifth fingers (40% bilateral). It is common in males aged 50–70 years. The fascia extends to the second phalanx, thus, if severe, the condition causes fixed flexion of MCPJs and PIPJs. It is associated with epilepsy, diabetes, and alcoholism, and usually is not painful.

## Investigation of wrist and hand disorders: adults
### Radiographs
- An AP view of the hand and wrist is a useful screening investigation to characterize a polyarthropathy and diagnose traumatic and metabolic bone lesions (Table 3.10).
- Radiographs may reveal soft tissue swelling around joints compatible with a diagnosis of synovitis.
- Radiographs are insensitive for identifying erosions in early autoimmune joint disease.
- An oblique view of the hand may add information about joint erosions if an erosive MCPJ arthritis is considered.
- Lateral and carpal tunnel views of the carpus can be obtained by varying the degree of X-ray projection angle; however, unless searching for evidence of fracture these views are rarely needed.

### Further imaging: US, MRI, and bone scintigraphy
- In experienced hands, US can be a useful way of looking for early synovitis and patterns of abnormality in association with median nerve entrapment.
- MRI may demonstrate a torn or avulsed triangular cartilage in patients with a post-traumatic painful wrist or with carpal instability.
- MRI images of the carpal tunnel are useful in confirming median nerve compression/tethering and soft tissue wrist pathology, particularly when symptoms recur after carpal tunnel release surgery.
- MRI can provide valuable information about the degree and distribution of inflammatory disease in joints and tendons, particularly in children and patients where history and examination are difficult.
- MRI is more sensitive than radiography in identifying joint erosions in RA. Choosing MRI over US depends on availability and sonographer experience.
- Bone scintigraphy is not specific for any single condition, but in young adults (after closure of epiphyses and before OA is likely) it may be useful for disclosing patterns of inflammation at and around joints and entheses. $^{99m}$Tc-labelled human immunoglobulin is more specific for detecting patterns of synovitis in children and adults.

**Table 3.10** Some conditions/features typically diagnosed on simple AP hand/wrist radiographs

| | |
|---|---|
| Bone conditions | Fractures (e.g. scaphoid, base of first metacarpal) |
| | Tumours |
| | Metabolic bone diseases (e.g. rickets, hyperparathyroidism—look for cortical loss and tunnelling in phalanges) |
| | Osteonecrosis (e.g. post-traumatic—lunate, sickle cell disease) |
| | Sarcoidosis (➲ Chapter 18)—typically bone cysts |
| Specific features | Cartilage damage (joint space loss and subchondral bone changes—primary or secondary OA) |
| | Articular erosions |
| | Osteophytes |
| | Infection (cortex loss, patchy osteolysis) |
| | Calcium deposition in joint (e.g. triangular ligament chondrocalcinosis in CPPD disease) |
| | Soft tissue swelling (e.g. over ulnar styloid in wrist synovitis) |
| | Periarticular osteoporosis (associated with joint inflammation) |
| | Carpal dislocation (e.g. lunate displacement in chronic carpal pain) |
| Polyarticular: overall patterns of radiological abnormality | OA (distribution of osteophytes and subchondral bone changes) |
| | RA (e.g. deformities, erosion appearance/distribution) |
| | Psoriatic arthritis (e.g. deformities, juxta-articular new bone, enthesophytes, erosion appearance—DIPJs) |
| | CPPD: carpal—particularly scapho-trapezial, trapezio-metacarpal and 2nd and 3rd MCPJs—degenerative changes, intense linear periarticular sclerosis and osteophytes |
| | Gout: erosion appearance—'punched out' bites, like Lulworth Cove. Bases of erosions sclerosed |

*Laboratory investigations*

- *FBC, ESR, CRP*: the characteristic, though non-specific, picture in patients with a systemic inflammatory condition such as RA is mild anaemia with normal (or slightly hypochromic, microcytic) red cell indices, high or high/normal platelets, and increased acute phase.
- Notably in PsA and in SpA the acute phase measures may be low, even normal, even when there is widespread pain/disease activity.
- Lymphopenia frequently accompanies autoimmune disease.
- Neutrophils are raised in infection, with steroids, with crystal-induced arthritis, and in adult-onset Still's disease (see ➲ Chapter 18).
- Blood urea, electrolytes, creatinine, and urate will detect hyperuricaemia and renal impairment associated with gout.
- Blood calcium, phosphate, albumin, vitamin D, alkaline phosphatase, and PTH will screen for metabolic bone disease. Test all components to interpret fully the metabolic picture.

- Rheumatoid factor (RF) and anti-cyclic citrullinated peptide (ACPA) are useful for diagnosing rheumatoid arthritis.
- Antinuclear antibody (ANA) and a screen of extractable nuclear antibodies (ENAs) may be helpful for the evaluation of a number of disorders, including SLE and scleroderma.
- Other investigations to consider: serum angiotensin converting enzyme (ACE) for sarcoidosis, glycosylated haemoglobin in diabetics, serum, and urinary protein electrophoresis for myeloma.

*Other investigations*
- Neurophysiology (EMG/NCS) is a useful adjunct to clinical examination in diagnosis of upper limb neuropathies.
- Joint/bursa fluid aspiration is mandatory in suspected cases of sepsis and should be sent for culture and microscopy (request Gram stain and polarized light microscopy of fluid from the lab).

## Treatment of wrist and hand disorders in adults

Treatments for specific diseases are considered in the relevant chapters in Part II of this book. Management of the soft tissue lesions in the hand and wrist, like elsewhere, combines periods of rest and splinting with active physical therapy, avoidance of repetitive activity, and analgesia. In most cases, the condition will resolve spontaneously, but severe or persistent pain and disability may warrant input from a hand occupational therapist, local steroid injections, or occasionally surgical soft tissue decompression:
- Conditions that respond to local steroid therapy (see ➲ Chapter 24):
  - tenosynovitis, e.g. De Quervain's.
  - tendon nodules and ganglia.
  - flexor tenosynovitis (and trigger finger).
  - Dupuytren's contracture.
  - carpal tunnel syndrome.
  - *synovitis:* radiocarpal and radioulnar at the wrist, MCPJs and PIPJs, first carpometacarpal.
- The accuracy of needle placement is likely to be improved by US guidance; however, greater efficacy from an US procedure versus blind injection has not yet been shown.
- The principles of steroid injection are dealt with in ➲ Chapter 24.
- Functional evaluation (from a physical and occupational therapist) is likely to be of use in cases of polyarthropathy. Early use of splints, orthotics, and exercises may lead to greater functional ability and a decrease in symptoms.
- Surgical options for the hand and wrist may include:
  - fusion or resection of the carpal bones.
  - ulna styloidectomy and wrist synovectomy (RA).
  - tendon repair and transfer operations (RA).
  - synovectomy of joints and/or tendons (RA).
  - fusion of small joints.
  - PIP/MCP joint replacements.
  - Dupuytren's release/fasciectomy.
  - carpal tunnel release.
  - trapeziectomy for thumb CMC joint OA.

Many of these procedures primarily reduce pain; function may not be restored.

# Wrist and hand pain in children and adolescents

## General considerations

Isolated MSK lesions in the wrist and hands of children are rare. A few notable conditions exist.

- Small swellings may be ganglia—resolve spontaneously in 50%.
- Congenital trigger thumb or finger is not rare and can affect 1 in 300 children. Spontaneous resolution occurs in up to 60% within 2 years.
- Swelling in wrists and fingers may denote JIA. US is a relatively easy and acceptable way of confirming synovitis is present in joints in young children, though older children may tolerate MRI.
- Wrist pain and swelling may be the key presenting feature of rickets, especially in a child or adolescent with a severely restricted diet.
- Digital vasomotor instability is more commonly seen in children with neurological conditions including cerebral palsy.
- Assessment of Raynaud's Disease, typically in adolescents, is similar to that in adults (see ➜ Chapter 13) and erythromelalgia, which causes marked redness of hand and feet associated with diffuse pain, swelling and distress, is more commonly seen in toddlers than older children.
- Digital ulcers and ischaemic lesions, Gottron's patches and nail bed vascular changes may indicate SLE, JDM or SScl.
- Although CRPS (see ➜ Chapter 22), is occurs in children, it is less common than in adults.
- Wrist pain may be the presenting feature of a skeletal dysplasia—a wrist radiograph should be obtained. Specialist centre radiologist input can be helpful in such cases (e.g. dREAMS: ℘ http://www.d-reams.org)
- Assessment of the wrist and hand in children and adolescents is essentially similar to the assessment in adults.
- For functional anatomy of the wrist see ➜ pp. 106–7, and for the hand, see ➜ pp. 112–15.

# Upper limb peripheral nerve lesions

### Background

- Upper limb peripheral nerve lesions are common. Most are entrapment neuropathies. Occasionally, nerve trauma may present to primary care providers or rheumatologists with (primarily) regional muscle weakness.
- Although not specific for its diagnosis, the combination of pain, paraesthesia, numbness, and weakness is suggestive of nerve entrapment. Features may be considered more specific for nerve entrapment if there is a history of acute or overuse trauma proximal to the distribution of the symptoms.
- Lesions may characteristically occur in association with specific activities, occupations, or sports (e.g. ulnar neuropathy in cyclists).
- Accurate diagnosis relies on demonstration of the anatomic lesion. Useful in this respect is knowledge of likely sites of entrapment or damage and, in the case of entrapment, the ability to elicit a positive Hoffman–Tinel sign (i.e. pressure or percussion over entraped nerve course eliciting sensory symptoms in the nerve distribution).
- Always compare examination findings in both upper limbs.
- Neurophysiologic examination is an adjunct to clinical diagnosis. It should not be relied on to make a diagnosis in the absence of good clinical assessment.
- MRI of nerve roots/spine and potential sites of distal nerve entrapment can be used, with clinical assessment and neurophysiology, to pinpoint with high accuracy, any nerve lesion in the upper limb.

### The long thoracic nerve

- Entrapment is in the differential diagnosis of painless shoulder weakness. The nerve origin is at C5–C7, and its course runs beneath the subscapularis and into the serratus anterior.
- Muscle paralysis is often painless and implies loss of the last 30° of overhead arm extension, disrupted scapular rhythm, and scapula winging. Winging is demonstrated by inspection from behind with the patient pressing against a wall with an outstretched arm.
- Damage to the nerve occurs typically from an anterior direct blow or brachial plexus injury. Damage sometimes occurs after carrying heavy backpacks (e.g. army recruits) or after surgical resection of a cervical rib.
- It can also occur spontaneously after infection. There is no specific treatment.

### The suprascapular nerve

- The nerve origin is at roots C4–C6; its course is lateral and deep to the trapezius, through the suprascapular notch, terminating in the supraspinatus and posteriorly in the infraspinatus. It carries pain fibres from the glenohumeral joint and AC joint.
- Impingement of the nerve at the suprascapular notch should be considered in a patient complaining of shoulder pain despite a normal examination and imaging tests.
- Injury to the nerve often gives diffuse shoulder pain, although painless paralysis of the muscles can occur.

- Injury is often thought to occur from repeated stretching of the nerve at the notch. Weightlifters are prone to bilateral injury and volleyball players prone to dominant side injury.
- Neuromyopathy (acute weakness, pain, CK+, muscle wasting on MRI?secondary to infection) of supraspinatus or infraspinatus is not uncommon.
- Compression by ganglia or tumours (and even possibly gout tophi) occurs and can be confirmed by MRI.

## Ulnar nerve

The ulnar nerve originates from C8 and T1. It lies along the medial side of the brachial artery in the upper arm, then above the medial humeral epicondyle where it passes posteriorly, piercing the medial intermuscular septum. It then runs behind the elbow in a groove between the olecranon and medial epicondyle, covered by a fibrous sheath and arcuate ligament (cubital tunnel). Following the line of the ulna in the flexor compartment of the forearm, branches supply the flexor digitorum profundus (FDP) and the flexor carpi ulnaris (FCU). The nerve enters the hand on the ulnar side dividing into superficial (palmaris brevis and skin over the medial one and a half digits) and deep (small muscles of the hand) branches:

- Lesions are usually due to entrapment.
- The ulnar nerve is occasionally damaged in the relatively exposed cubital tunnel (cubital tunnel syndrome) resulting in pain and paraesthesia along the medial forearm, wrist, and fourth/fifth digits. Damage may occur from direct trauma, compression, or recurrent subluxation. The Tinel test at the elbow may be positive and there might be sensory loss over the palmar aspect of the fifth digit.
- There are a number of sites where entrapment of the ulnar nerve may occur around the wrist, either proximal to the volar carpal ligament or beneath it or the pisohamate ligament. External compression, acute or recurrent trauma, and ganglia are the usual causes. Symptoms have been noted in cyclists, users of pneumatic or vibrating tools and in avid videogame players. Entrapment of the purely sensory cutaneous branch can occur from excess computer mouse use.
- Motor weakness may be most evident by observing general muscle wasting in the hand (hypothenar eminence, interossei, adductor pollicis) and flexion deformity of the fourth and fifth digits—the latter caused by third and fourth lumbrical weakness (see ➔ Plate 11).
- Flexion of the wrist with ulnar deviation (FCU) and thumb adduction may be weak (adductor pollicis weakness will be evident if you ask the patient to 'run the thumb across the base of the fingers' as normally it can sweep across touching the skin).
- Froment's sign also signifies weakness of the adductor pollicis, and is demonstrated by a weakness in holding paper between the thumb and the index finger when both are in the sagittal plane.
- Discrimination of a wrist site from an elbow site of nerve entrapment is helped by the site of a positive Hoffman-Tinel test, preservation of power of wrist flexion/medial deviation (FCU) in a wrist lesion, and electrophysiology.

- Rest, analgesia, and occasionally local steroids are helpful. A review of posture, repetitive activity, and a biomechanical assessment with changes in activities and technique are recommended. Surgical decompression may also be necessary.

## Radial nerve

The nerve origin is at roots C5–C8, and its course runs anterior to subscapularis then passes behind the humerus in a groove that runs between the long and medial heads of triceps. It then winds anteriorly around the humeral shaft to lie between brachialis and brachioradialis. In the flexor compartment of the arm it divides at the level of the lateral epicondyle into superficial branch (cutaneous/sensory) and the posterior interosseous nerve (PIN), which runs through the supinator muscle into the forearm to supply the extensor compartment muscles:

- Entrapment needs to be considered in those cases of shoulder or upper arm trauma, where subsequent presentation includes arm and wrist weakness.
- Compression of the radial nerve in the upper arm causes stiffness in the dorsal arm and forearm, weakness of the wrist, and little finger extension. The triceps is usually unaffected as the nerve supply to the muscle leaves the radial nerve proximally.
- Transient compression of the nerve at the site of the medial head of triceps has been described in tennis players.
- Compression can occur as the nerve pierces the lateral intermuscular septum just distal to the radial head and also where the PIN pierces the supinator.
- At this lower site, compression is often a consequence of trauma, may be associated with a positive Hoffman-Tinel test and local tenderness, and the pain may be reproduced by extreme passive forearm pronation combined with wrist flexion. Symptoms may mimic those of lateral epicondylitis. Surgical exploration may be necessary to confirm a diagnosis.

## Median nerve

The nerve origin is from C6–T1 nerve roots. Its course from the brachial plexus runs together with the brachial artery in the upper arm (supplying nothing) then enters the forearm between the two heads of pronator teres (from medial humeral epicondyle and coronoid process of the ulna). It runs deep in the forearm dividing into median and anterior interosseous branches. The median branch enters the hand beneath the flexor retinaculum on the radial side of the wrist. All pronator and flexor muscles in the forearm (except FCU and the medial half of FDP) are supplied by the two branches. The median supplies sensory nerves to the radial side of the hand:

- Entrapment syndrome at the wrist is very common; CTS.
- In the rare pronator syndrome, trauma, swelling, or masses between the two pronator heads can cause entrapment giving lower arm pain, paraesthesias, and weakness of forearm pronation. There is local tenderness and reproduction of pain from resisted forearm pronation or wrist flexion.

- Pain in CTS is often present at night and relieved by exercising the hand. Daytime symptoms can persist. Pain can be referred up the arm even to the shoulder. Sensory symptoms are confined to the radial three and a half digits.
- Clumsiness is a common early feature of CTS.
- Symptoms reproduced by a positive Tinel's sign (percussion over the volar aspect of the wrist) and Phalen's manoeuver (volar aspect of the wrist rested on the back of a chair and the hand allowed to fall loosely under gravity, held for 1 min) indicates nerve compression.
- A severe or chronic lesion is associated with sensory testing abnormality (Fig. 3.10) and motor weakness of the abductor pollicis brevis (APB), opponens pollicis, and the first and second lumbricals.
- NCSs are indicated if the diagnosis is uncertain, the condition is progressive, motor neuron disease is suspected (thenar muscle wasting marked/progressive with minimal sensory symptoms), dual pathology is suspected, surgical decompression is being considered, and in cases of surgical failure. False-negative results occur in 10% of cases.
- MRI appears to be more sensitive than US for detecting abnormalities involving the median nerve in or around the carpal tunnel.
- Aetiology of CTS is debated, but probably multifactorial. The following are associated: Colles' fracture, trauma, carpal OA, diabetes, inflammatory joint/tendon disease (e.g. RA, SScl), ganglia, menopause and pregnancy. Hypothyroidism, acromegaly, amyloid, and benign tumours are also associated with CTS.

*Treatment of carpal tunnel syndrome (CTS)*
(➲ Chapter 24 has further information on steroid injection techniques.)
- Night splinting may be curative, especially early in the condition.
- NSAIDs are helpful if there is underlying inflammatory disease.
- Local steroid injections are of value. If partial remission is achieved, consider repeating the injection (see ➲ Chapter 24).
- Surgical decompression is indicated when there is failure of conservative therapy, progressive/persistent neurological changes, or muscle atrophy/weakness.
- Failure of surgical release of the carpal tunnel requires further consideration of underlying causes such as a ganglion or other soft tissue lesion. Reconsider also whether there really is a mechanical/local or perhaps a subtler cause (e.g. mononeuritis or peripheral neuropathy, entrapment at the pronator or nerve root lesion).

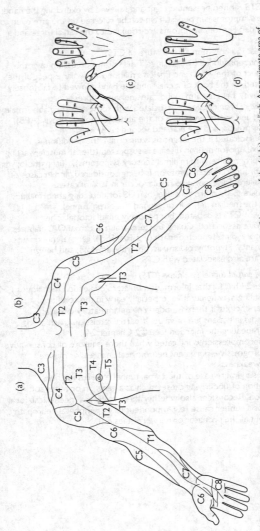

**Fig. 3.10** Approximate distribution of dermatomes on the anterior (a) and posterior (b) aspects of the (right) upper limb. Approximate area of sensory change in lesions of the median (c) and ulnar (d) nerves.

# Thoracic back and chest pain in adults

## Background

- The thoracic segment (T1–T12) moves less than the lumbar and cervical spine. Segmental movement in any direction is about 6°. However, given the number of segments this can add up to appreciable mobility overall. Less segmental movement results in reduced frequency of problems overall (only 6% of patients attending a spinal clinic have thoracic spine problems).
- Ribs (1–10) articulate posteriorly with vertebrae at two points: the articular facet of the rib head with the costovertebral facet on each vertebral body and the articular facet of the rib tubercle with the costotransverse facet on each vertebral lateral process. These are both synovial joints. Ribs 11 and 12 do not have costotransverse joints.
- The ribs, each continuous with its costal cartilage, articulate anteriorly by a synovial joint with the manubrium (1–2), sternum (2–7), each costal cartilage above (8–10), or do not articulate (11/12 'floating ribs').
- A massive block of spinal extensor muscles is responsible for maintaining the body against gravity. Some extend over some distance (e.g. the spinalis thoracis from the upper thoracic to the mid-lumbar spinous processes).
- Dermatomes are circumferential and extend from T2 at the clavicles to T10 at the umbilicus. However, up to five nerve roots may contribute innervation of any one point in a truncal dermatome.

## Taking a history in adults

The interpretation of cardiac, oesophageal, or pleural chest pain as MSK in origin can occur. It may result in missing a serious condition (Table 3.11 and Table 3.12). Similarly, the interpretation of neurogenic or MSK chest pains as cardiogenic, oesophageal, or pleural can occur and may lead to unnecessary investigations.

- A review of the quality and radiation of cardiac and oesophageal pain in the clinical context should always be considered.
- Pleuritic pain is common. Chronic pulmonary emboli may be underdiagnosed and have serious consequences. Any inflammatory, infective, or infiltrative pleural lesion will be painful.
- Lesions confined to pulmonary parenchyma do not produce pain.
- Pericardial pain can be misinterpreted as MSK or pleuritic.
- Mediastinal abnormalities can produce pain that is often referred.
- Thoracic spine lesions can result in referred anterolateral chest pain.
- Costovertebral and costotransverse joint dysfunction is relatively common and is generally age-related, but can occur in anyone with spinal deformity. It may produce thoracic spine pain alone or result in an extensive pattern of radiation of pain over the back, lateral, and anterior chest wall.
- Lower cervical spine lesions can refer pain to the anterior chest wall.
- Many painful chest conditions are associated with radiation of the pain down the left arm. This pattern is not specific for myocardial ischaemia.

**Table 3.11** Characteristics of chest pain in adults: from non-neurological and non-MSK pathology

| Process | Characteristics of pain |
|---|---|
| Angina | Gradual onset often related to exercise, a heavy meal, or emotion. Squeezing, strangling, or constriction in chest, can be aching or burning in nature. Commonly substernal, but radiates to any of anterior chest, interscapular area, arms (mainly left), shoulders, teeth, and abdomen. Reduces with rest and sublingual nitrates |
| Myocardial infarction | Similar to above regarding quality and distribution. Longer duration. Less easily relieved |
| Pericardial inflammation | Sharp or steady substernal pain. Can be referred to shoulder tip, anterior chest, upper abdomen, or back. Often has a pleural component and is altered by change in position—sharper more left-sided when supine but eased by leaning forward |
| Aortic dissection | Acute onset with extremely severe peak. Felt in centre of chest or back. Lasts for hours |
| Pleuritic inflammation | Common. Sharp, knife-like, superficial. Aggravated by deep inspiration, sneezing, or coughing. If accompanied by haemoptysis consider pulmonary embolism |
| Mediastinal conditions | Empyema or surgical emphysema may be intense and sharp and radiate from substernal to shoulder area. Associated with crepitus. Mediastinitis and tumour pain resembles pleural pain. May have constant feeling of constriction/oppression |
| Peptic disease | Penetrating duodenal ulcers can cause intense, persistent mid-thoracic back pain |
| Oesophageal reflux | Persistent retrosternal burning is typical. Often post-prandial, when lying or at night/early morning. Oesophageal spasm can be similar to angina and can cause mid-thoracic back pain, but reflux symptoms often coexist |

- Lower cervical pain may be referred to the inter-scapular region.
- Inter-scapular pain may also be associated with mechanical lumbar disorders. Unlike infection, tumours, and fracture, referred pain is eased or abolished by changes in position or posture.
- If there is thoracic back pain alone and it is acute and/or severe consider osteoporotic fracture, tumours, and infection.
- Osteoporotic vertebral collapse is common in postmenopausal women. An acute, non/minimal-trauma-associated severe pain is typical. Fractures occur in many other situations, e.g. AS or a neoplastic bone lesion.
- Spinal infections should not be missed. The most common are *Staphylococcus aureus*, *Brucella*, and *Mycobacterium tuberculosis*.

**Table 3.12** Painful neurological and MSK conditions of the thoracic spine and chest wall in adults

| | |
|---|---|
| Thoracic vertebral disease | Osteoporotic or pathological fracture |
| | Tumours, e.g. osteoid osteoma, metastasis |
| | Osteomyelitis |
| | Paget's disease |
| | Osteomalacia, rickets |
| | Costovertebral joint dysfunction |
| Nerve irritation | Root irritation/compression from disc prolapse or osteophyte at exit foramen, from structure distal to exit foramen, or from neuroma |
| Biomechanical/ degenerative | Scoliosis (non-structural compensatory, structural) |
| | Diffuse idiopathic skeletal hyperostosis (DISH) |
| | Calcium pyrophosphate dihydrate disease |
| Herpes zoster of intercostal nerve | |
| Chest wall/ superficial lesions | Rib fracture |
| | Other rib lesions, e.g. tumours, fibrous dysplasia, osteomalacia |
| | Costochondritis/enthesitis (e.g. PsA) |
| | Intercostal muscle tear/strain |
| | Mastitis or fibrocystic disease of the breast |
| | Myofascial pain and fibromyalgia |
| | Parietal pleural inflammation/infection/infiltration |
| Spondyloarthritis (SpA) | Spinal inflammation |
| | Acute discitis |
| | Chronic indolent discitis |
| Scheuermann's osteochondritis | In adolescents only |

*Ask about the quality of pain*
- MSK pain (local or referred) generally associates with specific movements, positions, or postures, and is reproducible.
- Pain that increases with coughing, sneezing, or deep inspiration, is suggestive of pleural lesions. Rib and intercostal lesions or costovertebral joint dysfunction may also cause this sort of pain.

*Ask about other symptoms and risk factors*
- The pain from a fracture/lesion (osteoporotic, malignancy, infection) is often localized and extreme, waking the patient at night.
- Acute or chronic thoracic spine lesions may be associated with cord compression. Ask about recent change in sphincter function and progressive lower limb stiffness or heaviness.

- Risks for osteoporosis (see ➲ Chapter 16).
- Systemic symptoms of fever (osteomyelitis).
- Bone pain elsewhere (metastases, osteomalacia, Paget's disease).
- Spinal pain in adolescence (for an adult with kyphosis/spinal pain).
- A positive family history is recognized in idiopathic scoliosis, osteoporosis, and generalized osteoarthritis (see ➲ Chapter 6).
- Depression and anxiety are important modulators of pain. However, although thoracic back and chest pains may be psychogenic, it is unwise to settle on this diagnosis without excluding MSK conditions and diseases of viscera that can cause referred pain.

## Examination of the (MSK) thorax in adults

### Visual inspection

Observe the patient (who has undressed down to their underwear) from the back and front. Look for deformity, asymmetry, swellings, and note the respiratory pattern:

- Any scoliosis should be noted. Non-structural scoliosis is frequently due to posture, severe back or abdominal pain, leg length discrepancy, and, rarely, can be psychogenic. Structural scoliosis may be due to various lesions at any age.
- There is a normal mild thoracic kyphos; however, marked kyphos in adults (particularly postmenopausal women) might suggest multiple osteoporotic vertebral fractures or degenerative disc disease. A loss of normal kyphosis (flat spine) may be seen in spondylitis or possibly severe muscle spasm.
- Loose folds of skin on the back can denote height loss from multiple vertebral fractures.
- Costochondral swelling occurs in some cases of costochondritis or SAPHO (synovitis, acne, pustulosis (palmoplantar), hyperostosis, and (aseptic) osteomyelitis) syndrome. Look for lesions of costosternal or sternoclavicular joints (which are also found in PsA).

### Palpation

Palpate over the vertebrae, paravertebral joints, and back musculature with the patient prone. Palpate the anterior chest wall:

- Spinal osteomyelitis may be associated with obvious skin swelling and erythema, exquisite focal tenderness, and extensor spasm. Tumours may give similar signs, though skin erythema is not likely.
- Costotransverse joints may be tender (4–5 cm from midline). Discomfort at any costovertebral joint and its referred pain can be elicited by individual rib manipulation (downward pressure on the rib lateral to its vertebral joints when the patient is prone).
- Identify any trigger points that reproduce myofascial pain in back muscles.
- Tender swelling of the sternoclavicular, costomanubrial, or sternocostal joints may suggest spondyloarthritis (axSpA) or SAPHO syndrome. See ➲ Chapter 8.
- Inflammation of costal cartilages is often associated with painful swelling and tenderness. Rib and intercostal lesions should be easily discriminated from referred pain by eliciting local tenderness.

*Check thoracic spinal movement*

Movements of the thoracic spine should be checked. Ask the patient to sit on the couch with their arms folded in front of them. Guided by movements of the spinous processes, gauge the range of thoracic spine movement:

- Approximate normal ranges of movement in the above-mentioned position are extension 30°, lateral flexion 30°, flexion 90°, and rotation 60°.
- Scoliosis is often associated with rotation that is accentuated, on examination, on flexion.
- Abnormal mobility will not be specific for any underlying condition, but may draw attention to the major affected spinal segment. Painful segments are 'guarded' and may appear hypomobile.
- AxSpA/ankylosing spondylitis (AS) may become obvious if there is extensive spinal hypomobility.
- Chest expansion should be measured from forced expiration to complete inspiration measuring at expansion, with a tape, at the level of the xiphisternum.

*Other examination*

- Given the range of serious conditions causing chest pains, a full medical examination is important and should always be considered.
- Neurological examination of the legs should be considered in anyone who is at risk of spinal cord compression. Look for increased tone, weakness, and brisk reflexes.
- Breast and axillary lymph node examination should be done.

## Investigations of thoracic conditions in adults

*Radiographs*

- Lateral view radiographs generally provide more information about thoracic spine lesions than anteroposterior views; however, together, both views should confirm osteoporosis, degenerative disease (e.g. previous Scheuermann's osteochondritis, ochronosis, DISH), and Paget's disease (see ➲ Chapter 16).
- Look for vertebral squaring (in axSpA/AS) and either marginal or non-marginal syndesmophytes as in psoriatic spondylitis or other SpAs (see ➲ Chapter 8).
- Discriminate enthesitis in SpA from DISH at the corners of vertebrae by the presence of erosions with bone reaction (enthesitis) compared with bone proliferation alone (DISH). Spondylodiscitis is part of the SpA spectrum of diseases.
- Radiographs of the spine, or CT images, are probably a better indicated of PsA in the spine compared with MRI.
- Normal radiographs do not exclude malignancy.
- Bone lesions can be well characterized by CT (e.g. osteoid osteoma).

### MRI
- MRI is important in discriminating tumour from infection.
- Disc lesions, spinal canal, and cord are well visualized with MRI.
- Fat suppressed or contrast-enhanced MR sequences may be necessary to detect enthesitis or spondylodiscitis associated with SpA.

### Bone scintigraphy ($^{99m}$Tc-diphosphonate-MDP)
- Bone scintigraphy is a sensitive test for infection and malignancy.
- In suspected cases of malignancy, it is more sensitive than radiographs, can often confirm the lytic or sclerotic nature of a lesion and will identify any other skeletal sites of disease.
- The pattern of abnormalities in SAPHO syndrome are characteristic.
- It is a useful investigation in patients with malignancy who present with back pain. A lack of additional lesions strongly suggests against a single spinal abnormality being malignancy-related.
- Scintigraphic tomography can detect abnormality in the pars interarticularis, facet joint, and disc/vertebral body.
- Scintigraphy sensitively identifies rib and, in most cases, inflammatory intercostal lesions. The differential diagnosis is of a metastasis, primary malignant or benign bone tumour, healed rib fracture, fibrous dysplasia, Paget's disease, hyperparathyroidism, or infection.

### Other investigations to consider in patients with chest pain
- CXR, then consider pulmonary ventilation-perfusion scan and spiral CT to evaluate for pulmonary embolism.
- CT of the chest in patients with unexplained pleural pain.
- ECG and an exercise stress test if possible cardiac ischaemia.
- Transthoracic echocardiography to show thickened pericardium or an effusion associated with pericarditis.
- Upper GI endoscopy in suspected cases of peptic ulceration.
- Diagnostic trial of a proton pump inhibitor in cases of reflux oesophagitis.

# Thoracic back and chest pain in children and adolescents

## General considerations

Chest pain is a common paediatric presentation to primary care and A&E in patients aged 10–21 years. *Acute* chest pain is cardiac in <6% of patients.

- Chest pain is often alarming to parents and patients, but rarely caused by a serious condition (Table 3.13).
- In a study of 300 patients with chronic chest pain there was a cardiac cause in just one patient.
- Differentiating cardiac pain and other serious parenchymal pathology, from musculoskeletal and other benign pain remains imperative.
- Paediatric chest pain can be classified into MSK, respiratory, GI, cardiac and other conditions (see Table 3.13).
- For assessment of: thoracic back pain in children and adolescents see ➜ Chapter 21 p. 618; low back pain in children see ➜ p. 154; and thoracic assessment in adults, see ➜ p. 130.

## History and examination

*General considerations*

- Focal chest pain in children is usually chest-wall (MSK) or pleural in origin.
- Diffuse chest pain is most likely to be referred from internal organ pathology.
- A third of adolescents with chest pains who present to outpatients have a history of stressful events. Their chest pain symptoms are typically associated with other somatic complaints and sleep disturbance. Hyperventilation, dyspnoea, dizziness, or paraesthesia may indicate panic attacks, unrecognized by the patient or parent.

**Table 3.13** Causes of chest pain in children and adolescents

| Tissue/organ | Diagnosis/syndrome | Frequency |
|---|---|---|
| Musculoskeletal | Trauma, injury | 15–30% |
| | Costochondritis/Tietze syndrome, xiphydinia | |
| | Slipping rib syndrome | |
| | Sickle cell disease | |
| Cardiac | Pericarditis, coronary arteritis (Kawasaki disease), aortic dissection, angina secondary to structural cardiac disease | Very rare (<2%) |
| Respiratory | Pleural inflammation (infection and sterile pleuritis (SLE)), pneumonia, PE, asthma, acute chest syndrome | 2–11% |
| Gastrointestinal | GORD, IBD, cholecystitis | 8% |
| Neurological | Herpes zoster | Rare |
| | Nerve root symptoms | |
| Other | Idiopathic | >50% |
| | Anxiety, panic-hyperventilation | |
| | Breast-related conditions | |

*Cardiac history and examination*

- Exertional chest pain with chest tightness and syncope might be due to atrial flutter or tachycardia which in turn may be due to structural cardiac disease (e.g. hypertrophic or dilated cardiomyopathy).
- Angina chest pain is usually associated with exertion, a feeling of tightness, and radiates to the neck, throat, jaw, teeth, or shoulder.
- Pericarditis presents as sharp retrosternal chest pain often radiating to the left shoulder, aggravated by lying supine or deep breaths and relieved by bending forward.
- Severe and tearing midsternal chest pain radiating to the back may be due to aortic dissection in Marfan syndrome, Turner's syndrome, Ehlers–Danlos type IV, and homocystinuria.
- Though non-specific, chest pain with fatigue and exertional dyspnoea or syncope can indicate pulmonary hypertension.
- Past medical history should be taken to note any previous Kawasaki disease or cardiac surgery.
- Take a family history for arrhythmias, to note familial sudden death, genetic conditions or hyperlipidaemia.
- Cardiac signs on examination: a harsh ejection systolic murmur radiating to the neck in aortic stenosis; an ejection click from a stenosed bicuspid aortic valve; abnormal peripheral pulses (e.g. previous Kawasaki disease).

*Musculoskeletal features*

- Chest wall pain exacerbated by deep breathing lasting seconds to minutes may be due to costochondritis (e.g. secondary to infection or intercostal muscle enthesitis in ERA or JSpA). Chest-wall tenderness may be present (usually unilateral along the upper two or more contiguous costochondral joints).
- Tietze syndrome is a term used to describe anterior chest wall pain usually in a single joint (commonly at the second or third rib articulation at the sternum or sternoclavicular joint). Differential diagnosis SAPHO syndrome in adolescent and enthesitis (see ➲ Chapter 16).
- Intense pain in the lower chest or upper abdomen may denote 'slipping-rib' syndrome, which is secondary to trauma and dislocation of ribs 8, 9, 10. Noting a history of physical strain, sports-related injury, or direct trauma is important.
- Slipping rib syndrome pain can be reproduced by hooking fingers under the inferior rib margin and pulling the rib edge outward and upward (hooking manoeuvre). This manoeuvre may produce a click.
- A history of sickle cell disease may be relevant given any MSK pains and pulmonary disease (e.g. thromboembolism).

*Pulmonary disease features*

- Pulmonary disease is chiefly identifiable from a history of dyspnoea, cough, and conventional respiratory symptoms.
- Severe pain, dyspnoea, and low oxygen saturations require both pulmonary embolism and pneumothorax to be excluded.

*Other*
- Abdominal pathology can present with chest pain (e.g. typical 'heartburn' symptoms in the throat; cholecystitis-related chest pain radiating to the right shoulder).
- Throbbing or burning focal chest pain locating to breast tissue is typical of mastitis, fibrocystic disease, or pregnancy.
- Burning pain or paraesthesia in a dermatomal pattern, preceding a rash by a few days suggests herpes zoster.

# Low back pain in adults

(See also ➔ Chapter 21.)

## Epidemiology

- The lifetime prevalence of back pain is 58% and the greatest prevalence is between 45 and 64 years of age.
- Most recent statistics report in the order of 12 million primary care consultations and over 2.4 million adult specialist consultations annually in the UK for low back pain (population 64 million). Low back pain is the fifth most common reason for all physician visits in the USA.
- 2% of the workforce in the USA is compensated for back injuries every year.
- Estimated annual cost to the UK National Health Service is £500 million with over £5 billion lost annually due to absence from work. The financial healthcare and indirect employment costs of low back pain in the USA are estimated to be more than $24 billion.

## Lumbar and sacral spine anatomy

- There are normally five lumbar vertebrae. Anomalies are not uncommon at the lumbosacral junction.
- The transition between the mobile lumbar spine (flexion, extension, and lateral flexion) and fixed sacrum together with high weight-loading combine to make the region highly prone to damage.
- The facet joints are sharply angled, effectively reducing rotation in lumbar segments.
- The sacroiliac joints (synovial) are held firmly by a strong fibrous capsule and tough ligaments. The amount of normal movement (essentially rotation) is normally inversely proportional to age.
- The spinal cord ends at L1/L2. Nerves then run individually, are normally mobile in the spinal canal, and together are termed the cauda equine.
- Each nerve exits its appropriate lateral intervertebral exit foramen passing initially superior and then laterally to the disc, e.g. L4 from L4/L5 exit foramen. However, in the spinal canal each nerve descends immediately posterior to the more proximal intervertebral disc before it exits. Thus, for example, L4 root symptoms can occur from either lateral herniation of the L4/5 disc or posterior herniation of the L3/L4 disc (or from both).
- Facet joint innervation is from posterior primary rami, each of which supplies the corresponding joint at its level, one higher and one lower.

## Basic principles of assessment

- Low back pain can arise from damage or inflammation of the thoracic or lumbar spines or from the posterior pelvis. Pathology in retroperitoneal abdominal and pelvic viscera can result in referred pain to the low back.
- A simple way of categorizing back pain is to consider its cause to be mechanical, inflammatory, neurologic, referred, or due to bone pathology (Table 3.14).

**Table 3.14** Common and/or serious causes of low back pain in adults

| | |
|---|---|
| Mechanical/degenerative (very common) | Intervertebral disc disease (annular tear, internal disruption, prolapse) |
| | Facet joint arthritis |
| | Spondylolisthesis |
| | Scoliosis/kyphosis |
| | Spinal stenosis |
| Inflammatory (common) | AS/axSpA (→ Chapter 8) including sacroiliitis |
| | DISH |
| Infection (rare) | Osteomyelitis (e.g. *Staphylococcus aureus*, TB, brucellosis) |
| Bone disease (common) | Osteoporotic fracture |
| | Paget's disease |
| | Osteomalacia |
| Neoplasia (rare) | Secondary metastases |
| | Multiple myeloma |
| Other | Sickle cell crisis |
| | Renal disease (e.g. tumours, infection) |
| | Gynaecological disease |
| | Fibromyalgia (→ Chapter 22) |

- Over 90% of episodes of low back pain in adults are mechanical, self-limiting, and do not require investigation.
- Indicators for further investigation include age >55 years, stiffness, focal pain, pain that disturbs sleep, nerve root symptoms, and chronic persistent (>6 weeks) pain.
- The low back is often a focus for those who may use pain (consciously or unconsciously) as a protective device in the face of domestic, emotional, or occupational stress. These stresses commonly influence the description and impact of pain but rarely act alone in causing pain—there is usually some underlying organic pathology.

### Taking a history of low back pain in adults

Differentiate whether the pain is likely to be primarily mechanical or inflammatory, due to bone pathology or referred:

- The site and extent of the pain does not easily discriminate the cause. All disorders may be associated with mechanical deformity and/or muscle spasm that may cause pain in a diffuse distribution.
- Generally, pain due to mechanical lesions is often acute in onset, while patients with pain from inflammatory lesions often present after symptoms have been present for some time.

- Inflammatory pain is often associated with morning stiffness that can last for several hours and is eased by movement. Mechanical lesions tend to worsen with use. Many 'mechanical' or 'degenerative' lesions may have an inflammatory component, e.g. internal disc disruption causing discogenic pain.
- Intrinsic bone pathology often causes severe, unremitting, focal pain. Sleep is disturbed. Pain does not ease substantially with movement.
- About 3% of patients presenting with back pain have non-MSK causes. A significant proportion of women have pelvic conditions such as ovarian cysts or endometriosis. Pain may be cyclical.
- For those aged >55 with no previous similar episodes of pain increase suspicion of an underlying neoplastic lesion. Investigation is required.
- Associated systemic symptoms are common in osteomyelitis and may be present if a malignancy has disseminated.

*Ask about pain radiation and symptoms in the legs*

- Progressive neurological leg symptoms suggest a worsening/expanding lesion such as a tumour, infection/vertebral collapse, Paget's disease, or lumbosacral spinal stenosis.
- Pressure on the cauda equina sufficient to cause a disturbance in perineal sensation and/or bowel/bladder paralysis is a neurosurgical emergency (cauda equina syndrome; see ⊃ Chapter 21).
- Leg pain caused by nerve root irritation/compression is often clearly defined and sharp, often accompanied by numbness or paraesthesias. The most commonly involved nerve roots are L4, L5, or S1. Pain generally radiates to below the knee and often, but not always, to the heel and big toe.
- Sciatic nerve entrapment at the piriformis muscle can produce identical radicular symptoms to L5 or S1 nerve root entrapment.
- Neurological symptoms in the distribution of the femoral nerve (primarily anterior thigh musculature) might suggest a high lumbar nerve root lesion (L1–L3, for example).
- Disc prolapse is the most common cause of nerve root pain, but bony encroachment at the nerve root exit foramen by vertebral end-plate or facet joint osteophytes, and/or soft tissue thickening or fibrosis can cause similar pain (foramenal stenosis).
- Annular disc tears and internal disruption (i.e. microfractures in vertebral end-plates) can cause a pattern of pain, termed discogenic pain, characterized by low back and referred buttock/posterior thigh pain aggravated by movement.
- Generally, all mechanical lesions of the lumbar spine can result in referred pain around the pelvis and anterior thighs. However, pain from lumbar facet joints and probably other segmental structures can be referred to the lower leg.
- Aching in the back and posterior thighs after standing is typical of, but not specific for, spondylolisthesis. There are often added spasms of acute pain, especially if there is segmental instability.
- The symptoms of spinal stenosis are often relieved by sitting bent slightly forward, since the spinal canal dimensions increase in this position.

- Sacroiliitis often causes referred pain to the buttocks and back of thighs. It occurs commonly in SpA (see ➡ Chapter 8).
- Sacroiliac pain can occur in multiparous women—the condition may be associated with hypermobility.

*Note the description of the pain*

- Pain may be 'severe' whatever the cause; however, note whether the patient's descriptors of it suggest non-organic influences.
- Sharp, lancinating leg pains suggest nerve root irritation/compression (radicular pain), whereas leg pain referred from other structures within a lumbar segment is generally deep and aching. The distribution may be similar (see earlier in section). More persistent, rather than episodic, radicular pain may denote stenosis of the nerve root exit foramen.
- A description of bilateral buttock/leg pain that worsens on walking is consistent with spinal stenosis, especially in those with normal peripheral pulses and no bruits.
- A change in the description of pain in someone who has an established diagnosis may be important, e.g. subacute, severe, unremitting localized pain in a patient with axSpA who normally has mild inflammatory pain might reflect a superadded discitis; or, acute severe unremitting sleep-disturbing pain in an elderly woman with known chronic mechanical pain associated with OA might suggest osteoporotic fracture.
- Florid descriptions of the pain and its severity are associated with psychological modulators of pain.

*Previous back pain and trauma, occupation, and family history*

- Scheuermann's disease (which is associated with irregular vertebral endplates) causes spinal pain in adolescence. It is a risk for spinal degeneration and kyphosis in adults. See ➡ p. 514.
- Previous trauma may have caused pars interarticularis fractures (an antecedent of spondylolisthesis), vertebral fracture (risk of further mechanical damage), or ligament rupture (subsequent segmental instability).
- It is generally accepted that the high prevalence of disc disease among manual workers at a relatively young age provides some evidence for a causal relationship.
- It is often the case that patients with chronic pain following (sometimes trivial) trauma may be dissatisfied with the quality of care received at the time of the injury. Be aware that many believe, and there is some evidence to support this, that the way in which spinal pain is handled at its onset significantly influences its subsequent course.
- Sacroiliitis is an early part of *Brucella* arthritis (20–51% of patients). Poor animal- or carcass-handling hygiene or ingestion of infected foodstuffs/milk can lead to infection. Spondylitis is a late feature and is characterized by erosions, disc infection, and abscesses.
- A positive family history of low back pain might, in context, suggest SpA or generalized OA.

## Examination of an adult with low back pain

*Inspect the undressed patient from the side and behind*

- Note the fluidity of movement when the patient is undressing.
- Check the skin for redness, local swelling, and skin markings. Redness and swelling occasionally accompany osteomyelitis.
- Lipoma, hairy patches, *café-au-lait* patches, or skin tags often reflect underlying structural nerve or bone abnormality, e.g. spina bifida, diastematomyelia, neurofibromatosis.
- Skinfolds often suggest an underlying significant structural change, such as osteoporotic fracture or spondylolisthesis.
- Note any deformity: hyperlordosis (associated with L5/S1 damage and weak abdominal musculature), prominent thoracolumbar kyphosis (multiple disc degeneration or vertebral fractures), scoliosis (degenerative, compensatory muscle spasm for unilateral pain).
- Look from the side. A gentle lordotic curve is normal. Flattening suggests muscle spasm or fusion in SpA. With major spondylolisthesis, a step between spinous processes can sometimes be seen.

*Observe active movements while the patient is standing*

Lumbar forward flexion ('. . . with your legs straight, slowly reach down to try and touch your ankles . . .'), lateral flexion ('. . . with your legs and back straight, tip sideways and run your hand down your leg towards your knee . . .') and extension ('. . . with your legs straight, slowly bend back-wards . . .'). Note: flexion can be mediated by the hip joints; extension can be affected by slight pelvic tilt and body sway. Ask what can be achieved normally and what is painful:

- Abnormal movements are not specific for any condition though they may help to localize a problem.
- Pain in extension is characteristic of retrolisthesis, facet joint arthritis, or impinging spinous processes. May be relieved by flexion.
- Failure of the spinous processes to separate in a patient who manages good forward flexion would be consistent with permanent spinal stiffness, e.g. axSpA/AS, with flexion mediated by the hip joints.
- Forward flexion can be measured using the modified Schöber test. When erect, mark the skin at the point midway between the posterior superior iliac spines (Venus' dimples) and again 10 cm above and 5 cm below. Measure the increase in distance between the outer marks at full forward flexion—in a young adult this is normally >6 cm.
- Ask the patient to stand on one foot then lift onto their toes a few times. Weakness might imply an L5 nerve root entrapment (gastrocnemius/soleus).

*Observe the gait pattern*

Abnormality of gait may reflect any spinal or lower limb problem:

- An antalgic gait; a self-protective limp due to pain, typically characterized by a short stance phase on the affected leg. The commonest cause is pathology at the hip.
- A wide-based gait suggests unsteadiness (due to dizziness, muscular weakness, proprioceptive, or cerebellar deficit, etc.).
- Leaning forwards/stiff legged—although not specific, in older people this may denote spinal stenosis.

- Shuffling, which could suggest parkinsonism (back pain/stiffness is a recognized early sign).
- Foot drop, which could suggest L5 or S1 nerve root compression.
- Flat feet, hind feet valgus, and genu recurvatum on stance phase, might suggest general hypermobility—associated with various low back lesions.

*Check extension and lumbar rotation (patient seated)*

With the patient seated on the couch, check lumbar extension and rotation (the pelvis is now fixed):

- Typically, combined rotation and extension can elicit pain from arthritic facet joints. It is a sensitive though not specific test.
- Slumping forwards (Fig. 3.11) stretches the dura. Increased lumbar pain may be elicited in cases of disc prolapse, but more importantly, leg pain can be elicited in cases of nerve root entrapment. A more provocative test can be done by gently extending each knee in turn in the slump position. Look for asymmetry.

*Examine the sacroiliac joints and hips (patient supine)*

With the patient supine, examination of the sacroiliac joints and an examination of the hips should be done to exclude pain arising from these structures:

- Test flexion and the rotational range of each hip by lifting the leg, flexed at the knee, so that the upper leg is vertical. Passive movement should normally be pain-free.
- No SI joint stress test is specific. Tests are designed to reproduce pain in cases of SI joint dysfunction or sacroiliitis. Here are two:
  - Press down/out reasonably firmly over both anterior superior iliac spines at the same time.
  - Lift one leg, flex, and abduct the hip slightly. Exert an axial force into the acetabulum at two or three different angles. This test is considered by many to be more useful and probably stresses both the joint and many of the sacral ligaments, but is less specific if the hip joint is abnormal.

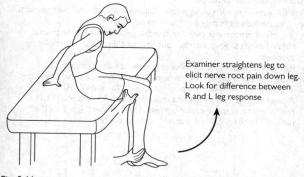

Examiner straightens leg to elicit nerve root pain down leg. Look for difference between R and L leg response

**Fig. 3.11** The (passive) slump test identifies pain from lumbar disc and nerve root irritation or compression. 'Active' leg extension can also trigger pain.

*Testing nerve root tension*

(Also see ➲ Chapter 21.) Use straight leg raise with the patient supine, Lasegue's test, and the slump test.

- The normal variation in straight leg raise ranges from 60° to more than 90° in adults. Compare sides:
  - Discomfort from normal tightening of the posterior thigh or calf muscles must be discriminated from a positive test.
  - A positive test (leg raising restricted to 40° or less by the radicular pain) is most specific in patients aged <30 years and for L5 or S1 nerve root lesions.
  - A crossed straight leg raise (pain elicited by raising the unaffected leg) is even more specific for nerve root entrapment.
- Lasegue's test is done by lifting the affected leg with knee fully flexed at first then with the upper part of the leg vertical, slowly extending the patient's leg at the knee (passive examination).
- A positive Lasegue's test is when pain is triggered in buttock or back as in the straight leg raise.
- Slump test is particularly useful when the patient is unable to lie supine for a straight leg raise or Lasegue's test. With the patient sitting, and slumped (Fig. 3.11) and legs hanging free off the ground, gradually extend the lower leg and ask if buttock or low back pain is triggered (a positive test).
- To identify more subtle cases of nerve root entrapment with all three tests, apply additional foot dorsiflexion at the maximum possible extent of leg raise/knee extension (pain-free).

*Neurological examination*

Neurological examination of the legs is essential in suspected cases of nerve root entrapment, cord compression, spinal stenosis, and cauda equina syndrome. Table 3.15 lists tests for muscle strength in the lower limbs—weakness may denote nerve root entrapment—and Table 3.16 lists the principal signs of lumbar nerve root lesions.

*Examination of the prone patient*

Ask the patient to turn to lie prone. Palpate low back and over sacrum:

- Diffuse tenderness may be due to muscle spasm.
- Superficial tenderness over the spinous processes or interspinous interval might suggest interspinous ligament disruption or impinging processes.
- Paravertebral bony tenderness may suggest facet joint arthritis.
- Costovertebral angle/loin tenderness could indicate renal pathology.
- Tenderness over the SI joints is not specific for sacroiliitis.
- A positive femoral stretch test reproduces L1–L4 (especially L3) radicular pain in the anterior or medial part of the thigh. Flex the patient's knee to 90° and passively extend the hip.

**Table 3.15** Testing muscle strength in the lower limbs (patient supine unless otherwise stated). Weakness may denote nerve root entrapment

| Muscle or muscle group | Nerve roots | Test* |
|---|---|---|
| Hamstrings (knee flexion) | L5, S1, S2 | Ask patient to flex the knee to 45°, hold patient's ankle and ask them to bend the knee further against your hold |
| Iliopsoas (hip flexion/internal rotation) | L1, L2, L3 | Ask patient to lift the leg with a bent knee, hold up the upper leg and resist your push. Try to push the leg down and slightly outwards |
| Quadriceps femoris (hip flexion, knee extension) | L2, L3, L4 | Hold the patient's relaxed upper leg above the couch (hold underneath above the knee). The lower leg should drop loosely. Ask them to raise the lower leg against your resistance |
| | | From patient standing test repetitive squatting for more subtle weakness |
| Tibialis anterior (ankle dorsiflexion). Tibialis posterior (ankle inversion and plantar flexion) | L4, L5 | With the knee straight ask the patient to pull back their foot (show them first) against your pull. Resist dorsiflexion |
| | | Standing or walking on heels tests for more subtle weakness. Note: if the hind foot rests in valgus or the patient significantly everts the foot during dorsiflexion, the test may also recruit peroneal muscles (L5, S1) |
| Extensor hallucis longus | L5, S1 | Ask the patient to pull their big toe back against your finger (at the base) |
| Gastrocnemius and soleus (ankle plantar flexion) | S1, S2 | Ask the patient to point their toes. Resist movement by pressing the ball of the foot |
| | | Standing or walking on the toes tests for more subtle weakness |

* Compare sides. Score according to scale, for example: 0 = no muscle contraction; 1 = contraction visible; 2 = active movement, gravity eliminated; 3 = active movement against gravity; 4–/4/4+ = active movement against slight/moderate/strong resistance; 5 = normal power.

*Other examination*

- In suspected cases of spinal stenosis or cauda equina syndrome, it is essential to check for sensory loss in the sacral nerve dermatomes. Also check anal sphincter tone by rectal examination (S5).
- In suspected cases of spinal stenosis, the patient can be asked to walk until limited by pain then re-examined. If there is any ischaemia of the cauda equina or of a nerve root (from foramenal stenosis), nerve root signs may become more obvious.

**Table 3.16** Principal combinations of signs used for identifying lumbar nerve root lesions

| Nerve root | Paraesthesias and sensory change | Muscle weakness | Tendon reflex changes |
|---|---|---|---|
| L2 | Upper thigh: anterior, medial, and lateral surfaces | Hip flexion and adduction | None |
| L3 | Anterior surface of lower thigh | Hip adduction and knee extension | Knee jerk possibly reduced |
| L4 | Anteromedial surface of lower leg | Knee extension, foot dorsiflexion, and inversion | Knee jerk decreased |
| L5 | Anterolateral surface of lower leg and dorsum/medial side of foot/toe | Hip extension and abduction. Knee flexion. Foot/toe dorsiflexion | None |
| S1 | Lateral border and sole of foot. Back of heel and calf | Knee flexion. Plantar flexion and eversion of foot | Ankle jerk decreased |

## Investigation of low back pain in adults

(Also see ➲ Chapter 21.)

There are two important initial steps in investigating low back pain. First deciding whether radiographs will help. Second, although relatively rare in practice, the possibility of infection, malignancy, and cauda equina compression always needs to be considered.

- Simple radiographic views are insensitive indicators of these conditions and, in most cases, are not specific although most radiologists would agree they are desirable in addition to CT or MRI. Laboratory tests are mandatory in all suspected cases of inflammation, infection, and malignancy.

*Radiographs: decision-making in requesting them*
(See Table 3.17.)

- Lumbar spine radiographs are not always helpful. Remember that nine out of ten cases of back pain in the primary care setting are mechanical and self-limiting. Features on a plain radiograph of the lumbar spine correlate poorly with the presence or pattern of pain.
- Spondylosis is common, age-related, and often isn't symptomatic.
- MRI best identifies a pars interarticularis fracture, any associated bone oedema and spondylolisthesis seen in young people and athletes (see ➲ p. 620). CT helps clarify the healing response (bridging of bone across the defect).
- Obtaining radiographs to help in the management of patients is a different issue to obtaining them to aid diagnosis and one that requires careful thought, e.g. is the patient likely to perceive that they have received suboptimal care if a radiograph is not requested?

**Table 3.17** Commonly reported patterns of radiographic abnormality in adults with spinal symptoms: the interpretation, and suggested reaction

| Radiographic abnormalities | Lesion suggested | Sensible further action |
|---|---|---|
| Lumbosacral anomalies | Risk for future back pain | May not be clinically significant. Risk for low back pain (esp. if hypermobile) |
| Generalized osteopenia | Osteoporosis | Measurement of bone density. Rule out secondary causes, e.g. myeloma |
| Narrowed disc space, marginal vertebral end-plate osteophytes or both | Intervertebral disc disruption | MRI if persistent symptoms or signs of same level nerve root entrapment, spinal or nerve root exit foramen stenosis |
| Localized lucent or sclerotic lesion, loss of cortex | Tumour, infection, or fracture | Discuss case with radiologist. MRI or CT may be advised. A bone scan may be helpful. Initiate appropriate laboratory tests immediately |
| Facet joint OA | Facet joint syndrome | Consider whether there is associated spinal/nerve root exit foramen stenosis (?radicular symptoms) or symptoms suggestive of spondylolisthesis. CT or MRI is then likely to be appropriate |
| Pars interarticularis defect | Spondylolysis/ ?spondylolytic | Further oblique film centred on suspected level or CT should confirm. Association with symptoms or signs of disc disease or spondylolisthesis. Flexion and extension lateral view radiographs may detail the lesion further. MRI characterizes bone stress, soft tissue involvement and nerve impingment. |
| Short lumbar pedicles | Spinal stenosis | Consider MRI if symptoms suggest spinal stenosis |
| Mixed patchy sclerosis and lucency in entire (enlarged) vertebra(e) | Paget's disease | Neurological leg symptoms suggest spinal/exit foramen stenosis or vascular 'steal' |

- Spondylolysis may be seen on a lateral view, but is seen better on oblique view. Oblique views may also show pedicle stress fractures.
- Spondylolisthesis may be identified and graded by a lateral film.
- Flexion and extension views may be helpful in delineating subtle cases, and instability (spondylolytic).
- General osteopenia is a risk factor for low bone mass; however, it is not a sensitive indicator of low bone mass.

- Look for vertebral squaring (in AS), non-marginal syndesmophytes (in other SpA, such as psoriatic—see ➲ Plate 13), or flowing syndesmophytes (in DISH—at least three contiguous vertebral bodies).
- Consider obtaining an AP view of the pelvis. Established (but not early) sacroiliitis can be ruled-out. A further 'coned' view is often helpful.
- Sacroiliitis (periarticular osteoporosis, erosion, sclerosis of bone, widening joint space) occurs in all types of SpA. It can be unilateral.
- Sclerosis of the SI joint on the lower iliac side alone suggests osteitis condensans ilii. Joint space is normal and joint margin well defined.
- Patterns of metabolic bone disease, Paget's disease and hip pathology are usually readily identifiable on a pelvic film.

### Bone scintigraphy (see ➲ Plate 16)

- Bone scintigraphy is a sensitive test for infection or malignancy. It is a useful investigation in patients with previously diagnosed malignancy who present with back pain, especially in those who have had no previous skeletal metastases. No additional lesions strongly suggests against a single spinal abnormality being malignancy related.
- It is not specific for the various degenerative lesions, but can help localize the site of a lesion.
- SI joint appearances can locate pathology but appearances may depend on both previous pathology and/or current inflammation.

### CT or MR?

The choice of imaging depends on local availability and likely differential diagnosis, although MRI is preferred in young people:

- For spondylolytic spondylolisthesis, CT shows bone bridging and size of defect whereas MRI shows bone stress of any recent fracture.
- Nerve impingement can be shown by CT or MRI.
- Intervertebral disc prolapse, both posterior and posterolateral, can be shown by either technique. Prolapse material is of similar CT density and MR signal to the disc, and well-defined against epidural fat.
- Changes in the normal disc signal pattern are associated with age-related disc degeneration. Discogenic pain has been associated with MRI abnormalities classified according to Modic.
- On T2-weighted MRI, disc material is usually of higher signal than 'scar' (e.g. fibrosis from a previous lesion), in which signal decreases with ageing. Recent scarring enhances immediately, but old scarring does so only slowly. This discrimination requires gadolinium-enhanced MRI.
- CT or MRI shows early sacroiliitis in axSpA when radiographs are normal though MRI will show current inflammation better than 'ever' involvement of SIJs—for which CT is better.
- The shape and outline of the spinal canal are ideally shown on CT, but are also seen with MRI. It is difficult for MRI to distinguish fibrous structures from sclerotic or cortical bone, though it shows intrathecal content more readily which is an advantage in identifying intradural tumours.
- Spondylodiscitis (part of axSpA), if chronic, may be difficult to discriminate from degenerative disc/vertebral end-plate disease. Fat-suppressed or gadolinium-enhanced sequences may show high signal at the anterior disc vertebral end-plate junctions.

*Screening for infection, malignancy, or metabolic bone disease*
- In cases where the history and examination suggest a mechanical condition, but where the clinician wishes to be more confident of excluding an inflammatory condition, ESR, and CRP are suggested.
- A raised ESR would point towards further laboratory investigation.
- An infection screen should include an FBC for anaemia and leucocytosis, CRP, blood, and urine cultures. If spinal tuberculosis is suspected a plain CXR should be taken and serial (over 3 days) early morning urine samples taken.
- Serum and urine protein electrophoresis (with immunofixation) are essential tests in the 'work-up' for myeloma. Urea and creatinine are also important as hypercalcaemia, and acute renal impairment have prognostic significance in this condition.
- Routine blood tests may point to an underlying metabolic bone disorder such as Paget's disease or osteomalacia. These tests are normal in postmenopausal osteoporosis.
- If osteoporosis is diagnosed (see ◑ Chapter 16) a screen for secondary causes should include ESR (and if raised, serum, and urine protein electrophoresis), calcium, phosphate, sex hormones, but also serum 25-hydroxyvitamin D, parathyroid hormone (PTH), thyroid function tests (TFTs), and liver function tests (LFTs).

## Treatment of low back pain: adults
(See also ◑ Chapter 21 for greater detail)
- An important therapeutic intervention in the case of acute pain is to take the patient seriously, take a positive view, and in the absence of sinister signs, e.g. nerve root pain, urge early mobility.
- Analgesics and muscle relaxants can be used in the short term, initially regularly, then as required.
- Physical therapy with graded-activity programmes may be of value, certainly early in disc disease or spondylosis.
- Cord compression due to bone collapse from a tumour is an acute emergency and should be discussed immediately with an oncologist or radiation oncologist, and a spinal orthopaedic or neurosurgeon.
- Cases with disc prolapse failing to respond to conservative therapy, or cases where there is ongoing or rapidly progressive neurological deficit, should be referred for surgery.
- Available surgical techniques for acute or persistent disc disease include decompression (e.g. nerve root decompression and partial facetectomy), prosthetic intervertebral disc replacement, intradiscal thermocoagulation, and intradiscal steroid injections, although evidence for long-term efficacy is lacking for all these procedures.
- Surgery for spinal stenosis is useful for relieving leg neurogenic features, but not indicated if there is no significant neurological compromise. Surgery is not usually done if the only effect of spinal stenosis is back pain.
- In chronic back pain, aerobic exercises combined with behavioural methods may be more effective than exercise alone and can help motivate the patient. Methods may also incorporate psychological and social assessment and management.

- The common treatments available for chronic back pain include:
  - analgesics and muscle relaxants.
  - antiepileptics/antidepressants for neuropathic pain.
  - local anaesthetic/steroid injections.
  - acupuncture.
  - transcutaneous electrical nerve stimulation (TENS).
  - physical therapy. See p. 609
  - ergonomic advice.
  - multidisciplinary programmes—counselling, cognitive therapy, education, relaxation, corsets and belts.
- Timely surgery for structural scoliosis can lessen spinal curvature.

# Low back pain in children and adolescents

## Synopsis

Children and young people present with a combination of back pain, deformity, limp, systemic or neurological features. Many of the features of adolescents overlap with young adults and the reader is referred to the assessment of adults on pp. 140–52. See also ➲ Chapter 21, pp. 618–21.

- Back pain in children and adolescents is common (lifetime prevalence up to 80% by 20y) and, as in adults, most cases are non-specific, self-limiting and do not present to the medical profession.
- Back pain is more common at times of rapid growth in girls and with high and low levels of activity. It is especially common in young athletes.
- Times of rapid growth are also associated with: progression of idiopathic scoliosis; other spinal deformities; and (if excessive) volume expansion of vertebrae which confers the potential for a discrepancy between bone size and bone mass (a reason for correcting DXA scan-derived BMD measures).
- The likelihood of finding underlying pathology (see ➲ Table 21.6, p. 618) is low, but more likely at younger ages (especially <4y old).
- Low back pain in adolescence is a significant risk factor for back pain in adulthood.

## Taking a history of low back pain in children

- It is important to consider back pain in relation to age and development. Loss of developmental milestones, refusal to walk, or irritability in a non-verbal child, especially if <4y, warrants immediate investigation.
- Systemic features, intractable or night pain in children <6y require assessment for infectious or neoplastic causes including TB in relevant populations.
- Back pain is more common at times of rapid growth in girls and with high and low levels of activity. It is especially common in young athletes. (see also ➲ Box 21.1).
- Trauma, especially sudden or repetitive twisting in adolescents may aggravate or cause a pars defect leading to spondylolisthesis.
- Disability (including school absence) disproportionate to examination findings may indicate pain amplification. Social history including stresses and sleep pattern should be elicited.
- Incongruence of history and examination raises suspicion of non-accidental injury.
- As in adults, differentiation between biomechanical and inflammatory clinical features should be elicited.

## Examination of back pain in adolescents

- Be opportunistic with a young child, observe play and review findings in context of developmental stage.
- Focal bony tenderness identified by palpation or percussion should be assessed further through radiological investigation.
- Examine gait (see ➲ pp. 37–9) and posture, for loss or exaggerated lordosis, pelvic tilt (from leg length discrepancy), neck jut, and kyphosis.
- Scoliosis is rarely painful.
- Reduced hamstring flexibility (determined by popliteal angle) and tight hip flexors (Thomas's test) are commonly associated with back pain.
- New, unilateral or persistent toe-walking suggests spasticity, tethered cord, or muscle weakness.
- Survey the skin for possible bruising, mid-line hairy patches, café-au-lait, axillary freckling (neurofibromatosis). Soft tissue swelling may denote extension of a spinal tumour.
- Neurological examination in 20% of children with bone or spinal cord tumours will show motor weakness.

## Investigations

- Investigations are the same as for adults see ➲ pp. 148–51.
- A general anaesthetic is commonly required for an MRI in young children.

# Pelvic, groin, and thigh pain in adults

## Anatomy

### Anatomy of the pelvis and hip region

- The bony pelvis consists of two innominate bones (ilium above the acetabulum and ischium below it) that articulate with each other at the anterior symphysis pubis and posteriorly with the sacrum at the SI joints (SIJs).
- SIJs are initially synovial but become fibrous with age. A few degrees of rotation can be demonstrated in children and young adults.
- Strong ligaments stabilize the posterior pelvis through sacroinominate, lumbo (L5)–sacral, and lumbo (L5)–iliac attachments.
- The symphysis pubis is a cartilaginous joint and normally does not move.
- When standing, weight is transferred through the head of the femur. The femoral head is stabilized in the acetabulum by the acetabular labrum and strong pericapsular ligaments.
- The ligamentum teres crosses the hip joint and carries blood vessels to the head of the femur in children and young adults. In old age, blood supply is largely via vessels that enter the femoral neck.
- Two bursae are found at the insertion of the gluteus maximus: one separates it from the greater trochanter, the other separates it from the vastus lateralis.
- The ischial bursa separates gluteus maximus from the ischial tuberosity and can become inflamed from overuse.

### Anatomy of pelvic musculature

- Three groups of muscles move the hip joint: the gluteals, the flexor muscles, and the adductor group.
- The major gluteal group muscles are:
  - *gluteus maximus (L5, S1/2):* arises mainly from ilium and sacrum, projects down posterolaterally and inserts into the posterior femur and the lateral tensor fasciae latae. It extends and externally rotates the hip (the hamstrings also extend the hip).
  - *gluteus medius (L4/5, S1):* lies deeper and more lateral. It inserts into the lateral greater trochanter and abducts and internally rotates the hip.
  - piriformis, obturator internus, and quadratus femoris arise deep in the pelvis and insert into the posterior greater trochanter. All externally rotate the hip.
- The major hip flexor, psoas major (L2/3), is a massive muscle that arises from the lateral part of the vertebrae and intervertebral discs (T12–L5) and lateral processes of the lumbar vertebrae. It runs anteriorly over the iliac rim, across the pelvis, under the inguinal ligament, and inserts into the lesser trochanter. The iliacus (L2–L4) arises from the 'inside' of the iliac blade, passes under the inguinal ligament medially to the lesser trochanter. Both flex, but the psoas also internally rotates the hip.
- The psoas is enveloped in a fascial sheath. Retroperitoneal or spinal infections that track along soft tissue planes sometimes involves the psoas sheath and can cause inflammation in the psoas bursa, which separates the muscle from the hip joint.

- All adductor muscles arise from the pubis or ischiopubic rami. The adductor longus and gracilis are the most superficial; they arise from the pubis and insert into the femoral shaft and pes anserinus ('goose's foot') below the knee, respectively. The adductor magnus (L4/5) is the largest of the deeper adductors; it inserts into the medial femoral shaft.
- Adductors stabilize movement around the hip towards the end of the stance phase of the gait. Body weight is transferred onto one leg during this action and, therefore, adductors need to be strong, especially for running.

*Functional anatomy of the hip*

- With a flexed knee, the limit of hip flexion is about 135°.
- Hip extension (at 30°), internal rotation (at 30–35°), and external rotation (at 45–55°) is limited by strong, pericapsular ligaments.
- Abduction is limited to 45–50° by contact between the greater trochanter and acetabular labrum rim. Adduction is limited to 20–30° with a fixed pelvis (see ➲ Plate 15). These are adult ranges.
- Greater femoral neck anteversion (angle of the neck compared to the distal femur) allows greater internal rotation of the hip (and reduced external rotation). Tibial torsion can compensate but this and hip anteversion results in a toe-in gait. Femoral neck retroversion (if the angle is posterior to the femoral intercondylar plane) allows greater external rotation of the hip, usually resulting in a toe-out gait.
- Normally infants have more anteversion than older children or adults (30–40° at age 2 years compared with 8–15° at age >18 years).

*Neuroanatomy*

- The femoral nerve is formed from L2–L4 nerve roots and supplies mainly muscles of the quadriceps group and some deeper hip adductors.
- With contributions from L4–S3 roots, nerves from the plexus converge at the inferior border of the piriformis to form the sciatic nerve. This is at a foramen formed by the ilium (above and lateral), sacrum (medial), sacrospinous ligament (below), and sacrotuberous ligament (posteromedial).
- In about 10% of people the sciatic nerve divides before exiting the pelvis. In some a branch exits above the piriformis muscle. Nerve entrapment and trauma at this site may give rise to piriformis syndrome, and may benefit from physical therapy.

## Taking a history

### Age

Age is a risk factor for some conditions:

- Unless there has been previous hip disease (e.g. osteonecrosis, synovitis), trauma, or a long-standing biomechanical abnormality (e.g. epiphyseal dysplasia) hip osteoarthritis (OA) is uncommon in adults <55 years old.
- Paget's disease of bone is rare in adults <50 years old except in familial disease.

*Distribution and type of bone and soft tissue pain*

- All mechanical lesions of the lumbar spine can result in referred pain around the pelvis and thighs. It is often bilateral, localizes poorly, and is aching in nature.
- Lateral pelvic pain is often referred from the lumbosacral spine. If pain localizes (i.e. the patient points) to the greater trochanter, it may be due to trochanteric bursitis, enthesitis, or meralgia paraesthetica (lateral femoral cutaneous nerve syndrome, see Table 3.18).
- Hip joint pain is felt in the groin, but it can be located deep in the buttock when ischial bursitis and sacroiliac pain should also be considered. It may be referred distally to the anteromedial thigh and knee.

**Table 3.18** Patterns of pain around the proximal leg and their major causes in adults

| Pattern of pain | Causes |
|---|---|
| Pain in buttock and posterior thighs | Referred pain from: lumbar spine, e.g. facet, OA, spondylolisthesis; SI joint inflammation; lower lumbar nerve root irritation; sciatic nerve entrapment (piriformis syndrome) |
| | Localized pain: ischial bursitis/enthesitis or fracture; coccidynia |
| | Diffuse muscular pain/stiffness: myositis or PMR |
| | Paget's or other bone lesion of sacrum |
| Lateral pelvic pain | Referred from lumbosacral spine |
| | Trochanteric bursitis/enthesitis |
| | Gluteus medius tear |
| | Lateral hip joint pain, e.g. osteophyte |
| Groin pain | Hip disease, e.g. OA, osteonecrosis, synovitis, femoroacetabular impingement |
| | Psoas bursitis |
| | Adductor tendonitis, osteitis pubis, pubis fracture |
| | Pelvic enthesitis |
| | Paget's disease (pelvis or femur) |
| | Femoral neck or pubic ramus fracture |
| | Hernia |
| Anterior thigh | Referred from: lumbar spine, e.g. facet OA, spondylolisthesis; upper lumbar nerve root; hip joint, femoral neck |
| | Myositis, PMR |
| | Meralgia paraesthetica (anterolateral) |
| | Adductor tendonitis, osteitis pubis |
| | Ischaemia (claudication) |
| | Lymph nodes |

- Groin pain on weight-bearing suggests hip pathology such as synovitis, osteonecrosis or OA, but it is not specific. Tendonitis of the adductor longus, osteitis pubis, a femoral neck stress fracture, osteoid osteoma, or psoas bursitis can give similar symptoms.
- Bone pathology typically gives unremitting pain. Sleep is often disturbed.
- Pain from deep MSK pelvic structures is typically poorly localized, although can be severe. If the pain appears to be 'catastrophic' consider pelvic bone disease (tumours, infection, Paget's disease, osteomalacia, osteoporotic fracture) (see ➲ Chapter 16) or an unstable pelvis (chronic osteitis pubis with diastasis/laxity of the symphysis pubis and sacroiliac joints).
- Enthesitis of the anterior pelvis and osteitis pubis associated with SpAs (see ➲ Chapter 8) are probably under-recognized.
- Aching in the back of the legs after standing is found with spondylolisthesis (i.e. anterior displacement of a vertebra).
- Sacroiliac pain and stiffness radiates to the buttocks and posterior thighs.

*Pain in a muscular distribution*

- Diffuse pain in the buttocks and thighs occurs in PMR. It is often sudden or subacute in onset, associated with stiffness, and may give similar symptoms to those caused by sacroiliitis but invariably occurs for the first time in a much older age group.
- Pain is not invariably present for all types of autoimmune myositis (see ➲ Chapter 14). When it does occur, it is unlikely to be confined to pelvic musculature or to be unilateral, but should be considered where acute or subacute onset diffuse pelvic girdle/thigh pain accompanies weakness.
- Multiple entheseal lesions—particularly of structures at the greater trochanter—can present with quite diffuse pain—interpreted by patients as 'muscular'.

*Quality and distribution of nerve pain*

- Nerve root pain is often clearly defined and sharp. It may be burning in quality and is often accompanied by numbness or paraesthesias. L5 or S1 lesions generally cause pain below the knee, but can also cause posterior thigh pain. L1–L3 root lesions can cause pain in the anteromedial thigh.
- Pain with paraesthesia on the anterolateral part of the thigh may be due to entrapment of the lateral cutaneous nerve of the thigh under the lateral part of the inguinal ligament (i.e. meralgia paraesthetica). Symptoms may be referred to this area with L2 or L3 nerve root lesions, since this is where the nerve originates.
- Diabetics with uncontrolled hyperglycaemia are at risk of diabetic amyotrophy. Acute unilateral or bilateral thigh pain with muscle wasting occurs. It should not be misdiagnosed as PMR (in which weakness or wasting do not occur) or inflammatory myopathy.
- Footballers are at risk of adductor tendonitis (often an adductor apophysitis) and osteitis pubis owing to substantial mechanical forces placed on pelvic structures during running and kicking.

- Although hip fractures are usually obvious, they can also present subacutely in a patient who continues to walk; this is particularly common among the elderly, who may develop stress fractures of the hip.

*Previous trauma, low back, and MSK problems*

- Previous trauma or disease causing permanent deformity of any lumbosacral or hip joint structure can be considered a risk factor for asymmetry, poor core stability and MSK pains (Table 3.19).
- Multiparity is a risk factor for osteitis pubis, sacroiliac, and pelvic pain, particularly where there is hypermobility.
- Trochanteric pain syndrome owing to enthesitis, bursitis or insertional tendonitis/tendon tear may coexist with referred back pain.
- Enthesitis of the gluteus medius can occur at its greater trochanter insertion and give similar symptoms to those caused by bursitis.
- Historically, tailors were at risk of ischial bursitis because of sitting on the floor continually crossing and uncrossing their legs, causing friction irritation of soft tissues overlying the ischial tuberosity.

## Examination of adults with hip and pelvic pain

The reader is referred to the sequence of examination for the low back, including the sacroiliac and lower limb neurologic examination elsewhere in this chapter (see ➋ 'Examination of an adult with low back pain', pp. 144–7). Always consider lower spinal, muscle, or neurological pathology when assessing weakness and pain around the pelvis.

**Table 3.19** Risk factors for painful pelvic or hip lesions

| Risk factor | Pelvic/hip pathology |
|---|---|
| Low back lesions (e.g. lumbar facet disease or intervertebral degenerative disc disease) | Referred non-dermatomal pain |
| | Sciatic pain |
| Hip joint structural lesion (e.g. Perthes' disease, slipped epiphysis, epiphyseal dysplasia) | Hip dysplasia, avascular necrosis or OA |
| Glucocorticoid use | Osteoporotic fracture |
| | Osteonecrosis of the femoral head (see ➋ Plate 17) |
| Autoimmune and autoinflammatory rheumatic joint disease (e.g. RA, JIA, axSpA, AS) | Synovitis hip |
| | Secondary OA of the hip |
| | Pyogenic arthritis of the hip |
| | Periarticular enthesitis |
| CKD3b–5 | CPPD/pseudogout of the hip joint |
| Multiple pregnancies | Osteitis pubis (± pelvic instability) |
| Sports | Adductor tendonitis/apophysitis |
| | Osteitis pubis |

*Observation and palpation*

For observation and palpation, the patient should be supine on a couch:

- Look for leg length discrepancy (hip disease, scoliosis) and a leg resting in external rotation (hip fracture).
- Psoriasis may be associated with pelvic enthesitis/sacroiliitis.
- Swelling in the groin may be a hernia (reducible, moves with cough), lipoma (soft/non-tender/diffuse), a saphenous varix, or lymphadenopathy (hard/rubbery and invariably mobile). A hip joint effusion cannot be felt.
- Tenderness over the hip joint in the groin is not specific for joint pathology: the joint is deep—muscles and psoas bursa overlie it.
- If the groin is very tender with slight touch, consider hip fracture or infection. Hyperpathia (and allodynia) is consistent with CRPS (see ➔ Chapter 22).
- Numbness over the anterolateral thigh suggests meralgia paraesthetica (Fig. 3.12).

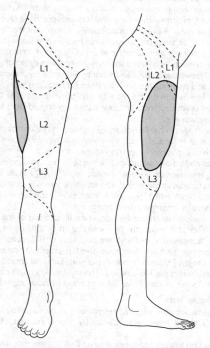

**Fig. 3.12** The approximate areas within which sensory changes may be found in lesions of the lateral cutaneous nerve of the thigh (hatched area) and high lumbar radiculopathy (broken line). Shaded area—sensory symptoms distribution from meralgia paraesthetica.

- The adductor longus tendon can be palpated at its insertion at the pubic tubercle and distally along the upper medial thigh. The pubic tubercle is found by palpating slowly and lightly downwards from umbilicus over the bladder until bone is reached.
- Pain from osteitis pubis or adductor apophysitis is often significant, with abdominal rectus contraction (ask the patient to slowly lift their head and shoulders off the couch keeping your finger on the pubic tubercle).

*Hip examination*

The patient is supine. Tests generally help to discriminate articular and extra-articular disease, but not the causes of articular disease:

- Measure and determine actual or apparent leg length discrepancy: measure from the anterior superior iliac spine to the medial tibial malleolus; by flexing hips and knees, the site of shortening should become apparent.
- A fixed loss of extension is a sign of intra-articular hip disease. The patient flexes the hip and knee on one side until normal lumbar lordosis flattens out (confirmed by feeling pressure on your hand placed under their lumbar spine during the manoeuvre). If the other hip flexes simultaneously, it suggests hip extension loss on that side (Thomas' test).
- Using the patella or tibial tubercle as pointers, test the rotational hip range in extension by rotating the straightened legs by holding the heels.
- Rotational movements are also tested by lifting the leg, flexed 90° at the knee, and swinging the foot out (internal rotation) or in (external rotation). Hip flexion can be tested in this position too (see ➲ Plate 15a). Patients without intra-articular pathology should have a pain-free range of movement.
- Rotational ranges in hip flexion and extension may differ between left and right in an individual. Also, variations in femoral neck anteversion contribute to variations in rotation range.
- To test hip abduction/adduction, fix the pelvis to avoid pelvic tilt by placing one hand firmly over the iliac crest (see ➲ Plate 15b). Occasionally, pain at the end of abduction or internal rotation occurs with a bony block (solid 'end-feel'). In an older patient this might suggest impingement of a marginal joint osteophyte.
- Barlow's manoeuvre checks for congenital dislocation of the hips in babies. Flex and adduct the hips exerting an axial force into the posterior 'acetabulum' to demonstrate posterior dislocation.
- Greater retroversion (allowing excessive hip external rotation) usually occurs in cases of slipped femoral epiphysis. External rotation is accentuated when the hip is flexed. The slip (usually inferoposterior) is thought to occur in association with a period of rapid growth.

*Muscle activation tests*

Specific muscle activation against resistance can be used to elicit pain, but results need to be interpreted cautiously in the context of known hip disease:

- Hip adduction against resistance (sliding their leg inwards towards the other against your hand) reproducing pain is a sensitive test for adductor longus tendonitis, but may be positive in osteitis pubis, hip joint lesions, and other soft tissue lesions in the adductor muscles.

- Test psoas by resisted hip flexion in slight internal rotation. Psoas bursitis or infection tracking along the psoas sheath is likely to give intense pain with minimal resistance.
- Hip abduction (sliding the leg outwards against your hand) may be particularly painful in cases of gluteus medius tears, but also in trochanteric bursitis or intra-articular pathology.

*Palpate posterolateral structures*

Ask the patient to lie on their side and palpate the posterolateral structures (Fig. 3.13):

- Tenderness over the greater trochanter is usually well-localized, although it may be anterior or posterolateral to the trochanter and refers a small way down the leg.
- The ischial tuberosity and its overlying bursa lie at the apex of the buttock.
- The soft tissues overlying the point where the sciatic nerve exits the pelvis is found midway between the ischial spine and the greater trochanter. There may be tenderness as a result of soft tissue lesions or trauma causing sciatic nerve entrapment (piriformis syndrome), which can lead to foot drop.
- A tender coccyx (coccidynia) can be palpated in this position. It can also be palpated (and the sacrococcygeal joint moved) from a bi-digital examination, though this requires the index finger to be placed inside the rectum, the thumb outside, the two digits then holding the joint.

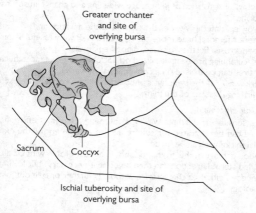

**Fig. 3.13** Bony anatomy of the posterior hip and pelvis, showing the position in which lesions around the greater trochanter and ischial bursa can be palpated.

### Investigation of an adult with hip and pelvis pain

#### Radiographs

An AP radiograph of the pelvis is a good initial screening test in patients with pelvic, hip, or thigh pain. AP and lateral lumbar spine films may be warranted:

- The pelvis is a common site of involvement in myeloma, metastatic malignancy, and Paget's disease of bone (see ➲ Chapter 16).
- Established, but often not early, sacroiliitis can be ruled out. The main differential diagnoses of the causes of sacroiliitis are AS, psoriatic or reactive arthritis, enteric arthropathy, brucellosis and other infections, hyperparathyroidism and osteitis condensans ilii (sclerosis of the SI joint on the lower iliac side).
- Widening of the symphysis in children may be a sign of congenital disorders of development (e.g. epispadias, achondrogenesis, chondrodysplasias, hypophosphatasia), trauma and hyperparathyroidism (see ➲ Chapter 16).
- Widening of the symphysis pubis, osteitis pubis (bone resorption and sclerosis) and osteitis condensans ilii are signs associated with chronic pelvic pain in multiparous women.
- General osteopenia is a risk factor for general low bone mass measured by densitometry; however, it is not a sensitive or specific indicator of osteoporosis (i.e. may be osteomalacia or rickets).
- Regional osteoporosis confined to the femur is non-specific: hip synovitis, infection, or transient osteoporosis of the hip are possible.
- Early synovitis and infection may be demonstrated through subtle radiological signs such as joint space widening and change in soft tissue fat planes.
- A 'frog leg' (lateral) view of the hip shows the anterior and posterior femoral head more clearly than an AP view (useful in early osteonecrosis/Perthes' disease, slipped epiphysis).
- The acetabulae are best visualized on 45° oblique views (acetabular fractures can be missed on a conventional AP view).
- 'Stork' views of the symphysis pubis (standing on one leg) are useful for confirming diastasis of the joint.

#### Diagnostic ultrasound

US is a sensitive and simple way of confirming a hip joint effusion. Using US, fluid can be aspirated for culture and an assessment of the extent of synovial thickening can be made.

- Tendon damage in the groin area should be identifiable with US alone (guided steroid injection can then be done if necessary) but MRI may be needed either to characterize pathology further or rule out joint pathology.

*Bone scintigraphy*

Characteristic, though non-specific, patterns of bone scan abnormality are recognized in the hip/pelvic area.

- The following conditions can be recognized: sacroiliitis, bone malignancy, myeloma, Paget's disease, hip fracture, femoral head osteonecrosis (see ➔ Plate 17), osteoid osteoma, OA, bursitis/enthesitis at the greater trochanter and synovitis of the hip.
- Visualizing osteitis pubis/adductor apophysitis requires special seated 'ring' view.

*CT and MRI*

- MRI of the high lumbar region should be considered to confirm a nerve root lesion causing groin or thigh pain.
- Specific patterns of X-ray attenuation or signal change around the SIJs occur in sacroiliitis with CT/MRI, although active and previous inflammation cannot easily be distinguished unless both modalities of imaging are arranged.
- A suspicion of bony malignancy from radiographs of the pelvis requires further characterization. CT is the technique of choice for characterizing bone lesions around the hip, such as femoral neck stress fracture, osteoid osteoma, or other bone tumours. CT may give more information about the lesion (and is valuable for 'guided biopsy'), but MRI is useful in checking for pelvic visceral lesions.
- MRI is the technique of choice if hip infection or osteonecrosis is suspected. In adults, patterns of signal change have been correlated with prognosis.
- During a single examination, the pattern of hip synovitis (vascularity and thickness), cartilage loss, and subchondral bone erosion can be documented.

*Laboratory investigations*

- ESR and CRP may be normal in inflammatory SIJs, lumbar vertebral disc, and pelvic enthesis disorders.
- PMR is invariably associated with an acute-phase response.
- Myeloma is unlikely if the ESR is normal.
- A high alkaline phosphatase is typically associated with an acute-phase response, although in the elderly, it might suggest Paget's disease.
- ANA and RF are unlikely to help diagnostically.
- Major metabolic bone disease, such as osteomalacia and hyperparathyroidism is usually excluded by a normal serum calcium and phosphate.

## Treatment of pelvic conditions in adults

Treatment of spinal and neuropathic pain is covered in the earlier section on ➔ 'Low back pain in adults', pp. 140–52 and in ➔ Chapter 21.

- NSAIDs may be required for a number of the conditions described earlier, particularly OA, hip synovitis, and tendon inflammation.
- Physical therapy and rehabilitation play a vital and early part in management, maintaining mobility, preventing tissue contracture, and re-strengthening/stabilizing the lower back, pelvis, and hip.

- Either physical therapists or podiatrists may help in accurately evaluating back and lower limb biomechanics. Asymmetry and muscular imbalance may be modifiable relatively simply with foot orthotics, for example.
- Steroid injections may be important in the following conditions:
  - meralgia paraesthetica.
  - osteitis pubis.
  - trochanteric bursitis/enthesitis.
  - ischial bursitis/enthesitis.
  - adductor tendonitis.
  - coccidynia.
  - hip synovitis (under imaging guidance).
  - sacroiliitis—in intractable pain and under X-ray or US guidance.
- Injection techniques are covered in ➔ Chapter 24.

*Surgery*
- When the hip has been damaged by an inflammatory arthritis or OA the principal surgical intervention is joint replacement. Osteotomy has been mainly superseded by more reliable replacement.
- Surgical synovectomy of the hip is a difficult procedure and opening the hip carries a risk of avascular necrosis. This procedure is very rarely done.
- Excision arthroplasty is only really necessary where infection or poor bone stock make reconstruction unwise. Power is often greatly reduced and even the previously fit young patient will not be able to ambulate without crutches.

# Pelvic, groin, and thigh pain in children and adolescents

## General considerations

Hip and pelvic problems in young children usually present with a limp noticed by a parent. In an older child or adolescent pain may be reported initially—in groin, around buttocks or greater trochanter areas.

- The commonest causes of pelvic, hip and upper thigh conditions in children are either due to developmental disorders, inflammatory lesions or trauma/overuse (see Table 3.20).
- If stress fracture of the femoral neck is suspected in a teenage girl then consider: amenorrhea, eating disorder and athletic over-training ('female triad syndrome').

## Examination

Examination begins with gait evaluation. Account for the developmental stage. Examine squatting, single-leg hopping, lunging, zig-zag running and abdominal curls/sit-ups (to disclose any symphyseal pain).

- Hip range of movement in children is similar to adults except the degree of femoral anteversion is greater in toddlers (30–40° at 2 years) reducing to 8–15° by 18 years of age.
- Reduced range of movement and irritability at end of range is typical of intraarticular pathology. Joint pain radiates into the groin.

**Table 3.20** Common causes of hip joint and pelvis area pains in children and adolescents

| Type of condition | Diagnosis | Incidence (per 10,000) |
|---|---|---|
| Developmental | Perthes' disease | 0.6 |
| | Slipped upper femoral epiphysis (SUFE) | 0.1–1 |
| Inflammatory or infection | Septic joint, osteomyelitis or pyomyositis | 1 (not known for pyomyositis) |
| | JIA | 0.3 |
| | Irritable hip (transient tenosynovitis) | 8 |
| | Idiopathic chondrolysis of the hip | <0.1 |
| Biomechanical and overuse injury | Snapping hip | ≈ 1 |
| | Tendinopathy /muscle strain | Common |
| | Enthesitis (apophysitis) | Uncommon (number due to SpA unknown) |
| | Stress fracture ("female triad syndrome") | Uncommon |
| Tumours | Osteoid osteoma | 0.1 |
| | Ewing sarcoma (femur) | <0.1 |
| | Leukaemia/neuroblastoma | <0.1 |
| Other | Intra-abdominal pathology | |

- Palpate for tenderness over ASISs, iliac crests, iliac tubercles, greater trochanters, SIJ region and pubic tubercles with the patient standing and lying on the side with hip flexed (when include posterior superior iliac spines too).
- Include joints above and below (lumbar spine, SIJ, knee) and try to reproduce the hip pain through palpation and manipulation.
- Also, examine groin nodes and masses and abdomen.

### Leg length discrepancy

Slight differences are normal and not associated with hip or knee restriction.

- Broadly, leg length discrepancy can be ascertained by assessment of pelvic tilt and knee crease symmetry when standing.
- Evaluation is then done with the patient lying prone measuring from anterior superior iliac spine to the medial malleolus and umbilicus to the medial malleolus. The latter may need to account for pelvic tilt, muscle contracture or spasm.
- Unless leg length discrepancy is idiopathic, the shorter leg is usually the abnormal one and usually due to either shortening of soft tissues, growth plate trauma, Perthes disease, SUFE, tumours, or infection and secondary degenerative changes.
- Radiographic evaluation assesses skeletal, joint and epiphyseal causes of leg length discrepancy.

### Specific examination tests

Some tests in children and adolescents are similar to those in adults though should be considered a guide to further tests/investigations as none are highly specific for pathology (Table 3.21).

**Table 3.21** Special tests: pelvis/hips in children and adolescents

| Test | Manoeuvre | Interpretation |
|------|-----------|----------------|
| Trendelenburg (patient standing) | Standing on one leg or the other. | The non-weight-bearing side of the pelvis drops with adjacent hip abductor or pelvic stabilizer deficiency (due to pain inhibition or true weakness) |
| Thomas test (patient supine) | Lift and flex one leg at the hip | As pelvis tilts the contralateral hip flexes: from a tight psoas, loss of hip joint extension or hip joint flexion contracture |
| Ober test (patient lying on side) | With the affected leg uppermost, the leg is abducted and knee flexed to 90°. Holding the hip joint in neutral with slight extension and external rotation, the leg is released | Failure of the knee to adduct (fall) is a positive test indicating contraction or tightness of the iliotibial band |
| Faber/Patrick test (patient supine) | At the hip bring one leg passively into flexion, abduction and external rotation with the foot resting on opposite knee. Press down gently but firmly on the flexed knee and the contralateral anterior superior iliac crest | Groin pain on the flexed hip side may indicate intraarticular hip pathology but also contralateral buttock pain may indicate an SI lesion on that side. |

# Knee pain in adults

## Anatomy of the knee

- The knee extends, flexes, and rotates.
- The main extensor quadriceps consists of four muscle segments—rectus femoris, vastus lateralis, medialis, and intermedius, which converge to form a tendon containing the patella that then inserts into the tibia. Rectus femoris arises from the pelvis and vastus muscles from the upper femur.
- The hamstring muscles (biceps femoris, semitendinosus, semi-membranosus) all arise from the ischial tuberosity and flex the knee. The biceps femoris inserts around the fibular head. The other two muscles insert into the tibia on the medial side and can externally rotate the femur.
- In the knee, the femoral condyles articulate within semicircular fibrocartilage menisci on the tibial condyles (Fig. 3.14). Only the peripheral 10–30% of the menisci is vascular and innervated and can potentially repair itself.
- As the knee approaches full extension, the femur internally rotates on the tibia (biceps femoris action) tightening each pair of ligaments relative to each other. This configuration confers maximum stability.
- As flexion is initiated, a small amount of femoral external rotation on the tibia occurs. This 'unlocking' is done by the popliteus—a muscle that arises from the posterior surface of the tibia below. It passes up obliquely across the back of the knee and inserts, via a cord-like tendon, into the lateral femoral condyle. The tendon partly lies within the knee joint capsule.
- Grooves on the femoral condyle articular surfaces allow tight congruity with the anterior horns of the menisci when the knee is extended. If full extension—and this optimal articulation configuration—is lost, then articular cartilage degeneration invariably follows. This is particularly important in inflammatory arthritis.
- The cruciate ligaments are the principal joint stabilizers. The anterior cruciate attaches above to the inside of the lateral femoral condyle and below to the tibia in front of the tibial spines though a slip attaches to the anterior horn of the lateral meniscus. Its main role is to control and contain the amount of knee rotation when the joint is flexed.
- The posterior cruciate attaches above to the inside of the medial femoral condyle. At the other end, it attaches in a (posterior) groove between tibial condyles. Its main role is to stabilize the joint by preventing forward displacement of the femur relative to the tibia when the knee is flexed.
- The cruciates are extra-articular and are covered by a layer of vascular synovium. Bleeding usually accompanies disruption.
- The tibial or medial collateral ligament (MCL) has superficial and deep layers (Fig. 3.15). It stabilizes the knee against valgus stresses, mostly during flexion.
- The superficial MCL overlies, and moves relative to, the deep part and is separated from it by a bursa. The lower part of the superficial MCL is covered by the long adductors, gracilis, semitendinosus, and sartorius muscles, as they merge into the pes anserinus before inserting into the tibia.

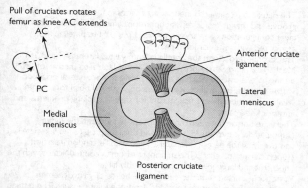

Pull of cruciates rotates femur as knee AC extends

AC

PC

Anterior cruciate ligament

Lateral meniscus

Medial meniscus

Posterior cruciate ligament

**Fig. 3.14** Axial section of the right knee joint (looking down on the tibial plateau, where the foot is fixed on the floor). The femoral condyles articulate within the menisci. As the knee extends the cruciate ligaments tighten and pull the femoral condyles acting to internally rotate the femur through the last few degrees of extension. The knee therefore 'locks' and is stable when the leg is straight.

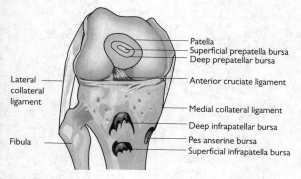

Patella
Superficial prepatella bursa
Deep prepatellar bursa

Anterior cruciate ligament

Lateral collateral ligament

Medial collateral ligament

Deep infrapatellar bursa

Pes anserine bursa

Superficial infrapatella bursa

Fibula

**Fig. 3.15** Anterior knee structures.

- The MCL and pes anserinus are separated by the anserine bursa. Deeper MCL fibres attach to, and stabilize, the medial meniscus.
- The fibular or lateral collateral ligament (LCL) joins the lateral femoral condyle to the fibular head and is separated from it by a bursa. It stabilizes the knee on its lateral side. It has no meniscal attachment. A small bursa separates it from the overlapping tendon insertion of biceps femoris.

- The patella is a seamed bone that articulates in the femoral condylar groove and makes quadriceps action more efficient. Patella articular facet configuration can vary; congenital bi/tripartite patellae are associated with anterior knee pain.
- The strongest force on the patella is from vastus lateralis (Fig. 3.16). Mechanical factors that increase the ratio of lateral to medial forces during patella tracking such as a wide pelvis, a more lateral origin of vastus lateralis, femoral neck anteversion, external tibial torsion, and a weak vastus medialis are risk factors for patella tracking problems and anterior knee pain.
- There are bursae between the quadriceps tendon and the femur (suprapatellar), the patellar tendon and tibial tubercle (deep infrapatellar), and overlying the patella (prepatellar) and patellar tendon insertion (superficial infrapatellar). The suprapatellar bursa communicates with the knee joint and large joint effusions invariably fill it.
- Posteriorly, bursae separate each of the heads of gastrocnemius (which arise from femoral condyles) from the joint capsule. The bursae communicate with the knee joint and can fill from joint effusions.

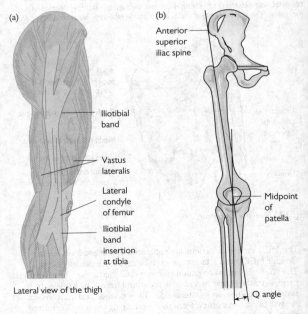

(a)

Iliotibial band

Vastus lateralis

Lateral condyle of femur

Iliotibial band insertion at tibia

Lateral view of the thigh

(b)

Anterior superior iliac spine

Midpoint of patella

Q angle

**Fig. 3.16** (a) The iliotibial band. (b) The patella Q angle (normal values—men 10°, women 15°).

## Taking a history of knee pain: adults

### Ask about the site of pain

Try to establish whether pain is from articular, soft tissue, or anterior knee structures. Is it referred pain?

- Bursa, tendon, and most ligament lesions cause well-localized pain.
- Localized tibiofemoral joint line pain suggests meniscal pathology.
- Localized medial knee pain has a number of possible causes: MCL tear or chronic inflammation (calcification of MCL origin termed the Pellegrini–Stieda phenomenon), medial meniscus tear, meniscal cyst, anserine tendonitis, bursitis, or enthesitis (semimembranosus insertion).
- Enthesitis of structures at their insertion to the patella margins can result in considerable pain.
- Overuse in runners and cyclists can cause localized inflammation and pain of the iliotibial band (ITB) or its underlying bursa over the lateral femoral condyle (as the band moves across the bone as the knee flexes).
- Anterior pain in adults invariably suggests an underlying mechanical abnormality. In older adults, the most common cause is patellofemoral OA (Table 3.22).
- Anterior knee pain may be referred from the hip or L3 nerve root. Hip pain is an aching pain; nerve root pain is sharp often with paraesthesia.
- Posterior knee pain associated with 'a lump' is often due to synovitis in the posterior knee compartment with popliteal cyst formation (Baker's cyst).

**Table 3.22** Causes of anterior knee pain in adults

| Common (non-inflammatory) | Patellofemoral OA (look for mechanical factors and generalized OA) |
|---|---|
| | Referred hip pain, e.g. hip OA |
| | Referred pain from lumbar spine, lateral pelvis, ITB, or greater trochanter lesions |
| | Tear/cyst of anterior meniscal horn |
| | Patellar ligament fat-pad syndrome |
| Common (inflammatory) | Patella ligament enthesitis (enteropathic SpA, PsA, or axSpA) |
| | Crystal-induced MSK inflammation |
| | Synovitis of anterior joint compartment (e.g. RA, PsA) |
| Uncommon (non-inflammatory) | Osteochondritis at patellar lower pole—overuse injury in jumping sports* |
| | Patellar fracture |
| | Enthesopathy at patellar margins (may be part of DISH) |
| Uncommon (inflammatory) | Bursitis (prepatellar, superficial/deep infrapatellar) |
| | Sepsis of joint or anterior joint structures |

* Sinding–Larsen–Johansson disease.

*Ask about injury*

Knee injuries are common; the most significant is anterior cruciate injury. Ask about injury and if the knee feels unstable or 'gives way':

- Anterior cruciate injuries are invariably associated with a haemarthrosis, thus a painful effusion will have occurred immediately. Meniscus tears can cause immediate pain, but synovitis and swelling are delayed for about 6 hours.
- Patients may volunteer that the knee 'keeps giving out on me'. This feeling may be the pivot shift phenomenon caused by reduced anterior cruciate stability against a valgus stress as the knee is flexing.
- Anterior cruciate and MCL injuries often coexist (since they are attached). Ask about medial knee pain originally and subsequently.

*Ask about knee locking*

Knee locking is a mechanical effect of disruption of normal articulation by 'loose bodies':

- Suspect meniscus damage in the middle aged or if the patient plays sports. A meniscus tear is the most common cause of the knee locking. In adolescents, locking may be due to a tear in a discoid meniscus (>98% lateral). Morphologically abnormal discs are prone to degeneration.
- Synovial chondromatosis is a rare cause.
- Some patients with anterior knee pain describe the knee locking or giving way. This is due to reflex quadriceps inhibition rather than true instability.

*Ask about the initial onset of pain*

- Acute pain is usual with injuries of cruciates and vertical meniscal tears.
- Acute onset pain without trauma (but always with swelling) suggests infection, crystal arthritis, or spontaneous haemarthrosis.
- In the very elderly, traumatic lesions may be missed, since the presentation is not always striking, e.g. intra-articular fracture with haemarthrosis.
- An insidious onset of pain is usual in cleavage tears of menisci (horizontal tears), which occur typically in adults where the disc is degenerate, in adolescents with discoid menisci, and in early osteochondritis dissecans.

*Ask about the pattern and type of pain*

- Pain from synovitis is often associated with stiffness and is often worse after a period of immobility. Almost without exception knee synovitis can occur in all forms of arthritis.
- Pain from subchondral damage (e.g. OA) is almost always worse on weight-bearing, but this association is not specific.
- Pain on kneeling/squatting is characteristic of anterior knee pain.
- Burning pain may be neurogenic, e.g. L3 nerve root or osteodystrophy pain or if focal may be enthesitic.

*Past medical, family, occupational, and leisure history*

- Knee synovitis and patellar enthesitis occur in all forms of SpA. Ask about previous uveitis, low back pain, urethral discharge, sexually transmitted disease, IBD-type symptoms, and psoriasis.

- Gout (see ➲ Chapter 7) is not uncommon around the knee. Ask about gout risk factors and whether the patient has ever had acute first MTPJ pain.
- There may be a family history of OA, an hereditary disease of connective tissue, or hypermobility in young adults with OA.
- Prepatellar bursitis classically occurred in housemaids, hence the nickname 'housemaid's knee'. Friction caused by repeated kneeling can cause it.
- Sports injuries are common. Anterior cruciate injury occurs characteristically in skiing. Meniscal injuries are common in soccer. Jumping events (e.g. high jump, basketball) can lead to patellar tendon apophysitis. Cycling is associated with anterior knee pain. MCL and meniscal injuries are common in skiing and weight-bearing activities where rotation and change of direction are frequent. Cycling and running are associated with ITB/bursa pain and inflammation.

## Examination of an adult with knee pain

### From front and behind, observe the patient standing

- Look for mechanical abnormalities that might be associated with knee lesions: patella asymmetry, prominent tibial tubercles from previous Osgood–Schlatter disease (anterior knee pain), flat feet, and hypermobility (patella dislocation, hyperextension of >10°).
- Check for mechanical abnormalities which might suggest specific pathology: genu varum (bowed leg, typical appearance with primarily medial compartment OA), obvious suprapatellar knee swelling (synovitis), psoriasis (associated synovitis or enthesitis), and genu valgum (knock-kneed).

### Examination of the sitting patient

Ask the patient to sit on the examination table with legs hanging, knees bent. Patellar tracking and pain from medial meniscus damage can be assessed. An alternative approach is with the patient supine. Observe any muscle wasting. Palpate anterior, medial, and lateral structures.

- In patients with anterior knee pain, look for symmetric patellar alignment.
- Observe active knee extension. Patellar movement should be smooth, pain free, and symmetric.
- Passively externally rotate each lower leg to its extreme. This is a reasonably sensitive test for conditions of the medial knee compartment (e.g. meniscus tear) and medial knee structures. Discomfort will be felt. If the MCL is totally deficient, an abnormally increased range of external rotation may occur.
- Quadriceps wasting (accentuated depression in muscle just above the patella) occurs with disuse after injuries and chronic arthritis.
- Sites of bursae, patellar tendon, and ligament insertions should be palpated in patients with localized pain (Fig. 3.17).
- Tibiofemoral joint line tenderness is likely to be due to either meniscus pathology or marginal osteophytes. Osteophytes give bony swelling.

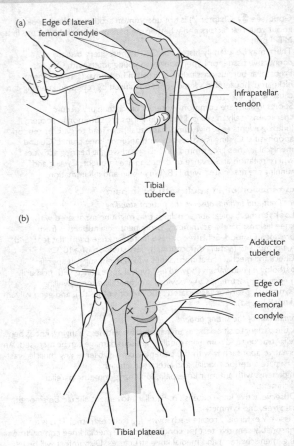

**Fig. 3.17** Position of the knee for palpation of most of its structures. Palpating for enthesitis at the patellar tendon insertion. (a) Palpation over the insertion of semimembranosus and pes anserinus under the tibial plateau (b) The site of the majority of osteochondritis lesions in the knee is shown by the 'X'.

- Anterior pain from patellofemoral joint disorders may be elicited by gentle pressure down on the patella. Mobilizing the patella sideways will give an impression of tissue laxity (possible underlying hypermobility).
- Factors that predispose to patellofemoral pain syndrome include: high or lateral patella, weak vastus medialis, excessive pronation, weak ankle dorsiflexors, tight hamstrings, reduced movement at the ankle, and a wide

Q-angle. The Q-angle is formed between a line from the anterior superior iliac spine to the centre of the patella, and a line extended upwards from the tibial tubercle through the centre of the patella. The larger the angle the greater the lateral tensile pull on the patella (Fig. 3.17).

- Localized tenderness of the femoral condyle is often the only sign of osteochondritis dissecans in adolescents. The most common site is on the inside of the medial femoral condyle (75%).

*Examine for joint synovitis (synovial inflammation giving synovial thickening and/or tenderness) and an effusion*

- The joint may be warm. Chronic synovitis doesn't always result in a warm joint, but infection, acute crystal arthritis, and haemarthrosis usually do.
- Gross synovitis can produce obvious effusions and/or synovial thickening most easily felt around the patellar edges.
- Effusions may be confirmed by the patellar tap test (see ➜ Plate 18).
- Small effusions can be detected by eliciting the 'bulge sign'. Fluid in the medial compartment is swept firmly upward and laterally into the suprapatellar pouch. Firm pressure on the lateral side of the joint may then push fluid back into the medial compartment, producing a bulge.
- Thickened synovium can be detected by experienced examiners in the absence of a detectable effusion. It is not always tender.
- Posterior compartment synovial thickening and popliteal cysts can be felt by wrapping the fingers around under the knee when it is slightly flexed.
- In contrast to adults, popliteal cysts in children are not usually associated with intra-articular pathology. Investigation is not always necessary.

*Test the knee for stability*

There are many tests for instability: instability may be straight or rotational and can be graded according to consensus criteria (consult orthopaedics texts).

- The Lachmann test (Fig. 3.18) is arguably the most sensitive test for eliciting anterior cruciate disruption: hold the knee flexed between 20–30°, grasped above and below the joint. Attempt to move the tibia forwards and backwards on the femur. Ask about pain and feel for laxity or a 'clunk'.
- The anterior draw test is not as sensitive as the Lachmann test for detecting partial anterior cruciate tears, but is easier to do. The patient lies flat, hip flexed, the knee flexed at 90°, with the foot flat on the table. Fix the foot by gently sitting on it and pull the top of the lower leg forwards in the line of the thigh. Ask about pain and feel for laxity.
- The posterior draw test identifies posterior cruciate disruption: with the knee flexed to 90°, press the top of the lower leg backwards in the line of the thigh, ask about pain and feel for laxity.
- Test medial stability at 0° and 30° of flexion (MCL stabilizes maximally at 30°) by holding the upper leg still and applying a valgus force to the tibia. Laxity associated with widening of the tibiofemoral joint (with or without pain) is a positive test and suggests MCL deficiency.
- Lateral (LCL and ITB) stability is similarly tested, though using a varus force on the lower leg.
- MCL tears can accompany anterior cruciate injuries and deep lesions are associated with simultaneous tears of the medial meniscus. Such complex pathology can make specific examination manoeuvers difficult to interpret.

**Anterior draw test**

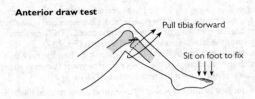

Pull tibia forward

Sit on foot to fix

**Lachmann test**

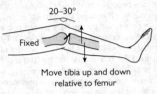

20–30°

Fixed

Move tibia up and down
relative to femur

**Fig. 3.18** Dynamic tests of anterior cruciate function. Patients should be relaxed lying supine on a couch. Excessive laxity is the most important sign.

*Test for meniscus damage*
- *McMurray test* (Fig. 3.19). Flex the knee, internally rotate the lower leg, then extend the joint. Repeat with the lower leg externally rotated. The fingers (over the joint line) may feel a 'clunk' as a femoral condyle passes over a torn meniscus. It is often positive (21–65% of cases) when surgery subsequently reveals no tear.
- Ask the patient to turn over. When prone, look and palpate for swelling in the popliteal fossa and proximal calf that may indicate a low lying popliteal cyst.
- Inflammation of the bursa underlying the ITB may result in tenderness over the lateral femoral condyle. The ITB may be tight. This is demonstrated using the *Ober test*. With the patient lying on their side and affected leg uppermost, the leg is abducted and knee flexed to 90°. Holding the hip joint in neutral with slight extension and external rotation, the leg is released. Failure of the knee to adduct/fall is a positive test—leg length inequality and foot over-pronation may be causative factors.
- Detecting specific structures in the posterior fossa is often difficult because of the lack of bony landmarks and overlapping soft tissue structures. Synovial cysts may form under pressure and are often hard and tender. Diffuse thickening suggests joint synovitis.

**McMurray test**

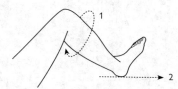

**Action:** Hold the knee and the heel.
Internally rotate the lower leg (1) then extend it (2)
**Positive test:** (Palpable) clunk at joint line

Fig. 3.19 Dynamic test designed to elicit signs of meniscus damage. 'Clunks', intra-articular pain, and coarse crepitus may indicate damage. The test is not specific and is open to misinterpretation.

*Relevant proximal MSK examination*

As always examine the immediate proximal structures at the end of the examination sequence—here examine the hip and gait.

- Gait examination—consider the lower limb as functionally inter-related from lower spine to toes.
- Hip examination can help determine ante/retroversion at the hip—and the configuration of such can have a bearing on lower leg pronation, in-toeing and pains at both knee and feet (see Fig. 3.20).

## Investigations of adults with knee pain

*Radiographs*

AP and lateral weight-bearing radiographs are suitable screening views if the diagnosis is unclear after clinical assessment:

- Early synovitis may only be evident from the presence of an effusion, periarticular osteopenia, or soft tissue swelling. Patterns of bone damage in chronic arthropathies may be recognized.
- Signs of joint infection, which may not necessarily present acutely, are patchy bone osteolysis and irregular loss of bone cortex.
- Osteonecrosis is uncommon in the knee although it is seen in femoral condylar bone, often without symptoms, in sickle cell anaemia.
- Loss of joint space, angulation deformity, osteophytes, subchondral bone sclerosis, and bone cysts are hallmark features of OA.
- Linear or vague intra-articular calcification suggests chondrocalcinosis (associated with calcium pyrophosphate dihydrate (CPPD) arthritis).
- Gross 'thumbprint' calcification is typical of synovial chondromatosis.

*Specialized radiographic views: tomographic views; 'skyline' (axial with knee bent) view; or lateral view taken with at least 30° of flexion*

- Tomography is useful for clarifying non-peripheral osteochondral defects.
- Skyline views demonstrate anomalous patellar facet configuration and can reveal patellofemoral incongruity though multiple views may be needed. Subchondral patellar pathology is seen more clearly than on lateral views.
- Patella alta is most reliably seen on a lateral view with 30° flexion.

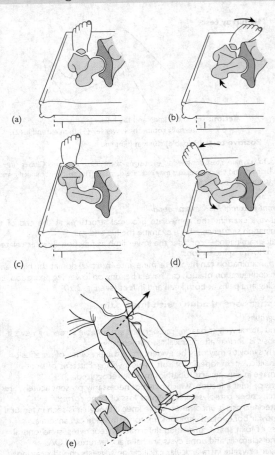

**Fig. 3.20** Femoral anteversion, retroversion, and tibial torsion. (a) Where the femoral neck angulates excessively forward relative to an imaginary axis through the femoral condyles, the hip is anteverted. (b) Femoral neck anteversion can lead to a greater than usual range of hip internal rotation and a toe-in gait. (c) and (d) Retroversion, where the femoral neck angulates posteriorly relative to a femoral condyle axis, can cause a toe-out gait. (e) In-toeing can also be caused by excessive medial tibial torsion. Normally the ankle mortise faces 15° externally relative to a sagittal plane axis through the tibial tubercle (arrow) but in medial torsion it faces forward or internally.

*Further imaging*

Further imaging depends on differential diagnosis and a discussion with your radiologist:

- Periarticular soft tissue lesions can be characterized with MRI, although with superficial lesions adequate information needed for further management may be obtainable with US alone.
- Patterns of meniscus damage are recognized on MRI, give an indication of prognosis, and aid the surgeon's decision to proceed to arthroscopy.
- MRI is essential if there is likely to be a combination of lesions, e.g. anterior cruciate, MCL, and medial meniscus lesions.
- In anterior knee compartment symptoms alone, US is a reasonable first option for imaging because inflammatory lesions can be injected with glucocorticoid if needed using imaging guidance.
- MRI is more sensitive than radiographs or US at identifying joint erosions in RA ('pre-erosions').
- The place of CT or MRI in investigating radiographically detected bone tumours depends on the nature of the lesion.

*Aspiration of joint and periarticular fluid collections*

- Early aspiration is essential if infection is suspected (see ➔ Plate 19).
- The knee is a common site of monoarthritis forms of systemic diseases (e.g. PsA, CPPD disease).
- Send joint fluid for cell count, polarized light microscopy, and culture.
- In adults, the usual differential diagnosis of sepsis of knee structures is gout, so fluid should be examined by polarized light microscopy for urate crystals.
- Blood-stained fluid either suggests a traumatic tap or chondrocalcinosis. Frank blood suggests haemarthrosis, the major causes of which are cruciate tear, bleeding diathesis, intra-articular fracture, and PVNS.
- Bursa fluid may be more successfully detected and aspirated using US guidance.

*Laboratory investigations*

These should be directed towards suspected underlying disease:

- FBC, acute-phase measures (ESR, CRP).
- Blood urea, electrolytes, creatinine, and urate.
- Blood calcium, phosphate, albumin, alkaline phosphatase, 25-OH vitamin D, and PTH to screen for metabolic bone disease.
- Autoantibodies: rheumatoid factor (RF), ACPA, antinuclear (ANA), and extractable nuclear antibodies (ENAs) to characterize an autoimmune process where synovitis is chronic.
- Serum angiotensin converting enzyme (ACE) for sarcoidosis.
- IgM *Borrelia burgdorferi* serology for acute arthropathy in Lyme disease, streptococcal antibodies for reactive streptococcal arthritis and parvovirus serology.

## Treatment of adults with knee pain conditions

- In general, most soft tissue lesions will settle with rest and NSAIDs.
- Anterior knee pain may respond well to isometric exercises, adjustments to foot alignment, e.g. with sensible shoes, orthotics (support insoles), and hamstring stretching exercises.

- The acute swollen knee requires aspiration, rest for 24 hours and gentle mobilization.
- If infection is considered, broad-spectrum antibiotics against staphylococcal and streptococcal agents should be started immediately while awaiting culture data. In infection, intra-articular antibiotics and steroids should be avoided. The patient should not bear weight on an acutely infected joint (see ➔ Chapter 17).
- Acute and chronic inflammation can lead to joint destruction and instability this is relevant for RA—early treatment may prevent long-term morbidity.
- Physical therapy and splinting play an important role in maintaining function and preventing contractures, etc.

### Address biomechanical factors

Input from a physical therapist may be helpful in cases of anterior knee pain. Success from McConnell (patellar) taping is more likely in non- patellofemoral OA-related anterior knee pain.

- Quadriceps strengthening exercises can be reviewed and reinforced by physical therapists in cases of knee OA.
- Knee pain, particularly anterior pain, may be linked to foot abnormalities (e.g. over-pronation), and hip alignment (Q-angle, above).
- Specific muscle strengthening exercises, foot orthotics, and knee braces should be considered.

### Local steroid injection

➔ Chapter 24 has more detail on local steroid injections.

Local steroid injections can be helpful in the following situations:
- Acute flare of non-infective inflammatory disease:
  - OA (especially when in inflammatory phase)—mild OA may also respond to hyaluronan injections.
  - autoimmune arthritis, e.g. RA.
  - intra-articular gout or CPPD/pseudogout.
  - SpA or more likely PsA effusion/monoarthritis.
- Bursitis (may be gout):
  - pre- and infrapatella (superficial and deep) bursa (the latter may require US guidance).
  - anserine.
- Baker's cyst (note: the knee joint is injected at the site of the pathology assuming there is intra-articular communication between joint and cyst. Direct popliteal cyst injection should be under US guidance only to avoid damage to vascular and nerve tissues).
- Enthesitis, e.g. semimembranosus insertion.
- Trauma, e.g. pain over MCL insertion.
- Other soft tissue: ITB syndrome.
- In patients with large joint effusions, merely aspirating the effusion may provide some level of symptomatic relief—this procedure may need to be done alone initially without steroid injection pending results from fluid microscopy and culture.

- Knee OA may respond transiently to an injectable steroid, such as methylprednisolone. Saline irrigation and injections with hyaluronan preparations are also used, but response is variable.
- Note: all intra-articular injection therapies are more effective when patient's knee is immobilized for 24 hours following the procedure.

*Drugs*
- NSAIDs will invariably be helpful in cases of inflammatory and septic arthritis.
- Colchicine 0.5 mg two to three times daily for 5 days is often useful in relieving pain from crystal arthritis in patients intolerant of NSAIDs.
- Paracetamol/acetaminophen may be as effective as NSAIDs for some patients.
- The effect of glucosamine and chondroitin for OA is debated. Although some studies demonstrate improved pain control and function, other studies indicate that these are no better than placebo.

*Surgery*
- Arthroscopy is often used as a diagnostic tool in cases of undiagnosed monoarthritis and to confirm and trim cartilage tears. Synovium and synovial lesions (e.g. PVNS, synovial chondromatosis) can be biopsied or excised (synovectomy) and the joint can be irrigated.
- In appropriate cases, joint replacement can be remarkably successful and is an important option to consider in OA and inflammatory arthritis, where pain is severe and present at rest, and when mobility is substantially restricted.
- Unicondylar osteotomy can aid realignment of the tibiofemoral joint, e.g. in metabolic bone disease, such as Paget's disease.

*Other*
- In OA, capsaicin cream applied three or four times daily to painful superficial structures, e.g. patellar margins or marginal tibiofemoral joint pain, can ease symptoms. Response is cumulative and may not occur for 6–8 weeks.
- Yttrium-90 radiation synovectomy has a long history of use for isolated knee synovitis occurring as a result of a number of conditions. Y-90 injection can be arranged to follow arthroscopic synovectomy aiming to maximize the effect of both procedures.
- Topical lidocaine patches may also be useful for control of pain limited to one joint.

# Knee pain and lower limb development in children and adolescents

## General considerations

In younger children, especially, knee, foot, and ankle problems need assessment in light of developmental stage and with reference to any developmental abnormalities.

### History

- Growing pains are common and occur typically in children <6 years. There is a nighttime predominance, hence the term 'benign nocturnal pain of childhood'. Knee is often identified as a key site but also thigh, shins, and feet.
- Osteochondroses of knee structures are common in the growing skeleton (see Table 16.11).
- Osteochondritis can affect the articular cartilage (e.g. medial/proximal tibia (Blount's)) or an enthesis or an epiphyseal plate.
- The osteochondritis lesion becomes more severe if the cartilage becomes separated as a fragment ('dissecans' lesion).
- Cause of osteochondritis at an enthesis is assumed to be traction-trauma in aetiology though the number of children with these lesions, who might have ERA, PsA, or JSpA is not known.
- Anterior knee pain at all ages is relatively common (the term 'chondromalacia patella' is a surgical finding which may or may not be associated with pain).
- The commonest cause of anterior knee pain in adolescents—termed patellofemoral syndrome (PFS)—is attributable to abnormal loading of the patellofemoral joint and patella mal-tracking. There is often underlying biomechanical imbalance including muscle tightness and vastus medialis obliqus (VMO) weakness.
- Anterior knee pain can be secondary to patella instability. This is a variable lesion which ranges from mild dynamic imbalance with lateral patellar compression to recurrent patella dislocation and chronic dislocation.
- Other causes of anterior knee pain in active children includes patella ligament origin or insertional enthesitis (in ERA, JSpA or JPsA), local bursitis or fat pad syndrome.
- Impingement of the infrapatellar fat pad—which is richly innervated—between patella and femoral condyle is amplified by mal-tracking of the patella, knee extension, prolonged standing and kneeling.
- The knee is a common presenting site for inflammatory disease particularly in IBD-related arthritis and JPsA.
- A swollen knee can be a presenting sign of JIA, PVNS, tuberculous/septic arthritis, and haemarthrosis (trauma).
- Pain is the main presenting features of tumours, which can occur around the knee (e.g. osteoid osteoma, chondroblastoma, Ewing sarcoma, leukaemia, neuroblastoma).

- Mechanical symptoms on movement (catching, knee giving way, painful clunks, etc.) may occur with patellofemoral instability or with an internal structural lesion—such as cruciate ligament deficiency or synovial plica.
- Synovial plicae are embryonic remnants, with a septated structure, which become tender and inflamed when trapped between patella and medial femoral condyle. Snapping and catching *during flexion* differentiate it from other biomechanical lesions.
- Finally ask about hip/groin pains given referred pain from the hip joint may be present and can denote Perthes disease or SUFE.

*Examination*

A general overview of relative MSK stiffness, hypermobility, functional movement ability, and muscle tone is helpful before a regional examination takes place.

- Functional biomechanics are assessed by evaluation of gait, and manoeuvres such as jumping, hopping, and squatting. This is followed by assessment of muscle group strength and stretch.
- Assess for the 'J' sign of patellar tracking. This is medial shift of the patella in early flexion as it enters the trochlea, suggestive of VMO weakness or tight lateral patella retinaculum.
- Fixed loss of extension or loss of full flexion is indicative of intraarticular pathology.
- A joint effusion is shown by sweep (or bulge) sign (see earlier).
- Other tests include patellar compression (Clarke test), Lachman test; anterior and posterior draw tests; McMurray and Trendelenburg tests— see ➲ 'Knee pain in adults', pp. 170–83.

# Lower limb developmental factors and variations

*Developmental factors*

- Developmental characteristics often imply that different age groups are prone to a different spectrum of conditions.
- Due to ligamentous laxity, when babies begin to walk, the midfoot is flat to the floor. A longitudinal arch usually develops by 5 years.
- During growth, tendon insertions (apophyses) are often weaker than the tendons themselves. Traction strain on tendons can lead to apophysitis (osteochondritis). This is a common pattern of injury in the foot in active older children.

*Femoral anteversion*

- This causes internal femoral torsion leading to a medially rotated patella and in-toeing.
- See Fig. 3.20.
- Femoral anteversion is present at birth in 40% but decreases with age and disappears by 10 years of age.
- Mild persistence with in-toeing does not usually result in functional disability.
- It may persist with patterns of sitting such as the 'W' position. Sitting crossed legged may encourage external rotation at the hips instead.

*Internal tibial torsion*
- This results in in-toeing and is normal in toddlers, resolving at 2–4 years.
- See Fig. 3.20.
- Thigh-foot axis angle of more than about −10° confirms the diagnosis, although treatment is only considered when greater than −45°.
- By contrast, external tibial torsion is a common cause of an out-toe gait and may lead to PFS.
- Osteotomy may be recommended for a thigh-foot axis angle of more than +40°.

*Genu varum (bow legs)*
- Bow legs are normal in toddlers and normal beyond 4 years if mild and symmetrical.
- Bow legs appear more pronounced in an overweight child and associated in-toeing may give appearance of a clumsy gait, but does not require intervention.
- Asymmetric or exaggerated bowing and reports of pain requires a full MSK assessment including metrology (of intercondylar distance and lateral thrust at the knee) and gait assessment.
- Radiographs may disclose Blount's disease (osteochondritis of the medial aspect of the proximal tibial physis).
- Bowing can occur in rickets (check vitamin D levels).
- A full leg AP radiograph assesses hip, knee, and ankle contribution and measures joint-to-diaphysis angles to identify which physis is contributing to the deformity.
- MRI, CT, and DXA are rarely useful.

*Genu valgum (knock knees)*
- Knock knees is physiological between 2 and 6 years of age and does not progress after 7 years. Intervention with braces or orthoses is unwarranted and meddlesome.
- Adolescent idiopathic genu valgum may be associated with circumducted gait, anterior knee pain and patellofemoral instability. Often hereditary, it may progress into adulthood to premature OA of the patellofemoral joint and lateral compartment of the knee.
- An angle of 12° of valgus or intermalleolar distance of >8 cm should prompt orthopaedic assessment for adolescent genu valgum.
- Other causes of genu valgum include local pathology from trauma or infection (usually unilateral), skeletal dysplasias, neurofibromatosis and vitamin D-resistant rickets.
- Genu valgum is best assessed using a full-length standing AP radiograph. The mechanical axis or centre of gravity (drawn from the centre of the femoral head to the centre of the ankle) should bisect the knee and lie within the intercondylar central area of the knee.

# Lower leg and foot disorders in adults

## Anatomy

*Anatomy of bones and joints*

- The leg absorbs six times the body weight during weight-bearing. Strong ligaments secure the ankle (formed by tibia above/medially and fibular malleolus laterally) and talocalcaneal (subtalar) joints and bones of the midfoot (Fig. 3.21).
- Anomalous ossicles in the foot are common. Some are associated with specific pathology. There are many potential sites, though the sesamoids in flexor hallucis brevis (FHB) are invariable.
- The foot is an optimal mechanical device to support body weight when walking or running over flat, inclined and uneven types of terrain. The configuration of bones at synovial articulations allows dorsal flexion (foot pulled up), plantar flexion (to walk on toes), inversion (foot tips in), eversion (foot tips out) and small degrees of adduction and abduction. Midfoot movements allow pronation and supination.

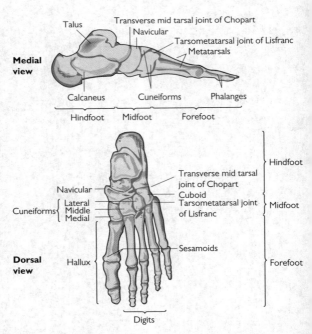

**Fig. 3.21** The bones of the foot.

- The normal ankle joint range is about 25° of dorsal flexion and 50° of plantar flexion from neutral (foot 90° to leg). The range of subtalar inversion–eversion is normally 10–15°.

*Anatomy of the long muscles and tendons*

- In the lower leg, a strong fascia connects the tibia and fibula. Lower leg muscles primarily move the foot. They are separated into compartments by fascia and are prone to pressure effects.
- The foot dorsal flexors—tibialis anterior, extensor digitorum longus (EDL), extensor hallucis longus (EHL), and peroneus tertius—lie adjacent to the anteromedial side of the tibia. Their tendons pass in front of the ankle in synovial sheaths held down by strong retinaculae (Fig. 3.22). The tibialis anterior, the bulkiest flexor, inserts into the medial midfoot (medial cuneiform).
- In the posterior lower leg, the gastrocnemius (and plantaris), which arise from the femur, plantar flexes the foot by pulling the back of the calcaneum. The soleus, which arises in the lower leg, merges with them in the Achilles tendon. This tendon has a deep and superficial bursa at its insertion site.

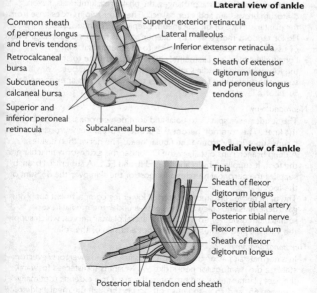

**Lateral view of ankle**

Common sheath of peroneus longus and brevis tendons
Retrocalcaneal bursa
Subcutaneous calcaneal bursa
Superior and inferior peroneal retinacula
Subcalcaneal bursa

Superior exterior retinacula
Lateral malleolus
Inferior extensor retinacula
Sheath of extensor digitorum longus and peroneus longus tendons

**Medial view of ankle**

Tibia
Sheath of flexor digitorum longus
Posterior tibial artery
Posterior tibial nerve
Flexor retinaculum
Sheath of flexor digitorum longus

Posterior tibial tendon end sheath

Fig. 3.22 Tendons, retinaculae, and bursae of the hindfoot.

- Plantar flexion is assisted weakly by long muscles, which arise in the lower leg, pass behind the medial malleolus in synovial sheaths (Fig. 3.22), and insert into the sole. They mostly invert the foot. Tibialis posterior, the bulkiest plantar flexor, inserts into the plantar surface of the navicular.
- The peroneus longus and brevis arise from the fibular side of the leg and pass around the lateral malleolus in a common synovial sheath held by a retinaculum. Longus passes into the sole and inserts into the medial cuneiform. Brevis inserts into the fifth metatarsal base. Both evert the foot.
- The tibial nerve and artery follow the course of the medial tendons under the flexor retinaculum (Fig. 3.22).

*Anatomy of intrinsic foot structure*
- Intrinsic foot structures have been greatly modified during evolution to combine provision of a flexible platform for support and a rigid lever for thrusting body weight forward when walking.
- In the sole of the foot, muscles are aligned longitudinally in four layers. The deepest layers include phalangeal interossei in the forefeet, tibialis posterior, peroneus longus, adductor hallucis, and FHB, which has two insertions into the proximal great toe phalanx, each containing a sesamoid.
- The superficial layers include flexor digitorum longus (FDL), which inserts into the lateral four distal phalanges, the phalangeal lumbricals, flexor digitorum brevis, and abductor hallucis. The latter two muscles arise from the plantar surface of the calcaneum deep to the plantar fascia.
- Flexor tendons merge with the deeper part of the plantar fascia, a swath of tissue that extends from os calcis to the metatarsal area.
- Longitudinal muscles, ligaments, and fascia contribute to stabilize the foot with a longitudinal arch—its apex at the talus, but also with some effect laterally. The foot arches transversely—its apex at medial cuneiform level.

*Neuroanatomy*
- The sciatic nerve splits into tibial and common peroneal nerves above the knee. The common peroneal is prone to pressure neuropathy as it runs superficially around the fibular head. The nerve then divides. A deep branch runs distally with EDL under the extensor retinaculum to the foot. It supplies tibialis anterior, EHL and EDL. A superficial branch supplies the peroneal muscles and most of the skin over the dorsum of the foot.
- The tibial nerve runs in the posterior lower leg compartment supplying gastrocnemius and soleus. It then passes under the medial flexor retinaculum dividing into medial and lateral plantar nerves, which supply the intrinsic plantar muscles of the foot and skin of the sole.

*Functional anatomy*
- In a normal gait pattern, the foot is dorsiflexed and invertors/evertors stabilize the hindfoot for heel strike. As weight is transferred forward, the foot plantar flexes and pronates, the great toe extends (optimally between 65° and 75°), and push off occurs through the medial side of the forefoot.

- All metatarsals bear weight and can suffer weight-bearing injury.
- Ligamentous attachments around the hindfoot are strong. A fall on a pronated inverted foot without direct trauma can result in a fracture of the distal fibula. This is probably a consequence of the relative strength of the talofibular ligaments compared with bone.

### Conditions of the lower leg

- Patients with lower leg conditions present with pain or deformity.
- Pains in the calf may be due to local soft tissue or muscle conditions, and are commonly due to referred lumbosacral pain. These pains are often described by patients as 'cramps'—suggesting a muscle problem at first. A detailed history may suggest nerve root pathology.
- Imbalance of muscles in the foot can lead to increased tension at tendon and fascial insertions in the calf and shin, resulting in 'shin splints'. Shin splints usually present after activity and are relieved by rest. Conditions to consider include:
  - stress fractures of the tibia or fibula.
  - tibialis posterior fasciitis—often with a flat, pronated foot.
  - compartment syndrome (soft tissue and vascular swelling).
  - popliteal artery stenosis.
  - referred nerve pain (spinal claudication).
  - peripheral vascular disease (intermittent claudication).

## Taking a history from an adult with lower leg or foot pain

### Ask about site and quality of pain in the lower leg

- Localized anterior pain occurs in bony lesions of the anterior tibia, e.g. stress fractures, periostitis.
- Burning pain suggests a neurogenic cause. Diffuse burning pain may be caused by peripheral neuropathy, CRPS (see ⊃ Chapter 22), or (rarely) erythromelalgia.
- Most commonly occurring in the elderly, bilateral leg pain with 'heaviness' or 'stiffness' limiting walking distance is typical of spinal stenosis. An alternative would be vascular claudication where often pain is more overt, and critical ischaemia can give night pain eased by hanging the legs over the side of the bed (gravity effects).
- Simultaneous knee problems may be relevant. Escape of synovial fluid from the knee into the soft tissues of the calf can present with acute pain and swelling and be misdiagnosed as a deep vein thrombosis (pseudothrombophlebitis). Often a history of preceding joint effusion can be elicited.

Low-lying synovial cysts connecting with the knee can cause calf pain (with or without swelling). This invariably occurs only with chronic synovitis.

### Establish possible causes of hindfoot pain

(See Table 3.23.)

Establishing the cause of hindfoot pain from the history alone is difficult. There are important clues, mainly from patterns of injury or overuse. Posterior heel pain has a few causes. Often clinically indistinguishable from Achilles tendonitis or retrocalcaneal bursitis, enthesitis is usually associated with axSpA (see ⊃ Chapter 8). An os trigonum may become damaged especially in soccer players and ballerinas (see later in section).

**Table 3.23** Conditions causing localized foot pain in adults

| Site of pain | Common lesions |
|---|---|
| Ankle region | Ankle or talocalcaneal joint: synovitis (e.g. gout), OA. L4/L5 root pain |
| Posterior heel | Achilles tendonitis. Retrocalcaneal bursitis. Achilles enthesitis. Osteonecrosis of os trigonum |
| Medial side of heel | As for ankle region. Calcaneal fracture. Tibialis posterior tendonitis. Plantar fasciitis |
| Lateral side of heel | As for ankle region. Calcaneal fracture. Peroneal tendonitis. Fifth metatarsal base fracture* |
| Underneath heel | Plantar fasciitis. Calcaneal fracture. Infra-calcaneal bursitis. Lateral plantar nerve entrapment |
| Top of foot | Midfoot joint synovitis (e.g. gout), OA. Navicular osteochondritis. Enthesitis. L5 root pain |
| Sole of foot | S1 root pain. Plantar fasciitis. Metatarsal stress fracture. Tibial/plantar nerve entrapment |
| Toes | MTP synovitis (e.g. RA, gout). MTP OA. Morton's metatarsalgia. Bursitis. Enthesitis/dactylitis |

* Robert–Jones fracture from an inversion–pronation injury.

- The origin of plantar heel pain is varied. Mechanical plantar fasciitis is thought to occur more frequently in people who are on their feet for long periods of time, those who are obese, have thin heel fat pads, or poor footwear. Symptoms of arthritis and enthesopathy elsewhere, low back pain (sacroiliitis), eye inflammation (iritis), psoriasis, or previous gut or 'urethral' infection, might suggest SpA.
- Less common causes of plantar heel pain include fracture through a calcaneal spur and lateral plantar nerve entrapment between the fascia of abductor hallucis and quadratus plantae muscles (causing pain/paraesthesias on the lateral side of the sole).
- In the elderly and postmenopausal women, calcaneal stress fractures are a recognized feature of osteoporosis and can present with heel pain.
- Ankle and talocalcaneal synovitis, OA, ankle osteochondritis dissecans, and tendonitis around the hindfoot may be difficult to distinguish from the history alone. Synovitis or an effusion often accompanies OA of these joints.

*Establish possible causes of midfoot and first MTPJ pain*

- Gout (see ➡ Chapter 6), OA (see ➡ Chapter 6), enthesitis, and referred L5 nerve root pain are the most likely diagnoses of midfoot and first MTPJ pain.
- Gout should always be considered a possible cause of painful lesions in the foot in people at risk. Gout is not always intra-articular, intra-bursal or intra-tendon. Local or diffuse soft tissue inflammation is common and often misdiagnosed as cellulitis.

- The first toe and midfoot are common sites for PsA; check radiograph for typical PsA periosteal new bone formation.
- L5 pain is referred to the dorsum and S1 pain to the sole, of the foot.
- In older adults OA of midfoot joints is common. Mild synovitis can occur with it and may be caused by CPPD disease (see ➋ Chapter 7).

### Establish possible causes of forefoot pain

- In those with forefoot pain, typically referred to as metatarsalgia, establish whether the condition is focal or due to arthropathy.
- Pain under the ball of the foot while walking is non-specific but might suggest any MTPJ abnormality, distal metatarsal stress fracture, Freiberg's disease, plantar nerve neuroma, or bursitis.
- Patients with RA often describe pain under the MTPJs and a feeling of 'walking on pebbles' (due to joint swelling and/or subluxation). Synovitis of the MTP joints is a common feature of early RA.
- Acute pain under the forefoot spreading into one or more (adjacent) toes and worse on walking suggests a plantar nerve neuroma (Morton's metatarsalgia) or intermetatarsal bursitis.
- Pain associated with paraesthesias or numbness under the forefoot might be due to S1 root irritation (common) or entrapment of the tibial nerve in the hindfoot (rare). Ask about back pain and other hindfoot problems.
- Non-traumatic toe pain associated with swelling of the entire toe suggests a dactylitis (associated with axSpA). Although many toes may be affected, dactylitis may be unilateral and affect just one toe.
- The development of hallux valgus is associated with tight footwear. The deformity is associated with altered weight-bearing and a second toe (hammer) deformity.
- Big toe pain might be due to hallux rigidus. It is usually due to OA and important to recognize as it may prevent toe dorsiflexion sufficiently to lead to a compromised gait pattern.
- Pain specifically under the hallux may be due to damage to the sesamoids in the flexor hallucis brevis tendon and be misdiagnosed as a joint problem.

### Ask for a description of the pain

- As in the hand, neurogenic pain is common and typical.
- Severe or unremitting pain when at rest suggests intrinsic bone pathology. Consider osteonecrosis, infection, fracture, and tumours, e.g. osteoid osteoma.
- Neurogenic pain may be sharp and well defined (e.g. in acute L5 or S1 root pain), deep, achy, and less well defined (e.g. chronic nerve root symptoms as in spinal or foramenal stenosis), or burning in quality. Paraesthesias and numbness may accompany both.
- If swelling accompanies neurogenic pain, consider a complex regional pain syndrome. There are numerous triggers, e.g. trauma and surgery. Patients may be unwilling to walk and apparent disability may appear profound.

*Weakness*

If true weakness is the major problem rather than pain, the diagnosis is usually between a myopathic process, but more likely is a spinal or peripheral nerve lesion (see ➔ 'Examination', p. 194).

## Examination of an adult with lower leg or foot pain

*Observation*

Observe the lower legs and feet from front and back, while the patient is standing. Note any swelling, deformities, or rashes:

- Lower leg deformities to note: tibia varum (or bow legs) in an older adult may be due to Paget's disease of the tibia. Muscle wasting might suggest disuse atrophy, old polio, or spinal stenosis (bilateral and subtle usually in older adults).
- Oedema or soft tissue swelling may be relevant to an underlying condition causing ankle synovitis. Although it may cause discomfort, oedema from cardiac failure, venous congestion, hypoproteinaemia, or lymphoedema is not painful unless there are ulcers or thrombophlebitis.
- Gout can cause swelling anywhere; gouty tenosynovitis can mimic the appearance of a cellulitis in the region of a joint.
- Calf swelling may be due to vein thrombosis or ruptured popliteal cyst.

Common patterns of foot deformity are: flat feet (pes planus), high-arched feet (pes cavus) with high medial arch, hallux valgus and rigidus, over-riding toes, hammer toes, or claw toes.

- Skin conditions from venous abnormalities are common in the elderly. Other skin lesions which may be relevant include purpura, panniculitis—which is often subtle and over the shins—and pyoderma gangrenosum.

*Ask the patient to walk in bare feet*

Gait patterns should be noted:

- An antalgic ('limp/wince') gait is a non-specific indicator of pain.
- A wide-based gait (>10 cm wider than normal) suggests instability: joint instability, muscle weakness, or neurological lesions may be the cause.
- A foot that slaps down or a high stepping gait suggests tibialis anterior weakness (L4 nerve root or common peroneal nerve lesion).
- Significant weakness of gluteus medius and gluteus maximus in L5 and S1 root lesions, respectively, can result in lurching during gait. In the former, as weight is taken on the affected side, gluteus medius may be weak in controlling the small 2–3 cm lateral displacement in the weight-bearing hip that normally occurs. This can be compensated for if the body centre of gravity is brought over the hip by lurching the upper body over the affected side. With gluteus maximus lesions (S1) extension of the hip, which helps mediate motion through the stance phase prior to toeing-off, may be weak. Thrusting the thorax forward with an arched back (forward lurch) compensates for the weakness and helps to maintain hip extension.
- A flat-footed gait with little or weak toe-off may suggest an S1 root lesion; however, 'flat-foot' (loss of the medial arch) with associated hind foot eversion and heel pain (plantar fasciitis) is extremely common. Often the arch weakness corrects when the patient is asked to walk.

*Examine the lower leg*

With the patient supine on the couch, examine the lower leg:

- After a ruptured popliteal (Baker's) cyst, calf tissues are often diffusely tender and swollen. Calf circumferences can be compared (e.g. 10 cm below tibial tubercle). There may also be mild skin erythema. Findings are not specific. Gout and infection are the main alternatives if there is marked tenderness.
- Check for bruising, swelling, and tenderness around the fibula head in patients with foot drop (possible peroneal nerve palsy). Neurological examination may be done at this point.
- Localized anterior tibial tenderness is often found in patients with stress fractures or with pseudo-fractures.
- Tibial deformity in adults may be associated with diffuse bony tenderness and heat (arteriovenous shunting) in Paget's disease.

*Examine the ankle and hindfoot*

At the ankle and hindfoot, examine for joint and tendon synovitis, palpate specific structures and test passive hindfoot joint mobility:

- Synovitis of hindfoot joints is not always easily detected. With ankle joint synovitis, thickened tissue may be felt anteriorly in the ankle crease (where there may be a 'springy fullness') or laterally around the malleoli.
- Posterior tibial and peroneal tendonitis are associated with soft tissue swelling of the medial and lateral hindfoot, respectively. Synovial thickening from ankle and talocalcaneal joints may also be felt here and synovitis of structures may coexist in RA or SpA. Pain from resisted movement of tendons may not be specific.
- Pathology of medial hindfoot structures may be associated with tibial nerve entrapment resulting in sensory symptoms on the sole of the foot. There may be a positive Tinel's sign.
- Posterior heel pain may be due to Achilles tendonitis, enthesitis and mechanical damage to the tendon, and retrocalcaneal bursitis. Deep tenderness may suggest an os trigonum lesion.
- The loss of passive hindfoot movements is not specific and can be associated with any cause of ankle or subtalar arthritis (20–30° of dorsiflexion and 45–55° of plantar flexion is average for the ankle and a 10–20° inversion–eversion range is average for the subtalar joint). Subtalar joint movement can be difficult to test accurately.
- The pain of plantar fasciitis may be elicited by firm palpation of the medial underside of the calcaneum. A negative test does not rule out pathology, as often the history is more sensitive. Full MSK examination is required to check for features of SpA, such as arthritis/enthesitis elsewhere and sacroiliitis.

*Examine for midfoot lesions*

Identifying specific midfoot lesions is difficult, though bony landmarks and discrete tender areas can be noted:

- Twisting the midfoot may elicit pain but locating the source in the midfoot may be difficult. Common lesions include PsA, OA, gout, and enthesitis or synovitis from SpA or RA respectively.

- Bony tenderness alone without soft tissue swelling does not rule out synovitis of an adjacent joint.
- The midfoot is a typical site for neuroarthropathy in diabetes.
- Bony exostoses that may have formed at sites of pressure are common in the foot (e.g. medial or dorsal aspect of the first MTPJ, base or head of the fifth metatarsal, distal talus, or over the midfoot).
- Both gout and infection result in swelling, skin erythema and local tenderness. Gout of the first MTPJ occurs at any one time in 70% of patients with the condition. It can occur anywhere in the foot.

*Examine the forefoot*

Check for bony or other swelling, digit separation, and examine the sole of the foot. Squeezing the whole forefoot at the line of the MTPJs is a non-specific, but useful screening test for painful forefoot lesions:

- Tender swelling of the whole toe (dactylitis) occurs in SpA, sarcoidosis (see ➲ Chapter 8), and HIV infection. Swelling is soft not bony. Tender bony swelling suggests a bunion and is common on the dorsal aspect of the toes and the first and fifth MTPJs.
- Forefoot splaying and interdigital separation suggests MTP synovitis or interdigital bursitis. MTPJs may be individually tender (simultaneously palpated with thumb below and finger above).
- Tenderness between metatarsal heads is typical in Morton's metatarsalgia. There may be a sensory deficit in the interdigital cleft. The differential diagnosis (in adolescents) may be osteochondritis of the second and third metatarsal head.
- Check for hallux rigidus. Passive hallux dorsiflexion should be >50°. Extending the hallux can reveal an ability to form a medial longitudinal arch in patients with flat feet (Jack's test).
- Discrete bony tenderness without swelling occurs with stress fractures.
- Uneven callus distribution under the forefoot may suggest an abnormally focused area of weight-bearing and an underlying mechanical abnormality.
- Rashes on the sole of the foot are uncommon but important to consider are pompholyx, pustular psoriasis, and keratoderma blennorrhagica ('reactive arthritis', see ➲ Chapter 8).
- Loss of sensation under the forefoot may be due to an S1 root lesion, peripheral neuropathy (e.g. diabetes), mononeuritis (e.g. vasculitis; see ➲ Chapter 15), Sjögren's syndrome (see ➲ Chapter 12), other AICTDs or, rarely, tibial nerve entrapment (examine hindfoot).

*Neurological examination*

Neurological examination of the feet is essential in cases where pain is neurogenic and likely to be referred or nerve root in origin or there is weakness, numbness, or paraesthesias (Table 3.24).

*Relevant proximal MSK examination*

As always examine proximally—here, the knee.

- Gait examination is important—consider the lower limb as functionally inter-related from lower spine to toes.
- Hip examination can help determine ante/retroversion at the hip—and the configuration of such can have a bearing on lower leg pronation, in-toeing and pains at both knee and in feet (see Fig. 3.20).

**Table 3.24** Patterns of common abnormal examination findings (primarily in the feet) in lower lumbar nerve root lesions

| Nerve root | Abnormal finding |
|---|---|
| L4 | Weakness of ankle dorsiflexion (tibialis anterior) |
| | Patient finds walking on their heels difficult (strong ankle dorsiflexon needed)* |
| | Reduced knee reflex (L3 and L4) |
| L5 | Weakness of big toe dorsiflexion (extensor hallucis longus) |
| | Weakness of foot eversion (peroneal muscles, also S1) |
| | Sensory deficit over dorsum of foot |
| | Reduced ankle reflex (L5 and S1) |
| S1 | Weakness of ankle plantar flexion (gastrocnemius and soleus) |
| | Patient finds walking on, or repeatedly rising onto, tiptoe difficult* |
| | Sensory deficit over sole of foot |
| | Reduced ankle reflex |

* Manoeuvres may be affected by pain, making interpretation difficult.

## Investigations of an adult with lower leg or foot pain

### Imaging of the lower leg

- Suspected tibial abnormalities such as stress fractures and pseudofractures in osteomalacia and Paget's disease have characteristic radiological appearances.
- Periosteal changes occur in trauma, psoriatic arthritis (above ankle), HPOA, and pachydermal periostitis.
- In athletes with exercise-related pain, three-phase bone scintigraphy is part of the work-up for anterior shin pain.
- In suspected (but radiograph-negative) cases of bony disease, such as cortical stress fracture, periostitis, or cortical hyperostosis, bone scintigraphy may be useful to identify subtle pathology.
- MRI is needed in suspected cases of myopathy though imaging may b done more usefully of the upper leg.

### Imaging of the foot

Information available on radiographs of the hindfoot includes:

- Increased soft tissue attenuation around the tendon insertion in cases of Achilles tendonitis or retrocalcaneal bursitis.
- Erosions or periostitis at the Achilles tendon insertion in enthesitis associated with SpA.
- Erosions in gout and RA-associated retrocalcaneal bursitis.
- Axial radiographs of the hindfoot are useful in showing talocalcaneal joint abnormalities, e.g. in RA.
- If radiographs are normal in patients with posterior heel pain, US can show patterns of tendon and bursal inflammation. MRI can further characterize any discrete pattern of tendon injury.

- Osteonecrosis of an os trigonum or posterior talar process or tarsal navicular may be identified by radiographs. It is invariably located by bone scintigraphy and can be characterized further, usually with soft tissue swelling, by MRI.
- A plantar spur may denote recurrent plantar fasciitis.
- Plantar heel pain may be due to a fracture in a spur. Erosions just above the spur may be seen. The thickness of heel fat pad can be gauged from its X-ray attenuation (thin = risk for plantar fasciitis). A fat pad >23 mm thick in men and >21.5 mm thick in women is associated with acromegaly.
- Calcaneal fractures or an osteoid osteoma can be seen in some cases with radiographs alone. Bone scintigraphy/CT are more sensitive.
- Patterns of joint, enthesis, and tendon inflammation can be documented using MRI or bone scintigraphy. This is useful information when characterizing an arthropathy.
- Bony abnormalities in the mid and forefoot are generally revealed by radiographs alone, though metatarsal stress fractures may be missed. MRI can discriminate a plantar neuroma from interdigital bursitis and MTPJ synovitis. The former are probably best initially demonstrated by US.

*Other investigations*

- Neurophysiology (NCS) is a useful adjunct to clinical examination in diagnosis of lower limb neuropathies, and can help discriminate between peripheral (common peroneal or sciatic) or nerve root causes of foot drop, and also S1 root or tibial nerve entrapment causes of paraesthesias of the sole of the foot.
- Joint/bursa fluid aspiration is mandatory in suspected cases of sepsis and should be sent for culture (remember to consider gonococcus in young adults and TB in patients from endemic or inner-city areas). Fluid should be sent for polarized microscopy if a crystal-induced disease is suspected.
- Laboratory tests requested should reflect suspicion of specific infective, inflammatory, metabolic, or malignant pathology.

## Treatment of lower leg and foot conditions: adults

*Lower leg disorders*

- Anterior shin pain should be treated according to cause. If there is also a problem of foot alignment, then orthoses that support both the hind foot and mid arch may be very useful. Patients may volunteer that good walking shoes or 'trainers' ('sneakers') help (as is the case with plantar fasciitis).
- Exercise-induced lower leg pain has a number of causes and includes shin splints and compartment syndrome. The latter may require further investigation with pressure readings or exercise scintigraphy ($^{99m}$Tc-MIBI). In cases resistant to rest, analgesia, and modification of triggering factors, decompressive surgery may be required.
- Patients with Paget's disease of the tibia may require treatment with IV zoledronate and will need a biomechanical assessment.

*Ankle and hindfoot disorders*

- Tendonitis around the ankle should respond to treatment of its underlying cause. Chronic posterior tibial tendonitis left untreated will eventually accelerate the development of hindfoot valgus. Consider heel and arch support orthotics early.

- Steroid injection of inflamed ankle, subtalar and (both posterior tibial and peroneal) tendons can be done easily (though with subtalar injection, image guidance is advisable). See ➲ Chapter 24.
- Plantar fasciitis may respond to a number of measures:
  - Hind and midfoot orthotics and/or supportive shoes.
  - NSAIDs.
  - Modification of weight-bearing activity.
  - Achilles tendon stretching.
  - Hindfoot strapping.
  - Resting night splint (preventing ankle plantar flexion).
  - Steroid injection around the medial calcaneal tubercle.
  - surgery.
  - Disease modifying anti-rheumatic drugs/immunosuppressants (e.g. sulfasalazine or methotrexate) if part of PsA or SpA.
  - External beam radiotherapy.

## Forefoot disorders

- Localized forefoot pain (e.g. metatarsalgia) may respond to support pads and a change to a wider, more supportive, low-heel shoe. A podiatry/chiropody opinion should be sought as required.
- Forefoot stress fractures and metatarsal head osteochondritis require rest, supportive footwear and time to heal.
- Patients with chronic forefoot pain may benefit from a podiatric assessment. 'Stress offloading' foot orthoses for metatarsalgia and other biomechanical abnormalities (e.g. hallux rigidus) can be individually moulded using thermoplastic materials.

## Steroid injections

Steroid injections may be of value in the following:

- Ankle joint inflammation (e.g. RA, PSA, OA, acute CPPD and gout) (see ➲ Plate 20a).
- Subtalar joint inflammation (imaging guidance needed).
- Tarsal tunnel syndrome.
- Achilles peritendinitis (steroid injections for Achilles nodules should be avoided as the risk of rupture is high. The same concern, though probably lesser risk, applies to Achilles peritendinitis).
- Calcaneal apophysitis (Sever's disease—Achilles tendon insertion).
- Retrocalcaneal bursitis.
- Plantar fasciitis.
- Gout/OA/enthesitis at first MTPJ.
- Initial treatment of a Morton's neuroma.

## Surgery

- Minor surgical techniques can be curative in tarsal tunnel syndrome and in excising an interdigital (Morton's) neuroma.
- Consider excision of painful exostoses and troublesome rheumatoid nodules and amputation of deformed or over-riding toes.
- Major surgical procedures with good outcomes in appropriate patients include fusion of hindfoot joints and forefoot arthroplasty in chronic inflammatory arthritides.
- Osteotomy realignment of a hallux valgus deformity can be successful in the long term.

# Lower leg and foot disorders in children and adolescents

## General considerations

Foot and ankle problems are common in children and adolescents and most are attributable to minor trauma or repetitive stress. Concerns can arise from over-interpretation of common developmental variation or congenital anomalies (see ➋ Table 2.1) and failure of conditioning or rehabilitation after acute injury.

## Taking a history in children and adolescents

- Overuse and acute trauma is common: tendinopathy, stress fractures, osteochondritis and apophysitis. Taking an accurate history of trauma is important.
- If stress fracture is suspected (e.g. second, third, or fifth metatarsals or navicular or calcaneal) in a teenage girl then amenorrhea, eating disorder and overtraining (in an athlete) needs to be considered ('female triad syndrome').
- A history of initial trauma then chronic symptomology is recognized with some lesions—particularly lateral tibiofibular ligament injury, 'turf-toe' and tarso-metatarsal joint injury.
- Pes cavus or planus, tarsal coalitions (stiffness and sometimes pain in the hind-mid foot), and metatarsus adductus presenting in young children are primarily developmental/congenital in origin. Symptoms may have been present since the child started walking though not always and a history of discomfort may have evolved over a long period of time.
- Pain under the heel or a reluctance to heel strike can disclose plantar fasciitis (e.g. traction apophysitis).
- Tendonitis may not be an isolated lesion. For example, posterior tibial tendonitis can often accompany an accessory navicular and peroneal tendonitis is associated with excessive pronation.
- Osteochondritis of different structures present across somewhat differing but broad age ranges: fifth metatarsal base enthesis (9–15 years), Achilles insertional apophysitis (6–17 years), navicular articular chondritis (3–7 years old).
- A dissecans osteochondritis lesion of the dome of the talus presents with hindfoot pain ± catching/locking of the hindfoot. Severe lesions can develop osteonecrosis.
- JIA and pain amplification syndromes can present with foot symptoms though it is wise to rule out all trauma and developmental lesions initially. Dual pathology of course may exist.

### Examination

Examination should begin with functional assessment of gait, jumping, hop-ping, toe walking, walking on heels and in inversion, and figure-of-8 running. Major problems will become apparent.

- Observe when standing and look for pelvic tilt, hindfoot valgus, subtalar and forefoot position, medial longitudinal foot arch, claw toes and a Morton's foot (first ray shorter than second).

- Palpate and move the foot to reproduce pain and assess range of movement.
- Be aware that if the subtalar is only examined offloaded, abnormalities of the joint may not be apparent.
- Test heel rise to assess rigid or flexible pes planus.
- Check thigh–foot angle to screen for tibial torsion (see ➲ 'Internal tibial torsion', p. 180).
- Other examination: is there correctable forefoot adduction? Is there pain on hindfoot external rotation suggesting a deficiency to the anterior talofibular ligament?.
- Check strength (active movement against resistance) of ankle dorsiflexion and plantar flexion, subtalar inversion (tibialis posterior), subtalar eversion (peroneal tendons), first MTPJ dorsiflexion (EHL) and plantar flexion (FHL).
- Finally examine the knee (see ➲ p. 185).

## Common foot conditions in children and adolescents

### Metatarsus adductus (MTA)

This is a common exaggerated turning in of the forefoot typically identified when the child starts to walk.

- MTA may be detected at birth, when attributed to an *in utero* foot position.
- Most MTA configurations are flexible and asymptomatic and require no intervention.
- Stretching may help the foot move into a straighter position and may be supported by the use of a boot, although evidence for this is limited. Casting and surgery are rarely required—only in severe cases.

### Calcaneovalgus

This excess dorsiflexion and valgus of the hindfoot, detected in neonates, is typically identified when the child starts to walk.

- The position of the foot is usually correctable by the examiner.
- There is no dislocation or bony deformity.
- Muscle imbalance due to neurological disturbance may result in weakness of the plantar flexors and unopposed action of tibialis anterior and foot extensors.
- Radiographs typically show posteromedial bowing of the tibia and the first metatarsal lining up with a vertically held talus.
- The condition differs from rocker bottom feet which are not correctable—when the talus is plantar to the first metatarsal.
- Prognosis is good with spontaneous resolution. Passive stretching exercises may expedite resolution.

### Pes planus

Pes planus (flat feet) is a normal variant in young children unless the foot is rigid from a neurological deficit (diplegia) or bony changes.

- Associations of pes planus include hind foot valgus, tightening of the Achilles tendon, and inward rotation of the forefoot to balance the heel position (or the foot may begin to slant outwards from the middle of the foot).

- Hypermobile pes planus corrects if the child rises on tip-toe. Radiographs need only be done for *rigid* flat feet or if pain suggests a tarsal coalition, congenital vertical talus, or accessory navicular.
- Usually no treatment is needed and the patient should be encouraged to walk barefoot as much as possible.
- The value of arch supports is debated as this does not improve the dynamic support of the foot and may make things worse, although can provide pain relief.

*Pes cavus*

A high medial longitudinal arch that does not flatten when weight-bearing is termed pes cavus. It is present in 10% of the population.

- A full neurological history (including of motor milestones) and examination is wise.
- Pes cavus may rarely indicate neuromuscular disease (hereditary motor sensory neuropathy, Friedrich's ataxia, muscular dystrophy, or cerebral palsy).
- If pes cavus is unilateral or rapidly progressive, then consider there may be a spinal tumour.
- Associated clawing of the toes, contracture of the plantar fascia, and dorsiflexed great toe may cause midfoot pain.
- May also affect footwear.
- Physiotherapy, foot orthoses, and foot wear modifications for pain or instability should be considered.
- Surgical treatment is reserved for cases where conservative measures have failed. Surgery includes tendon transfers, soft tissue manipulation, osteotomy and arthrodesis

*Talipes equinovarus (clubfoot)*

- The flexible variant is a common congenital deformity and requires physiotherapy guidance alone.
- The rigid form, which is of genetic aetiology, typically responds to the Ponseti method of manipulation without invasive surgery.

*Tarsal coalition*

A tarsal coalition is a congenital anomaly where there is an abnormal fibrous, cartilaginous or osseous connection between hindfoot bones.

- Coalitions are usually asymptomatic.
- Pain occurs when there is decompensation of supporting musculature, a rigid flat foot, hindfoot valgus, or peroneal spasticity.
- The commonest coalitions are calcaneonavicular (presenting at 8–12 years old) and talocalcaneal (presenting in 12–15-year-olds).
- Radiographs confirm the lesions but MRI is helpful in characterizing fibrous variants and assessment of bone stress (bone oedema).
- Management includes 'determined' physiotherapy working on gait and muscle support of the foot, which, if successful avoids surgery.
- Overall surgery is rarely required and not desired.

*In-toeing*

Clumsiness or regular tripping after 2 years of age is common. Mild in-toeing may be a normal variant. However, assessment requires a thorough examination of potential contributing factors which might be modifiable with physiotherapy and/or foot orthoses (e.g. femoral anteversion, MTA, or any condition resulting in muscle weakness).

*Toe anomalies*

- Congenital curly toes result from shortening of flexor tendons as child starts to walk. Surgical tendon release can be considered in cases where there are painful blisters or rubbing.
- A hammer toe is a tendon contracture with progressive PIPJ flexion and compensatory extension at the MTPJs and DIPJs. Management, including for pain, is usually conservative.
- A mallet toe is a contracture of the DIPJs.
- A claw toe is formed from dorsal toe subluxation at the MTPJs and flexion deformities at the PIPJs and DIPJs.
- Toe instability (dorsal subluxation of the proximal phalanx over the metatarsal head) is rare in young people. Often there is a history of repeat tearing (pain) and swelling of the plantar plate with local tenderness and swelling.
- Polydactyly occurs 1 in 500 live births with radial, ulnar, or central extra digits. There is a high likelihood of syndromic genetic anomaly and chance of multiple genetic defects. A referral to a geneticist is recommended.
- Syndactyly is an embryonic failure of apoptosis of the digit webbing at about 16 weeks' gestation. Most lesions are isolated defects but there may also be an association with genetic defects.

# The spectrum of disorders associated with adult rheumatic and musculoskeletal diseases

# Skin disorders and rheumatic disease

## The importance of examining the skin

- The skin is the most accessible organ to examine.
- Pattern recognition of skin symptoms and lesions is valuable in aiding diagnosis (e.g. acute or chronic sarcoid) and prognosis of rheumatic diseases (e.g. nodules and vasculitis in RA).
- MSK abnormalities may be mirrored by skin abnormalities (e.g. joint hypermobility and skin laxity with bruising, scarring, and striae).
- Some antirheumatic drugs produce specific and potentially serious cutaneous reactions that require prompt management.
- Some rare autoinflammatory conditions associated with MSK symptoms can manifest primarily with skin pathology (see ➲ Chapter 18).

## Regional abnormalities

*The scalp*

Scalp symptoms and lesions may be subtle.

- Scalp tenderness is a sign of GCA.
- C2 root/occipital neuropathy (e.g. in C1–C3 facet joint OA or crowned dens syndrome/CPPD disease) or shingles may be associated with dysaesthesia over the scalp and occipital neuralgia.
- Alopecia may be localized (areata) or diffuse (e.g. in SLE or iron deficiency). Scarring alopecia is typical of discoid lupus.
- Scalp psoriasis may be patchy and discrete, and often affects the hairline.

*Face and ears*

Face and ears are in sun-exposed areas. Consider ultraviolet (UV) skin sensitivity.

- A variety of patterns of SLE-associated, UV-sensitive rashes may occur. The rash is often diffuse. Shaded areas (e.g. nasolabial folds) may not be affected (see ➲ Chapter 13).
- As in SLE, rosacea can present with an erythematous facial rash. Distinction is sometimes difficult without biopsy.
- Periorbital oedema occurs in dermatomyositis, angio-oedema (which may be a presenting feature of SLE), and in nephrotic syndrome.
- Heliotrope rash refers to violaceous oedema/erythema of the eyelids in dermatomyositis (see ➲ Chapter 14).
- The cutaneous infiltration of chronic sarcoid (lupus pernio) (see ➲ Chapter 18) across the nose and cheeks may be overt (papular) but also may be quite subtle (see ➲ Plate 21).
- Saddle nose deformity/nasal cartilage destruction has a number of causes: PR3-positive ANCA-associated vasculitis (AAV; see ➲ Chapter 15), relapsing polychondritis (➲ Chapter 18), hereditary connective tissue disease (e.g. Stickler's syndrome; see ➲ Chapter 19), and lethal midline granuloma. Nasal septal perforation can occur from cocaine use.
- Oral aphthous ulcers are common. Oral ulceration may follow disease activity (e.g. in SLE). Ulcers in reactive arthritis are typically painless. Oral aphthous ulcers are frequently idiopathic, and not associated with systemic disease.
- Large punched-out and numerous tongue and buccal ulcers that scar are a hallmark of Behçet's disease (see ➲ Chapter 18). They may remain for several weeks.

- Strawberry erythema of the tongue and lips should not be missed in children. It may denote self-limiting streptococcal infections but may also herald the desquamating palmar (and sole) rash of Kawasaki disease (KD; see ➋ Chapter 15).
- Lacy white streaks on the buccal mucosa suggest lichen planus.
- The pinna is a common site for gouty tophi and discoid lupus. Relapsing polychondritis typically causes softening and distortion of cartilage (but is lobe-sparing).
- Lipid skin deposits around the eye occur in hyperlipidaemia and multicentric reticulohistiocytosis.

### Hands and nails

Hands and nails should be examined closely.

- A photosensitive eruption spares the finger webs and palms.
- Erythema on the back of the fingers may help distinguish dermatomyositis from SLE.
- In patients with Raynaud's disease (RD), finger ulceration, finger pulp atrophy (with smooth tapering of the finger tips), induration, and tethering of the skin indicate scleroderma (see ➋ Chapter 13).
- Unlike normal skin, the skin of scleroderma does not form fine wrinkles when pinched.
- Onycholysis, nail-pitting, salmon patches, and subungual hyperkeratosis are typical of psoriasis (see ➋ Chapter 8).
- Subungual splinter haemorrhages may be associated with trauma, infective endocarditis, vasculitis, or thromboangiitis obliterans.
- Nailfold capillaries can be examined with an ophthalmoscope at 40 dioptres after applying a drop of oil (or surgical lubricant) to the cuticle. Enlarged (dilated) capillary loops and capillary 'dropout' suggests an underlying autoimmune connective tissue disease (AICTD), particularly systemic sclerosis (SScl).
- Nailfold vasculopathy is non-specific, and can occur with vasculitis, dermatomyositis and infective endocarditis.

## Types of eruption

### Macular rashes

Macular rashes are flat (non-palpable) areas of altered skin colour. Papules are lumps <1 cm in diameter.

- Maculopapular rashes are typical of viral infections.
- A short-lived, pinkish, maculopapular eruption occurs on the trunk and limbs in systemic-onset JIA (soJIA; see ➋ Chapter 9) and adult-onset Still's disease (see ➋ Chapter 18). It is often prominent in the late afternoon, and coincides with temperature spikes. If scratched, the rash may blanch (Koebner phenomenon).
- Erythema that enlarges to form erythematous patches with pale centres suggests rheumatic fever ('erythema marginatum').
- A 'bulls-eye' erythematous lesion around a tick bite may be the erythema migrans of Lyme disease.
- Maculopapular eruptions can occur from NSAIDs, gold, sulfasalazine, azathioprine hypersensitivity, and leflunomide (see ➋ Chapter 23).

*Pustules and blisters*

Blisters may be vesicles (<0.5 cm) or bullae (>0.5 cm).

- The most common pustular rash is due to folliculitis.
- Pustules confined to the hands and feet suggest reactive arthritis or SAPHO, although local forms of psoriasis may be indistinguishable. Psoriasis can also occur as 'raindrop' erythematous lesions, also known as guttate lesions.
- Generalized pustular rashes can occur in vasculitis, the neutrophilic dermatoses, intestinal bypass syndromes, Behçet's disease, and gonococcal bacteraemia.
- Bullous eruptions may be due to SLE and drug reactions, pemphigus, and pemphigoid.

*Plaques*

Plaques are slightly raised, circumscribed areas—often disc shaped.

- Plaques are the hallmark of psoriasis. Skin may be scaly and flake off easily. Lesions are often red.
- Psoriatic plaques can occur anywhere on the skin, but typical sites are over the extensor surfaces of the joints, in the intergluteal cleft, at sites of skin friction (e.g. under waistbands of trousers or underwear) and the umbilicus.
- Scaling may be a feature of discoid lupus; scaling tends to occur at the periphery of the lesion.

*Vascular lesions*

Bleeding into the skin that does not blanch is called purpura. It may sometimes be palpable. Telangiectases are dilated small vascular lesions that blanch on pressure.

- Non-palpable purpura may be due to thrombocytopenia, platelet dysfunction, trauma (± capillary/skin fragility, e.g. chronic steroid use), haemophilia, anticoagulation, and hereditary connective tissue diseases (e.g. EDS; see ➾ Chapter 19).
- Palpable purpura suggests vasculitis, including drug-induced disease (see ➾ Chapter 15).
- Widespread telangiectasia occurs in limited cutaneous scleroderma (lcSScl; see ➾ Chapter 13), hereditary haemorrhagic telangiectasia, and dermatomyositis.
- Livedoid rashes can be subtle, occur mainly over the legs, can occur in smokers but are also associated with SLE and antiphospholipid syndrome (APS).
- Lumpy erythema on the lower legs especially, which can be tender, may be panniculitis (e.g. erythema nodosum), and related to systemic disease (e.g. sarcoid, Crohn's)

*Ulcers and ulcerating rashes*

Ulcers are defined as a loss or defect of dermis and epidermis produced by sloughing of necrotic tissue.

- Cutaneous ulceration may have more than one cause in autoimmune diseases. For example, vasculitis, venous stasis in an immobile patient, and ulceration over nodules or pressure points may all contribute to the same set of lesions. Trauma may be an important cause of cutaneous ulcers in a patient who is already predisposed towards forming these lesions.

- An indurated, expanding, plum-coloured plaque or acneiform pustule that then ulcerates suggests pyoderma gangrenosum. The ulcer has irregular, bluish margins.
- Neurotropic ulcers are classic sequelae of diabetes, but they can also occur in association with mononeuritis multiplex (from vasculitis) and other rheumatic diseases.
- Vasculitic ulcers in the context of livedo reticularis and antibodies to phospholipids (e.g. cardiolipin) may denote APS (see ➲ Chapter 11).

*Textural abnormalities*

Abnormalities of the texture of the skin may be difficult to discern. Atrophy and thinning, laxity, thickening, and induration may all be associated with disease.

- Generalized skin atrophy and thinning is an age-related process, but this can be accelerated by chronic steroid use; hereditary diseases of connective tissue should also be considered.
- Skin laxity can best be demonstrated over elbow and knee extensor surfaces. Generalized laxity of connective tissue may result in varicose veins and internal organ prolapse.
- True acral and digital puffiness in a patient with Raynaud's disease is suggestive of SScl. Skin thickening has a variety of causes (see later in this topic and ➲ Chapter 13).
- Scleroderma and scleroderma-like skin may be localized, limited, or diffuse—this distinction is important (Table 4.1).

## Diagnostic issues in patients with skin thickening

- Raynaud's disease (RD) invariably precedes the onset of SScl, but is not a characteristic of morphea or linear scleroderma.
- In patients with RD, abnormal nailfold capillaries on capillaroscopy may indicate SScl (see ➲ Plate 9).
- The specificities of autoantibodies are often predictive of SScl subtype. In patients with RD, ANA has predictive value for identifying patients who may progress to SScl; anticentromere antibody can predict progression to limited cutaneous SScl; anti-topoisomerase I (SCL-70) and anti-RNA polymerase antibodies are linked with progression to diffuse cutaneous SScl (dcSScl).
- Patients with dcSScl have a preponderance of visceral organ involvement in the first 5 years of disease; screening investigations are usually useful, and should include cardiovascular screening tests (refer to ➲ Chapter 13).
- Eosinophilic fasciitis (see ➲ Chapter 18) may occur as a paraneoplastic syndrome, and is associated with haematological malignancies.
- Linear scleroderma in children can produce lifelong deformities because limbs fail to develop correct length and bulk.

**Table 4.1** Pattern recognition in patients with skin thickening

| Classification | Skin features |
|---|---|
| Morphea may be localized (guttate) or generalized | Early small skin areas affected (itchy). Progression to hidebound skin, typically on trunk (areola spared) and legs. Lesions become waxy and hypo/hyper-pigmented guttate (small <10 mm) papules usually on neck and anterior chest |
| Linear scleroderma | Linear band-like pattern often in dermatomal distribution. Atrophy of muscles is common. Fixed joint deformities and growth abnormalities can occur |
| 'Coup de sabre' | Linear scleroderma on the face/scalp can be depressed; ivory in appearance. Hemi-atrophy can occur |
| SScl (early) | Early morning 'puffiness' in hands and feet, facial 'tightness'. Non-pitting oedema of intact dermal and epidermal appendages. High degree of suspicion needed |
| SScl (classic) | Firm, taut, hidebound skin proximal to MCP joints. Skin may be coarse, pigmented, and dry. Epidermal thinning, loss of hair, and sweating can occur. Telangiectasia and skin calcinosis become obvious. Skin creases disappear. Such change proximal to elbows or knees in the limbs or below the clavicles (in those with face and neck involvement) classifies disease as diffuse as opposed to limited systemic sclerosis |
| SScl (late) | 2–15 years after onset of classical phase, skin softens, but pigmentation changes remain. Skin becomes atrophic and can ulcerate |
| Eosinophilic fasciitis | *Phases:* early—pitting oedema; progressive—*peau d'orange*; late—induration ('woody feel') with venous guttering when limb elevated. Arms and legs most commonly affected, but fingers mainly spared. Synovitis and low-grade myositis may occur. Eosinophilia is usually striking, but not always present |
| Lipodermato-sclerosis | Hyperpigmentation and induration of lower legs associated with venous stasis ('champagne-bottle legs') |
| Diabetes | Waxy thickening of extremities. Insidious progression. Joints of the hands become stiff, the tendons can thicken. Skin changes proximal to wrist and on the face very unlikely, but stiffening of elbow and shoulder joints not uncommon |
| Dependent lymphoedema | Feet/ankles/lower legs. Often pitting. Chronic presence may give hyperkeratosis. Main causes: R- or L-sided heart failure, renal failure, nephrotic syndrome, and low-protein states |

# Skin vasculitis in adults

## Background

There are a variety of ways in which systemic vasculitis may present, including fever of unknown origin, organ infarction, gastrointestinal (GI) bleeding, and high acute phase in a generally unwell patient. A vasculitic skin rash is one of the most common presenting features of systemic vasculitis, and is an important diagnostic clue (see ➔ Chapter 15).

## When to consider a diagnosis of vasculitis

- Primary systemic vasculitis is rare.
- Cutaneous vasculitis, however, is not rare; it can follow viral or bacterial illness, can be triggered by drugs, and is associated with malignancy. Biopsy generally demonstrates degranulation of neutrophils ('leucocytoclasis') and evidence of vessel destruction.
- The list of causes is long (Table 4.2); however, in about 50% of cases no cause may be found.
- Cutaneous vasculitis may also occur in association with another autoimmune disease not normally characterized by vasculitis, such as SLE, RA, and Sjögren's syndrome.

**Table 4.2** Precipitants and associations of leucocytoclastic small vessel vasculitis

| | |
|---|---|
| Drugs | Sulphonamides, for example (there are many). Some drugs may cause a lymphocytic vasculitis without leucocytoclasis |
| Infections | Hepatitis B, hepatitis C, HIV |
| | β-haemolytic *Streptococcus* |
| Foreign protein | E.g. serum sickness |
| Autoimmune disease | Rheumatoid arthritis |
| | Sjögren's syndrome (anti-Ro positive) |
| | SLE (though livedoid vasculitis may occur in association with secondary APS, and this may be lymphocytic without leucocytoclasis) |
| Inflammatory diseases | Sarcoid |
| | Crohn's disease, ulcerative colitis, chronic active hepatitis |
| Malignancy | Myelo- and lymphoproliferative disorders |
| | Solid tumours |
| Cryoglobulinaemia | |

## Important considerations

The following important points of clinical assessment should be followed in patients with possible vasculitic rashes.

- Determine whether the patient has been taking a new drug. Many antibiotics, including penicillins, sulfonamides, and cephalosporins, cause cutaneous vasculitis. Biologics may too, notably anti-TNFα.
- Evaluate the patient for evidence of chronic infection: hepatitis B, hepatitis C, and HIV are worth considering. Endocarditis should also be considered (e.g. the elderly, or patients who use IV drugs).
- Look for evidence of a primary autoimmune disorder that may be associated with cutaneous vasculitis. IBD, for example, can occasionally cause a leucocytoclastic vasculitis in addition to oral ulcerations and pyoderma gangrenosum. Because SLE is common, check ANA and serum complement C3/C4.
- Look for evidence of cryoglobulinaemic vasculitis. Serum cryoglobulins tests are often mishandled, leading to false-negative results, primarily because the sample needs to be kept warm (usually by simply holding in the closed palm of the hand) and should be taken straight to the laboratory.
- RF is detected in 80% of patients with mixed essential cryoglobulinaemia, and may be a better screening test than the latter.
- Age-appropriate screening for malignancy should be done. Serum and urine electrophoresis with immunofixation may be of value.
- Urinalysis may demonstrate 'active sediment'; evidence of haematuria, proteinuria, or red blood cell casts may be the first clue that a patient has a systemic vasculitis.

## Systemic vasculitis

- Untreated primary systemic vasculitis is generally characterized by general inflammation; many patients will complain of B-type symptoms, including fevers, weight loss, and night sweats. Patients with cutaneous vasculitis alone, on the other hand, often feel quite well.
- The extracutaneous signs and symptoms may provide clues to the correct diagnosis:
  - Henoch–Schönlein purpura (HSP): colicky abdominal pain.
  - Eosinophilic granulomatosis with polyangiitis: adult-onset asthma, eosinophilia.
  - PR3-positive AAV: chronic sinusitis, pneumonitis.
  - Microscopic polyangiitis: haemoptysis, red blood cell casts.
- Mononeuritis multiplex, which presents as a 'wrist drop' or 'foot drop', is suggestive of systemic vasculitis in a non-diabetic patient.

## Investigations

### Skin biopsy

- Discuss the case with a histopathologist.
- Punch biopsy is simple, and may be sufficient to yield a diagnosis. Elliptical biopsy provides more tissue, and may increase yield.
- Use a needle to lift the skin sample. Avoid forceps-induced damage.

- Biopsy should extend to the subcutaneous fat, which generally includes the arterioles and venules affected by primary systemic vasculitis. Idiopathic leucocytoclastic vasculitis affects the capillaries but generally spares the arterioles and venules.
- Biopsy should be sent for routine histology and for direct immunofluorescence, which may yield important clues regarding the underlying cause:
  - IgA: HSP.
  - IgM, C3: cryoglobulinaemic vasculitis.
  - IgG, IgM, IgA, C3: SLE.
  - Low immunoreactant staining: AAV.
- Samples for immunofluorescence should be snap frozen in liquid $N_2$ or dry ice or transported immediately to the laboratory. Immunofluorescence cannot be done on samples treated with formalin.
- See Table 4.3 for a list of laboratory investigations to be carried out in patients with suspected vasculitis.

**Table 4.3** Laboratory tests in patients with suspected vasculitis

| Haematology | FBC, ESR, lupus anticoagulant |
|---|---|
| Biochemistry | Electrolytes, urea, creatinine, LFTs, ACE, CRP, serum and urine protein electrophoresis |
| Microbiology | Urine microscopy for red cell casts, blood culture, Hep B and C serology, consider HIV, streptococcal antibodies. Also, save 10 mL of clotted blood for viral serology and repeat in 2–3 weeks for paired titre analysis |
| Immunology | Immunoglobulins (include IgG subsets if IgG4 disease being considered), cryoglobulins, ANA, ENAs, RF, anti-cardiolipin antibodies, ANCA, Complement (C3, C4, CH50/CH100, anti-C1q antibodies if considering urticarial vasculitis)) |

# Cardiac conditions

Subclinical cardiac involvement is found in many rheumatic MSK diseases, and it is not uncommon for a cardiac abnormality to be discovered incidentally. As our ability to treat the underlying rheumatic diseases improves, our ability to identify and to treat the cardiac complications of these diseases becomes increasingly important.

## Pericardium

- Pericardial effusion has been reported in association with a large number of rheumatic diseases, including SScl, Sjögren's syndrome, polymyositis, mixed connective tissue disease (MCTD), RA, SpAs, and systemic vasculitides.
- In the majority of cases, effusions are discovered incidentally, are often small, clinically asymptomatic, and require no specific therapy.
- Pericardial effusions can also occur in the setting of non-rheumatic illness. When a patient with a known rheumatic disease presents with a symptomatic effusion, it is important to consider other possible explanations, such as infection (e.g. TB, viral), malignancy, and other unrelated conditions (uraemia, hypothyroidism).
- Pericardial effusions are common in SLE and are due to immune complex deposition into the pericardium. Effusions can be serous, serosanguinous, or haemorrhagic. Analysis of the pericardial fluid generally demonstrates evidence of complement, immune complexes, and leucocytes, consistent with an active inflammatory state.
- Although pericardial effusions are common with SLE, they are generally trivial. Cardiac tamponade is found in <1% of patients with SLE. Since the effusion tends to reflect the overall disease, generally treatment of the underlying disease is adequate to resolve the effusion. Rarely, therapeutic pericardiocentesis may be required.
- Pericardial effusions are found in up to 30% of patients with RA, although only a small number of these patients will present with pericarditis or evidence of tamponade.
- Pericardial effusions are more common in RF-positive patients with a history of rheumatoid nodules. Chronic pericardial effusions can become infected, and in rare cases lead to constrictive pericarditis.
- For both groups of patients, the presence of a symptomatic pericardial effusion is associated with increased mortality. In one study of patients with SLE who presented with cardiac tamponade, the 5-year survival was only 46%.

## Myocardium

- Myocarditis is an uncommon feature of rheumatic diseases. Myocarditis can be found among patients with active SLE and RA, although it generally does not lead to clinically significant dysfunction.
- Cardiomyopathy among patients with RA and SLE is more likely to be due to premature coronary artery disease, followed by the development of ischaemic heart disease.
- Although uncommon, the possibility of hydroxychloroquine-induced cardiomyopathy should be considered in patients who develop congestive heart failure in the absence of coronary artery disease. The diagnosis can be confirmed with myocardial biopsy, and the condition responds to drug cessation.

- Eosinophilic granulomatosis with polyangiitis (EGPA; formerly Churg–Strauss vasculitis) can lead to an acute eosinophilic myocarditis that can be life-threatening if not treated promptly.
- One-third of patients with AAV may have cardiac dysfunction as a consequence of the underlying vasculitis. The majority of these patients will have wall motion abnormalities on echocardiography, but valvulitis and ventricular aneurysm have also been reported. The majority of these lesions will be asymptomatic, but the 5-year survival rate for patients with cardiac lesions attributable to AAV is 57%.

## Valvular disease

- Aortic regurgitation is an important potential consequence of aortitis, which can occur with any of the large-vessel vasculitides (including Takayasu arteritis, GCA, and Behçet's disease). The aortitis leads to aneurysms, which create valvular incompetence.
- Aortic regurgitation can also occur as a consequence of AS. Unlike the vasculitides, in AS there is inflammation at the aortic root leading to dense scarring of the aortic valves. Although the mechanism is unique to this disease, it should be monitored and treated like any form of aortic insufficiency.
- Mitral regurgitation and mitral valve prolapse are common manifestations of SLE.
- Mitral valve prolapse may also be a feature of Ehlers–Danlos syndrome.
- A more serious valvulitis can occur in association with SLE or APS. In the process of healing, the valves become scarred and calcified, a process that can eventually lead to clinically significant valvular disease.
- Libman–Sacks endocarditis is a classic manifestation of SLE. In this disease, vegetations form from immune complexes, mononuclear cells, and fibrin, which attach to the valves. Although not infectious, these vegetations can embolize.
- Haemodynamically insignificant valve lesions have also been reported in association with RA, MCTD, SScl, and Sjögren's syndrome.

## Coronary artery disease

- Surprisingly, the primary vasculitides rarely lead to coronary artery inflammation, although coronary artery vasculitis has been reported in association with PAN and AAVs.
- APS is associated with a substantial increased risk of myocardial infarction, even in the absence of true coronary artery disease.
- Both RA and SLE are strongly associated with coronary artery disease. This may be the result of systemic inflammation or a response to chronic immunosuppression. Regardless, patients with these diagnoses should undergo early cardiac evaluation to address modifiable risk factors for coronary artery disease.
- Accelerated atherosclerosis may be an important consequence of glucocorticoid exposure. Even chronic low-dose prednisone may place some patients at increased risk of cardiovascular disease.

## Conduction abnormalities

- Clinically insignificant dysrhythmias and conduction defects are common among patients with inflammatory myopathies (dermatomyositis, polymyositis) and scleroderma.
- Clinically significant abnormalities (including heart block) can be seen in patients with SpAs as a result of the same scaring process that leads to the valvular abnormalities noted earlier.

# Pulmonary conditions

## Pleura

- An exudative pleural effusion is found in up to 50% of patients with SLE. These effusions can be unilateral or bilateral, and frequently are found in association with a pericardial effusion.
- Pleural disease is a common manifestation of RA, which is associated with pleural effusions and pleural thickening. Effusions are generally asymptomatic, and are found in the setting of active disease.
- Asymptomatic pleural effusions can also be found in 10–30% of patients with AAV.
- Pleural effusions are classified as transudates, typically arising as a consequence of left ventricular, renal and hepatic failure, and SLE; or exudates, usually due to infection, malignancy or pulmonary embolism.
- By the 'Light' criteria (with a 75–80% sensitivity) a transudate is:
  - clear.
  - specific gravity <1.012.
  - fluid protein <2 g/dL.
  - fluid:serum protein ratio <0.5.
  - fluid:serum LDH ratio <2/3.
  - cholesterol <45 g/dL.
- In the same criteria, an exudate is defined as:
  - cloudy.
  - specific gravity >1.020.
  - fluid protein >2.9 g/dL.
  - fluid:serum protein ratio >0.5.
  - fluid:serum LDH ratio >2/3.
  - cholesterol >45 g/dL.
- If an exudate is identified fluid should be examined for:
  - *amylase*: in oesophageal rupture, pancreatitis.
  - *glucose*: decreased in infection, malignancy and RA.
  - *pH*: low in empyema.
  - Gram stain.
  - polymerase chain reaction (PCR) for tuberculosis.

## Pulmonary nodules/masses

- Both PR3-positive AAV and sarcoidosis are often diagnosed incidentally, after the discovery of lung masses. Sarcoidosis is associated with hilar lymphadenopathy, while PR3-positive AAV generally presents with multiple peripheral pulmonary nodules that can be mistaken for lung cancer.
- In a patient with a known rheumatic disease who presents with a lung mass, it is always important to consider the possibility of malignancy. Lung cancer risk is increased among patients with RA and SScl, and many rheumatic diseases are associated with an increased risk of lymphoma.
- PR3-positive AAV (and less commonly, AS and RA) can lead to cavitating apical lesions that can be mistaken for TB.

## Interstitial lung disease (ILD)

- ILD and pulmonary fibrosis (with a predilection for the lung bases and periphery) is a common feature of both dcSScl and the inflammatory myopathies.
- Pulmonary fibrosis is found in 20–65% of patients with SScl. Radiographically, the lesions take on the appearance of ground glass ILD infiltrates that gradually lead to honeycombing and fibrosis.
- ILD may be the initial manifestation of an inflammatory myopathy, and pulmonary symptoms may precede clinical evidence of muscle involvement.
- RA is also associated with ILD.
- Apical fibrosis can be found in 1% of patients with AS. Apical fibrosis is also an uncommon feature of rheumatoid lung.
- Pulmonary fibrosis can also occur as the long-term sequelae of pulmonary capillaritis, which may occur in patients with AAV.
- ILD in primary Sjögren's syndrome can be subtle and evolve insidiously. The usual pattern is non-specific (NSIP).
- Bronchiolitis obliterans organizing pneumonia (BOOP) has been associated with autoimmune rheumatic and connective tissue diseases but the association is not frequent.

## Vasculature

- Haemoptysis can be the result of pulmonary capillaritis, which can be found in association with the so-called pulmonary renal syndromes: SLE, AAV (predominantly microscopic polyangiitis), and anti-glomerular basement membrane syndrome. Acute or severe pulmonary vasculitis may require prompt plasmapheresis.
- Cryoglobulinaemic vasculitis can also cause pulmonary capillaritis, although this is not one of its more common manifestations.
- Pulmonary artery hypertension (PAH) is most commonly associated with lcSScl. Isolated PAH can also be seen with dcSScl, although it generally appears as a consequence of pulmonary fibrosis.
- SScl causes PAH by narrowing of the small arteries and arterioles that gradually leads to obliteration of the pulmonary vascular bed.
- RA, SLE, inflammatory myopathy, MCTD, and Sjögren's syndrome can also be associated with PAH, but it is considered an uncommon feature of these diseases.

## Airways

- RA can lead to laryngeal obstruction when it affects the cricoarytenoid joints. It usually presents with hoarseness or odynophagia.
- Subglottic stenosis is a common feature of PR3-positive AAV, which can lead to significant stridor.
- Uncontrolled relapsing polychondritis can cause tracheomalacia, which is a significant cause of morbidity for this disease.
- Any part of the airway can become symptomatic in primary Sjögren's syndrome: xerotrachea, xerostomia, sinus symptoms.

# Renal conditions

### Evaluation of renal failure: overview

The kidneys are an essential component in the evaluation and management of the rheumatic MSK diseases.

- In terms of time course, renal failure may be secondary to acute kidney injury (AKI) or chronic kidney disease (CKD). AKI can occur in patients with stable CKD.
- AKI (grade 1) is defined when one of the following criteria is met:
  - Serum creatinine rises by ≥26 μmol/L within 48 hours.
  - Serum creatinine rises ≥1.5× from the reference value, which is known or presumed to have occurred within 1 week.
  - Urine output is <0.5 mL/kg/hour for >6 consecutive hours.
- The above-listed indices are the minimum required for definition (grade 2 and 3 AKI have definitions: http://www.renal.org/guidelines/modules/acute-kidney-injury).
- Urgent urinalysis and renal ultrasound should be obtained in all AKI patients.
- Glomerular filtration rate value (mL/min/1.73m$^2$) classifies renal function as WHO stage: normal (grade 1; >90), mild (grade 2; 60–89), moderate (grade 3; 30–59), severe (grade 4; 15–29), severe failure (grade 5; <15).
- The presence of red blood cells and protein, or red blood cell casts (i.e. 'an active sediment') implies glomerulonephritis, which can occur with vasculitis and SLE.

### Pre-renal azotaemia

- Hypovolaemia is an important cause of pre-renal AKI. Dehydration and anaemia can both lead to pre-renal azotaemia (e.g. the elderly RA patient).
- Renal hypoperfusion can also be caused by diminished blood flow to the kidneys. Diseases involving the renal artery (such as renal artery stenosis or thrombosis or PAN affecting the renal artery) may cause pre-renal azotaemia. This may be acute leading to AKI or slowly evolving causing CKD.
- Conditions associated with low cardiac output (including shock, congestive heart failure, myocarditis, tamponade, and pulmonary arterial hypertension) may all predispose the patient to pre-renal AKI.
- Hyperviscosity, which is seen with type I (monoclonal) cryoglobulinaemia, is a very rare cause of pre-renal azotaemia.
- All of these conditions may be exacerbated by drugs that decrease renal perfusion, including NSAIDs and ACE inhibitors.
- With pre-renal azotaemia, the fractional excretion of sodium [FENa = (UNa × PCr)/(PNa × UCr)] is <1.0; this test is not reliable in patients treated with diuretics.

## Post-renal azotaemia

- Nephrolithiasis is not a common cause of post-renal azotaemia, but should be considered in a patient with gout: 5–10% of renal calculi in the United States are caused by uric acid; this is particularly common among patients with gout who have been treated with uricosuric agents (e.g. probenecid).
- Sarcoidosis can cause hypercalcaemia and hypercalciuria, which in turn can lead to nephrolithiasis and nephrocalcinosis, both of which can rarely cause post-renal azotaemia.
- Methotrexate and trimethoprim/sulfamethoxazole can cause crystalluria and renal obstruction.
- Ultrasound is a useful modality to evaluate both for the presence of obstruction leading to hydronephrosis and renal calculi.

## Intrinsic renal failure: 'active sediment'

- Intrinsic renal disease from a rheumatological conditions can present acutely (AKI) or insidiously as evolving CKD.
- The nephritic syndromes are an important cause of moderate/severe AKI among patients with rheumatic diseases, particularly vasculitis and SLE.
- The presence of haematuria, proteinuria, and red blood cell casts strongly suggests the presence of glomerulonephritis.
- A renal biopsy is crucial to determining the underlying diagnosis and the severity/chronicity of the disease.
- Nephritic syndromes can be divided into 'focal proliferative' and 'diffuse proliferative' based on histology.
- Causes of focal proliferative glomerulonephritis include SLE, HSP, and other forms of small vessel vasculitis.
- Diffuse proliferative glomerulonephritis is caused by cryoglobulinaemia, SLE, anti-glomerular basement membrane disease (Goodpasture's syndrome), and small-vessel vasculitis (including AAV and renal-limited vasculitis).
- Direct immunofluorescence can also provide valuable information regarding the correct diagnosis: SLE biopsy demonstrates multiple immunoreactants ('full house' staining pattern); IgA deposition implies HSP; cryoglobulinaemic vasculitis leads to IgG and C3 deposition; sparse or absent immunoreactants on biopsy is sometimes called 'pauci-immune', and implies an AAV.

## Intrinsic renal failure: 'bland sediment'

- A bland sediment refers to a urine sample that is acellular; transparent hyaline casts may be seen.
- A bland sediment is also seen in pre-renal and post-renal azotaemia.
- Acute tubular necrosis (ATN) reflects acute, intrinsic renal failure associated with a urine sediment that has muddy brown casts and tubular epithelial cells.
- Nephrotoxic tubular injury from drugs is a common cause of ATN in patients with rheumatic disease.

- Prolonged pre-renal azotaemia can lead to permanent kidney damage; therefore, diseases of the renal artery (including polyarteritis nodosa and renal artery thrombosis from APS) should be considered.
- Interstitial nephritis is most commonly seen as a drug reaction (e.g. gold, penicillamine).
- Interstitial nephritis can also be seen as a manifestation of several rheumatic diseases, including Sjögren's, SLE, sarcoidosis, and EGPA.
- NSAIDs cause renal vasoconstriction and interstitial nephritis, both of which can eventually lead to a chronic analgesic nephropathy.
- Unlike the other forms of AAV, the mechanism of renal failure among patients with the EGPA is an interstitial nephritis; glomerulonephritis is relatively rare with this diagnosis.
- The most common causes of secondary renal amyloidosis are AS, RA and FMF. Glomerular deposits of amyloid lead to proteinuria (which can be nephrotic range) and progressive renal failure.

## SScl renal crisis

- SScl renal crisis is a rheumatologic emergency characterized by AKI and malignant hypertension (see ➲ Chapter 25, p. 720).
- Patients with dcSScl are at greatest risk.
- SScl renal crisis generally occurs within the first 4 years after diagnosis, but it can occur at any time. Patients who are treated with high-dose glucocorticoids and are anti-RNP positive are at highest risk.
- Urinalysis generally demonstrates a bland sediment. Kidney biopsy demonstrates evidence of a thrombotic microangiopathy that histologically cannot be distinguished from malignant hypertensive nephrosclerosis, haemolytic–uraemic syndrome, SLE, or APS.
- The cornerstone of therapy is escalating doses of ACE inhibitors, followed by angiotensin II receptor blockers (ARBs) and calcium channel blockers if adequate blood pressure control is not achieved.

## Renal tubular acidosis

- Renal tubular acidosis (RTA) is a non-anion gap metabolic acidosis caused by a failure of the renal tubules to maintain acid–base status.
- Type I RTA, caused by an inability to excrete acid, is found with Sjögren's syndrome and SLE.
- Type IV RTA is most commonly caused by hyporeninaemic hypoaldosteronism, can occur as a result of treatment with NSAIDs, ACE-inhibitors, and ARBs. This is commonly associated with hyperkalaemia.

# Endocrine conditions

Well-characterized MSK conditions occur in many endocrine disorders. Some are specific for certain disorders; others are non-specific, but occur with greater frequency among patients with endocrine disease. MSK features occur either as a result of metabolic disturbances or are influenced by a common link in autoimmune pathophysiology.

## Diabetes

- Dupuytren's contracture, trigger finger, carpal tunnel syndrome, diffuse idiopathic skeletal hyperostosis (DISH), and adhesive capsulitis all occur with greater frequency among patients with diabetes.
- Some form of tissue or joint hypomobility/stiffness is common among patients with diabetes (Table 4.4); in some cases, this can appear similar to scleroderma. These scleroderma-like skin changes are more prevalent among patients with type I diabetes.
- Hand weakness may be due to diabetic neuropathy and may be mistaken for carpal tunnel syndrome. Neurophysiology tests help discriminate between these two diagnoses.
- Calcification of soft tissues around the shoulder occurs in approximately 20% of diabetics, and is associated with variable symptoms and disability.

**Table 4.4** Patterns of joint and tissue hypomobility/stiffness in diabetes by reported series. Tissue changes are thought to occur from changes in hydration properties/kinetics of glycosaminoglycans (consequence of an excess local production of sugar alcohols)

| Patient series | Major abnormalities | Associations |
| --- | --- | --- |
| Diabetics overall | In about 30–40% mainly in long-standing disease: slow decrease in hand mobility; waxy skin thickening ('scleroderma-like') | Occasional lung fibrosis. Microvascular diabetic complications |
| Adults | 55–76% prevalence of joint hypomobility in type 1/type 2 diabetes, respectively | Not associated with diabetic complications |
| Mature-onset diabetes (mean 61 years) | Stiffening of connective tissue (assessed in hands) | Diabetic nephropathy |
| Children with type 1 diabetes | 31% have limited joint mobility | None with glycaemic control, retinopathy, or proteinuria |
| Juvenile and young adult onset (age 1–24 years) diabetes | 34% had skin thickening. Changes rarely proximal to MCPs and never proximal to wrists. Joint contractures in >50%, often third or fourth fingers | No flexor tendon rubs (as seen in scleroderma) |

- Diabetic amyotrophy is uncommon. It presents acutely with pain, weakness, and wasting of the proximal lower limb muscles. It may be unilateral. Differential diagnosis includes myositis (see ➲ Chapter 14) and PMR. It is associated with uncontrolled hyperglycaemia. The aetiology is unknown, but it is probably a neuromyopathy.
- Though rare (1:500 diabetics), neuropathic arthritis can occur in advanced disease. Most patients are aged 40–60 years and have poor glycaemic control. Tarsal and metatarsal joints are most frequently affected (60%). The usual presentation is of swelling of the foot with no or little pain. Trauma may have occurred. Early radiographic changes can resemble OA.
- Asymptomatic osteolysis can occur at the distal metatarsals and proximal phalanges with relative joint sparing: aetiology unknown.
- Osteomyelitis is not uncommon and needs to be discriminated from cellulitis and neuropathic arthritis (Charcot's joint). A triple-phase bone scan should be helpful. Osteomyelitis is usually disclosed by prominent blood flow in the dynamic (first) phase and increased uptake of tracer by soft tissue and bone in later stages. Cellulitis is associated with minimal uptake of tracer in bone in the delayed (third) phase. Neuropathic joints display minimal first-phase abnormalities but prominent tracer uptake in the third phase.
- Diabetic muscle infarction can present as a painful muscle mass and is a result of arterial narrowing. Often mistaken for thrombophlebitis, myositis or vasculitis, this is a late complication of diabetes. Biopsy may be needed to confirm this diagnosis.
- Diabetes may be associated with a 'metabolic syndrome' (diabetes + hypertension, hyperuricaemia, obesity).

## Hypothyroidism

- Over 25% of patients with hypothyroidism have an arthropathy—cross-sectional data. The likeliest explanation is coincidental arthritis disease: generalized OA, CPPD-related (see next bullet point) or an autoimmune arthritis (e.g. RA). Whether a specific arthritis occurs directly as a result of thyroid abnormality, is debatable.
- Radiographically-defined chondrocalcinosis is only marginally increased compared with controls (17% vs 10%). About 1/10 patients with acute CPPD are hypothyroid.
- Thyroid disease may also be autoimmune and the serum ANA positive, again often mistaken for assuming the presence of a primary rheumatic condition.
- Carpal tunnel syndrome is common (7%). Up to 10% of patients with carpal tunnel syndrome may have hypothyroidism.
- Hyperuricaemia is common, but gout attacks are rare. However, screening for hypothyroidism in patients with gout is recommended. Treated hypothyroidism then requires review of the need for uric acid-lowering therapy.

- Myopathy is relatively common. About 1 in 20 cases of acquired myopathy are due to hypothyroidism. The presentation can mimic polymyositis with elevation of muscle enzymes, but muscle biopsy typically shows no inflammatory cell infiltrate. Improvement with thyroxine replacement is sometimes complicated by muscle cramps, but these should resolve in a few weeks.
- The combination of weakness, muscular stiffness, and an increase in muscle mass in an adult with myxoedema is termed Hoffman's syndrome. Muscle mass increase is sometimes striking and can take many months to resolve on treatment.
- Lymphocytic thyroiditis (Hashimoto's) is an autoimmune condition characterized by hypothyroidism and autoantibodies to thyroglobulin and thyroid microsomes. These antibodies are found in 40% of patients with primary Sjögren's syndrome, but only about 10% are or have been overtly hypothyroid.

## Thyrotoxicosis

- Hyperthyroidism can cause a proximal myopathy (70%), shoulder periarthritis (7%), acropachy (thickening of extremities), and osteoporosis.
- Graves' disease is frequently associated with fatigue and muscular weakness. It is associated with autoimmune rheumatic and connective tissue diseases.

### Thyroid acropachy

This is rare (<2% of patients with thyrotoxicosis) and most often occurs in treated patients who are hypo/euthyroid.
- There is clubbing, and painful soft tissue swelling of hands and feet.
- Periosteal new bone occurs on the radial aspect of the second and third metacarpals.
- Acropachy occurs most frequently in patients who have the ophthalmopathy or dermopathy associated with autoimmune thyroid disease.

## Hyperparathyroidism

See ⊃ Chapter 16.
The following points refer to both primary and secondary disease:
- MSK symptoms are the initial manifestation in up to 16% of patients with primary hyperparathyroidism.
- Hyperparathyroidism, chondrocalcinosis, and CPPD frequently coexist. Acute CPPD can be triggered by parathyroidectomy.
- Chronic CPPD arthropathy can mimic RA. Unlike RA, synovial proliferation is absent. Radiographically, erosions have a predilection for the carpus, mid-feet and second/third MCPJs. Pericapsular calcification is often present.
- An erosive polyarthritis favouring the large joints can occur with renal osteodystrophy in patients with chronic renal failure on dialysis. It may relate to a number of different, or combination of, crystal induced inflammatory-based mechanisms (hydroxyapatite, basic calcium phosphate, pyrophosphate, urate).

- Hyperparathyroidism is associated with a specific shoulder arthropathy characterized by intra/periarticular erosions of the humeral head. This may be sub-clinical.
- Subjective muscle weakness and fatigability are common complaints. Typically, muscle enzymes are normal and biopsy shows type II fibre atrophy; the features of an inflammatory myopathy are generally absent.
- The hallmark of radiographic changes is bone resorption: sub-periosteal (typically on the radial side of second and third phalanges), intracortical, subchondral, trabecular, sub-ligamentous, and localized (Brown's tumours) resorption patterns are seen. Bone sclerosis, periostitis, and chondrocalcinosis also occur.
- Fragility fracture is common and often precedes a diagnosis of primary hyperparathyroidism. Although significant and fast accretion of bone occurs after surgery, bone mass often remains low long term.

## Acromegaly

- Over-stimulation of bone and connective tissue cells from excessive growth hormone can result in several features: bursal and cartilage hyperplasia, synovial and bony proliferation, an OA-like picture, backache, and hypermobility.
- Joint complaints usually manifest about 10 years after the onset of clinical acromegaly. Knees are frequently affected.
- Joint symptoms are not typical of an inflammatory arthritis. Morning stiffness is not prominent and joint swelling is present in <50%.
- Carpal tunnel syndrome affects >50% and is frequently bilateral.
- Back and neck pain and radicular symptoms from nerve root compression or spinal stenosis are not uncommon and are related to axial bony proliferation.
- A painless proximal myopathy occurs infrequently.
- Radiographs characteristically show widened joint spaces (e.g. >2.5 mm in adult MCPJs) and a thickened heel pad (>23 mm in men and >21.5 mm in women).
- Diagnosis relies on demonstration of a failure of growth hormone to be suppressed by a glucose tolerance test, but a lateral skull radiograph is a good screening test as 90% have enlargement of the pituitary fossa.

# Gut and hepatobiliary conditions

MSK features frequently occur in patients with gut or hepatobiliary disease (Table 4.5).

- Data on the frequency of rheumatological features are largely based on studies of hospital patients with clinically overt gut or biliary disease—leading to an underestimate of the frequency of association.

**Table 4.5** Associations between gastrointestinal (GI) and rheumatic disorders

| GI disorder> | Rheumatic disorder | Association |
|---|---|---|
| Enteric infection | Reactive arthritis: self-limiting in most | Arthritis in 2% who get *Shigella, Salmonella, Yersinia, Campylobacter, Clostridium difficile* overall but in 20% of infected who are HLA-B27+ |
| Crohn's disease | Arthritis 20%. AS 10%. Sacroiliitis in 26% | 60% of spondyloarthritis patients have histological evidence of bowel inflammation. See also below in table |
| Ulcerative colitis | Arthritis 20%. AS 7%. Sacroiliitis 15% | See also above in table. Severity of gut and joint inflammation varies in its association but SI joint/pine inflammation does not |
| Whipple's disease | Migratory arthritis in >60% | *Tropheryma whipplei* identified in small bowel. Diarrhoea occurs in >75% ultimately |
| Intestinal bypass surgery (blind loop syndrome) | Polyarticular symptoms 50% in scleroderma | Intestinal bacterial overgrowth in small bowel? Associated with joint symptoms |
| Coeliac disease | Arthritis is rare | ?Increased intestinal permeability |
| Viral enteritis | Rare (<0.5%) | Most common: Coxsackie or echo |
| Hepatitis A | Arthralgia 15%. Vasculitis rare | Causal association |
| Hepatitis B | Arthralgia 10–25%. PAN | Aetiological |
| Hepatitis C | Sialadenitis in >50%. Vasculitis (cryoglobulinaemic) | ?Aetiological in Sjögren's syndrome. Hepatitis C identified in 27–96% of patients with cryoglobulinaemia |
| Primary biliary cirrhosis | Polyarthritis 19%. Scleroderma 18%. Sjögren's 50% | Autoimmune 'overlap'. Features may be subclinical |
| Chronic active hepatitis | Polyarthralgia or arthritis in 25–50% | Autoimmunity |
| Haemochromatosis | OA 50% | Iron storage disease |
| Wilson's disease | OA in 50% adults. Chondrocalcinosis | Copper storage disease |

- Well-established associations include:
  - toxic effects of medications (e.g. NSAIDs; see ➲ Chapter 3).
  - irritable bowel syndrome and fibromyalgia.
  - functional GI motility disorders (e.g. SScl, EDS).
  - sacroiliitis, arthritis, and enthesitis in patients with SpA and IBD.
  - degenerative arthritis in haemochromatosis and Wilson's disease.
- The frequency of enthesitis in patients with IBD may be underestimated. Enthesitis may be detected at the medial/lateral humeral epicondyles, Achilles' tendon insertion, calcaneal plantar fascia origin and insertion, greater trochanters, and the patellar tendon origin and its insertion at the tibial tubercle.
- Radiology studies in patients with IBD suggest that sacroiliitis is under-recognized by clinicians.

*Severity of rheumatologic manifestations*

- Optimal surveillance strategies for the MSK manifestations of gut or biliary disease are not known in many instances.
- Faecal calprotectin is a sensitive measure for IBD screening in patients with SpA, but modest elevations can occur in a number of scenarios.
- Life-threatening vasculitis may occur from chronic viral infection. Hepatitis B is associated with polyarteritis nodosa, and hepatitis C may lead to cryoglobulinaemic vasculitis.
- In most patients who develop joint inflammation or enthesitis after bacterial dysentery, the condition is self-limiting. Chronicity and severity may be linked to HLA-B27. Progressive spondylitis is rare.

## Gut and hepatobiliary conditions in patients with rheumatic diseases

(Tables 4.6 and 4.7; also see ➲ Chapter 15, 'Vasculitis')

- The most common problem among patients with RA is dyspepsia associated with gastroduodenal erosions or ulcers due to NSAIDs. Peptic lesions may be clinically silent and may present with dropping haemoglobin levels or an acute bleed.
- RA may be the most common cause of AA amyloidosis. Biopsies of the upper GI tract will demonstrate amyloid deposits in 13% of patients. There are numerous GI manifestations of amyloidosis, including GI haemorrhage, malabsorption, obstruction, and hepatosplenomegaly.
- In SLE, serious gut and hepatobiliary manifestations are relatively uncommon (5%), but nausea, anorexia, vomiting, and diarrhoea are quite frequent.
- SScl has numerous GI manifestations including refractory gastro-oesophageal reflux disease, gastric antral vascular ectasia ('watermelon stomach'), oesophageal dysmotility, bacterial over-growth, and faecal incontinence.
- The reflux associated with SScl often requires treatment with high-dose proton pump inhibitors.
- 'Watermelon stomach' can lead to significant acute and chronic haemorrhage.
- In SScl, bloating and abdominal distension caused by bacterial overgrowth may respond to cyclic courses of antibiotics.

Table 4.6 Gut and hepatobiliary manifestations of rheumatological diseases I: general

| Disease | Abnormalities | Presentation with |
|---|---|---|
| Rheumatoid arthritis (see ⊃ Chapter 5) | TMJ arthritis. Oesophageal dysmotility | Impaired mastication Dysphagia, reflux |
| | GI vasculitis (0.1%) | Ulcers, pain, infarction |
| | Portal hypertension | Splenomegaly (Felty's) |
| | Liver involvement (Felty's) | Enzyme abnormalities |
| | Hepatosplenomegaly | Palpable viscera |
| Systemic lupus (see ⊃ Chapter 10) | Oesophageal dysmotility | Dysphagia, reflux |
| | GI vasculitis | Ulcers, pain, perforation |
| | Protein-losing enteropathy | Hypoalbuminaemia |
| | Peritonitis | Ascites (10%), serositis |
| | Hepatosplenomegaly (30%) | Palpable viscera |
| Scleroderma (see ⊃ Chapter 13) | Oesophageal dysmotility | Heartburn/dysphagia |
| | Delayed gastric emptying | Aggravated reflux |
| | Intestinal dysmotility and fibrosis (80%) | Malabsorption, pseudo-obstruction (<1%) |
| | Pseudo- and wide-mouth diverticula | Haemorrhage, stasis, bacterial overgrowth |
| Polymyositis and dermatomyositis (see ⊃ Chapter 14) | Muscle weakness | Aspiration, dysphagia |
| | Disordered motility | Dysphagia, constipation |
| | Vasculitis (rare) | Ulcers, perforation |
| MCTD | Hypomobility | Dysphagia, reflux, pseudo-obstruction |
| Sjögren's syndrome (see ⊃ Chapter 12) | Membrane desiccation | Xerostomia, dysphagia |
| | Oesophageal webs (10%) | Dysphagia (>60%) |
| | Gastric infiltrates/atrophy | Masses, dyspepsia |
| | Pancreatitis | Pain, amylasaemia |
| | Hepatic dysfunction | Hepatomegaly (~25%) |
| | Hepatic cirrhosis | Primary biliary cirrhosis |
| Spondyloarthritis (see ⊃ Chapter 8) | Ileocolonic inflammation | May be asymptomatic |
| Adult-onset Still's disease | Hepatitis, peritonitis, hepatosplenomegaly | Pain or abnormal enzymes (~75%) |
| Systemic JIA (see ⊃ Chapter 9) | Serositis | Abdominal pain |
| | Hepatomegaly | Abnormal enzymes |
| Marfan syndrome, joint hypermobility syndrome, Ehlers–Danlos syndrome(see ⊃ Chapter 19) | Defective collagen | Hypomotility, malabsorption, visceral rupture/laxity |
| | | Functional GI disorders |

**Table 4.7** Gut and hepatobiliary manifestations of rheumatic diseases II: vasculitis. See also ➔ Chapter 15

| Disease | Frequency of GI vasculitis and features |
| --- | --- |
| Polyarteritis nodosa | 80% (mesenteric). Buccal ulcers, cholecystitis (15%), bowel infarction, perforation, appendicitis, pancreatitis, strictures, chronic wasting syndrome |
| Henoch–Schönlein purpura | 44–68%. Abdominal pain, melena, haematemesis, ulcers, intussusception, cholecystitis, infarction, perforation, appendicitis |
| EGPA | ~40%. Haemorrhage, ulceration, infarction, perforation |
| Behçet's disease | Buccal and intestinal ulcers, haemorrhage, perforation, pyloric stenosis, rectal ulcers |
| Systemic lupus erythematosus | 2%. Buccal ulcers, ileocolitis, gastritis, ulceration, perforation, intussusception, volvulus (1%), pneumatosis |
| Kawasaki disease | Abdominal pain, intestinal obstruction, non-infective diarrhoea |
| AAV | <5%. Cholecystitis, appendicitis, ileocolitis, infarction |
| Juvenile dermatomyositis | Well recognized. Perforation, pneumatosis |
| MCTD | Rare. Ulceration, perforation, pancreatitis |
| RA and JIA | 0.1%. Buccal ulcers, abdominal pain, peptic ulcers, acalculus-cholecystitis, gut infarction, and perforation |
| Polymyositis and dermatomyositis | Very rare. Mucosal ulcers, perforation, and pneumatosis |
| Cryoglobulinaemia | Rare. Ischaemia and infarction |

- Mesenteric vasculitis is classically caused by polyarteritis nodosa, but can be seen with a variety of rheumatic illnesses, including Takayasu arteritis, AAV, and (rarely) with SLE. Although mesenteric angina is the symptom most strongly associated with mesenteric vasculitis, the earliest sign of intestinal ischaemia is diarrhoea.
- HSP is an IgA-mediated small vessel vasculitis that presents with colicky abdominal pain and purpura (adults and children). Although generally mild and self-limited in children, it can occasionally cause intussusception and bowel necrosis.

## Gut and hepatobiliary side effects from drugs used in treating rheumatic and bone diseases

(See also ➔ Chapter 23.)

The main rheumatology drugs causing side effects are:
- NSAIDs—which are a common cause of GI distress. COX-2 inhibitors were developed to decrease the risk of peptic ulcer disease; most have been withdrawn from the market due to concerns regarding increased risk of cardiovascular events and those remaining may be no more effective than taking a conventional NSAID with a proton pump inhibitor.

- Glucocorticoids may cause gastritis, peptic ulcer disease, and GI haemorrhage. Although the absolute increase in events is small, the combination of steroids and NSAIDs results in a synergistic increase in the risk of GI sequelae.
- Methotrexate (MTX) may cause stomatitis, which may respond to supplemental folate. Nausea, emesis, and dysgeusia may respond to dose reduction. MTX can cause a transaminitis; it is therefore recommended that patients minimize alcohol intake.
- Sulfasalazine gut and hepatobiliary side effects are common and may occur in up to 20% of patients. The most frequent are mild: indigestion, nausea, vomiting, anorexia, and abdominal pain. Gut ulceration, bloody diarrhoea and serious liver problems are rare; in 65% of patients, side effects occur in the first 3 months of treatment.
- Azathioprine (AZA) can cause nausea (15%), vomiting (10%), and abdominal pain (8%). Diarrhoea is rare (5%). Liver enzyme abnormalities are often mild and may remit on lowering the dose. The GI side effects can occur in patients with normal levels of thiopurine methyltransferase.
- Penicillamine causes altered taste (25% within the first 3–6 months), nausea or vomiting (18%), and stomatitis/mouth ulcers (5%). Hepatotoxicity and haemorrhagic colitis are rare.
- Chloroquine and hydroxychloroquine, can cause non-specific GI intolerance (10%). The onset is often insidious.
- Ciclosporin causes gingival hyperplasia, nausea, diarrhoea, and elevation in hepatic enzymes.
- Effects of cyclophosphamide on the gut are frequent: nausea, vomiting, diarrhoea, and stomatitis. Serious hepatotoxicity is rare.
- Leflunomide can cause nausea (8–13%), diarrhoea (up to 25%), and abnormal liver enzymes. In studies, most rises in transaminases have been mild (<2-fold) and are reversible on drug withdrawal.
- Oral bisphosphonates (such as alendronic acid and risedronate) and strontium ranelate can cause nausea, dyspepsia, and diarrhoea. Oesophageal ulceration has occasionally been noted with alendronate, although it is thought this occurs only in people who do not follow the instructions for taking them. Myalgias and arthralgias can also occur with bisphosphonates.
- Calcitonin either given as subcutaneous injection or as nasal spray can give abdominal pains and diarrhoea.

## Malignancy

# Malignancy

Rheumatic MSK features may be clues to the existence of cancer. Symptoms may arise directly from neoplastic tissue invasion or indirectly as a paraneoplastic phenomenon.

## Primary and secondary neoplastic diseases of bone and joints

- Synovial tumours are rare. Sarcoma (synovioma) is more common in men than women and unusual in those >60 years. It usually occurs in the legs (70%) and can occur around tendon sheaths and bursa. At diagnosis, pulmonary metastases are common.
- Para-articular involvement by bone tumours may give a monoarticular effusion. Invasion of synovium may occur and malignant cells can be detected in joint fluid. Breast, bronchogenic carcinoma, GI tumours, and melanoma can all metastasize to joints.
- Lymphomas and leukaemias may simulate various conditions especially in children and cause synovitis in a single or in multiple joints.
- Arthritis complicating the presentation of myeloma or an acute leukaemia is most likely to be polyarticular and asymmetric.
- In adults, arthritis complicating leukaemia is rare (5% of cases).
- Leukaemia is the most common cause of neoplastic skeletal symptoms in childhood and adolescence (15% of leukaemia cases).
- Neuroblastomas are the most frequent cause of a solid tumour metastasizing to the skeleton in children.

## Clues that may lead to a suspicion of malignancy directly causing MSK symptoms

- Constitutional symptoms without evidence for vasculitis.
- The coexistence of bone pain from metastases (see ➔ Plate 16). Also, consider metabolic bone diseases, sarcoid, SAPHO syndrome, and the SpA conditions.
- Haemorrhagic joint fluid (also consider trauma, PVNS, chondrocalcinosis/pseudogout).
- Radiographs that show adjacent bone destruction, perhaps with loss of cortex (also consider infection).
- Radiographic calcification in soft tissue mass (consider synovioma).

## Paraneoplastic idiopathic inflammatory myopathy (IIM)

- IIMs may be due to carcinomatous neuromyopathy.
- Polymyositis, dermatomyositis, Eaton–Lambert myasthenic syndrome (ELMS), and hypophosphataemic (oncogenic) osteomalacia are all found in association with malignancy (Table 4.8).
- Carcinomatous neuromyopathy is characterized by symmetric muscle weakness and wasting and can pre-date the malignancy.

**Table 4.8** Myopathy and links with malignancy

| Condition | Typical pattern of weakness | Common cancer associations | Other features |
|---|---|---|---|
| Carcinomatous neuromyopathy | Pelvic girdle—symmetric | *Lung:* 15% men, 12% women. *Ovary:* 16%. *Stomach:* 7% men, 13% women | Wasting, EMG abnormality, and increase in muscle enzymes are not invariable |
| Dermatomyositis (+?PM) | Proximal limb. Truncal | Reflects underlying cancer frequency in local population | Response to steroids is usual |
| Myasthenia gravis (MG) | Frequently ocular and bulbar muscles involved | Thymus. Any | Muscle strength fluctuates (fatiguability). Responds to anti-cholinesterases |
| Eaton–Lambert myasthenic syndrome (ELMS) | Pelvic girdle muscles. Altered gait. Ocular muscles not affected | Small cell lung. Can occur up to 2–3 years after ELMS | Autonomic disturbances. EMG + poor response to anticholinesterase distinguish from MG |
| Oncogenic osteomalacia | Generalized. Develops insidiously | Small, discrete mesenchymal tumours in bone, soft tissues, and sinuses. Neurofibromatosis | Bone pain and osteomalacia. High FGF23, hypophosphataemia and low $1,25(OH)_2$-vit-D |

## Non-myopathy paraneoplastic syndromes

- The non-myopathic paraneoplastic syndromes are rare.
- Hypertrophic pulmonary osteoarthropathy consists of clubbing, periostitis of diaphysis of long bones, and an arthropathy (varies from arthralgias to diffuse polyarthritis). Suspicion of HPOA should be investigated with bone scintigraphy, which typically shows increased radionuclide uptake in affected bones. Radiographs often show periosteal elevation.
- HPOA complicates 20% of primary lung tumours, but it is associated with other malignancies.
- Polyarthritis may be the presenting feature of cancer. Most cases occur >60 years old. The arthritis associated with malignancy tends to be asymmetric, and does not cause erosions.
- Eosinophilic fasciitis, severe bilateral palmar fasciitis (often mistaken for scleroderma), and fasciitis associated with panniculitis have been associated with malignancy.
- Cases of 'shoulder–hand' syndrome (a form of osteodystrophy; see ➲ Chapter 22) have been reported in association with malignancy.

## Rheumatological diseases associated with an increased incidence of malignancy

A number of rheumatic MSK diseases are associated with an increased incidence of malignancy compared with healthy populations.

- Non-Hodgkin's lymphoma is most strongly associated with RA. Myeloma and paraproteinaemia are also found in RA patients.
- The relative risk of colon cancer among RA patients is 0.77; this may be due to the use of chronic NSAIDs in this patient population, which may be protective.
- Non-Hodgkin's lymphoma develops in a subset of patients with Sjögren's syndrome (4%). Its onset may be indicated by rapid enlargement of salivary glands, the appearance of a paraprotein, or decrease in circulating immunoglobulins or RF titre.
- SScl has been associated with an increased risk of both lung cancer and non-Hodgkin's lymphoma.
- Dermatomyositis is probably associated with malignancy in adults, though as convincing evidence for an association of polymyositis with malignancy is lacking. Gonadal tumours are relatively common among such patients.
- Eosinophilic fasciitis may be associated with malignancy.

## Rheumatological drugs and malignancy

(See also → Chapter 23.)

- Chronic azathioprine use is associated with an increased risk of skin cancer so patients taking azathioprine long term should be counselled regarding sun protection and monitoring for skin cancer.
- Use of cyclophosphamide is associated with an increased risk of lymphoma and bladder cancer.
- Anti-TNFα drug therapy is theoretically associated with a risk of malignancy. However, patient disease registries have not identified an excess incidence in patients treated long-term with the therapy.
- If malignancy develops while a patient is taking anti-TNFα then usually its correct to stop the therapy.
- There is incomplete data on whether starting anti-TNFα increases the risk of relapse of malignancy in patients previously treated successfully for their cancer.
- Though very high dose per weight teriparatide is associated with sarcoma development in rats, there is no evidence, at doses used in humans, that there is an increased risk.
- The following have not been associated with an increased risk of malignancy (as of 2016): sulfasalazine, leflunomide, rituximab, abatacept, apremilast, ustekinumab, secukinumab, belimumab, and denosumab.

# Neurological conditions

Entrapment neuropathies and radicular lesions are discussed in ➋ Chapter 3. Also, radiculopathy is included in ➋ Chapter 21.

## Inflammatory peripheral neuropathy

- Inflammatory neuropathies can occur as part of any AICTD, though are probably most likely to occur in association with SLE and Sjögren's syndrome.
- Vasculitis (and probably APS) can cause small vessel vascular lesions which compromise peripheral nerve function and cause sensory, and if severe, motor features of nerve damage.
- Nerve conduction studies may form part of the investigations at the outset of characterizing systemic vasculitis and severe AICTDs.
- Mononeuritis occurring as part of RA is possible but nowadays is very unlikely unless severe RA disease is left untreated.

## Entrapment neuropathies

- Entrapment neuropathies are common in rheumatological practice. Symptoms arising from these lesions include paraesthesiae, a feeling of swelling, numbness and a burning quality to pain in the distribution of the trapped nerve.
- Median nerve irritation/entrapment may be secondary to carpal OA or inflammation secondary to inflammatory arthritis.
- Ulnar nerve irritation (fourth and fifth finger territory symptoms) is most commonly associated with medial elbow lesions.

## Spinal cord lesions

Spinal cord lesions usually arise due to intrinsic spinal canal or extrinsic compression or inflammation.

- Tumours and ischaemic spinal cord lesions often present acutely with upper motor neuron features distal to the affected level and issues of bladder and bowel sphincter control.
- Some tumours and syrinxes (thoracic, neck) can cause subacute evolution of pyramidal features in the legs (often not pain but stiffness and motor function problems).
- Extrinsic cord compression can occur secondary to tumours, osteoporotic vertebral and a combination of (usually degenerative) lesions. In the latter, spinal cord compression is rarely acute and because it evolves very slowly is often overlooked in the elderly.
- Transverse myelitis causes acute focal back pain and distal spinal cord symptoms and features including acute lower limb motor symptoms. It is a feature of SLE and APS.

## Cerebrovascular lesions

- Acute cerebellar or stroke-like symptoms can be a presenting feature of ischaemic lesions secondary to APS. If occurring in the non-elderly <60 years then screening for APS and SLE is mandatory.

- Cerebral lupus can be present with profound symptoms of confusion and brain function decompensation or may be subtler presenting with mild cognitive or frontal cortex dysfunction.
- Conventional stroke disease is a complication of many inflammatory rheumatic diseases, probably most associated with APS and ongoing poorly controlled inflammatory disease and in the context of other risk factors (e.g. smoking, metabolic syndrome in PsA, glucocorticoid-associated hyperlipidaemia).

## Headache

- Among the causes of headache in rheumatological practice, neurological causes are probably rare.
- The hemicranial headache (with scalp sensitivity) of GCA and drug-induced headache are the most likely causes of headache encountered in rheumatology patients.
- Other causes of headache occasionally encountered are the global headache from cranial sinus thrombosis in Behçet's disease, and meningeal lesions (e.g. in neurosarcoid).

## Neuromyopathy

- Neuromyopathies may present to rheumatologists with focal pain or generalized pain and weakness.
- Focal neuromyopathies can occur after nerve trauma or infection. Marked acute wasting with pain, often with raised CK and a myositis-type signal on MRI, can be seen.
- Fluctuating neuromyopathic effects can occur in myasthenia gravis. There may be a variation of effects over a day with muscle fatigue influencing the timing, characteristics, and severity of weakness. Symptoms can be focal—as in orbital muscle myasthenia, which can present initially with diplopia—or general involving larger muscle groups.

# Ophthalmic conditions

Blepharitis, conjunctivitis, uveitis, and ischaemic lesions can all occur with rheumatic MSK diseases.

### Dry eye (xerophthalmia)

- Xerophthalmia often presents with sore or gritty eyes and sensitivity in certain atmospheric environments (e.g. air-conditioning). Oddly patients can get epiphorae if tear film is not drained because of inferior orbital duct blockage through to the sinuses.
- Blepharitis is often a consequence of dry eye—lids can get 'sticky'.
- Xerophthalmia is most severe in primary Sjögren's syndrome but can occur in SOX syndrome and all autoimmune joint and connective tissue diseases (secondary Sjögren's syndrome).

### Uveitis

- Anterior uveitis can be acute or chronic. Symptoms include ocular pain and photophobia. The eye becomes visibly erythematous.
- The most common associations of anterior uveitis include SpAs, sarcoid Behçet's disease, and JIA.
- All children and adolescents diagnosed with any form of JIA, regardless of ANA status, should have an eye examination to rule out uveitis.

### Ischaemic ophthalmic lesions

- Retinal examination is the most direct and accessible way to visualize blood vessels *in vivo*.
- Ophthalmic examination is valuable in the assessment of systemic vasculitis.
- The input of an experienced medical ophthalmologist is essential in departments that offer a service to manage vasculitis patients.
- The ischaemic lesions of GCA can present variably but most typically with amaurosis symptoms (visual field curtaining).

### Scleral and corneal disease

- Lesions of the sclera and cornea are rare in rheumatology patients except in severe (usually high-titre seropositive) RA patients.
- Scleral or corneal disease in an RA patient should prompt consideration of the presence of systemic RA vasculitis.

### Other

- Proptosis is a recognized feature of AAV and is usually due to granulomatous inflammation in the retro-orbital space.
- Conjunctivitis can accompany many diseases but is an acute lesion in some cases of (SpA-associated) reactive arthritis.
- Ophthalmoplegia is a recognized presenting feature of mononeuritis associated with systemic vasculitis. Cerebrovascular disease (thus APS and GCA also) should be considered as possible in relevant patients also.

# Part II

# The clinical features and management of rheumatic diseases

# Rheumatoid arthritis

# Introduction

### Epidemiology

Rheumatoid arthritis (RA) is the most common inflammatory arthritis, with an incidence in the general UK population of 1.5 and 3.6 per 10,000 people per year, for male and females respectively.

- RA affects people worldwide and affects females more frequently than males, with a F:M ratio of ~3:1.
- RA most commonly occurs at age 45–65 years although it can occur at any age—occurring as a distinct disease in childhood.

### Classification

The updated ACR/EULAR 2010 classification criteria (Table 5.1) have been designed to identify early RA. However, they should not be used to exclude the diagnosis if all criteria are not met; clinical judgement should be used.

### Pathogenesis

RA is an autoimmune inflammatory disease, manifest primarily in synovial tissues, mediated by interaction between T lymphocytes, B lymphocytes, and synovial fibroblasts, leading to dysregulation of the inflammatory cascade.

- Smoking increases the risk of developing RA.
- Familial RA does exist but the odds ratio of developing RA if there is a first-degree relative with the disease is only 1.1.

### Immunopathology

Overproduction of inflammatory cytokines, in particular tumour necrosis factor-$\alpha$ (TNF$\alpha$) and interleukin-6 (IL-6), is central to the pathology of RA.

- Persistent inflammation leads to increased vascularity and inflammation of the synovial lining of joints (synovitis), and secondary cartilage degradation (joint space narrowing) and bone erosion.
- Autoantibodies are seen in 50–80% of RA cases, in particular rheumatoid factor (RF) and anticitrullinated peptide antibodies (ACPA).
- The sensitivity and specificity of ACPA for identifying RA is greater than that of RF (67% and 95% for ACPA vs 69% and 85% for RF, respectively).[1]
- Positivity for both RF and ACPA has a near 100% positive predictive value for subsequent development of RA.
- Genetics also contribute to the risk of developing RA. HLA-DRB1 is most commonly associated with RA, and is often referred to as the 'shared epitope'.

### Synovial pathology

The exact reason why synovium is targeted is unknown. Synovium in joints and tendons becomes inflamed and local tissue damage of cartilage, bone, and surrounding tissues ensues.

- There is increased synovial vascularity, influx of monocytes and plasma cells, and activation of tissue macrophages and fibroblasts.
- Synovial plasma cells are numerous and produce antibodies which will have a proinflammatory local effect.
- Cellular activation of cytokines locally results in bone resorption activating osteoclasts causing bone erosion.

**Table 5.1** ACR/EULAR 2010 classification criteria for rheumatoid arthritis

Target population is patients who have ≥1 joint with definite clinical synovitis (swelling)* with the synovitis not better explained by another disease.

*Classification criteria for RA. Add score of categories A–D; a score of ≥6/10 is needed for classification of a patient as having definite RA.‡*

| | Score |
|---|---|
| **A. Joint involvement**§ | |
| 1 large joint¶ | 0 |
| 2–10 large joints | 1 |
| 1–3 small joints (± involvement of large joints)** | 2 |
| 4–10 small joints (with or without involvement of large joints) | 3 |
| >10 joints (>1 small joint) | 5 |
| **B. Serology (at least 1 test result is needed for classification)** ‡‡ | |
| Negative RF and negative ACPA | 0 |
| Low-positive RF or low-positive ACPA | 2 |
| High-positive RF or high-positive ACPA | 3 |
| **C. Acute-phase reactants (at least 1 test result is needed)**§§ | |
| Normal CRP and normal ESR | 0 |
| Abnormal CRP or abnormal ESR | 1 |
| **D. Duration of symptoms** | |
| <6 weeks | 0 |
| ≥6 weeks | 1 |

* Criteria are aimed at classification of newly presenting patients. Patients with erosive disease typical of RA plus history compatible with fulfilment of the 2010 criteria and patients with long-standing disease, should be classified as having RA.

‡ Although scores < 6/10 are not classified as having RA, criteria may be reassessed and fulfilled cumulatively over time.

§ Joint involvement refers to any swollen or tender joint, which may be confirmed by imaging evidence of synovitis. DIPJs, 1st CMC and 1st MTP joints are excluded.

¶ 'Large joints' are shoulders, elbows, hips, knees, and ankles.

** 'Small joints' are MCPJs, PIPJs, 2nd to 5th MTPJs, thumb IPJs and wrists.

‡‡ 'Negative' refers to international unit (IU) values that are ≤ to the upper limit of normal (ULN) for the laboratory assay; low +ve refers to IU values that are higher than the ULN but less than 3× the ULN for the laboratory and assay; high +ve refers to IU values that are more than 3× the ULN for the laboratory and assay. If only +ve or −ve RF information is available, a +ve result = low-positive for RF.

§§ Normal/abnormal determined by local laboratory standards.

ACPA, anti-citrullinated protein antibody; CRP, C-reactive protein; ESR, erythrocyte sedimentation rate

Guidelines reproduced from Aletaha D et al. 2010 'Rheumatoid Arthritis Classification Criteria' (2010) *Arthritis & Rheumatism* 62:9 2569–2581 with permission from John Wiley and Sons.

- In severe cases, cellular aggregation can lead to lymphoid follicles forming in the synovial tissue.
- Extra-synovial inflammation includes rheumatoid nodule formation and inflammation of lung and cardiac tissue.

## Reference

1. Nishimura K, Sugiyama D, Kogata Y, et al. Meta-analysis: diagnostic accuracy of ACPA and RF for RA. Ann Intern Med 2007;146:797–808.

# Clinical features

RA is characterized by swelling, pain, and stiffness of synovial joints, systemic features, and involvement of extra-articular organs and tissue.

## Joints and tendons

RA typically affects the small joints of the hands and feet, but can affect any joint (bursa or tendon) where there is synovial tissue (e.g. elbows, shoulders, ankles, knees, hips, and TMJs).

- Symptoms characteristically include stiffness worse in the morning, and lasts for >30 min.
- Joint symptoms develop over weeks, but can also do so over a few days. Occasionally symptoms can have a migratory onset over months, with temporary periods of resolution/improvement.
- Movement of the affected joints often alleviates stiffness and discomfort in the early stages of the disease.
- Active movement of an inflamed joint can cause 'gelling' where the patient describes an abrupt momentary 'paralysis' of movement.
- The functional impact of joint symptoms should be assessed. The Health Assessment Questionnaire (HAQ) is helpful to provide a standardized assessment of disability.
- Examination should focus on any affected joints, assessing for the degree of swelling, warmth, and range of movement.
- Joint or tendon synovitis may not be detectable clinically in the early/mild stages of disease. Boggy swelling over the joint line is indicative of joint synovitis. Ballotable joint effusions can be present if larger joints are involved.
- In the early stages of the disease, deformities are not seen; however, in aggressive, longstanding, or untreated disease, deformity can occur and lead to significant disability.
- Deformities seen in RA include:
  - ulnar deviation at the wrist, often accompanied by a depressible prominent ulna styloid (piano-key sign).
  - swan-neck and boutonniere deformities may be identified in the fingers in advanced disease.
  - fixed loss of extension deformities.
  - limited shoulder movement, due to joint erosion, effusion, or ligament rupture.
  - lateral deviation of the toes.
  - subluxation of the metatarsal heads leads to discomfort when walking. Callosities, skin degradation, soft tissue infection, and osteomyelitis may ensue.
- At the atlanto-axial joint, erosion of the odontoid can lead to an unstable C1–C2 articulation, with potentially life-threatening consequences from cord or brainstem compression.
- Symptoms of atlanto-axial joint involvement can include occipital pain, syncope, and headaches.
- The consequences of small cervical facet joint involvement can be upper limb radicular symptoms and hand weakness, and if the spinal cord is affected, stiffness (including of legs).
- The differential of lower cervical radiculopathy is carpal tunnel syndrome—also a secondary lesion in RA from wrist joint disease.

## Extra-articular features

- Rheumatoid nodules are associated with seropositivity (RF and ACPA) and can occur anywhere in the body, but are most commonly found on the hands, feet, and elbows. When a small mass/nodule is identified in any internal organ in a RA patient, cancer must be excluded before attributing the lesion to a rheumatoid nodule.
- RA is associated with pulmonary fibrosis, exudative pleural effusions, and pleurisy.
- Splenomegaly is common, and may be part of Felty's syndrome (RA, neutropenia, and splenomegaly).
- Lymphadenopathy can be due to RA but patients also have a greater likelihood of developing lymphoma compared to the general population, so investigation of 'B symptoms' is very important.
- Neurological examination may reveal nerve impingement due to synovitis, tenosynovitis (e.g. carpal tunnel syndrome), joint damage, or bony impingement (e.g. spinal nerve root impingement).
- Rheumatoid vasculitis can present as a mononeuritis multiplex.
- Leucocytoclastic rashes are rare but may cause skin ulceration.
- The most common ophthalmic manifestation is dry eyes (sicca).
- Painful scleritis, leading to scleromalacia, is a serious sight-threatening condition. Scleral thinning may manifest as a darkening of the sclera, and requires urgent ophthalmic input.

## Systemic features and assessment

- Fatigue is often a prominent symptom and is challenging to manage.
- Disease activity should be assessed using a standardized clinical outcome measure at each clinical review. The most commonly used measure is the Disease Activity Score of 28 joints (DAS28).
- Other disease activity measures include the Clinical Disease Activity Index (CDAI), and the Simplified Disease Activity Index (SDAI).

## Associated clinical manifestations

- Patients with RA have an increased risk of developing septic arthritis due to pre-existing joint damage and use of immunosuppressants.
- Active RA commonly is associated with muscle atrophy, primarily due to reduced use, but also due to systemic inflammation.
- Osteoporosis is more common in RA than the general population, due to systemic inflammation, reduced mobility, and steroids.
- Osteoporosis risk should be assessed in patients >40 years using FRAX® (℗ http://www.shef.ac.uk/FRAX) and in postmenopausal women and men >50 years using FRAX® and DXA scanning.
- Patients with RA have an increased cardio- and cerebrovascular risk profile due to chronic inflammation promoting atherosclerosis. Active risk management is important.
- Secondary amyloidosis is increasingly uncommon, but should be considered in patients with long-standing active disease.

# Investigations

RA is primarily a clinical diagnosis. However, a set of baseline investigations can assist in making the diagnosis, and provide a point of reference for monitoring disease progression, drug response, and toxicity.

- Laboratory tests should be done to aid diagnosis, as a baseline before and when monitoring disease-modifying antirheumatic drugs (DMARDs; Table 5.2).
- Imaging can confirm a clinical diagnosis and characterize synovitis in joints and tendons, evaluate joint and bone damage from joint inflammation, and can help exclude alternative diagnoses (Table 5.3).
- Key to diagnosis is detection of ACPA and RF. ACPA are as sensitive for diagnosis of RA as RF but are more specific.

**Table 5.2** Suggested baseline laboratory investigations for RA

| Investigation | | Interpretation |
|---|---|---|
| Full blood count | Hb ↓/↔ | Due to chronic inflammation/bone marrow suppression. Often low MCV and MCH owing to poor utilization of iron into erythrocyte precursors |
| | Platelets ↑/↔ | Due to inflammatory response |
| | WCC ↑/↔ Neuts ↑/↔ Lymph ↓ Eos ↑/↔ | Total WCC/neut count often ↑ from inflammatory response, with infection and in haematological malignancies.GCs cause ↑ neuts (↓ vascular margination). Mild ↑ in eosinophils. If persistent ↑ then investigate alternative causes (e.g. EGPA, parasitic or helminth infection). |
| Renal tests | Creat ↑/↔ GFR ↓/↔ Urea ↑/↔ K ↔; Na ↔ | NSAIDs can cause renal impairment. Many DMARDs are renal-excreted ∴ baseline renal function important. If unexplained renal dysfunction, consider amyloidosis or drug cause. |
| Liver function tests | ALT ↔ ALP ↔ Albumin ↔ INR ↔ | Most DMARDs are metabolized in liver. If ↑ consider drug effect |
| Inflammatory markers | CRP ↑ ESR ↑ | Typically elevated in active RA, although normal inflammatory markers do not exclude a diagnosis of RA |
| Autoantibodies | RF ACPA ANA | One/both/neither may be present but if both negative be rigorous about making a correct diagnosis (differential inflammatory OA, CPPD polyarthritis, PsA). The autoantibody titres are not related to disease activity. ANA positivity can occur with overlap (SLE or primary Sjögren's) |

ALP, alkaline phosphatase; ALT, alanine aminotransferase; AST, aspartate aminotransferase; CPPD, calcium pyrophosphate dihydrate disease Cr, creatinine; CRP, C-reactive protein; EGPA, eosinophilic granulomatous with polyangiitis; ESR, erythrocyte sedimentation rate; GFR, glomerular filtration rate; Hb, haemoglobin; K, potassium; Na, sodium; WCC, white cell count.

**Table 5.3** Baseline imaging investigations useful in RA

| Investigation | | Interpretation |
|---|---|---|
| Radiographs | Hands and feet<br>CXR<br>Other | Hands (including wrists) and feet to assess for erosions, periarticular osteopenia and soft tissue swelling<br>CXR to assess for pulmonary fibrosis prior to starting DMARDs<br>Flexion/extension sagittal C-spine films to assess for C1/C2 instability |
| Ultrasound | Hands and wrists, feet and other joints | Helpful for assessing for synovitis, hyper-vascularity, effusion, and early erosions. Can aid diagnosis if little clinical synovitis present, or if it is unclear if joint pain is due to inflammation or structural damage. Effective at providing dynamic joint imaging (e.g. shoulder, ankle, wrist) |
| MRI | C-spine, specific joints | Essential to assess for cervical myelopathy if C1/C2 instability suspected<br>Joint MRI helpful to confirm joint and tendon synovitis, identify pre-erosions and erosions, and rule out other MSK lesions at (symptoms/sign-affected) sites |
| DXA | | RA is a risk factor for osteoporosis. DXA (hip and spine) should be done at any age if the patient is on steroids or has had a fragility fracture, and in all postmenopausal women and men >50 yrs old |

CXR, chest X-ray; MRI, magnetic resonance imaging.

# Management

### General considerations

Intensive target-driven treatment of RA, aiming for disease remission, is recommended.[2, 3] All patients with RA should have access to regular meetings with a rheumatologist. Patient involvement and shared decision-making is essential in treatment planning. For example, for a guide to RA management by auditable standards, see NICE Clinical Guideline 79.[2]

- Remission is defined depending on the disease activity score used (e.g. <2.6 using DAS28).
- Early institution of DMARD therapy, usually with conventional synthetic DMARDs (csDMARDs) initially before the onset of joint damage, is essential (see ➲ Chapter 23 for DMARD nomenclature).
- A 'treat-to-target approach' has been shown to improve outcomes in RA and involves setting a realistic treatment target (e.g. remission) with the patient and escalating treatment until the goal is reached. This approach can be intensive and requires frequent patient meetings or contacts to assess treatment response until the target is achieved.
- While remission is an appropriate target in early disease, patients with long-standing disease may require a more pragmatic target, such as low disease activity.
- A multidisciplinary approach is essential when managing RA:
  - Early and regular specialist practitioner consults can help both disease and medicines management, as well as self-management through education and a deeper understanding of the patient of their RA.
  - Early referral to physiotherapy and occupational therapy is recommended to advise patients on appropriate exercises to maximize joint movement, function, and strength.
  - Living aids, pacing, coping skills, and self-management of disease activity flares/fatigue can also be learned through therapy and practitioner input.
  - Early institution of strategies to help patients to continue to participate in work and social activities is essential to maintaining a good quality of life for individuals with RA.
  - Podiatric or foot orthotics input can be helpful to alleviate foot symptoms and deformity.
  - RA can lead to problems with low mood and depression so screening for psychological dysfunction and referral for specialist input is very important.
- Patients with RA have a higher risk of developing cardiovascular and cerebrovascular disease. An annual review and management of risk factors is therefore mandatory.

**First-line*:**
**Combination synthetic DMARD (assess response over 3–6 months) + glucocorticoids if needed:**
– Methotrexate (first line) plus at least one of:
– Hydroxychloroquine
– Sulfasalazine
– Leflunomide  (prescribed at 10 mg daily if concomitantly with methotrexate, and with closer monitoring)

**Second-line*:**
**Continued severe disease (DAS28 >5.1 at two time-points ≥1 month apart) unresponsive to combination synthetic DMARDs at maximum tolerated dose (or significant side effects/intolerance to DMARDs).**
Combination methotrexate + biologic DMARD:
– anti-TNFα
– tocilizumab
– abatacept
Assess response over 3–6 months (see specific NICE guidance if patient is methotrexate intolerant).

**Third-line*:**
**Continued severe disease after 6 months (DAS28>5.1, or no reduction in DAS28 >0.6 from baseline – classed as 'EULAR moderate response'), loss of response, or significant side-effects or intolerance to the first biologic DMARD.**
Switch to methotrexate + second-line biologic DMARD:
– alternative anti-TNFα
– rituximab
– tocilizumab
– abatacept
Assess response over 3–6 months (see specific NICE guidance if methotrexate not tolerated).

**Ongoing management and monitoring:**
Analgesia:
   Paracetamol or weak opiates as required.
   NSAIDs as required at lowest dose and for the shortest time possible
Glucocorticoids:
   Either oral/IM/IA/IV on an 'as required' basis
MDT involvement with education & counselling:
   Rheumatology specialist nurse, physiotherapy, occupational therapy, podiatry, primary care, psychological support, and social services. Patient advice line for flare management.
Comorbidity and lifestyle optimization:
   Cardio/cerebrovascular disease risk management, diabetes, hypertension, optimise body weight, smoking cessation, and fragility fracture risk/osteoporosis management.

**Figure 5.1** Summary of UK National Institute for Health and Care Excellence (NICE) guidance for the management of RA *This summarizes UK (NHS care) NICE guidelines. Local/regional guidelines may vary. Guidelines adapted from NICE https://www.nice.org.uk/guidance/cg79.

## General pain-relieving measures and analgesia

Analgesia can help manage symptoms while csDMARD and/or biologic DMARD therapy (bDMARD) takes effect, and to treat flares of disease activity.

- Paracetamol and/or weak opiates (or in combination) will reduce pain and can be well tolerated.
- Concomitant NSAIDs (preferentially selective COX-2 inhibitors are invariably effective though they are tolerated variably).
- NSAIDs should be prescribed at the lowest effective dose and for the shortest time possible.
- A proton pump inhibitor to reduce the risk of gastrointestinal (GI) ulcers and to reduce GORD symptoms should be considered, especially in patient aged >65 years, or with a history of GI disease.
- When choosing a NSAID/COX-2 inhibitor, consider a patient's individual risk factors, and choose a drug which least increases these risks. Patients should be counselled about the possible cardiorenal, GI, and liver side effects.
- Transcutaneous electrical nerve stimulation (TENS) can be a helpful measure to manage local/regional pain, and poses few side effects. Broken skin and areas with reduced sensation (i.e. diabetic neuropathy) should be avoided.

## Synthetic DMARD medications (sDMARDs)

For a more detailed discussion, see ➔ Chapter 23.

RA immunotherapeutics need planning with each patient. Objectives and a time-frame for achieving objective should be set by agreement. There needs to be a baseline safety assessment (Box 5.1) and careful monitoring of disease activity, any disability, comorbidity, and drug effects (Box 5.2).

- Methotrexate (MTX) is the first-line conventional sDMARD of choice. sDMARD doses should be escalated rapidly if tolerated.
- All sDMARDs and bDMARDs have a variable time to onset of efficacy, between 3 and 6 months.
- Combination therapy (>1 sDMARD), ideally including MTX, is recommended if tolerated.
- There is good quality evidence that using low-dose GC therapy during the first 6 months (e.g. 'COBRA-lite' 30 mg prednisolone daily initially), in order to achieve early disease control, reduces long-term structural joint damage.
- Once disease control is achieved, GCs should be tapered and stopped as quickly as possible.
- Intra-articular (IA) GC injections can be efficacious for particularly swollen joints. IM and IV GCs can be helpful to manage flares of joint pain/disease activity.
- If combination sDMARD therapy is ineffective, early escalation to biological therapy should be considered.
- MTX should be co-prescribed with biologic therapy (particularly with anti-TNFα) where possible, as it improves anti-TNFα response and persistence.
- If first-line biologic therapy is inefficacious, switching to another biological agent is recommended.

## Box 5.1 Investigations and assessments to consider before starting sDMARDs for RA

### Height, weight, blood pressure

Some sDMARDs cause ↑ blood pressure, so a baseline measure is required. Height and weight are required for drugs prescribed by ('ideal') bodyweight.

### Laboratory tests and imaging

See Table 5.2 and Table 5.3, respectively.

### Comorbidities

Review comorbidities, especially any respiratory, hepatic, or renal conditions that may affect sDMARD choice. Consider screening for occult viral infection (such as hepatitis/HIV).

### Pregnancy, fertility and breastfeeding

Discuss current and future plans for pregnancy and breastfeeding and tailor treatment accordingly.

### Vaccinations

Vaccinations against pneumococcus and influenza before starting sDMARDs or biologics are recommended. Live vaccines are not recommended (except with hydroxychloroquine or SSZ). The shingles vaccine is a live vaccine and evidence is limited on the use in immunocompromised individuals. Local recommendations and clinician discretion should guide decisions. Prior to commencing anti-TNFα, hepatitis B vaccination should be considered in at-risk individuals.

Data from Ledingham J et al. BSR and BHPR guideline for the prescription and monitoring of non-biologic disease-modifying anti-rheumatic drugs. *Rheumatology* 2017;56(6):865–8.

### Methotrexate (MTX)

- Once-weekly oral preparation, or subcutaneous (SC) injection. Folic acid co-prescription, often the day after MTX administration.
- Therapeutic range is approximately 10–25 mg weekly and time to therapeutic effect: 8–12 weeks.
- Toxicity (stomatitis, GI disturbance, dysphoria-lassitude effects, and alopecia) may be addressed by the addition of folic acid daily (apart from day of MTX dosing).
- SC administration is a useful option if oral treatment is not tolerated. There is some evidence of improved efficacy with SC compared with oral administration, due to the higher bioavailability.
- Mild drug-induced hepatitis is relatively common and is often corrected by the addition of folic acid. Routine liver biopsy is not necessary, but can be helpful in patients with other liver disease or persistent low-grade liver function abnormalities.
- Liver function abnormalities fluctuate and may require the drug to be stopped for a short period if transaminase levels rise above 2–3 times the upper limit of normal, with re-introduction after a period of time when levels have normalized, with close monitoring.
- Myelosuppression is rarely severe. Antifolate drugs such as trimethoprim and folate deficiency increase the risk of toxicity.
- Renal impairment reduces MTX clearance and may lead to toxicity.
- Concomitant NSAID use is not contraindicated, but monitoring for hepatotoxicity is recommended.

## Box 5.2 Managing and monitoring sDMARDs: British Society for Rheumatology UK recommendations

### Methotrexate (MTX)

Co-prescribed with weekly folic acid (e.g. 5 mg/day after MTX).

Teratogenic. Not safe in breastfeeding. Advise low alcohol intake. Rarely causes pneumonitis (caution with pre-existing lung disease/poor respiratory reserve). Rarely causes myelosuppression.

*Monitoring*: FBC, Cr/GFR, ALT, albumin all 2-weekly until dose/results stable then monthly for 3 months then 3-monthly thereafter.

### Sulfasalazine (SSZ)

GI side effects early in treatment course generally mild and do often subside. Very rarely causes leucopenia, pancytopenia, haemolysis, and aplastic anaemia in early treatment. Reduced potency in men.

*Monitoring*: FBC, Cr, ALT, albumin all 2-weekly until dose/results stable, then monthly for 3 months, then 3-monthly until 12 months and no routine monitoring required thereafter.

### Hydroxychloroquine (HCQ)

Cumulative dose should not exceed 6.5 mg/kg of body weight.

*Monitoring*: no routine lab monitoring required. Eye screening within 1 year of starting and then annually if on drug for >5 years.

### Leflunomide (LEF)

Diarrhoea relatively common side effect. Can cause hypertension so avoid if BP uncontrolled. Not recommended in pregnancy or breastfeeding. Long half-life drug and requires active washout if there is severe toxicity (e.g. 10-day cholestyramine). Rarely causes pneumonitis.

*Monitoring*: FBC, Cr, ALT, albumin: all 2-weekly until dose/results stable then monthly for 3 months then 3-monthly thereafter. BP monthly.

### Azathioprine (AZA)

Assess thiopurine methyltransferase (TPMT) genotype before treatment. If likely absent TPMT activity do not prescribe AZA. Avoid co-prescription with allopurinol (blocks excretion of AZA). GI disturbance relatively common but often mild. Relatively safe in pregnancy.

*Monitoring*: FBC, Cr, ALT, albumin: 2-weekly until dose/results stable, then monthly for 3 months then 3-monthly thereafter.

### IM gold

Can cause bone marrow and liver disturbance. Contraindicated in pregnancy/breastfeeding. Rarely: hypersensitivity reactions from injections. Long-term treatment can cause chrysiasis (grey/blue skin pigmentation).

*Monitoring*: FBC, Cr, ALT, albumin: all 2-weekly until dose/results stable then monthly for 3 months then 3-monthly thereafter. Urinalysis for blood and protein prior to each dose.

Data from Ledingham J et al. BSR and BHPR guideline for the prescription and monitoring of non-biologic disease-modifying anti-rheumatic drugs. *Rheumatology* 2017;56(6):865–8.

### Sulfasalazine (SSZ)

- Daily oral preparation. Therapeutic range 1.5–3 g daily in twice-daily doses.
- Time to therapeutic effect: 12 weeks.
- Toxicity: may cause leucopenia, pancytopenia, haemolysis, aplastic anaemia, and hepatic transaminitis. Bone marrow toxicity unusual.
- SSZ can rarely cause a hypersensitivity reaction characterized by LFT abnormalities, lymphadenopathy, and rash.
- Spermatogenesis and libido can be affected by SSZ, but it is reversible. No apparent adverse effect on female fertility.

### Hydroxychloroquine (HCQ)

- Daily oral preparation with usual therapeutic dose 200 mg twice daily.
- Time to therapeutic effect: about 12 weeks.
- Retinal toxicity and maculopathy are rare. The risk increases with abnormal liver or kidney function; after a cumulative dose >1000 g; and treatment duration >5–7 years.

### Leflunomide (LFN)

- Daily oral preparation. Therapeutic dose 20 mg daily.
- Time to therapeutic effect: 12 weeks
- LFN is an inhibitor of the enzyme dihydro-orotate dehydrogenase and shows antiproliferative activity, inhibiting pyrimidine synthesis. It has a long half-life of 2 weeks.
- Initially, it was administered with a loading dose of 100 mg daily for 3 days followed by maintenance therapy with 10–20 mg daily. The loading dose was associated with diarrhoea in many patients, and clinicians now use maintenance therapy dose from the start.
- Side effects include myelosuppression, elevation of liver transaminases, diarrhoea, and hypertension. Severe hepatitis is uncommon and usually occurs in the first 6 months of treatment.
- The long half-life has implications for drug withdrawal. If rapid washout is required, cholestyramine for between 14 days to 6 weeks should be prescribed, followed by two blood tests to ensure drug levels are below 0.02 mg/L.

### Azathioprine (AZA)

- Daily oral preparation dose range 2–2.5 mg/kg/day in twice-daily or three times a day doses.
- Time to therapeutic effect: 12 weeks.
- Infrequently used for RA as therapeutic effect relatively weak.
- Toxicity: may cause leucopenia, pancytopenia, haemolysis, and aplastic anaemia; especially in individuals with low/absent thiopurine methyltransferase (TPMT) activity. AZA should not be prescribed for patients with 'low-activity'-associated TPMT alleles.

### Gold (myocrisin)

- IM preparation with loading doses then usually 50 mg monthly.
- Time to therapeutic effect: variable.
- Infrequently used for RA nowadays (and auranofin, the oral gold salt preparation, is even less seldom used).
- Toxicity: hypersensitivity to injections, permanent blue/grey skin discoloration, renal and liver dysfunction can occur uncommonly.

*Glucocorticoids (GCs)*
- Oral, IM, IV, or IA use.
- Time to therapeutic effect: depends on the mode of administration; hours/days.
- IM and oral GCs can be very effective to manage flares and as a bridge to sDMARDs taking effect.
- IA injections are of value in symptom control, in both early disease and flares. However, their effect is transient, with little impact on the overall process of RA, and should not be repeated any more than 3-monthly.
- Caution should be exercised if considering IA injection in anticoagulated patients as the risk of haemarthrosis is increased.
- There is no evidence to suggest an increased risk of joint infection, as long as an aseptic technique is used.
- Long-term systemic GCs can have sequelae, including cataracts, premature coronary artery disease, osteoporosis, muscle atrophy, insulin resistance/diabetes, and osteonecrosis. Appropriate fracture prevention therapy should be given to patients expected to be on glucocorticoid therapy for >6 weeks at a dose ≥7.5 mg.

*Anti-tumour necrosis factor α therapy (anti-TNFα)*
Baseline assessment is advisable (Box 5.1 and Box 5.3).
- Given SC (e.g. etanercept, adalimumab) or IV (e.g. infliximab).
- Time to effect: 2–24 weeks.
- TNFα is a potent pro-inflammatory cytokine whose levels are elevated in RA.
- Anti-TNFα therapies are available as originator or biosimilar drugs—mainly either monoclonal antibodies or receptor fusion proteins (infliximab, etanercept, adalimumab, certolizumab, golimumab).
- Common adverse effects include infection, headache, nausea, and injection-site reactions, and increased risk of infection.
- Rarely can trigger a (ANA-positive) lupus-like syndrome responsive to therapy withdrawal.
- Very rarely can cause demyelination.
- Withdraw if cardiac failure worsens.
- Consider withdrawal if interstitial lung disease develops or worsens.
- Can cause psoriasis when used to treat RA and even worsens psoriasis in PsA patients ('paradoxical psoriasis'). This is a class effect and will re-occur if an alternative anti-TNFα is tried.
- Antibodies can develop versus the therapeutic antibody/fusion protein. Such antibodies can be detected by specific immunoassays. MTX therapy may reduce anti-anti-TNFα drug antibody formation.

*B-cell depletion (anti-CD20): rituximab (RTX)*
Baseline assessment is advisable (Box 5.1 and Box 5.3).
- Given IV. A dose consists of 1g given twice by infusions given 2 weeks apart. Most rheumatologists advocate a minimum of 6 months between subsequent doses, but often required less frequently. Usually co-administered with IV GCs.
- Time to therapeutic effect: 12–24 weeks.

## Box 5.3 Investigations and considerations before starting biologic therapy

### TB infection

All patients should be screened (history, CXR, T-spot/IgRA test) for presence of active or latent mycobacterial infections and treated according to current guidelines before starting biologic therapy.

### Hepatitis

Screen all patients starting a biologic for hepatitis B and C. Increased risk of infusion reactions in patients with hepatitis C treated with RTX.

### HIV

A thorough history is required and if any risk factors are present, HIV testing should be undertaken.

### Malignancy

See ➓ 'RA-associated cancer risk', p. 260.

### ANA testing

Anti-TNFα therapy has been associated with development of lupus-like syndrome in rare cases. Obtain a baseline test of ANA.

### Demyelination (including optic neuritis)

Anti-TNFα therapy has been associated with demyelination, and it should not be prescribed to patients with a history of demyelination.

### Cardiac failure

Anti-TNFα is not recommended with NYHA grade 3/4 cardiac failure.

### Interstitial lung disease (ILD)

There is mixed evidence on the association of anti-TNFα therapy and ILD. Monitoring lung function should be considered.

### Uveitis

Anti-TNFα should be used cautiously in patients with pre-existing uveitis. Some studies have identified an increased risk of uveitis.

### Fasting lipids

Patients starting on tocilizumab (TCZ) should have a baseline fasting lipid profile. A repeat profile is recommended after 3 months of treatment. If worsening lipid level, consider reviewing treatment. Ongoing monitoring should be in line with local guidelines and individual risk factors.

### Immunoglobulins

Immunoglobulins should be checked in patients starting RTX, 4–6 months after an infusion, and before each treatment. There's an increased risk of infection with IgG <6 g/L.

ANA, antinuclear antibodies; NYHA, New York Heart Association; RTX, rituximab.

Information summarized from Ding T, et al. BSR and BHPR rheumatoid arthritis guidelines on safety of anti-TNF therapies. *Rheumatology* 2010;49:2217–9.

- B cells play an important role in the pathogenesis of RA and administration of rituximab leads to rapid CD20 positive B-cell depletion in the peripheral blood. Normal B-cell repopulation occurs within the next 3 months.
- The best responses are seen in RF-seropositive patients, and when co-prescribed with MTX. If patients are unable to take MTX then consider LFN or RTX monotherapy.
- RTX is contraindicated if there is hypogammaglobulinaemia.
- Very rarely causes progressive multifocal leucoencephalopathy.

*CTLA4-Ig: abatacept (ABA)*
Baseline assessment is advisable (Box 5.1 and Box 5.3).
- Given SC (125 mg weekly) or IV (maintenance dose every 4 weeks according to weight).
- Time to effect: 12–24 weeks.
- Abatacept disrupts the CD80/86 co-stimulatory signal required for T-cell activation by competing with CD28 for binding.
- Co-prescription with MTX is advisable.

*Anti-interleukin-6 receptor blocker: tocilizumab (TCZ)*
Baseline assessment is advisable (Box 5.1 and Box 5.3).
- Given SC (162 mg weekly) or IV (8 mg/kg every 4 weeks).
- Time to effect: 12–24 weeks.
- IL-6 is a potent pro-inflammatory cytokine. High levels have been found in serum and synovial fluid of RA patients, and levels correlate with disease activity.
- Tocilizumab binds specifically to both soluble (sIL-6R) and membrane-bound IL-6 receptors (mIL-6R).
- Best results are when it is co-prescribed with MTX, but is licensed as monotherapy.
- Use with caution in patients with a history of diverticulitis due to increased risk of gut perforation. Risk is elevated if patient taking GCs and/or NSAIDs. Patients need counselling about the risk.

## Biologic DMARD biosimilars

The European Medicines Agency defines biosimilars as 'a biological medicine that is similar to another biological medicine that has already been authorised for use'. This usually occurs after a patent expires on an originator drug. See Box 5.4.
- Since biologic therapies are derived from yeast or bacterium, biosimilars are not identical to the originator drug and as such, cannot be classed as a generic drug.
- For this reason, caution should be exercised if switching between originator and biosimilar compounds.
- At the time of writing, three anti-TNFα biosimilar therapies were available. Experience in the widespread use of biosimilars is lacking.
- There are currently no long-term data on the use of biosimilars. If starting or switching a patient into a biosimilar drug, consider enrolling the patient onto a patient (national) registry.
- Guidance regarding usage (including switching) of biosimilars varies widely, so it is advised to follow local policies.

**Box 5.4 The British Society for Rheumatology consensus guidelines for biologic therapies for RA**

*Anti-TNFα\**

Local guidelines vary on blood monitoring requirement for anti-TNFα. It is prudent to check FBC with WCC regularly to screen for neutropenia and malignancy such as lymphoma.[4]

*Anti-IL-6 receptor (TCZ)*

Check WCC and neutrophil count monthly for 6 months. If no neutropenia occurs in the first 6 months, monitoring can be reduced to 2-3 monthly. For TCZ monotherapy, check LFTs monthly for the first 6-months, then every 2-3 months if results are stable. For TCZ co-prescribed with sDMARDs, monthly LFT monitoring is recommended.[5]

*Abatacept (ABA)*

None available. For safety and monitoring, see information on its SPC at ℬ http://www.medicines.org.uk

*Anti-CD20 (RTX)*

Check immunoglobulins 4–6 months after each infusion. If there is active infection, IgG levels <6g/L or very low CD4/CD8 counts, withhold treatment.[6] See also its SPC at ℬ http://www.medicines.org.uk

FBC, full blood count; LFTs, liver function tests; RTX, rituximab; WCC, white cell count.

\* 2010 BSR Guidelines to be updated in 2017. Please see BSR website: ℬ https://www.rheumatology.org.uk/

## Novel medications on the horizon

- In addition to currently licensed drugs, numerous drugs are in development for use in RA. Most notable of these are small molecules that target intracellular processes involved in RA.
- Small molecule drugs can be administered orally.
- Janus kinase (JAK) inhibitors have been extensively investigated and one JAK inhibitor (tofacitinib) is currently available in the USA for the treatment of RA.
- Further biologic therapies continue to be developed and trialled in RA, including IL-17 inhibitors and variations on IL-6 blockade.

## Managing infections while on immunosuppression

The main risk of immunosuppression is infection. 'Serious infection' is generally defined as an infection that requires hospitalization or parenteral antimicrobial treatment.

- See references 4 and 7 at the end of the chapter for full details.
- Generally, all sDMARDs (with the exception of HCQ) should be stopped during any serious infection, and until recovery is complete.
- Biologic DMARDs should be discontinued during serious infection.
- Anti-TNFα therapy increases the risk of getting a serious infection, and infection can present atypically, so vigilance is required.

- A careful review of the risks and benefits of anti-TNFα therapy should be undertaken, especially in patients with:
  - chronic infected leg ulcers.
  - septic arthritis of a native joint within the last 12 months.
  - sepsis of a prosthetic joint within the last 12 months (if removed) or indefinitely (if joint remains *in situ*).
  - persistent/recurrent chest infections.
  - indwelling urinary catheter.
  - bronchiectasis.
  - hypogammaglobulinaemia.

*Tuberculosis (TB)*
- If a patient develops symptoms suggested of TB infection while on anti-TNFα, anti-mycobacterial treatment should be initiated.
- If the patient remains systemically well, anti-TNFα therapy may continue while the TB infection is treated.
- Patients on anti-TNFα therapy are more likely to develop extra-pulmonary TB.
- Non-TB mycoplasma infections are rare and require expert advice.
- Evidence for the occurrence of TB with other biologic agents is limited, but appears to be less than for anti-TNFα.

*Opportunistic infection risk issues*
- While rare, monitor for opportunistic bacterial (e.g. *Listeria, Salmonella*) and fungal (e.g. histoplasmosis, candidiasis, aspergillosis, *Coccidioides, Pneumocystis jirovecii*) infections in patients treated with anti-TNFα.
- Consider treatment with varicella zoster immunoglobulin in all immunocompromised RA patients who have had significant contact with an individual with varicella zoster.
- Treat shingles and herpes zoster according to standard guidance.

## RA-associated cancer risk

There is an increased risk of malignancy with RA, with a standardized incidence ratio (SIR) of 1.1. The risk is greatest for Hodgkin's (SIR 3.21) and lung cancer (SIR 1.64).[8]
- A recent study from the BSR Biologics Register for RA reported no increased risk of solid tumours with anti-TNFα therapy when compared to RA patients treated with sDMARDs.[9]
- There is some evidence that skin cancers (both non-melanoma and melanoma) may be more likely.
- There is a theoretical increased risk of cancer in patients treated with anti-TNFα therapy who have previously had a cancer, or have risk factors for cancer (e.g. smoking). Treatment decisions should be made on a case-by-case basis. However, because patients with previous cancer have been excluded from most RCTs, little is known about the risk in this context.
- Data on cancer risk are scarce for other biologics; primarily due to smaller numbers of patients taking these drugs and shorter exposure times since drug licensing.

## Pregnancy and breastfeeding with RA

The topic has been extensively reviewed quite recently.[10]

- RA often improves in pregnancy, particularly in the third trimester.
- Preconception counselling is essential, as many sDMARDs are contraindicated in pregnancy and breastfeeding, and some sDMARDs can affect fertility.
- Ideally, conception should be planned and medications optimized prior to conception.
- The management of RA in pregnancy should be discussed with all women of childbearing age, and men considering having children.
- It is important to review how the pregnancy and birth are likely to proceed. If possible, early referral to a specialist obstetric clinic with expertise managing pregnant women with RA is recommended.
- If RA affects the hip, pelvis, or spine, an obstetric review is necessary to discuss birth plans and analgesia.
- RA may make certain tasks more difficult for the new mother or father with RA (e.g. changing nappies, bathing the baby). Planning and addressing these problems prospectively is recommended.
- Patients should have a method of contacting the rheumatology team (e.g. telephone advice line) should difficulties arise. A management strategy should be agreed with the patient and obstetric and primary care team should the RA flare in the perinatal period. Arrangement for an early rheumatology review in the postnatal period, to ensure optimal disease management, is recommended.
- Drug use in pregnancy needs careful planning. Guidelines updating practice have been recently published (Box 5.5).
- Paracetamol is safe in pregnancy and breastfeeding. Intermittent use might be reasonable given restrictions on NSAID use (see Box 5.5). Avoid regular paracetamol use during weeks 8–14 of pregnancy as there is a small risk of cryptorchidism. There are no data on paternal exposure, but paracetamol is likely to be safe.
- Biologic therapy experience is emerging for a number of the therapies but for abatacept there are still very few data on its safety.

## Surgery in RA patients

A thorough perioperative plan should be made for all patients.

- Inform the surgical and anaesthetic team of the diagnosis of RA and any relevant complications/comorbidities.
- Spinal involvement should be highlighted to the anaesthetist, to inform intubation, positioning, and spinal anaesthesia.
- Respiratory involvement may make artificial ventilation challenging, and increase the risk of postoperative infection.
- Postoperative occupational and physiotherapy will need to be tailored to accommodate the patient's RA.
- For elective procedures, advance assessment and preparation of the home environment should be undertaken to facilitate rehabilitation.
- Generally, sDMARDs should be continued throughout the perioperative period, to minimize the need for GCs (as the latter increase risk of surgical site infection and non-healing).

## Box 5.5 The British Society for Rheumatology 2016 guidelines for prescribing NSAIDs, GCs, sDMARDs, and bDMARDs in pregnancy and breastfeeding

*NSAIDs (including COX-2 selective NSAIDs)*
Limited evidence. Possible ↑ risk of miscarriage and fetal malformation ∴ caution in first trimester. Stop NSAID by 32 weeks' gestation to avoid premature closure of ductus arteriosus. NSAIDs are excreted in breast milk but no evidence of harm. Compatible with paternal exposure.

*Glucocorticoids (GCs)*
Compatible with pregnancy and breastfeeding.

*Hydroxychloroquine (HQC)*
Compatible with pregnancy and breastfeeding.

*Methotrexate (MTX)*
Contraindicated in pregnancy and breastfeeding. Stop MTX >3 months before conception. In accidental pregnancy, stop MTX and start folic acid (5 mg/day). Low-dose MTX paternal exposure probably not risky.

*Sulfasalazine (SSZ)*
Compatible with pregnancy (use folic acid 5 mg/day) and breastfeeding.
May ↓ fertility in men, however, don't stop SSZ to improve fertility unless conception is delayed >12 months.

*Leflunomide (LEF)*
Not recommended in pregnancy or when breastfeeding. Women considering pregnancy should undergo cholestyramine washout prior to conception. If accidental conception occurs, cholestyramine washout should be instituted until LEF plasma levels are undetectable.

*Azathioprine (AZA)*
Compatible with pregnancy at doses ≤2 mg/kg/day and in breastfeeding and with paternal exposure.

*Anti-TNFα*
Infliximab: stop after 16 weeks' gestation. Compatible with paternal exposure. Etanercept: stop by third trimester. Compatible with paternal exposure. Adalimumab: stop by third trimester. Compatible with paternal exposure. Certolizumab pegol: compatible with all trimesters of pregnancy. Compatible with paternal exposure. Breastfeeding probably safe on any anti-TNFα therapy, although evidence is limited.

*Rituximab (RTX)*
Stop 6 months before pregnancy. No evidence on RTX during breastfeeding. Second/third trimester exposure associated with neonatal B-cell depletion. Limited evidence on paternal exposure—likely not harmful.

*Tocilizumab*
Stop 3 months <conception. No data on breastfeeding.

Data from Flint J et al. BSR and BHPR guideline on prescribing for rheumatological conditions in pregnancy and breastfeeding. Part 1 and II. ♫ https://www.rheumatology.org.uk/Knowledge/Excellence/Guidelines

- For high-risk ('dirty'/lengthy) procedures and when patients have comorbidities, sDMARDs may need to be stopped.
- Close monitoring of renal function is essential in the perioperative period, to monitor for sDMARD-related toxicity.
- Anti-TNFα therapy should be stopped before surgery. 'Washout' times for biologics vary depending on half-life of the drug.
- Biologics can be restarted after surgery once good wound healing has progressed and there is no evidence of infection. Please refer to local guidelines, but a typical current practice is to stop biologic therapy 2 weeks prior to surgery, and restart 2 weeks after surgery.

## Complementary therapies for RA

- Some patients will want treatment from complementary therapists, either in advance or during their long-term management of RA.
- Some commonly used complementary therapies include acupuncture, chiropractic, homeopathy, aromatherapy, and faith healing.
- Patients often find treatments beneficial, and provided they do no harm, there is generally no reason to advise patients to stop treatment.
- It is important to highlight the absence of robust evidence for these treatments, and they are not a substitution for standard management.
- Spinal/neck manipulation is generally not recommended, especially if RA is known to affect the spine.
- Inquire about any supplements, herbal, or other medication use that might interfere with the metabolism of analgesics and sDMARDs.
- Please refer to ➔ Chapter 9 for information on juvenile RF-positive polyarthritis.

## References

2. NICE. *Rheumatoid Arthritis in Adults: Management* (Last updated: December 2015). London: NICE. ℬ http://www.nice.org.uk/guidance/cg79
3. Smolen JS, Landewé R, Bijlsma J, et al. EULAR recommendations for the management of RA with synthetic and biological disease-modifying antirheumatic drugs: 2016 update. *Ann Rheum Dis* 2017;76:960–77. ℬ http://ard.bmj.com/content/early/2017/03/06/annrheumdis-2016-210715
4. Ding T, Ledingham J, Luqmani R, et al. BSR and BHPR RA guidelines on safety of anti-TNF therapies. *Rheumatology* 2010;49:2217–9.
5. Malaviya AP, Ledingham J, Bloxham J, et al. The 2013 BSR and BHPR guideline for the use of intravenous tocilizumab in the treatment of adult patients with rheumatoid arthritis. *Rheumatology* 2014;53:1344–6.
6. Bukhari M, Abernethy R, Deighton C, et al. BSR and BHPR guidelines on the use of rituximab in rheumatoid arthritis. *Rheumatology* 2011;50:2311–3.
7. Ledingham J, Gullick N, Irving K, et al. BSR and BHPR guideline for the prescription and monitoring of non-biologic DMARDs. *Rheumatology* 2017;56:865–8.
8. Simon TA, Thompson A, Gandhi KK, et al. Incidence of malignancy in adult patients with rheumatoid arthritis: a meta-analysis. *Arthritis Res Ther* 2015;17:212.
9. Mercer LK, Lunt M, Low AL, et al. Risk of solid cancer in patients exposed to anti-tumour necrosis factor therapy: results from the British Society for Rheumatology Biologics Register for Rheumatoid Arthritis. *Ann Rheum Dis* 2015;74:1087–93.
10. Flint J, Panchal S, Hurrell A, et al. BSR and BHPR guideline on prescribing for rheumatological conditions in pregnancy and breastfeeding. Part 1 and II. ℬ https://www.rheumatology.org.uk/Knowledge/Excellence/Guidelines

# Osteoarthritis

# Introduction

Osteoarthritis (OA) is a chronic disorder characterized by cartilage loss, bone remodelling, joint deformity, and synovial inflammation. It is the most common joint disease in humans.

# Epidemiology

- It is estimated that 8.5 million people in the UK have joint pain attributable to OA, and that 15% of the UK population aged >55 years have symptomatic knee OA.
- The prevalence of radiographic hand OA in the UK is estimated at 4.4 million people, significant radiographic knee OA at 0.5 million people, and significant radiographic hip OA at 0.2 million.[1]
- By 2020, OA is expected to be the fourth leading cause of disability in the world.
- OA poses a significant economic burden on the UK economy, using 1% of gross domestic product, and causing 36 million working days to be lost each year.[2]

## References

1. Arthritis and Musculoskeletal Alliance. *Standards of Care for People with Osteoarthritis.* London: ARMA, 2004.
2. NICE. *Osteoarthritis: Care and Management of Osteoarthritis in Adults.* Clinical Guideline 59. London: NICE, 2008.

# Pathology

- Although there are recognized associations between OA, age, and trauma, advances in knowledge of cartilage biochemistry and the recognition of crystal-associated disease have renewed interest in OA as a dynamic condition of cartilage loss (chondropathy) with periarticular bone reaction.
- At present, OA is assessed and managed clinically as a structural, rather than physiological condition, with an emphasis on established disease and disease prevention.
- Chondrocyte dysfunction leads to changes in the extracellular matrix, and metalloproteinase enzyme release.
- Proteoglycan degradation leads to oedema and micro-fissures in the cartilage. Micro-fissures progress to subchondral cysts and erosions.
- Cartilage degradation products stimulate synovial inflammation and the production of pro-inflammatory cytokines (e.g. IL1 and TNFα).
- Macroscopic changes in OA include cystic bone degeneration, cartilage loss, and growth of bone at joint margins (osteophytes).
- Microscopic changes include flaking and fibrillation of articular cartilage with variations in vascularity and mineralization of subchondral bone, leading to sclerosis and new bone formation.
- Most surveys of OA rely on radiographic features for definition and severity—this is problematic because of poor correlation of radiographic change with clinical status, symptoms, or function.
- Radiographic staging is best done at the hip and knee, but is poorest in the hand and spine. The correlation between pathology and radiology is shown in Table 6.1.

**Table 6.1** Radiographic–pathology correlates in OA

| Pathological change | Radiographic abnormality |
| --- | --- |
| Cartilage fibrillation, erosion | Localized joint-space narrowing |
| Subchondral new bone | Sclerosis |
| Myxoid degeneration | Subchondral cysts |
| Trabecular compression | Bone collapse/attrition |
| Fragmentation of osteochondral surface | Osseous ('loose') bodies |

# Aetiology

- Females are at higher risk of OA (relative risk (RR) 2.6) and tend to develop structural damage more quickly, and are more likely to proceed to a total hip arthroplasty.
- Hip OA is more common in Europeans than in Asians or in African Americans.
- The Framingham study found that 27% of people aged 63–70 years, and 44% of people aged >80 years had radiographic knee OA.
- A UK study showed that 50% of adults aged >50 years with radiographic knee OA had symptoms. Similar figures are seen in hip OA.
- Notably only 3–7% of people with radiographic features of hands OA, are symptomatic.
- Risk factors associated with OA include the following:
  - Family history; particularly with generalized nodal OA.
  - Genetics: increased concordance for OA in monozygotic vs dizygotic twins, and particularly for nodal OA.
  - Genome-wide association studies have identified genetic loci associated with OA: hand OA with chromosomes 1, 7, 9, 13, and 19; knee OA with the LRCH1 gene on chromosome 13; hip OA with chromosome 11 (RR 1.4–1.6).
  - Genetics of bone or articular cartilage structure (COL2A1 gene).
  - High bone density.
  - Calcium crystal deposition disease and acromegaly.
  - Obesity (close association with onset and progression of knee and hand OA, but not hip OA).
  - Femoral dysplasia (hip OA).
  - Trauma (repeated or single event).
  - Low vitamin C and D levels (progression of knee OA).
- Factors with less, or no, evidence for there being a risk for OA:
  - For hip OA: previous hip disease (e.g. Perthes disease), acetabular dysplasia, avascular necrosis of the femoral head, severe trauma, generalized OA, and occupation (e.g. farming).
  - There is little evidence to link OA with repetitive injury from occupation or sports, such as running in those with normal joints, except perhaps knee-bending in men.

## Clinical Features

# Clinical features

The symptoms, and to a degree, most features of OA (Table 6.2), often do not correlate with functional or anatomical change judged radiographically.

- Several potential mechanisms may be responsible for the pain associated with OA.
  - Since cartilage is aneural, pain may arise from a number of other sites: inflammatory mediators causing intra-articular hypertension, capsular distension, and/or stimulation of synovial and subchondral bone nerve fibres.
  - Concomitant enthesopathy or bursitis may lead to pain.
- Morning stiffness of <30 min is common in OA.
- Muscle weakness and atrophy due to altered joint use is common.
- Several subsets of OA exist, with migration between patterns:
  - Primary OA.
  - Generalized nodal OA (GNOA).
  - Inflammatory/erosive OA (iOA).
  - Large joint OA (knee and hip).
  - Spinal OA.
  - Secondary OA (Table 6.3).

## Generalized nodal OA (GNOA)

- This common condition (see ➔ Plate 7d), more common in women than in men, is characterized by polyarticular involvement.
- It is characterized by Heberden's nodes (DIPJ) and Bouchard's nodes (PIPJ).

**Table 6.2** Clinical features of osteoarthritis

| Parameters | Features |
|---|---|
| Symptoms | Pain often worse after use, better with rest |
| | 'Gelling' after inactivity |
| | Without significant inflammatory features |
| | Minimal stiffness, evenings > mornings |
| Signs | Bony enlargement |
| | Crepitus |
| | Reduce range of movement |
| | Tenderness on palpation |
| | Malalignment or instability |
| Site | 1st carpometacarpal joint (CMCJ) |
| | Proximal (PIPJ) and distal interphalangeal joints (DIPJ) |
| | 1st metatarsophalangeal joint (MTPJ) |
| | Large joints: hip, knee |
| | 1st metatarsal joint |
| | Cervical or lumbar spine |

- GNOA predisposes to OA of knee, hip, and spine.
- The is often a strong family history.
- There is often MCPJ involvement, particularly the second and third. If there is MCPJ involvement, further investigation to exclude causes of secondary OA are recommended.

## Inflammatory/erosive OA (iOA)

- Sometimes called erosive OA, iOA is characterized by interphalangeal joint involvement, flares of inflammatory symptoms with rapid progression, and a tendency to joint ankylosis.
- Central joint subchondral erosions and associated bony remodelling.
- The peak onset is around the menopause.
- Functional impairment is more likely than with nodal OA.
- The key differential diagnosis is psoriatic arthritis. Unfortunately, the two conditions can be indistinguishable on plain radiographs in the early stages and on ultrasound unless there are other psoriatic disease features such as skin/nail psoriasis or tenosynovitis.

## Large joint OA

- The knee is commonly affected; most often the patellofemoral and medial tibiofemoral compartments.
- Severe bone and cartilage loss leads to instability and varus (bow) deformity.
- Instability and 'giving way' of a knee may be exacerbated by quadriceps weakness.
- Hip OA tends to present as groin, buttock, or anterior thigh pain on weight bearing, rather than lateral hip discomfort.
- Differential diagnosis for hip and groin pain include iliopsoas dysfunction, ischial bone lesions, symphysis, and trochanteric pain syndrome.
- Subdivision of hip OA is usually made on the basis of acetabular cartilage loss patterns:
  - Superior pole: common pattern, often unilateral, more common in men, and likely to progress.
  - Central (medial): less common, usually bilateral, more common in women, and less likely to progress.
  - Indeterminate acetabular-concentric patterns are also described.

## Secondary OA

Secondary OA is associated with a wide variety of disorders as listed in Table 6.3.

**Table 6.3 Secondary OA**

| Trauma | Inflammatory arthritis |
|---|---|
| Metabolic/endocrine: | Crystal deposition disease: |
|   Haemochromatosis |   Calcium pyrophosphate |
|   Acromegaly |   Uric acid |
|   Hyperparathyroidism |   Hydroxyapatite |
|   Ochronosis (alkaptonuria) | |
| Neuropathic disorders: | Anatomical abnormalities: |
|   Diabetes mellitus |   Bone dysplasia |

# Investigation

- The diagnosis of OA is based on clinical and radiological findings. There are no specific laboratory tests.
- As the disease progresses, other findings may appear and aid diagnosis, including osteophytes, subchondral bone sclerosis, and subchondral cysts.
- Radiographs correlate poorly with symptoms and clinical function. Many older patients will have radiographic changes consistent with OA, but will be asymptomatic.
- MRI is better at identifying early articular cartilage loss, subchondral bone oedema, and low-grade synovitis, but it is rarely used.
- Laboratory tests (including synovial fluid analysis) may be useful to exclude other causes of joint pain, such as RA, though abnormalities and pattern of acute phase may be similar for PsA and calcium pyrophosphate deposition disease.
- There are biomarkers of tissue destruction and inflammation that may eventually translate from research settings to clinical use, including:
  - cartilage oligomeric matrix protein (COMP).
  - pyridinoline and bone sialoprotein.
  - metalloproteinases.
  - hyaluronan.
  - C-terminal cross-link telopeptide of type II collagen (CTX-II).
- Optical coherence tomography (OCT) imaging: uses infrared light (in a similar way to sonography) to produce high-resolution dynamic images. This research tool may translate to clinical practice.

# Management

Management is based on symptoms and the impact of symptoms and joint structural changes including the effect on quality of life, function, occupation, leisure, and sleep.

- Functional requirements are addressed by therapists following therapy assessment (occupational and physiotherapy).
- Occupational therapy can provide splints, aids, safe environment, and joint protection techniques.
- Exercise is a key treatment in many cases as it improves muscle strength, joint proprioception, and aerobic fitness.
- Patient expectations influence the use of analgesia and referral for surgical procedures.
- Weight is associated with a number of types of OA in weight-bearing joints and is linked to poor prognosis. Weight loss is therefore important as a key intervention.
- Psychosocial factors (mood and relationships) may influence symptoms and impact of OA and require therapeutic input occasionally.
- A multi-disciplinary approach is sensible. In the UK, NICE has produced guidelines for management of OA in adults that emphasize a holistic approach tailored to the patient's specific needs.[3]
- NICE identifies core treatments that should be offered to all patients, in addition to the use of pharmacological and adjunctive treatments based on patient needs (Box 6.1).

## Pharmacotherapies

- NSAIDs and COX-2 inhibitors may can be effective for use in short periods during inflammatory disease flares.
- UK NICE guidance emphasizes NSAID use for the shortest time and at the lowest dose possible and with caution in older patients.
- Cardiovascular adverse events appear equal between conventional NSAIDs and COX-2 inhibitors.
- The addition of local anaesthetic to intra-articular GC injection does not improve efficacy, but may reduce pain from the injections.
- Asymptomatic effusions do not require intra-articular injection.
- Most joint injection data are for knee OA. Infection is rare (<1:10,000), but care should be taken to clean overlying skin and avoid injecting through infected skin or psoriatic lesions. Patients should be warned of the risk of skin depigmentation and fat atrophy. It is advised that patients receive no more than 3–4 injections per year, each ≥3 months apart
- Intra-articular injection of hyaluronic acid derivatives (viscosupplementation) is not supported by robust data and is not supported by UK NICE guidance.
- Oral glucosamine and chondroitin sulphate supplements have been shown in RCTs and meta-analyses to be no better than placebo, and are not recommended by NICE in the UK.
- Evidence that avocado/soybean unsaponifiable supplementation, evening primrose oil, rose hip extract, blue-lip mussel extract, and omega-3 fish oils improve pain is limited.

## Box 6.1 OA: Disease management principles

### Core treatments
- Holistic, patient-centred care plan.
- Provision of written and verbal information.
- Advice on footwear.
- Exercise.
- Weight loss.

### Adjunctive treatments
- TENS machine.
- Braces, walking aids, and insoles.
- Thermotherapy: cold/warm measures to reduce symptoms.

### Pharmacological treatments

#### Initial
- Regular paracetamol 1 g 3–4 times daily.
- Topical anti-inflammatory gels (NSAIDs).
- Topical capsaicin cream.

#### Subsequent
- Oral NSAIDs/COX-2 inhibitors ± proton pump inhibitor.
- Intra-articular glucocorticoids (useful during flares; duration of benefit variable).

#### Rarely
- Codeine–paracetamol combination analgesics.
- Buprenorphine.
- Gabapentin or pregabalin.

#### Surgical
- Arthroscopic lavage/debridement if mechanical locking.
- Joint replacement for activity-limiting symptomatic OA—may reduce pain rather than increase function.

## Future therapeutic strategies

Current OA research is focusing on disease-modifying anti-osteoarthritis drugs (DMOADs), with the aim of preventing joint damage. Approaches include:
- Inhibition of RANK ligand-mediated subchondral bone resorption using monoclonal antibodies.
- Bisphosphonates reducing bone loss—putatively anti-(subchondral bone) resorption.
- Inhibition of cathepsin K, a potent protease involved in degradation of type I collagen in bone matrix.
- Vitamin D supplementation, which will optimize calcium absorption and reduce PTH, slowing bone resorption. Studies are yet to be done.
- Diacerein, an IL1 blocker, has been shown to reduce joint space loss in hip OA over 3 years in one RCT. Further studies need to be performed.
- Mesenchymal stem cell therapy—precursor cells capable of differentiating into osteogenic, chondrogenic, or adipogenic cells. Several clinical trials are ongoing in early phases.

## Reference

3. NICE. *Osteoarthritis: Care and Management*. Clinical Guideline 177. London: NICE, 2014. https://www.nice.org.uk/guidance/cg177

# Prognosis

## Knee OA

- Progression in the knee may take many years. Cohort studies have found that radiographic deterioration occurs in one-third of cases.
- BMI predicts progression of patellofemoral OA.
- For tibiofemoral compartment OA, patients with contralateral knee OA, a baseline index knee OA grade of 1, higher body mass index (BMI) and higher baseline Western Ontario and McMaster Universities arthritis index total scores are more likely to develop Kellgren & Lawrence grade of 3 or 4 within 5 years.

## Hip OA

- Progression of hip disease is variable. A Danish study found that 66% of hips worsened radiologically over 10 years, although symptomatic improvement was common.
- Heterogeneity of prediction factors is found across studies and within study populations.
- Clinical characteristics (higher comorbidity count and presence of knee OA), health behaviour factors (no supervised exercise and physical inactivity), and sociodemographics (lower education) have been found to predict deterioration of pain (weak evidence).
- A higher number of comorbidities have been found to predict deterioration of physical functioning (strong evidence).

# Crystal-induced musculoskeletal disease

# Gout and hyperuricaemia

Gout is a common, painful, and potentially destructive rheumatologic disorder, related to hyperuricaemia. The clinical consequences of uric acid or urate (monosodium urate (MSU)) crystal deposition include acute and chronic arthritis, tophus formation, nephrolithiasis, and gouty nephropathy.

## Epidemiology

- Several epidemiologic studies from different countries suggest that the incidence and prevalence of gout is increasing, perhaps related to better recognition, and changes in lifestyle and diet.
- In the UK, gout affects 25 per 1000 of the population, and accounts for 250,000 GP consultations per year. Prevalence data from the USA on self-reported estimate that 13.6 per 1000 adult males and 6.4 per 1000 adult females are affected.
- Gout is more common in middle-aged and elderly people.
- The risk factors for gout are the same as those for hyperuricaemia (Table 7.1).

**Table 7.1** The causes of hyperuricaemia and risk factors for gout

| | |
|---|---|
| Primary gout | Male gender |
| | Increasing age (in women) |
| | Ethnicity |
| | Being overweight |
| | Diet (purine rich diet)—particularly red meat, oily-fish, shellfish, sugary drinks, and fructose-rich foods |
| | Alcohol use (beer appearing to pose the highest risk) |
| | Renal insufficiency |
| | Hypertension |
| Inherited metabolic syndromes | X-linked HPRT deficiency (Lesch–Nyhan), X-linked raised PRPP synthetase activity. Autosomal recessive G6P deficiency (von Gierke's disease) |
| Uric acid overproduction | Cell lysis: tumour lysis syndrome, myeloproliferative disease, haemolytic anaemia, psoriasis, trauma. Drugs: alcohol, cytotoxic drugs, warfarin |
| Uric acid underexcretion | Renal failure |
| | Drugs: alcohol, salicylates, diuretics, laxatives, ciclosporin, levodopa, ethambutol, pyrazinamide |
| Lead toxicity | Renal impairment and altered purine turnover |

G6P, glucose-6-phosphatase. G6P deficiency leads to increased activity of aminophosphoribosyl transferase and purine formation; HPRT, hypoxanthine guanine phosphoribosyl transferase—a salvage enzyme converting hypoxanthine back to precursors and therefore competing with its conversion to xanthine and then uric acid; PRPP, phosphoribosylpyrophosphate synthetase—a component enzyme in purine ring synthesis.

## Classification criteria

- The current ACR/EULAR guidelines stipulate, for the classification of gout, the occurrence of ≥1 episode ('attack') of joint or bursal swelling, pain or tenderness.
- MSU crystals in (symptomatic) synovial fluid or from a tophus is sufficient for diagnosis of gout.
- The domains of the criteria include:
  - clinical (pattern of joint involvement, characteristics, and time course of symptomatic episodes).
  - laboratory (serum uric acid (SUA) levels).
  - synovial fluid (aspirate analysis for crystals).
  - imaging (radiographic gout-related erosion, double-contour sign on ultrasound, or MSU crystals on dual-energy CT).

## Clinical features

- The first stage of the condition is usually asymptomatic hyperuricaemia (SUA >680 mg/L) often starting years before symptoms develop.
- This concentration marks the physiological point above which urate salts are no longer soluble in the serum at physiologic pH and temperature. Not everyone with hyperuricaemia develops gout, however.
- Inflammation to MSU crystals is typically sudden and severe and is often referred to as an 'attack' of gout.
- The initial attack commonly occurs in the fourth to sixth decade of life in men, and in postmenopausal women.
- The initial attack is usually monoarticular, affecting the first metatarsophalangeal joint (podagra) in up to 60% of patients.
- Other frequently involved joints include the ankle, midfoot, knee, wrist, elbow (olecranon bursa), and the small joints of the hands.
- Axial and large joints and spinal structures are rarely involved.
- With an attack, pain reaches its maximum intensity in 4–12 hours, with marked limitation of physical function. Symptoms usually resolve in 3–14 days.
- 70–80% of individuals will have another attack(s) within 2 years.
- The initial attacks are usually separated by asymptomatic inter-critical period, lasting months to years.
- As the disease progresses, acute attacks may become more polyarticular, with associated joint damage and deformity. Intervals between attacks tend to shorten. Disability, chronic pain, and tophi formation can be observed if treatment is suboptimal (see ➔ Plate 7).
- Tophi are deposits of MSU embedded in a matrix composed of lipids, proteins, and calcific debris:
  - Tophi are usually subcutaneous, but have been reported to occur in bone, eyes, and other organs.
  - Classic sites for tophi formation include ear pinna, elbow and knee bursae, Achilles tendon, and dorsal surface of the MCPJs.
  - Tophi are usually painless, although the overlying skin may ulcerate and become infected.
  - Those most at risk of tophi are patients with prolonged severe hyperuricaemia, polyarticular gout, and the elderly with primary nodal OA on diuretics.

- Some clinicians will treat asymptomatic hyperuricaemia to prevent the onset of 'urate nephropathy'; but this is controversial.
- Hyperuricaemia and gout are associated with the metabolic syndrome (dyslipidaemia, hypertension, obesity, and insulin resistance).

### Investigation

- Synovial fluid analysis is the most important investigation.
- Negatively birefringent, needle-shaped crystals on polarized light microscopy confirms the diagnosis.
- Crystals may be extra- or intracellular. However, the absence of crystals does not rule out the diagnosis.
- MSU crystals are identifiable in the synovial fluid from previously affected joints and about 70% of those receiving SUA-lowering therapy during the asymptomatic inter-critical period.
- SUA concentrations may be normal during an acute attack in up to 30% of cases, and may not reflect pre-flare levels. Therefore, SUA concentration cannot be used to exclude the diagnosis during an acute flare.
- SUA concentrations are of value in assessing the patient only once the acute flare has subsided; either to confirm hyperuricaemia or to monitor the effectiveness of therapy.

### Imaging

- Imaging findings vary at different stages of gout.
- Plain radiographs are often normal during the early phase of the disease, but soft tissue swelling can be apparent.
- Radiographs are useful to assess for other conditions such as trauma or infection (Box 7.1). Subcortical bone cysts may be suggestive of tophi or erosions. Para-articular erosions with 'overhanging edges' of bone are characteristic of gout.
- Later in the disease, radiographs may demonstrate tophi near joints, tissue swelling, para-articular erosions, periosteal new bone formation, and joint deformity. Many features mimic RA.

---

### Box 7.1 Clinical conditions that can mimic gout

- CPPD disease (pseudogout)
- Basic calcium phosphate (BCP) arthritis
- Cellulitis
- Infectious (septic) arthritis
- Trauma (can coexist with gout)
- Rheumatoid arthritis (polyarticular)
- Psoriatic arthritis (monoarthritis/dactylitis)
- Erythema nodosum
- Reactive arthritis (monoarthritis/dactylitis).

- US can be useful to detect early disease and monitor treatment. Diagnostic features include a linear density parallel to the joint surface (double-contour sign), or tophaceous deposits which appear as oval stippled signal (hyperechoic cloudy area).
- Dual-energy CT specifically identifies MSU deposits and distinguishes them from calcium deposition.

## Management

The management of gout should be approached in two phases: the treatment of the acute attack and the treatment of chronic or tophaceous gout (Fig. 7.1).

### The acute attack of gout

- Rest, elevation, and ice packs can partly ease symptoms.
- The principal therapies are NSAIDs, colchicine, and oral and intra-articular (IA) glucocorticoids (GCs).
- SUA-lowering drugs are ineffective in acute gout. Patients already on SUA-lowering drugs, should continue without interruption.
- NSAIDs decrease pain, swelling, and duration of gout attacks.
- All NSAIDs, including COX-2 selective NSAIDs, have potentially similar efficacy for gout.

| Management of the acute attack | Management of chronic or tophaceous gout | Lifestyle and comorbidity modifications |
|---|---|---|
| 1. NSAIDs and PPI, rest, ice, elevation. | 1. Allopurinol. *Titrate dose up for SUA reduction to target (<360 μmol/L [6 mg/dL] or <300 μmol/L [5 mg/dL] for severe gout) | 1. Weight loss |
| 2. Colchicine 0.5 mg 2 to 4 times daily orally. | | 2. Dietary modification: reduce/stop consumption of alcohol, red meat, shellfish, and high-sugar drinks. |
| 3. Glucocorticoids (GCs) orally or IM if >4 joints affected. | 2. Febuxostat in patients who do not reach target SUA target level* with allopurinol, or have significant renal impairment. | 3. Drink low-fat milk daily. |
| 4. Intra-articular GC injections if 1–3 joints affected. | 3. Uricosuric drugs: sulfinpyrazone or benzbromarone. Avoid in patients with renal stones or impairment. | 4. Optimize management of hypertension, renal disease, any hyper-triglyceridaemia and cardiovascular comorbidities. |
| 5. Interleukin-1β inhibitor (anakinra or canakinumab) in patients with repeated gout attacks, refractory disease, or where there are contraindications to other medications. | 4. Pegloticase/rasburicase: reserved for patients with severe gout where other medications are ineffective. | 5. Consider stopping diuretic where permissible |

**Fig 7.1** The management of gout. GC, glucocorticoid; IM, intramuscular; NSAID, non-steroidal anti-inflammatory drug; PPI, proton pump inhibitor; SUA, serum uric acid.

- NSAIDs are most effective when initiated within 48 hours of symptom onset. The dose may be reduced after a reduction in symptoms, and discontinued 1–2 days after complete resolution of signs.
- The typical duration of NSAIDs required for an acute attack is 5–7 days. NSAIDs are contraindicated in renal insufficiency (e.g. CKD3b–5). NSAIDs should be used with caution in the elderly and patients with GI risk factors.
- Colchicine can be very effective in acute gout, and have a rapid onset of action. Oral colchicine 0.5 mg, two to four times daily, for 5 days can be effective but may cause diarrhoea at higher doses.
- Colchicine is often given in addition to NSAIDs, although there is no evidence to support this. IV colchicine is no longer used due to high risk of bone marrow suppression and death.
- Oral prednisone 10–30 mg daily is effective for immediate relief of gout, with dose then tapered over 7–10 days.
- Parenteral GCs maybe used in individuals unable to take oral form and with polyarticular gout. A study comparing intramuscular triamcinolone with oral indometacin found no significant difference in time to recovery.
- IA GCs are useful if ≤4 joints are affected. A systematic review on the safety and efficacy of IA GCs for acute gout could not identify any RCTs of their use.
- IA GCs should be avoided if septic arthritis is possible.
- IL-1 inhibitors are under study for acute gout. IL-1β is the predominant mediator of acute inflammation.
  - Anakinra 100 mg SC daily has been used until symptoms improve with good effect.
  - Canakinumab 150 mg SC is licensed for acute gout in Europe.
  - In one study comparing SC canakinumab with IM triamcinolone, canakinumab achieved better outcomes in terms of pain relief, joint swelling reduction, and patient-assessed global response.
  - Canakinumab is effective in patients either with multiple gout 'flares' or whose disease is refractory to other treatment or have contraindications to other medications.
  - However, canakinumab is associated with increased infections, and at the time of writing is 5000× the cost of triamcinolone.

*Treatment of chronic or tophaceous gout*
- Addressing adverse lifestyle factors and comorbidities should be a priority, including to:
  - attain a normal BMI (20–25)/reduce centripetal obesity.
  - reduce, or preferentially stop, consumption of alcohol, red meat, shellfish, and sugary drinks.
  - manage hypertension and associated hypertriglyceridemia.
  - encourage to drink low-fat milk daily (a natural uricosuric).
  - remain well hydrated.
  - consider how best to minimize treatments which can aggravate hyperuricaemia (e.g. thiazide, furosemide, indapamide, ciclosporin, levodopa, theophylline).
- The target SUA with all drug therapy is <360 μmol/L (6 mg/dL) or <300 μmol/L (5 mg/dL) where there is severe gout. Gout attacks are very unlikely where SUA is below target.

- Drugs that decrease SUA levels are indicated in individuals with frequent or disabling attacks of gout, clinical or radiological evidence of chronic gouty arthropathy, tophaceous disease, with secondary renal impairment, or urolithiasis.
- SUA-lowering drugs are initiated 2–4 weeks after an acute flare subsides, as they may prolong or worsen the acute flare.
- Allopurinol (a xanthine oxidase inhibitor) is the first-line treatment:
  - Allopurinol is initiated at 100 mg daily with incremental dose titration every month, aiming to lower SUA to ≤300 mg/L.
  - The dose range of allopurinol is 100–900 mg daily.
  - Most patients respond to 400 mg daily of allopurinol.
  - Dosing should be adjusted for renal impairment.
  - Allopurinol takes 4 days to 2 weeks to take effect.
  - Approximately 5–10% of patients develop significant drug intolerance: nausea, diarrhoea, elevated transaminase levels (3–5%).
  - Severe hepatic disease including granulomatous hepatitis, cholestatic jaundice, and hepatic necrosis are rare.
  - About 2% of patients develop a pruritic, maculopapular rash. Pruritis alone can herald the onset of rash.
  - Bone marrow suppression occurs rarely—at high doses.
  - HLA-B*5801 status increases the risk of developing allopurinol drug reaction eosinophilia and systemic symptoms (DRESS).
  - In mild to moderate intolerance, allopurinol can be reintroduced at very low levels (e.g. 10 mg daily) and titrated up slowly.
  - Allopurinol can interfere with the metabolism of azathioprine and warfarin, increasing the risk of side effects.
  - Concomitant colchicine (0.5 mg twice daily orally) is recommended as prophylaxis against acute flares for the first 3–6 months of allopurinol treatment.
- Febuxostat is a non-purine xanthine oxidase inhibitor:
  - Febuxostat is more effective at lowering SUA than allopurinol, and may be used in patients allergic to allopurinol, patients not attaining target SUA at maximal allopurinol dose, and in patients with moderate renal insufficiency.
  - Doses range from 40 to 120 mg/day.
  - Dose reduction is required in patients with renal dysfunction.
  - Side effects include nausea, liver dysfunction, arthralgia, and rash.
  - Some studies have shown a higher incidence of cardiovascular side effects with febuxostat compared with allopurinol.
  - Febuxostat is substantially more expensive than allopurinol.
- Some patients may respond to allopurinol and a uricosuric agent (e.g. probenecid) when either alone has been ineffective.
- Uricosuric drugs should be avoided in patients with renal insufficiency or a history of nephrolithiasis.
- Fenofibrate decreases SUA by increasing renal uric acid clearance. It may have an unlicensed role in patients resistant or intolerant to other treatments. It should be avoided in hepatic and biliary disease, hypothyroidism and pregnancy. Side effects include myoarthralgias.

- Sulfinpyrazone is a uricosuric drug which is effective and well tolerated, but is contraindicated in patients with renal stones and is ineffective in those with renal insufficiency.
- Benzbromarone is a uricosuric agent available in Europe. It is effective in patients with renal insufficiency. Liver function must be monitored for drug-induced hepatitis (fulminant liver failure reported).
- Pegloticase is a porcine uricase reserved for patients with severe gout, in whom other gout treatments have been ineffective. Administration is 8 mg IV every 2 weeks. Concomitant colchicine prophylaxis is recommended for the first 6 months of use. Anti-pegloticase antibodies have been reported.
- Rasburicase is a non-pegylated recombinant uricase. It may be more immunogenic than pegloticase.
- Patients with uric acid stones are best managed with adequate hydration, urinary alkalization, and allopurinol. This regimen is also effective in preventing calcium oxalate stones.
- Gouty tophi may be amenable to surgical removal.

# Calcium pyrophosphate deposition disease

# Calcium pyrophosphate deposition disease

- See Box 7.2 for an overview of EULAR definitions and clinical presentations.
- Precipitation of calcium pyrophosphate (CPP) crystals in tissues is extremely common and arguably the most common reason why previously ill hospitalized patients develop MSK problems when unwell in hospital.

---

**Box 7.2 EULAR definitions of calcium pyrophosphate (CPP) deposition (1–3) and clinical presentations of CPP deposition (CPPD) disease**

*1. CPP crystals*
Simplified term for calcium pyrophosphate crystals.

*2. CPPD*
The umbrella term for deposition of CPP crystals.

*3. CC*
Cartilage calcification, identified by imaging or histology—but not always due to CPPD.

*Asymptomatic CPPD*
May be of no clinical consequence; but the degree to which cartilage or other soft tissue CPP crystals increase the risk of significant MSK lesions (e.g. osteoarthritis, intervertebral disc degeneration, chronic enthesopathy, spinal stenosis) is largely unknown.

*Acute CPPD arthritis*
Acute self-limiting synovitis.

*CPPD disease with osteoarthritis (OA)*
CPP crystals in a joint which is osteoarthritic.

*Chronic CPPD arthritis*
Typically affects wrists, 2nd/3rd MCPJs, hips, knees (mimics RA but is ACPA negative).

*Spinal CPPD disease types*
Inflammation proven or suspected around the odontoid ('crowned dens syndrome'), causing or complicating intervertebral disc disease or associated with ligament flavum thickening contributing to spinal and/or lateral recess stenosis.

*Other CPPD (possibly all CC)-related lesions*
Tendon insertion/enthesis-based inflammation associated with CPPD; boxing-glove-like hand/wrist swelling features of acute disease.

- The spectrum of CPP crystal deposition disease includes acute and chronic arthropathy, inflammation and symptoms at entheses or within/ involving tendons, soft tissue and bursal inflammation, asymptomatic cartilage calcification, and symptoms from spinal canal and intervertebral disc crystals.
- The risk of CPPD-related disease increases with age. Presentation in a young adult <50 years old should prompt a search for an associated metabolic cause.
- Definite associations with CPPD disease and chondrocalcinosis (i.e. calcification of fibrocartilage and hyaline cartilage typically of the knee and wrist) include:
- Hypomagnesaemia (check Mg, PTH, vitamin D, bone profile and renal function).
- Hypophosphatasia (low ALP, raised serum pyridoxal-5 phosphate and increased urinary phophoethanolamine).
- Haemochromatosis (positive family history, abnormal LFTs, raised haemoglobin, ferritin and transferrin saturation, and disease-associated HFE genotype).
- Wilson's disease (neurological disease, abnormal LFTs, eye disease, and abnormally low serum caeruloplasmin).
- Hyperparathyroidism (primary, secondary, and tertiary in renal disease). So check PTH, bone profile, renal function/estimated GFR, and vitamin D).
- Vitamin D deficiency—chronic (through causing secondary hyperparathyroidism). Check as for hyperparathyroidism.
- Possible CPPD disease associations include gout, ochronosis, hypocalciuric hypercalcaemia, diabetes, DISH, and XLHR.
- The main precipitants of an acute CPPD disease episode (if in a joint historical term was 'pseudogout') are listed in Box 7.3.

---

**Box 7.3 Factors that may trigger acute CPPD-induced inflammation**

- Acute illness (e.g. chest or urinary infection).
- Direct trauma (e.g. joint cartilage damage or tendon tear/strain).
- Post-surgical.
- Especially post-parathyroidectomy.
- Blood transfusion or IV fluids.
- Commencement of thyroxine replacement.
- Joint lavage.

## Investigation

- CPPD disease is defined by the presence of positively birefringent, rhomboid-shaped crystals under polarized light microscopy of synovial fluid. Crystals may be intra- or extracellular.
- Radiographs of the affected joints may not be helpful in establishing the diagnosis. However, the presence of chondrocalcinosis increases the likelihood of CPPD disease. Radiographic clues that may help to distinguish CPPD disease from OA include:
  - axial involvement.
  - sacroiliac erosions.
  - cortical erosions of the femur.
  - osteonecrosis of the medial femoral condyle.
  - associated hyperparathyroid disease signs: endocortical erosions of long bones in the hands and feet, cortical tunnelling, and osteopenia in phalanges.
- US features indicative of CPPD include a thin hyperechoic band along the cartilage, running in parallel to the bony cortex ('tram-lines'). Sites can include the MCPJs, wrists, knees, and tendons. Nodular deposits in bursae, entheses, and hyperechoic lines parallel to tendons can also be observed.
- Both CT and MRI may be needed to disclose disease in spinal structures: MRI to show inflammatory changes and CT to disclose the distribution of calcification (see ➔ Plate 22).

## Management

### Acute CPPD-related arthritis

- The management of acute CPPD disease is summarized in Fig. 7.2.
- Rest, ice, and splinting in the acute phase will help symptoms.
- NSAIDs in the acute phase.
- Oral colchicine (0.5 mg, two to four times a day) can be used in patients in whom NSAIDs are contraindicated in the acute setting or as prophylactic use to prevent recurrent flares (see Fig. 7.2).
- Joint aspiration and IA GC injection for acute joint inflammation, once joint infection has been excluded (see ➔ Chapters 24).
- Oral GCs will undoubtedly help in the acute setting but the dose should be reviewed and minimized to avoid long-term use and steroid dependency.
- Anakinra has been used in polyarticular acute CPPD disease, unresponsive to other medications.
- As in all CPPD cases, identify and manage associated metabolic abnormalities.

| Management of the acute inflammatory episode | Management of chronic CPPD arthritis | Non-pharmacological management |
|---|---|---|
| 1. NSAIDs and PPI | 1. NSAIDs and PPI | 1. Rest, ice, and consider splinting of *acutely* inflamed joints |
| 2. Joint aspiration and IA glucocorticoid (GC) injection. | 2. Colchicine 0.5 mg twice daily (can be used as ongoing treatment or as prophylaxis against acute inflammatory episodes) | 2. Identify and treat any underlying metabolic abnormality (e.g. hyperparathyroid disease) |
| 3. Short course of oral GCs (e.g. prednisolone 15 mg daily for 2 weeks tapered over 4 weeks) if IA GC unfeasible. | 3. Low-dose oral GCs (e.g. 5–10 mg daily) | 3. Identify and manage risk of GORD if using NSAIDs, renal disease, and osteoporosis risk if using steroids |
| 4. Colchicine 0.5 mg 2 to 4 times daily if NSAIDs are contraindicated | 4. Hydroxychloroquine (resistant disease). | |
| 5. Interleukin-1β inhibitors (e.g. anakinra) in patients with repeated flares and refractory disease. | 5. Methotrexate (resistant disease). | |

Fig. 7.2 Management of calcium pyrophosphate deposition (CPPD) disease. GC, glucocorticoid; GORD, gastro-oesophageal reflux disease; IA, intra-articular; NSAID, non-steroidal anti-inflammatory drug; PPI, proton pump inhibitor.

### Chronic CPPD arthritis/disease

- Disease may mimic RA if polyarticular and can cause persistent inflammatory-type spinal symptoms.
- Ongoing metabolic influences of CPPD disease may need addressing. Renal disease, hyperparathyroidism (primary, secondary, or tertiary (but for secondary also consider vitamin D deficiency)), and chronic dehydration may all play a role.
- Hydroxychloroquine (200–400 mg daily in twice-daily doses for trial period of 4 months for example) or methotrexate (e.g. 15 mg weekly for trial period of 6 months initially) may be tried in patients with resistant disease.
- Arguably there is more evidence to support the use of methotrexate than hydroxychloroquine.[1]

### Reference

1. Zhang W, Doherty M, Pascual E, et al. EULAR recommendations for calcium pyrophosphate deposition. Part II: management. *Ann Rheum Dis* 2011;70:571–5.

# Basic calcium phosphate crystal-associated disease

- Basic calcium phosphate (BCP) crystals include hydroxyapatite, octacalcium phosphate, and tricalcium phosphate.
- BCP and associated crystals are associated with several rheumatological diseases (Table 7.2).
- The treatment of these conditions is as per CPPD disease, with NSAIDs and colchicine (see ➔ Chapter 23, for further details).

Table 7.2 BCP crystal-associated conditions

| | |
|---|---|
| Articular disease | Milwaukee shoulder syndrome (severe degenerative arthropathy, more common on the dominant side and in elderly women) |
| | Osteoarthritis (synovial fluid crystals found in 60% of OA patients) |
| | Erosive arthritis |
| | Mixed crystal deposition |
| Periarticular disease | Pseudopodagra, calcific tendonitis, and bursitis |

# Calcium oxalate arthritis

- Crystals are positively birefringent and bipyramidal under polarized light microscopy of synovial fluid.
- Radiographs and laboratory tests are not diagnostic.
- Most labs will not have the expertise to specifically identify these crystals on synovial samples.
- Treatment is as for CPPD disease.
- Several conditions are associated with calcium oxalate arthritis (Box 7.4).

---

**Box 7.4 Conditions associated with calcium oxalate arthritis**

- End-stage renal disease on dialysis.
- Short bowel syndrome.
- Diet rich in rhubarb, spinach, and ascorbic acid.
- Thiamine deficiency.
- Pyridoxine deficiency.
- Primary oxalosis: recessive trait, early renal failure (in the third decade of life), arthritis, tendonitis.

# The spondyloarthritides including psoriatic arthritis

# Introduction

All spondyloarthropathies (SpAs) are commonly characterized by inflammatory back and axial skeletal pains, enthesitis, and an association with HLA-B27.

- The SpAs are:
  - Axial spondyloarthritis (axSpA).
  - Ankylosing spondylitis (AS; encompassed by axSpA definition).
  - Psoriatic arthritis (PsA).
  - Reactive arthritis (ReA).
  - Inflammatory bowel disease-related SpA.
  - Juvenile SpA/enthesitis-related arthritis (ERA; see ➲ Chapter 9).
- Considered together the SpAs are the most common form of chronic inflammatory arthritis; more common than RA.
- All SpAs are potentially manifest by:
  - enthesitis.
  - inflammatory back pain.
  - asymmetric peripheral arthritis.
  - inflammatory bowel lesions.
  - psoriasis.
  - dactylitis.
  - osteitis.
  - sterile urethritis.
  - uveitis (typically acute anterior uveitis).
  - aorta/aortic valve lesions (rare).
  - abnormal antigen presentation associated with HLA-B27.
- Similarities exist between SpAs and the SAPHO (synovitis, acne, palmoplantar pustulosis, hyperostosis, aseptic osteomyelitis) syndrome; SAPHO is not considered to be a SpA; see ➲ Chapter 16.
- Pathological changes are mainly at entheses but also in tissues of the gut, uveal tract, urethra, aorta, bone, synovium, and skin.
- A common inflammatory 'target' or precise common reason why such tissues might be affected is postulated though not yet proven.
- Lines of immunopathology research currently focus on general and local tissue resident Th17 cell activation by Il-23 and subsequent activating effects specific to the local tissue environment.

# Spondyloarthritis (SpA): a paradigm shift

Key to classifying all SpAs is the presence of inflammatory back pain (Box 8.1) and, for day-to-day clinical recognition—the presence of enthesitis (Box 8.2).

- Sadly, there is still a 7–10-year delay in a sizable number of patients between symptom onset and diagnosis of ankylosing spondylitis (AS)— similar data to data derived >30 years ago. One reason is that it takes many years in some patients to confirm AS as it is based partly on radiographic criteria (of SIJs) which can take years to evolve (Box 8.3).
- The classification of axial spondyloarthritis (axSpA; see the Assessment of Spondyloarthritis International Society (ASAS) working group criteria: ℘ http://www.asas-group.org) *includes* classical AS as well as earlier stages and abortive courses of the disease, in which structural alterations have not yet occurred.
- ASAS has facilitated classification of SpA in terms of axial or peripheral predominant disease.
- The new ASAS criteria (for axSpA; Box 8.4) potentially allow all patients, who will ultimately develop AS, to be identified earlier in their disease compared with the modified New York (mNY) criteria.
- However, it is likely that not all ASAS axSpA classifiable patients will progress to an AS phenotype classifiable by the mNY criteria.
- Previously, early SpA disease was recognizable formally only through a definition (ESSG) of 'undifferentiated SpA' (USpA). Many such patients would now be classifiable by the newer ASAS working group criteria for (peripheral) SpA (Box 8.5).
- Recently, classification criteria for PsA have also been developed (CASPAR; see ➔ 'Psoriatic arthritis', pp. 308–13).

---

### Box 8.1 Inflammatory back pain (IBP)

A history of IBP is key to considering axial symptoms as secondary to SpA—for people in whom it starts at <40 years of age. Applicable for back and/or posterior pelvic symptoms. A number of descriptions exist (e.g. after Calin, Rudwaleit, or ASAS). Typically, IBP:

- comes on gradually over time (insidious onset).
- is improved with exercise.
- does not improve with rest.
- causes pain at night with improvement on getting up.
- is reported by patients as occurring with "stiffness".
- improves with a ('once-daily') modified-release NSAID taken at bedtime.

## Box 8.2 Enthesitis

An enthesis is the name given to specialized tissue which attaches a ligament or tendon to a bone. Examples include the attachments of the Achilles tendon to os calcis, the origin of the finger extensor tendons at lateral humeral epicondyle, the gluteus tendon insertion at the greater trochanter, or the attachments of the patella ligament.

## Box 8.3 Modified New York (mNY) criteria for classifying AS

*Clinical criteria*

- Low back pain and stiffness for >6 months, improving with exercise, but not relieved by rest.
- Limitation of lumbar spine movements in sagittal and frontal planes.
- Limitation of chest expansion relative to normal values for age and sex.

*Radiological criteria*

- Greater than or equal to grade 2 bilateral sacroiliitis.
- Grade 3 or 4 unilateral sacroiliitis

*Combined diagnostic criteria*

- Definite AS if radiological and clinical criterion.
- Probable AS if three clinical criteria or a radiological criterion without signs or symptoms satisfying the clinical criteria.

Adapted from Van der Linden et al. 'Evaluation of diagnostic criteria for ankylosing spondylitis.' *Arth Rheum*, 1984;27:361–368 with permission from Wiley.

# Axial SpA including ankylosing spondylitis

The diagnosis of axial spondyloarthritis (axSpA) includes classical ankylosing spondylitis (AS) as well as earlier stages and abortive courses of the disease, in which (radiological evident) structural alterations have not yet occurred. Cases of the latter might be also classified as non-radiographic axSpA (nr-axSpA).

For a comparison of the ASAS criteria for classification for axSpA and peripheral SpA, see Box 8.4 and Box 8.5.

## Epidemiology of AS (on modified New York criteria or earlier definitions)

- There is an extensive wealth of data on the epidemiology of AS defined on mNY and earlier criteria.
- Patients are typically <40 years of age with a M:F ratio of 3:1.
- The condition occurs most frequently in Caucasians.
- In Pima American Indians, where HLA-B27 prevalence is high, AS is particularly frequent, whereas the condition is less common in African Americans, and rarer still in sub-Saharan Africans, reflecting the low prevalence of HLA-B27 in these groups.
- Prevalence estimate is 0.5–0.8/100,000 in Caucasian adults.
- Epidemiology data necessarily depend on patients satisfying criteria for diagnosis that necessarily means they have had their disease a relatively long time (to have radiographic changes at SIJs).

---

### Box 8.4 ASAS criteria for classification of axial SpA

In patients with ≥3 months' back pain and age at onset <45 years:
*either*
Sacroiliitis on imaging plus ≥1 SpA feature
*or*
HLA-B27 plus ≥2 other SpA features.

*SpA features*: IBP, arthritis, enthesitis (heel), uveitis, dactylitis, psoriasis, Crohn's/colitis, NSAID response, family history of SpA, HLA-B27, CRP+

*Sacroiliitis on imaging*: either active (acute) inflammation on MRI highly suggestive of sacroiliitis associated with SpA, or definite radiographic sacroiliitis according to the mNY criteria

Information from Rudwaleit M et al. The development of Assessment of SpondyloArthritis international Society classification criterial for axial spondyloarthritis (part II): validation and final selection. *Ann Rheum Dis* 2009;68:777–783.

---

---

### Box 8.5 ASAS criteria for peripheral SpA

Arthritis or enthesitis or dactylitis
(clinically assessed)

*plus*

≥1 SpA feature
(uveitis, psoriasis, Crohn's/colitis, preceding infection,
HLA-B27, sacroiliitis on imaging)

*or*

≥2 other SpA features
(arthritis, enthesitis, dactylitis, IBP (ever),
family history for SpA)

Information from Rudwaleit M et al. The development of Assessment of SpondyloArthritis international Society classification criteria for peripheral spondyloarthritis and for spondyloarthritis in general. *Ann Rheum Dis* 2009;70:25–31.

---

## Epidemiology of axSpA

- One implication of this paradigm shift is that a definition of axSpA results in a defined patient prevalence much higher than has been accepted for AS (based on mNY criteria, for example).
- There is an evolving understanding of the prevalence of axSpA based on ASAS criteria.
- Studies of modelling disease prevalence suggest that axSpA is considerably more common than AS.
- It is likely that the frequency of axSpA patients in any given cohort of IBP or chronic back pain patients, is higher than previously defined for an AS definition (e.g. 29% of patients with IBP met the criteria for nr-axSpA and 39% of patients with chronic low back pain had IBP).[1]

## Pathogenesis

### HLA-B27 and genetics

- HLA-B27 is associated with the SpAs in 50–95% of patients. In most populations, HLA-B27 is prevalent in about 10%.
- HLA-B27 is inherited as autosomal co-dominant: 50% of first-degree relatives of probands with HLA-B27 possess the antigen.
- 5–10% of HLA-B27-positive people develop AS over time.
- 20% of people with HLA-B27 develop a reactive arthritis after bacterial infection with *Chlamydia* or *Salmonella*.
- About 50% of patients with psoriatic or inflammatory bowel disease-related spondylitis are HLA-B27 positive.
- 50% of non-Caucasians with AS are HLA-B27 positive (< the prevalence of HLA-B27 in Caucasians with AS; 95%).
- Concordance in monozygotic twins is 70% vs 13% in dizygotic twins.
- HLA-B27 is found in up to 40% of cases of uveitis, even in the absence of underlying rheumatic disease.
- There is an excess of HLA-B27 prevalence in patients presenting with isolated aortic root or valve insufficiency.
- HLA-B27 has been found in 90% of males with a combination of aortic regurgitation and conduction system abnormalities.

- Genotyping studies have shown two AS susceptibility loci in addition to HLA-B27: ERAP1 and the gene encoding the IL-23 receptor. The former codes for an aminopeptidase of the ER involved in trimming peptides to an optimal size for binding to MHC class I molecules.
- HLA-B27 is probably relevant to pathogenesis by (possibly non-exclusive) mechanisms currently summarized as either:
  - allowing abnormally restricted T-cell immune responses to self-antigens or arthritogenic peptides.
  - itself misfolding during assembly and leading to endoplasmic reticulum stress and autophagy responses.
  - itself triggering innate T-cell, NK cell pro-inflammatory responses by presenting on the cell surface as homodimers and being recognized by these cells.

*Immunopathology*

- There is debate over whether one or a number of microorganisms contribute to pathophysiology.
- Increased faecal carriage of *Klebsiella aerogenes* has been reported in patients with established AS and may relate to exacerbation of both joint and eye disease.
- There is increasing evidence that axSpA and AS are due to an abnormal host response to the intestinal microbiota with involvement of Th17 cells, which play a key role in maintaining mucosal immunity.
- This leads to production of various inflammatory cytokines including Il-12, Il-23, Il-17, and TNFα which play key roles in the pathogenesis of enthesitis and other inflammatory lesions.
- Th17 cells may be resident in tissues and activated there causing local tissue inflammation and triggering local tissue changes.

## Clinical features of axSpA and AS

- Hallmark features of axSpA are IBP, fatigue, and enthesitis.
- Most axSpA lesions occur at entheses, subenthesial bone (osteitis), in tendons and synovium (see ➲ Plate 24).
- Typical entheses affected include plantar fascia origin at os calcis medial calcaneal tubercle, Achilles insertions at os calcis, extensor digit tendon origin at lateral humeral epicondyle, and gluteus medius insertion at greater trochanter (see also Table 8.4).
- Synovitis can occur, typically in the larger peripheral joints (hips and knees in particular). Though 20–40% of patients have peripheral joint disease at some stage, studies have not previously shown whether the features are synovitis or enthesitis or both.
- About 50% of patients with adult AS will develop hip arthritis.
- The standardized mortality ratio for AS is 1.5, due to cardiac valve and respiratory disease, amyloidosis, and fractures.
- AS patients are high risk for having to alter or give up work.
- Although recognized as typical of AS, few patients progress to the classical late 'bamboo spine'.
- When spine segments do fuse in AS (syndesmophytes bridging the gap between vertebral bodies), microfractures can occur leading to acute episodes of severe pain.

- Spondylodiscitis is an uncommon though severe lesion: acute aseptic disc and end-plate inflammation.
- The burden of spinal disease is typically variable chronic low-grade IBP and stiffness with evidence of reduction in spinal mobility.

## Non-musculoskeletal clinical features

- Constitutional features of fatigue, weight loss, low-grade fever, and anaemia are common. Fatigue is often the most troublesome symptom for many patients.
- IBD lesions are present in about 50% of AS patients though lesions are not symptomatic in all patients.
- Uveitis occurs in up to 40% of cases, but has little correlation with disease activity in the spine.
- There are no known triggers for uveitis and although self-limiting, topical, or systemic steroids may be required in severe cases. The uveitis is predominantly anterior and mostly unilateral.
- Upper lobe, bilateral pulmonary fibrosis is a recognized but rare feature of AS. Occasionally, the fibrotic area is invaded by *Aspergillus* with changes mimicking tuberculosis.
- In late AS, fusion of the thoracic wall leads to rigidity and reduction in chest expansion. Ventilation is maintained by the diaphragm; however, there is a threefold increased risk of death from a respiratory cause compared with the normal population.
- Cardiac involvement includes aortic incompetence, cardiomegaly, and conduction defects. Of the 20% of AS patients with aortic valve disease, the majority are clinically undetectable.
- Neurological lesions are a rare consequence of spinal MSK disease: nerve root entrapment and cauda equina syndrome.
- Sterile urethritis is an under-recognized SpA lesion.
- Renal involvement is rare but can be due to NSAID use (interstitial nephritis) or renal amyloidosis.
- Osteoporosis is an under-recognized finding:
  - AS patients are at high risk of vertebral fracture.
  - Micro-fractures may occur with trauma and fractures can occur through syndesmophytes.
  - Systemic osteoporosis occurs and is identifiable through hip and forearm BMD measurement.
  - Estimates of osteoporosis prevalence range from 20–60%, increasing with age and disease duration.
  - DXA evaluation of lumbar spine BMD will be inaccurate in advanced AS due to the presence of syndesmophytes.
  - Studies suggest that bone loss occurs early and during the acute inflammatory stage of the disease.

## Investigations in axSpA

- Systemic measures of acute-phase response are often detected though typically also can be normal despite symptoms.
- Plain AP, or 'coned' view radiographs of the posterior pelvis are conventionally used to detect established sacroiliitis.

- Radiographic SIJ changes may initially be asymmetric. Late changes include subchondral sclerosis, erosions, and finally ankylosis.
- Conventional axial skeletal signs on spine and pelvis radiographs include squaring of vertebrae, syndesmophytes, spinal ligament ossification, Romanus lesions, pelvic enthesophytes, and osteitis pubis.
- Radiograph detection of syndesmophytes requires a distinction to be made between DISH and AS syndesmophytes. Generally, DISH patients present later than AS patients, have paramarginal syndesmophytes, frequently asymmetric in thoracic spine and have OA (DISH may be associated with chondrocalcinosis and CPPD disease).
- $^{99m}$Tc-MDP bone scintigraphy is sensitive for SIJ inflammation, and scans can identify significant peripheral skeletal lesions from a single study through obtaining 'spot' peripheral views.
- CT provides excellent images of the SIJs and sensitively detects previous SIJ lesions but cannot date the lesions and is not an investigation to use to detect current inflammation.
- MRI of SIJs show active inflammatory lesions but subtle previous SIJ pathology can be missed.
- MRI discriminates spinal DISH from AS in doubtful cases.
- Both fat-suppressed MRI and US can detect inflammation at entheses though the absence of inflammatory 'signal' on MRI or Doppler signal on US, does not rule out enthesis disease as part of SpA.

### Disease status and prognostic indicators in axSpA/AS

There are validated instruments measuring disease status in AS including Bath indices, ASAS response criteria, and quality of life indicators.

- Historically, for staging and monitoring AS, the Bath indices have been used (devised in Bath, UK by Andrei Calin's group):
  - Bath Ankylosing Spondylitis Functional Index (BASFI).
  - Bath AS Disease Activity Index (BASDAI; Box 8.6).
  - Bath AS Metrology Index (BASMI).
  - Bath AS Radiology Index (BASRI) (see Table 8.1).
- The AS disease activity score (ASDAS) combines simplified self-reported clinical indices with a measure of ESR or CRP. The performance of ASDAS to discriminate low and high disease activity and cut-off values are quite similar in patients with AS and axSpA ( http://www.asas-group.org/clinicalinstruments/asdas_calculator/asdas.html).
- ASAS have defined response criteria for therapies used in AS.[2] These measures (ASAS 20, ASAS 40, ASAS 5/6; see Box 8.7) incorporate some Bath measures, are increasing used and more widely validated (in an axSpA definition of disease), and may update the BASDAI (alone) as favoured disease (treatment) response measures.
- A number of quality of life measures can be used (e.g. ASQoL[3]).
- A number of enthesitis indices have been developed (Table 8.1). In clinical practice, either MASES or SPARCC are most useful:
  - The most frequently used radiographic index of skeletal spine changes is the Modified Stoke AS Spinal Score. It is based on the degree of vertebral erosion, sclerosis, and squaring and the presence of syndesmophytes and their degree of vertebral bridging.
  - MRI spinal osteitis scoring for research purposes: SPARCC index.

## Box 8.6 Measuring disease activity in AS and axSpA: Bath AS Disease Activity Index (BASDAI) and AS disease activity score (ASDAS)

### BASDAI description

The assessment comprises six questions. Patients score each as 0–10 on a linear scale. Scores are weighted and a composite score is generated.

### ASDAS description

On a 0–10 scale, the patient scores back pain, duration of morning stiffness, their assessment of global disease, a score of peripheral pain and stiffness, then a contribution of either CRP or ESR is added and a composite score is generated.

### Availability

A BASDAI calculator is available online at ℘ http://basdai.com/
    ASDAS is available online at ℘ http://www.asas-group.org/clinical-instruments/asdas_calculator/asdas.html

### Performance of indices

- In AS, BASDAI has long since been shown to have validity in discriminating high and low disease activity in different populations and is responsive to change over a practical duration of disease. BASDAI has historically been adopted widely as a useful index of AS disease activity.
- ASDAS-CRP and ASDAS-ESR have similar performance to BASDAI in discrimination of high and low disease activity, and change in disease activity generally and with anti-TNFα therapy, both in AS and in axSpA.

---

Table 8.1 Enthesitis indices (EIs) for AS assessment

| Enthesitis index (reference) | Comments |
| --- | --- |
| MANDER (Ann Rheum Dis 1987;46:197–202) | The original EI. Scores tenderness at 66 entheses. Impractical and used little in research |
| MASES (Heuft-Dorenbosch. Ann Rheum Dis 2003;62:127–32) | Relatively well validated. Scores 13 entheses as either 'tender' or non-tender'. Includes ASIS, PSIS, iliac crest, Achilles insertion, sternal attachment 1st and 6th/7th rib and over upper sacrum |
| SPARCC (Maksymowych. Ann Rheum Dis 2009;68:948–53) | Scores 18 entheses as either 'tender' or 'non-tender' (superiomedial greater trochanter, quadriceps insertion at patella, inferior patella pole, tibial tuberosity, Achilles insertion, plantar fascia origin, medial and lateral epicondyles and supraspinatus insertion) |
| BERLIN EI (Braun. Lancet 2002;359:1187–93). | Not extensively validated. Scores 12 entheses. |
| UCSF EI (Gorman. N Engl J Med 2002;346:1349–56). | Scores 17 entheses. Performs well in assessment of anti-TNFα in AS |

## Box 8.7 ASAS response criteria

ASAS improvement criteria (ASAS-IC). Four domains, based on the discrimination between treatment (originally NSAID) and placebo:

- Physical function, measured by the BASFI.
- Spinal pain, measured on a 0–100 mm visual analogue scale (VAS).
- Patient global assessment in the last week, on a 0–100 mm VAS.
- Inflammation, measured as the mean of the last two BASDAI questions

ASAS 20% response criteria (ASAS20). Treatment response defined as:

- ≥20% and ≥10 mm VAS on a 0–100 scale in at least 3 of 4 ASAS-IC domains, and no worsening of ≥20% and ≥10 mm VAS on a 0–100 scale in 4th domain.

ASAS 40% response criteria. Treatment response is defined as:

- ≥40% and
- ≥20 mm VAS on a 0–100 scale in at least 3 of 4 ASAS-IC domains, and no worsening of ≥40% and ≥20 mm VAS on a 0–100 scale in 4th domain.

ASAS 5 out of 6 response criteria (ASAS 5/6). Developed for use in trials of anti-TNFα therapy. Treatment response defined as improvement in 5 of 6 domains without deterioration in the 6th domain, using predefined percentage improvements:

- Pain
- Patient global assessment
- Function
- Inflammation
- Spinal mobility
- C-reactive protein (acute-phase reactant).

- The main predictive factors of poor outcome in AS are to be:
  - hip involvement, early loss of lumbar spine mobility.
  - oligoarticular disease; low social–educational background.
  - sporadic disease rather than familial; onset <16 years; ESR >30.
  - poor initial response to NSAIDs; presence of dactylitis.

## The treatment of axSpA including AS

### General treatment

- UK NICE guideline for management of axSpA 2017.[4]
- Treatment principles are indicated and include the following:
  - Patient education.
  - Exercises (see ♒ http://www.nass.co.uk).
  - Other physical therapy and hydrotherapy.
  - Avoid smoking given its pro-inflammatory effects.
  - NSAIDs for IBP and enthesitis.
  - Oral glucocorticoid (GC) or IM methylprednisolone.

- With exercise the emphasis is placed on the need to maintain posture and physical activity. Spinal extension exercises are important as the natural history of the disease otherwise leads to spinal 'stoop', lack of back extension, and loss of height.
- Physiotherapy provides benefit in the short term. Spa treatment improves function for up to 9 months and reduces health resource use.
- Fatigue is not easily treated though some effort to improve sleep health and maintain some aerobic exercise may play a positive role.

### NSAIDs and synthetic DMARDs (sDMARDs)

- For the majority of patients, NSAIDs remain the treatment of choice. Regular full-dose NSAID use is often required.
- Continuous, rather than intermittent NSAID (including COX-2 selective NSAIDs) may slow radiographic progression of axial skeletal changes but the research evidence overall is weak.
- Sulfasalazine (SSZ) has been shown in a meta-analysis to be efficacious when compared with placebo for peripheral joint disease only. However, improvement in symptoms and quality of life is not dramatic.
- Mixed results have been found with methotrexate. A Cochrane meta-analysis concluded that there is insufficient evidence to support its use in AS. Benefit may be limited to patients with peripheral disease.
- Joint inflammation can be managed in acute, severe cases with IA GC injections.
- Care should be taken injecting GC around tendons, as rupture can occur if the injection is placed into the tendon itself.
- Steroid injection around the Achilles tendon can help/is safe if there is paratenon inflammation alone (preceding imaging advisable).
- Topical GC eye drops should be used to treat uveitis. If the symptoms persist for >3 days an ophthalmological opinion should be sought.
- IV bisphosphonates can help spinal osteitis symptoms. Pamidronate 90 mg monthly can be used. Zoledronic acid can resolve osteitis lesions for 3 months in a majority of patients.

### Biologic DMARDs (bDMARDs)

- Anti-TNFα bDMARDs are effective in AS in reducing symptoms and inflammation though there is debate on whether they can reduce the progression of structural skeletal changes (infliximab, etanercept, adalimumab, certolizumab, and golimumab).
- In the UK, NHS anti-TNFα is recommended for treating 'severe active' AS in adults whose disease has responded inadequately to, or who cannot tolerate, NSAIDs. Infliximab is recommended only if treatment is started with the least expensive infliximab product.
- Infliximab is licensed to treat AS at a dose of 5 mg/kg (compared with 3 mg/kg used in RA), though published data suggest AS can be frequently treated to remission with 3 mg/kg dosing.
- Remission of disease following anti-TNFα treatment is more common the earlier in the disease course anti-TNFα is used. These consistent findings highlight the need for early identification of AS and prompt treatment plan implementation.

- Evidence overall now supports the efficacy and safety of anti-TNFα in nr-axSpA. Secukinumab is the first drug targeting the Il-17 pathway in radiographic-axSpA (AS) that has shown efficacy.
- Anti-TNFα therapy recommendations in UK (NICE TA383)[5] are now available based on the ASAS definition of nr-axSpA.
- Secukinumab (monoclonal anti-IgG1,) is the first drug targeting the Il-17 pathway (it targets Il-17A) and is licensed to treat AS and PsA. At a dose of 150 mg (monthly SC after 4 initial weekly disease) it has shown efficacy in two phase III RCTs (NNT to achieve ASAS40 response: 3–4).
- Ustekinumab (monoclonal antibody targeting the common subunit of both Il-12 and Il-23) and tofacitinib (JAK inhibitor) have shown positive results in phase II/proof-of-concept trials.

## References

1. Burgos-Vargas R, Wei JCC, Rahman MU, et al. The prevalence and clinical characteristics of non-radiographic axial spondyloarthritis among patients with inflammatory back pain in rheumatology practices: a multinational, multicenter study. *Arthritis Res Ther* 2016;18:132.
2. Zochling J, Braun J. Assessment of ankylosing spondylitis. *Clin Exp Rheumatol* 2005;23(Suppl 39):S133–41.
3. Doward L, Spoorenberg A, S Cook S, et al. Development of the ASQoL: a quality of life instrument specific to ankylosing spondylitis. *Ann Rheum Dis* 2003;62:20–6.
4. NICE. *Spondyloarthritis in Over 16s: Diagnosis and Management.* [NG65] London: NICE, 2017. ℘ https://www.nice.org.uk/guidance/ng65
5. NICE. *TNF-alpha Inhibitors for Ankylosing Spondylitis and Non-Radiographic Axial Spondyloarthritis.* [TA383] London: NICE, 2016. ℘ https://www.nice.org.uk/guidance/ta383

# Psoriatic arthritis

### Epidemiology

Psoriasis (Ps) affects up to 3% of the population. The heterogeneity of clinical features of psoriatic arthritis (PsA), the numerous classification criteria existing for it historically, and until recently poor understanding of its lesions and their detection, have implied great uncertainty in knowing the true prevalence of PsA (see Box 8.8).

- Historic estimates of the prevalence of PsA suggest it is present in up to 40% of patients with Ps. More conservative estimates suggest PsA occurs in about 10–20% of the Ps population (i.e. 0.5–1% of the whole population).
- However, estimates have not adequately considered the overall likely prevalence of PsA in all its forms, and given obvious difficulties in identifying PsA sine Ps and defining disease without peripheral joint synovitis (e.g. enthesopathic forms and forms characterized by tendonitis and/or enthesitis and/or spinal disease alone).
- The condition affects women and men equally with usual onset between the ages of 20 and 40 years.

### Pathophysiology

*Genetics*
- Ps is familial. There are about 40–50 genes which are associated with an increased odds ratio of developing psoriasis.
- Genetic factors also have an important role in PsA and family studies have suggested that the heritability may exceed 80%.
- Variants in the HLA-B and HLA-C genes are the strongest genetic risk factors but other variants exist.

---

### Box 8.8 CASPAR classification criteria for PsA

CASPAR updates previous criteria: Moll and Wright 1973; Vasey and Espinoza 1984; Gladman 1987, McGonagle 1999, Fournie 1999.

Inflammatory articular disease (joint, spine or enthesis)

with ≥3 points from the following:
(1 point each unless stated)
- Current Ps (scores 2 points)
- History of Ps in 1st- or 2nd-degree relative
- Psoriatic nail dystrophy
- IgM RF negative*
- Current dactylitis
- History of dactylitis
- Juxta-articular new bone.**

* By any method except latex.

** Ill-defined ossification near joint margins (excluding osteophytes) on radiographs of hands or feet.

*Immunopathogenesis*

- Many variants overlap with those implicated in Ps where there may be >40 susceptibility loci, and lie within or close to genes in the IL-12, IL-23, and NFκB signalling pathways.
- It is thought that an environmental trigger, probably a microorganism, triggers the disease in genetically susceptible people, leading to activation of dendritic and T cells.
- CD8+ T cells, which recognize antigen presented in the context of HLA class I, are more abundant than CD4+ T cells within the joint which is in keeping with the genetic association between PsA and HLA-C and -B variants.
- II-23/II-17 pathway plays a pivotal role in PsA.
- A triggering stimulus may cause over-production of II-23 by dendritic cells, which then promotes differentiation and activation of Th17 cells which produce II-17A.
- II-17A and Th1 cytokines such as IFNγ and TNFα, act on macrophages and tissue-resident stromal cells at entheses, in bone, and within the joint to produce additional proinflammatory cytokines and other mediators which contribute to inflammation and tissue damage.

## Clinical features

- Ps-related MSK symptoms can present with, before, or after the onset of Ps. The situation for nail disease is the same. In some cases, gaps between presentations of the different aspects of Ps disease can be many years. Some patients can go through life with their PsA and never get Ps.
- MSK imaging research has shown lesions exist at entheses of tendon and ligaments, in the nail bed, in bone, and on bone surfaces (adjacent to entheses, probably periostea). Synovial may well be a secondary lesion due to adjacent enthesitis and by no means an essential lesion of PsA.
- Nail lesions are not always present but distinctive. Nail lesions occur in 40% of patients with Ps alone. See ➔ Plate 8.
- Fatigue is a consistent and often severe symptom of Ps-related disease.
- Dactylitis, swelling of the whole finger, occurs in over one-third of classically defined PsA patients.
- In about 20% of PsA cases there is a chronic, progressive, and deforming arthropathy with an often-asymmetrical pattern including DIPJ involvement, or arthritis mutilans, and/or polydactylitis and/or large joint deterioration.
- Some clinical patterns of PsA that have been written about historically are listed as follows. However, it is probable that patterns do not always persist in any individual and as yet no distinct genotype or immunopathological features segregate in association with these descriptive patterns of disease:
  - DIPJ predominant disease.
  - Asymmetric oligoarthritis.
  - Symmetrical polyarthritis.
  - Spine predominant disease (estimates 2–40%).
  - Enthesopathic predominant disease.
  - Arthritis mutilans is a classic but uncommon manifestation of PsA. Bone resorption leads to collapse of the soft tissue in the digits, creating 'telescoping fingers'.

- It is not clear, however, if the patterns of disease have any prognostic significance in themselves.
- Adverse prognostic factors in the 1995 Toronto cohort were polyarthritis, greater HAQ, and increase in use of sDMARDs.
- Persistent dactylitis is a marker of associated digit small joint deterioration.
- The radiological features associated with PsA that help to differentiate it from RA and inflammatory generalized OA include:
  - absence of juxta-articular osteoporosis.
  - absence of subchondral plate changes in early disease.
  - DIPJ disease (with marginal changes initially and an absence of early subchondral plate changes).
  - 'whittling' (lysis) of terminal phalanges.
  - asymmetry of joint involvement.
  - 'pencil-in-cup' deformities.
  - ankylosis.
  - periostitis (often 'fluffy' juxta-articular periosteal new bone—see ➔ Plate 23).
  - spondylitis (asymmetric 'floating' syndesmophytes, spondylodiscitis, facet joint (FJ) changes—though FJ appearances in PsA are not at all well-defined given a presumed common finding of OA affecting FJs and poor definition to date of juxta-articular new bone in PsA FJs).

## Clinical assessment in PsA

- The variation in clinical features between patients, the potential for multiple MSK lesions, and involvement of spine structures has historically led to a difficulty in establishing agreed and universal classification criteria for PsA and consequently in designing applicable treatment outcome assessment tools for PsA.
- Typically, assessments have been adopted from their use in RA. Some salient points are:
  - DAS68 should be used rather than DAS28 for assessing joint tenderness and swelling.
  - Though all have been developed for AS, different enthesitis indices (see Table 8.4) can be applied to PsA.
  - Though representing some methodological challenges, the PASI remains the best assessment of Ps skin response to treatment.
- Comprehensive PsA assessment requires an index (indices) to allow measurement of the response of joint, tendon, enthesis, nail, spine, and skin disease to treatment, but also to measure general health and function changes capturing the effects of fatigue and mood.
- Composite indices have been proposed. DAPSA: Disease Activity for Psoriatic Arthritis; PsAJAI: Psoriatic Arthritis Joint Activity Index; CPDAI: Composite Psoriatic Disease Activity Index. Indices have been summarized.[6]
- The only enthesitis index which has been developed specifically for PsA is the Leeds Enthesitis Index (LEI). It scores six entheses scoring tenderness (1) or no tenderness (0) at lateral humeral epicondyles, over medial femoral condyles, and at Achilles insertions.

- An index of minimal disease activity (MDA) has been proposed.[7]
  A patient with PsA is defined as having MDA when 5 of 7 of the
  following are present:
  - Tender joint count ≤1.
  - Swollen joint count ≤1.
  - PASI ≤1 or BSA ≤3.
  - Patient pain VAS ≤15/100.
  - Patient global activity VAS ≤20/100.
  - HAQ ≤0.5.
  - Tender entheses ≤1.

## The extended psoriasis-related disease comorbidities

- Comorbidities, which require screening for in Ps patients, include
  arterial hypertension, dyslipidaemia, obesity, diabetes mellitus, metabolic
  syndrome, non-alcoholic steatohepatitis (NAFLD), depression,
  nicotine abuse, alcohol abuse, chronic inflammatory bowel disease, and
  lymphoma.
- In the UK, screening Ps patients for PsA using PEST is currently
  recommended (⌖ http://www.bad.org.uk/library/).
- The association of metabolic syndrome with PsA in patients with or
  without Ps is unknown.
- Hyperuricaemia is associated with Ps and PsA. An association of PsA
  with gout has been recognized for a long time.

## Treatment of PsA

### General treatment

- Patient education about the various lesions of PsA, their relapsing and
  remitting nature, and about the risk of long-term comorbidity risk is of
  increasing importance.
- Encouraging patient group participation may be helpful (e.g. in the
  UK: PAPAA (⌖ http://www.papaa.org).
- Localized lesions may respond to rest, ice, and physiotherapy.
- Comorbidities need to be addressed: obesity, cardiovascular risk,
  hyperuricaemia, depression (e.g. screen with HADS).
- Physiotherapy assessment particularly if there is IBP.

### NSAIDs and synthetic DMARDs (sDMARDs)

- Treatment is tailored to the site and number of MSK lesions.
- NSAIDs would be expected to help.
- sDMARDs have conventionally been reserved for patients who have
  inflammatory disease threatening joint integrity; however, with multiple
  site and/or severe symptoms, fatigue, Ps, and a potential impact from
  multiple symptoms on function and contributing to comorbidities, many
  specialists regard sDMARD therapy introduction wholly reasonable
  when based on such symptom-based and 'holistic-view' criteria.
- Evidence for unequivocal sDMARD efficacy is not strong though
  some evidence exists for methotrexate (MTX), leflunomide (LEF),
  and ciclosporin. Evidence is weaker still for SSZ, hydroxychloroquine
  (HCQ), gold, penicillamine, and azathioprine (AZA).

- The first-line sDMARD choice of many rheumatologists for PsA remains MTX. This is reflected in the EULAR guideline for managing PsA.[8]
- Essentially, the EULAR guide advocates:
  - Phase 1: NSAIDs and GC injections.
  - Judge phase 1 response against treatment target.
  - If target not reached: phase 2—start MTX.
  - If contraindications to MTX: start LEF.
  - If target not reached: phase 3—start anti-TNFα.
  - If axial disease alone, on failure of phase 1: start anti-TNFα.
- Many clinicians would advocate relevant efficacy only occurs at the higher weekly doses of MTX (20–25 mg/week).
- HCQ can aggravate psoriasis (see Summary of Product Characteristics for the drug).
- Oral and IM GCs might be generally avoided in patients with Ps because although the skin disease responds, after the steroids there can be a rebound worsening of skin disease.
- Good efficacy on joint disease in PsA is established with all anti-TNFα drugs; however, criteria for study recruitment and judging outcome with all anti-TNFα drugs has been set fairly conventionally and has focused on *joints*, and therefore to a significant degree, on *synovial* disease (i.e. using ACR 20/50 outcome criteria or DAS28—both adopted from their development in assessing RA, not PsA).
- In the UK, etanercept, infliximab, adalimumab and golimumab (see NICE Technology appraisal guidance TA199 and TA220)[9, 10] are approved by NICE for the treatment of PSA. All have positive effects on skin, as well as joint disease.
- For UK NHS funded anti-TNFα treatment, PsA patients need to have peripheral arthritis with ≥3 tender and ≥3 swollen joints and have not responded to, or failed to tolerate, at least two standard sDMARDs alone or in combination.
  - Essentially merging UK NICE requirements and EULAR guidance suggests UK clinicians need to choose MTX first then LEF second, pre-anti-TNFα.
  - In the UK, NICE requires anti-TNFα treated PsA patients are assessed at 12 weeks using validated outcome measures such as Psoriatic Arthritis Response Criteria (PSARC) measurements.
  - NICE rules do not require PsA patients to be simultaneously treated with MTX while receiving anti-TNFα.
- For patients with significant nail disease for whom topical (GC ± calcipotriol) therapy has failed, treatment with adalimumab, etanercept, intralesional steroid, ustekinumab, MTX and acitretin are recommended
- Certolizumab pegol has shown efficacy in PsA also with specific effect demonstrated on different MSK lesions and nail disease; however, it is not authorized for treatment in UK by NICE. Some concern has been raised[11] that this anti-TNFα drug is associated with greater risk for adverse effects compared with other anti-TNFα drugs.

- Ustekinumab, a monoclonal antibody which binds to, and neutralizes IL-23 (specifically binds the p40 subunit common to Il-12 and Il-23 preventing receptor binding) has been licensed to treat Ps for some years.
- Efficacy of ustekinumab in PsA importantly shows significant responses in joint, dactylitis, and enthesitis extending to a year after treatment in phase III trials.
- In the UK, NICE has authorized use of ustekinumab for PsA patients who have failed anti-TNFα.
- The finding that Il-23 stimulated Th17 cell activation (including generating Il-17) in SpAs and psoriasis has heralded a new approach to developing bDMARDs targeting this immune activation pathway (e.g. the anti-Il-17A monoclonal secukinumab in phase III development).
- Apremilast, an orally available small molecule inhibitor of phosphodiesterase 4 (PDE4), was licensed by the FDA in the USA in 2014 and in the European Union for treating PsA.
- In the UK, NICE has not authorized the use of apremilast (in the USA marketed as Otezla® for Ps and PsA) for both Ps and PsA.
- Apremilast compares favourably to placebo in patients failing previous sDMARD therapy in PsA but has not directly been compared with high-dose MTX therapy alone. Apremilast is associated with frequent mild to moderate adverse effects but also weight loss, worsening depression, and suicidal ideation.

## References

6. Wong PC, Leung YY, Li EK, et al. Measuring disease activity in psoriatic arthritis. *Int J Rheumatol* 2012;2012:839425.
7. Coates L, Fransen J, Helliwell PS. Defining minimal disease activity in psoriatic arthritis: a proposed objective target for treatment. *Ann Rheum Dis* 2010;62:48–53.
8. Gossec L, Smolen JS, Gaujoux-Viala C, et al. European League Against Rheumatism recommendations for the management of psoriatic arthritis with pharmacological therapies. *Ann Rheum Dis* 2012;71:4–12.
9. NICE. *Etanercept, Infliximab and Adalimumab for the Treatment of Psoriatic Arthritis.* [TA199] London: NICE, 2010. ℘ https://www.nice.org.uk/guidance/ta199
10. NICE. *Golimumab for the Treatment of Psoriatic Arthritis.* [TA220] London: NICE, 2011. ℘ https://www.nice.org.uk/guidance/ta220
11. Singh JA, Wells GA, Christensen R, et al. Adverse effects of biologics: a network meta-analysis and Cochrane overview. *Cochrane Database Syst Rev* 2011;2:CD008794.

# SpA-associated reactive arthritis

## Background and clinical features

- SpA-associated reactive arthritis (ReA) is a ('lesion-aseptic', i.e. lesions not directly infected) inflammatory condition affecting spine and axial skeletal structures, joints, tendons, and entheses triggered by infection with certain bacteria including *Chlamydia*, *Campylobacter*, *Salmonella*, *Shigella*, *Yersinia*, and possibly also *Clostridia*, *Ureaplasma*, and *Mycoplasma*.
- The risk of developing ReA after having one of these infections is ~1–4% generally but 20–25% in people who are HLA-B27 positive.
- Non-SpA-associated ReA can occur after viruses (particularly parvovirus) and *Streptococcus* (β-haemolytic), gonococcus, HIV, *Borrelia* (Lyme disease), *Mycobacterium* (Poncet's disease) and possibly other pathogens but the characteristics of ReA following these infections are not SpA-like in clinical features nor immunopathology and have no association with HLA-B27.
- SpA-associated ReA is basically an acute form of SpA. Indeed, it is possible that ReA is the triggering event in developing long-term SpA—a semantic issue perhaps when considering the alternative—'chronic ReA', which historically is regarded to occur in a small minority of patients with acute ReA.
- A high index of suspicion of sexually acquired ReA (SARA) is required particularly in women where genital *Chlamydia* infection can be asymptomatic in up to 50%.
- The onset of reactive arthritis is usually acute with systemic symptoms and inflammatory MSK symptoms.
- Differential diagnosis includes septic arthritis, gout, and other SpAs.
- Non-MSK symptoms worth noting are mucocutaneous features including painless circinate balanitis of the glans penis, conjunctivitis, and pustular psoriasis of the palms or feet (keratoderma blennorrhagica).
- In GI infection-triggered ReA, the acute GI symptoms may precede the MSK symptoms by 1–4 weeks:
  - Initial GI symptoms may be so mild as to be ignored by the patient and often the provoking bacterium has cleared from the gut before the MSK symptoms arise.
  - Persistent bowel symptoms, particularly pain and diarrhoea should raise suspicion of inflammatory bowel disease.
- Recurrent or repeated infections do not always lead to a recurrence of ReA MSK lesions and, in the case of SARA, may occur in the absence of further sexual intercourse.

## Investigation of SpA-associated ReA

- Acute-phase response measures are invariably high.
- If SARA is suspected from symptomatic urethritis, prostatitis, or cervicitis, or if suspicion of SARA is high based on MSK and non-genitourinary (GU) symptoms alone, referral for rigorous GU investigation is recommended.
- With triggering bowel infections, often by the time ReA is apparent, then stool culture will likely be negative.

- Serological evidence of recent *Yersinia* or *Campylobacter* can be sought (IgM+) but often delays from initial infection to ReA issues with assay specificity impede use. For example, recent parvovirus B19 infection leads to false-positive ELISAs for a number of these pathogens.
- Serology for *Chlamydia* infection—*C. pneumoniae* or *C. trachomatis*—is not recommended.
- Radiographs are of limited use. The distribution of inflammatory lesions at SIJs, joints, and entheses can be confirmed with bone scintigraphy.
- Lumbar spinous processes and posterior pelvis MRI may show typical SpA inflammatory lesions (osteitis, sacroiliitis, enthesitis).
- Regional MSK US may be useful in selected cases (e.g. of 'hindfoot' may show enthesitis at Achilles insertion, plantar fascia origin, any synovitis, and its site and fluid can be aspirated under US guidance for Gram stain and culture and for polarized light microscopy examination, to rule out gout).

## Management of SpA-related ReA

- NSAIDs and local joint or enthesis GC injections are the mainstay of therapeutic intervention.
- If symptoms persist >6 months and there is clinical evidence of ongoing synovitis and joint destruction, then a synthetic DMARD (sDMARD) such as SSZ or methotrexate may be considered.
- Physiotherapy should be considered if there is persistent IBP.
- The majority of patients are in complete remission at the end of 2 years of sDMARD therapy, most within 6 months.
- Balanitis and keratoderma may persist—predictors of poor prognosis. Other factors that may be predictive of poor outcome include arthritis of the hip, persistently raised ESR, B27 positivity, poor response to NSAIDs, dactylitis, and lumbosacral spine involvement.
- Aseptic urethritis and early conjunctivitis resolve quickly and spontaneously.
- Antibiotic therapy will clear underlying infections, but this may not have any effect on the duration of ReA disease.
- Uveitis should be treated in the usual way with topical steroid drops and a referral to an ophthalmologist if there has been no response within 3 days.
- Patient education, particularly in the context of food hygiene and prevention of exposure to sexually acquired infection, is important. Contact tracing is vital in cases of sexually transmitted infection.
- Anti-TNFα is reserved for cases of sDMARD failure. In the UK, there are no specific NICE guidelines for treating SpA-related ReA.

# Inflammatory bowel disease-related SpA

## Clinical presentation

- The clinical characteristics of inflammatory MSK symptoms presenting in patients with active Crohn's disease and (ulcerative) colitis are often typical of SpA lesions and occur, broadly speaking considering all studies, in a sizeable minority of IBD patients.
- Epidemiology data depend on whether patient groups are defined first by their IBD or by their SpA.
- In one series of IBD patients, sacroiliitis was present in 17% detected by MRI; though of note, non-inflamed, non-current SIJ disease may be missed by MRI.
- By contrast, when AS or axSpA patients are investigated for IBD rigorously, bowel lesions are seen in about 50% of patients.
- Whether IBD-related SpA is distinct from axSpA (new ASAS definition) will need to be established; however, pre-ASAS axSpA definition, many, if not all IBD-related SpA patients might be classified using the ESSG criteria for SpA.
- In summary, there is still some uncertainty as to whether all cases of IBD-related arthritis are true SpAs.
- The association of the inflammatory arthritis with IBD is arguably stronger with Crohn's disease than with UC. The association might be more visible given the likelihood that the correlation between activity of IBD and severity of MSK symptoms is greater for Crohn's than it is for UC.
- In Crohn's-associated inflammatory arthritis/SpA, the arthritis tends to remit after surgical removal of diseased bowel tissue or tight control of enteric inflammation.
- It is observed that MSK symptoms associated with IBD are greater if the integrity of the ileocecal valve is lost. Speculatively, then, it may be that bacterial colonization of previously bacteria-free small bowel is a key trigger in pathogenesis of the SpA.
- Lesions can be discordant by some years. IBD can evolve (sometimes years) following the onset of SpA (e.g. see reference 12).
- Non-MSK extra-intestinal features of IBD include:
  - aphthous stomatitis.
  - fatigue.
  - anaemia.
  - uveitis, (in about 10%).
  - erythema nodosum.
  - pyoderma gangrenosum.

## Management of IBD-related SpA

- NSAIDs are usually contraindicated if there is known IBD.
- IA or IM GCs are used relatively early in the disease course given the avoidance of NSAIDs.
- Mesalazine and AZA, used to treat IBD, is not recognized for its effect on MSK symptoms but SSZ and MTX do have effect. Their use may require liaison with the gastroenterologist as mesalazine/AZA needs to be discontinued in most cases.
- Anti-TNFα choices need to be made carefully given both SpA and IBD lesions in relevant patients. Etanercept has no efficacy in IBD.
- The use of anti-TNFα in UK NHS patients with IBD-related SpA requires qualification for funding for treatment based on either AS, PsA, or IBD criteria alone.

## Reference

12. Vavricka SR, Rogler G, Gantenbein C, et al. Chronological order of appearance of extraintestinal manifestations relative to the time of IBD diagnosis in the Swiss Inflammatory Bowel Disease Cohort. *Inflamm Bowel Dis* 2015;21:1794–800.

# Juvenile spondyloarthritis

### Epidemiology and classification

- Juvenile SpA (JSpA) is an 'umbrella' term encompassing a group of diseases with shared genetic predisposition that affect children <16 years of age.
- The classification of JSpA (International League of Associations for Rheumatology (ILAR); Table 8.7) accepted by most is:
  - enthesitis-related arthritis (ERA).
  - juvenile psoriatic arthritis (JPsA), which can be sub classified into SpA similar to PsA in adults or peripheral arthritis similar to ANA-positive JIA.
  - undifferentiated SpA (if ERA and JPsA features are present).
- Juvenile PsA and ERA are classifiable using the ILAR classification endorsed by WHO in 1999 (see ➲ Table 8.2, p. 318).
- Other JSpAs not specifically accounted for in the ILAR classification include juvenile AS (JAS) who fulfil the mNY criteria before they are 16 years, reactive arthritis, and IBD-related SpA.
- Estimates of JSpA prevalence are based on data for JIA and do not include JAS.
- ERA and JPsA together account for 10–20% of JIA, which gives an estimated 2–60 cases per 100,000 children.
- Of adults with AS, 8–15% have onset in childhood.

**Table 8.2** ILAR classification of JIA—SpA relevant criteria

|  | Inclusion criteria | Exclusion criteria |
|---|---|---|
| JPsA | Arthritis plus psoriasis (Ps) or arthritis plus ≥2 of: <br> • dactylitis; <br> • nail pitting/onycholysis; <br> • psoriasis in a 1st degree relative. | • Arthritis in a HLAB27 positive male >6y. <br> • AS, ERA, or IBD with sacroiliitis, reactive arthritis or acute anterior uveitis or history of one of these disorders in a 1st degree relative. <br> • Presence of IgM RF on ≥2 occasions >3 months apart. <br> • Systemic-onset JIA. |
| ERA | Arthritis plus enthesitis or arthritis or enthesitis plus ≥2 of: <br> • Presence or history of SIJ tenderness and/or IBP; <br> • HLAB27 positive; <br> • onset of arthritis in boy >6y; <br> • acute symptomatic anterior uveitis; <br> • history of: AS or ERA or sacroiliitis with IBD or reactive arthritis or anterior uveitis - in a 1st degree relative. | • Psoriasis or a history of psoriasis in the patient or a 1st degree relative. <br> • Presence of IgM RF ≥2 occasions at least 3 months apart. <br> • Systemic JIA. |

- JSpA mostly occurs in late childhood or adolescence with peak onset at 12 years; 60% are male.
- Approximately 50% of JSpA patients are HLA-B27 positive and 20% have a family history of HLA-B27-associated disease.
- Rheumatoid factor and ANA characteristically are negative.

## Clinical presentation

- Arthritis is usually oligoarticular, asymmetric, and primarily of the lower extremity.
- Hip and midfoot arthritis are suggestive of JSpA and dactylitis is typical of JPsA.
- Enthesitis is present in 66–82% of JSpA patients, affecting mainly the inferior pole of the patella, Achilles tendon insertion, plantar fascia origin and insertions at metatarsal heads, and gluteus medius insertion into the greater trochanter.
- Axial involvement at onset occurs in 10–24% of children frequently presenting as sacroiliac pain and stiffness.
- Two-thirds of MRI-positive sacroiliitis may be asymptomatic.
- By age 10 years, two-thirds of JSpA patients have axial disease.
- Other manifestations include acute anterior uveitis (unilateral painful red eye with photophobia in 25% of children over time), bowel inflammation, psoriasis, nail pitting, and, rarely, cardiac disease.

## Approach to diagnosis

- There is no standardized enthesitis index for paediatric patients.
- Recent evidence suggests a role for whole-body MRI as enthesitis can be overestimated in children by physical examination.
- Typical clinical findings in JSpA include:
  - insidious onset of low back pain with morning stiffness of >30 min that improves with exercise.
  - tenderness on direct compression over the SIJ.
  - decreased lumbar flexion.
  - positive FABER (Patrick) test (ℜ http://www.physio-pedia.com/FABER_Test).
- MRI utility in asymptomatic and symptomatic disease is unclear. Correlation of positive MRI findings with symptomatic improvement on bDMARD therapy has yet to be shown. Gadolinium enhancement of MRI is preferred by some paediatric centres.
- Where JSpA fulfils the New York criteria for AS, a diagnosis of juvenile AS is made.

## Management of JSpA

- JSpA conditions, like all forms of JIA, can be severely debilitating and places a heavy physical and psychological burden on children and families affected by the disease. Multidisciplinary team (MDT) support is essential.
- The principles of treatment include patient and parental education, physical therapy, splints, orthotics, NSAIDs, and IA GC for peripheral arthritis.

- With joint involvement, there is a high risk of permanent joint contractures with persistent disease. Intensive physiotherapy and judicious use of IA steroid is important.
- Treatment guidelines for JIA, including JSpA, have been published by the American College of Rheumatology.
- MTX, SSZ, and LEF are used for peripheral arthritis, but efficacy for enthesitis and axial disease has not been fully assessed in ERA.
- Response to anti-TNFα therapy appears to be similar to that of AS and axSpA in adults. It is not clear whether treatment halts progression of structural damage.
- Drugs that target Il-12/23 and Il-17 may have a role in JSpA treatment but are not yet approved in JSpA or JIA.

## Outcome of JSpA

- JSpA may have a poorer overall prognosis than JIA and <20% of patients experience disease remission within 5 years.
- Persistent disease activity is associated with midfoot arthritis/disease, hip arthritis with 6 months of disease onset, family history of AS, HLA-B27, and HLA-DRB1*08.

## Further reading

Colbert RA. Classification of juvenile spondyloarthritis: enthesitis-related arthritis and beyond. *Nat Rev Rheumatol* 2010;6:477–85.

Gmuca S, Weiss PF. Juvenile spondyloarthritis. *Curr Opin Rheumatol* 2015;27:364–72.

Hugle B, Burgos-Vargas R, Inman RD, et al. Long-term outcome of antitumor necrosis factor alpha blockade in the treatment of juvenile spondyloarthritis. *Clin Exp Rheumatol* 2014;32:424–32.

Rachlis AC, Babyn PS, Lobo-Meuller E, et al. Whole body magnetic resonance imaging in juvenile spondyloarthritis: will it provide vital information compared to clinical exam alone? *Arthritis Rheum* 2011;63:S292.

# Juvenile idiopathic arthritis

# Introduction

Inflammatory arthritis, resulting in stiffness, swelling, joint restriction and damage, was characterized in children in 1896 by GF Still and is now recognized as one of the commonest causes of disability in childhood. Juvenile idiopathic arthritis (JIA) is the 'umbrella' term, accepted by the international community, for several forms of arthritis (summarized into subtypes for practical terms in Table 9.1; for JSpA conditions there are many similarities with adult presentations, see ⟴ Chapter 8).

## Epidemiology

- JIA affects 1 in 1000 children and young people up to 16 years of age, from best available UK estimates and has similar prevalence to diabetes (1 in 700). More recent international studies indicate a higher prevalence of 167–400 per 100,000 person-years.
- The annual incidence of JIA is ~1 in 10,000 children/young people.
- A majority of patients with JIA have a phenotype distinct from adult inflammatory arthritis which includes an association with uveitis.
- The diagnosis of JIA requires the presence of arthritis for 6 weeks to distinguish it from reactive arthritis etc.; however, the treatment of JIA and referral to ophthalmology should not wait 6 weeks.

**Table 9.1** The classification of JIA subtypes

|  | Diagnosis | Peak age-range(s) | Extra-articular features |
|---|---|---|---|
| Oligo-JIA | ≤4 joints | 2–4 yrs | Uveitis |
| Poly-JIA (RF or ACPA +ve) | >4 joints | >9 yrs | Nodules, malaise, weight loss |
| Poly-JIA (RF and ACPA −ve) | >4 joints | 2–4 yrs 7–12 yrs | Uveitis, poor growth |
| SoJIA | Fever, rash, hepatomegaly splenomegaly | 4–7 yrs | Serositis, carditis, coronary ectasia, MAS |
| ERA | Enthesitis, asymmetrical large joint arthritis and SIJs | >6 yrs | Acute uveitis |
| JPsA | Psoriasis ± in 1st-degree relative, nail pitting, dactylitis | 9–11 yrs | Psoriasis, bone oedema, panuveitis |

Information from Petty RE et al. International League of Associations for Rheumatology classification of juvenile idiopathic arthritis: second revision, Edmonton, 2001. J Rheumatol 2004;31:390–2.

- In most forms of JIA, there is inflammation of the joint lining (synovium). Circulating activated lymphocytes migrate into joints and the resulting generation of pro-inflammatory cytokines leads to activation of macrophages and joint stromal cells (e.g. fibroblasts) similar to that seen in adult RA. In affected joints, there is excess cytokine production, of TNFα, IL-6, and IL-17.

## Classification

The classification of JIA was radically changed in 2001. For years, there was confusion between North America and European conventions for naming the different forms of juvenile arthritis.

- Classification has been subsequently complicated in practice by the evolving understanding of the breadth of effects in the spondyloarthritis (SpA) conditions.
- We include juvenile SpA also in ● Chapter 8.

# Management of JIA

## National guidelines to aid management

The following key documents promote best practice in JIA and paediatric rheumatology:

- National service specification for paediatric rheumatology (E03/S/b): ℜ http://www.england.nhs.uk/commissioning/spec-services/npc-crg/group-e/e03/
- NHS Commissioning Quality Dashboard: ℜ http://www.england.nhs.uk/commissioning/spec-services/npc-crg/spec-dashboards/
- British Society of Paediatric and Adolescent Rheumatology (BSPAR) guidelines: ℜ http://www.bspar.org.uk/clinical-guidelines
- Arthritis and Musculoskeletal Alliance (ARMA) Standards of Care for JIA: ℜ http://www.arma.uk.net/resources/standards-of-care
- BSPAR website www.bspar.org.uk
- Interim Clinical Commissioning Policy Statement: Biologic Therapies for the treatment of Juvenile Idiopathic Arthritis (JIA): ℜ http://www.engage.england.nhs.uk/consultation/specialised-services-policies/user_uploads/biolgcs-juvenl-idiop-arthrs-pol.pdf
- NICE—abatacept, adalimumab, etanercept, and tocilizumab for treating JIA: ℜ http://www.nice.org.uk/guidance/TA373

## Diagnosing arthritis in children

There are no diagnostic tests for JIA. Diagnosis requires a thorough history and examination to distinguish JIA from other causes of joint pain or swelling (Table 9.2).

Table 9.2 The differential diagnosis of JIA conditions

| Condition | Examples | Investigations |
|---|---|---|
| Monoarticular disease | Septic arthritis, TB, PVNS, foreign-body synovitis, sickle cell disease, haemophilia, leukaemia, non-bacterial osteomyelitis | Blood and synovial fluid culture, Mantoux, IGRA, US, MRI, synovial biopsy, blood film, genetics, coagulation factor assays |
| Arthritis following infection | Lyme disease, viral arthritis, post-streptococcal arthritis, HSP, Kawasaki disease | AI serology, ASOT, anti-DNAse B, throat swab, transthoracic echo |
| Inflammatory back pains conditions | HLA-B27-associated reactive arthritis, ERA, IBD-associated SpA, enthesitis | |
| Biomechanical and orthopaedic conditions | Trauma, haemarthrosis, NAI, patellofemoral pain, osteochondroses, osteochondritis dissecans, osteonecrosis, osteoid osteoma, tarsal coalition, biomecanical imbalance from deconditioning, muscle tightness and hypermobility conditions | Radiographs, MRI |
| Pain conditions | Complex regional pain syndrome (CRPS), chronic widespread pain | |

- Inflammatory arthritis in children is characterized by prolonged morning stiffness (typically >20 min), swelling, restriction, and loss of joint function.
- JIA should be considered when:
  - joint swelling from presumed trauma (including knee and ankle) persists beyond 2 weeks.
  - there is involvement of several joints.
  - aspirated joint fluid is shown to be aseptic.
  - there is morning stiffness.
  - there is joint restriction in the absence of a mechanical lesion.
- Careful examination aims to confirm swelling, which may be subtle, identify joint restriction (typical of actively inflamed joints in children) and establish the distribution of affected joints.
- Quick and methodical assessment of other joints is achieved using pGALS (see ➲ Chapter 1, 'The paediatric GALS screen').
- The examination technique of specific joints uses a systematic approach identified in pREMS (⌘ http://www.pmmonline.org).
- Abnormal signs which might reveal JIA summarized from a typical detailed regional examination are shown in Table 9.3.
- Involvement of multiple joints increases the likelihood that arthritis is JIA, especially in the absence of systemic symptoms.
- Juxta-articular changes in JIA include muscle atrophy, leg length discrepancy due to limb overgrowth from knee involvement, reduced limb length from early closure of growth plates adjacent to inflammation during adolescence, and synovial cysts.
- SoJIA presents with systemic features and the differential diagnosis is wide so a broad approach to assessment and investigations is essential (Table 9.4).

Table 9.3 Key signs compatible with a diagnosis of JIA, summarized from a (necessarily) detailed regional MSK examination

| Joint | Abnormal signs to identify in JIA conditions |
|---|---|
| Wrist | Volar displacement, reduced grip strength, poor or difficulty in handwriting |
| Fingers | Dactylitis, nail pitting, nodules, handwriting (as for wrist) |
| Elbow | Flexion deformity, inability to touch shoulder |
| Shoulder | Loss of abduction, difficulty dressing |
| Neck | Loss of normal cervicothoracic spine lordosis, reduced rotation |
| Spine | Loss of lumbar spine lordosis, positive Schöber test, midline or sacral bony tenderness, reduced or asymmetric lower limb muscle length |
| Hips | Apparent leg length discrepancy, Trendelenburg gait, loss of hip swing on gait, pain at end of range of (passive) rotation, positive FABER test, positive Thomas test |
| Knees | Loss of extension (especially if asymmetrical), synovial (including popliteal) cysts, vastus medialis wasting |
| Ankle and foot | Abnormal/antalgic gait: no/abnormal heel strike, foot pronation/inversion, calf muscle length asymmetry, midfoot rigidity |
| TMJ | Restricted or asymmetric jaw opening, TMJ crepitus |

**Table 9.4** Conditions and investigations to consider when suspecting SoJIA

| Conditions | Investigations |
|---|---|
| Acute lymphoblastic leukaemia | Blood film, bone marrow aspirate, whole-body MRI (including fat-suppressed sequence) |
| Neuroblastoma | Urine or blood adrenaline/noradrenaline |
| Lymphoma | CXR, abdominal US, whole-body MRI or CT |
| Sepsis, TB | Blood cultures, serology, PCR, Mantoux, IFNγ release assay, joint aspiration, MRI |
| SLE, APS | Coagulation, complement C3 and C4, autoantibodies, urinalysis |
| Juvenile DM | Quadriceps MRI, CK, LDH |
| Reactive arthritis, rheumatic fever | Lyme, *Bartonella* and *Brucella* serology, ASOT/anti-DNAaseB and throat swab, transthoracic echocardiogram (TTE) |
| Vasculitides | TTE, ECG, urinalysis, ANCA, detailed history, angiography, biopsy |
| Viruses | Serology (EBV, CMV, *Parvovirus*, *Rubella*) |
| Travel-associated diseases | Tests according to suspicion |
| Periodic fever conditions and porphyrias | Genotyping (see ➲ Chapter 18), IgD, urinary mevalonic acid, urinary porphyrins |
| Inflammatory bowel disease | Faecal calprotectin, endoscopy, barium swallow |

### Differences from adult arthritis

- Arthritis in children directly affects limb growth and may have an overall effect on height and weight attainment.
- Joint restriction is often a more sensitive sign of inflammatory joint disease activity in children than it is in adults.
- With effective disease control and before puberty there is a likelihood of repair of joint damage.
- Medication has to account for body size and different pharmacodynamics and pharmacokinetics.
- Blood monitoring of medications use is frequently different.

### Investigations

At presentation, investigations help distinguish differential diagnoses since there are no diagnostic tests for JIA.

- ESR and CRP do not correlate well with the extent or severity of inflammation and may be normal.
- A particularly high ESR may indicate the presence of inflammatory bowel disease (IBD) or (very rarely) leukaemia.
- A low haemoglobin may indicate anaemia of chronic disease rather than iron deficiency.

- ANA positivity occurs in 40–75% of JIA patients and indicates an increased risk of eye disease. It is not a diagnostic test or predictive of outcome.
- Rheumatoid factor (RF) positivity is rare in JIA and difficult to interpret in oligoarticular JIA. High titre ANA and RF may indicate SLE.
- US is the radiological investigation of choice to corroborate arthritis and evaluate tenosynovitis and joint damage. Its false-negative rate is higher in foot and ankle disease than for other joints.
- Radiographs may show soft tissue swelling, periarticular osteopenia. and erosions in long-standing arthritis.
- Arthroscopy should be avoided unless a biopsy is required as in PVNS.
- Synovial fluid aspiration, but not arthroscopy, is essential when considering sepsis and TB.
- To monitor disease activity, drug therapy and tissue damage:
  - ESR and CRP frequently do not reflect the extent or severity of inflammation.
  - A falling ESR and haemoglobin with climbing ALT/AST may indicate macrophage activation syndrome (see ➔ Chapter 25) as may a ferritin level >10,000 ng/mL.
  - US is used to monitor changes in synovial inflammation and joint damage but contrast-enhanced MRI may provide more useful images including the presence of bone oedema.
  - Monitoring of drug side effects includes the measurement of FBC and LFTs.

## Treatment

The overall approach to treatment in JIA is to gain early rapid control of inflammation, minimize the adverse effects of treatment, and support the general physical and mental health of the patient. This patient-centred holistic approach requires the participation of a full multidisciplinary team—each member with dedicated experience of JIA.

### Treatment of the acute swollen joint

The management of the acute swollen joint should primarily focus on ruling out sepsis (see ➔ Chapter 25, pp. 708–9).

- Ibuprofen, naproxen, diclofenac, or other NSAIDS, should be used, especially when waiting for a paediatric rheumatology review.
- For an effective NSAID response (managing inflammation as opposed to simply pain), the recommended dosing frequency should be continued for >2 weeks +/– gastroprotection.
- IA glucocorticoids (GCs) can be considered for:
  - limp, disability, joint restriction, other complications of arthritis.
  - persistently marked joint swelling.
  - a bridging strategy whilst awaiting long-term medication to become effective.
- Oral or IV GCs should be used to supplement, or as an alternative, to IA GC, if there are many joints involved or joint injections therapy is not immediately feasible or the effect of IA GCs has been tried and was limited.

*Long-term management of JIA*
- Long-term management of JIA requires close collaboration between members of the MDT with effective communication both within the service and across the regional network.
- Members of the MDT include a clinical nurse specialist, physiotherapist, occupational therapist, orthotist or podiatrist, ophthalmology colleagues, musculoskeletal radiologist, psychologist, social work, and dietetic support.
- Medication forms only a part of the long-term management of JIA.
- Fundamental is the promotion of physical activity which encourages a return of the strength and stamina lost from active arthritis, and correction of muscular imbalances that result in pain, injury, and loss of joint protection.
- Provision of information and education for parents and patients is a constant requirement. This is critical for their participation in joint decision-making and adherence to agreed treatment plans and helps dissipate lingering anxiety.
- Pain management frequently involves strategies other than the use of medication.
- Vaccination advice is usually given at the outset and changes in national guidelines (August 2017) indicate that it is safe to give live vaccines to patients before treatment or whilst on low to moderate doses of GCs and csDMARDs (⌖ http://www.gov.uk/government/uploads/system/uploads/attachment_data/file/655225/Greenbook_chapter_6.pdf).
- In individual cases, giving live vaccines even if immunosuppression is being taken far outweighs the risks. All routine non-live vaccines may be given without complication.
- Effective liaison is required with schools, primary care, and community services.
- Effective transition, which includes age-appropriate services for young people from puberty onwards, is also an essential requirement to optimize the well-being and self-efficacy of this age group. This should continue well after transfer to adult services.
- A healthy diet avoids some of the problems of growth restriction or delay and excess weight gain from low physical activity or GC use.
- Although close collaboration with orthopaedics ensures timely referral of patients and good medical management of orthopaedic conditions, the rate of surgical intervention in JIA has greatly diminished.
- Surgical synovectomy, soft tissue release (tenotomies and capsulotomies) and joint replacement are now rare.

*Long-term medication in JIA*
The aim of medication in the long term is to reduce the frequency and impact of flares of arthritis and uveitis.
- Long-term medications in the form of (synthetic) disease-modifying antirheumatic drugs (sDMARDs) are used for:
  - Persistent arthritis or uveitis refractory to, or incompletely controlled by, IA or periocular GCs.
  - Presence of chronic complications or tissue damage.
  - Extension to other joints or eye.
  - Joint-specific effects on the wrist and hand function, the hip and mobility, or jaw.

- sDMARD treatments typically take a few weeks to become effective and may require a bridging course of GCs either IA, orally, or IV.
- Given the extensive support and experience required, sDMARDs are best instituted by a specialist service or delegated responsibility to secondary care within a clinical network.
- There is now extensive experience of the valuable role of primary care in monitoring treatment with the back-up of an accessible secondary or tertiary service.
- The standard sDMARD used in JIA and uveitis is methotrexate (MTX).
- MTX in SC form, rather than tablets or liquid preparations, is typically used in the young child and where there is extensive or severe inflammation.
- Alternative sDMARDS for arthritis include leflunomide (LEF), sulfasalazine (SSZ), and hydroxychloroquine (HCQ).
- Azathioprine (AZA) and ciclosporin may have a role in both arthritis and uveitis, whereas mycophenolate and tacrolimus are considered to have a specific role in uveitis.
- The value of sDMARD combinations is not well studied in JIA but are used with good effect in some patients and have not been shown to have increased levels of adverse effects.
- Biologic DMARD (bDMARD) therapies including anti-TNFα therapies have been shown in high-quality studies to be effective in JIA and are now a standard treatment in the presence of refractory disease to or intolerance of MTX or other sDMARDs:
  - In the UK, there is NHS (NICE) approval for the use of abatacept (a fusion protein of the extracellular domain of human cytotoxic T-lymphocyte-associated antigen 4 (CTLA-4) linked to a modified Fc portion of IgG1), the anti-TNFα therapies adalimumab and etanercept, and tocilizumab (an anti-IL-6 receptor monoclonal bDMARD) in JIA. In England there is also an agreement with NHSE to use anakinra, infliximab and rituximab under certain conditions.
  - bDMARD use in England is directed by NICE and NHSE (ℛ http://www.england.nhs.uk/commissioning/wp-content/uploads/sites/12/2015/10/e03pd-bio-therapies-jia-oct15.pdf).
- Supplementary medications include those for pain, gastritis, and nausea and to optimize bone density and strength in the presence of GCs or reduced physical activity.

## Outcome and prognosis

Given the progress in management strategies and advent of bDMARD therapies, old published outcome data will no longer be applicable. Current paediatric rheumatologist consensus is that there has been a marked improvement in outcome and many patients.

- The incidence of joint replacement has reduced considerably from reports in the early 2000s when 80% of patients with RF-positive JIA followed up over a period of 20 years required arthroplasty.
- There is strikingly little high-quality data measuring long-term remission off medication.
- About 50–75% of patients with persistent oligo-JIA will achieve long-term remission by their early teens but may still experience flares at any time in adulthood.

- About 20–30% of patients with (RF and ACPA) seronegative polyarticular-JIA achieve drug-free long-term remission into adulthood.
- The concept of minimal disease activity has only recently been validated in JIA and may be a better outcome variable for those patients who do not achieve complete remission.
- Despite changes in treatment strategies and outcome, suboptimal outcomes do occur and are associated with:
  - delayed diagnosis.
  - delayed referral to a specialist MDT.
  - suboptimal control of active disease.
  - inadequate engagement and collaboration with the patient, parent, or other carers (see psychology support later in this list).
  - presentation with uveitis and ocular damage.
  - ongoing disease activity in systemic-onset JIA (SoJIA) at 6 months.
  - SoJIA in males.
  - young age of onset in oligoarticular and polyarticular disease.
  - psoriatic arthritis.
  - hip involvement.
  - rapid early onset of JIA in small joints of hands and feet.
  - in association with early radiographic changes.
- Psychology support improves outcome by:
  - reducing the impact of MTX-associated nausea.
  - reducing the impact of fear and anxiety around diagnosis and treatment.
  - identifying, managing, and referring any mental health concerns.
  - alleviating factors that adversely impact on quality of life and engagement with school.
  - addressing adverse body image concerns.
  - managing the frustration or disappointment of persistent or flaring disease activity and side effects from medication.

# Transition services

'Transition' means, and hopes to achieve, the seamless and appropriate care transfer from paediatric/adolescent services to a young-adult or adult service. The development of age-appropriate clinics is a well-regarded strategy to reduce the barriers to effective treatment.

- A transition service is achieved through optimizing engagement of adolescents or young adults, promotion of self-efficacy, and enhancement of self-advocacy and adherence to agreed management plans.
- Many centres now offer adolescent clinics for patients aged from 10–13 years to 17–18 years and young adult clinics for those aged 17–25 years.
- The implementation and optimization of adolescent and young persons' clinics requires:
  - close collaboration between paediatric and adult clinicians.
  - age-specific nursing expertise.
  - age-appropriate environment and information resources.
  - that the patient be seen (first) without parents present.
  - the promotion of an understanding of confidentiality and consent (or assent).
  - the promotion of effective health-related behaviours including joint decision-making, self-advocacy, and self-efficacy.
  - support for the attendance and performance at school, college, and university and when seeking employment.
  - the early identification of mental health problems that may be a barrier to care.
  - respect for developing body awareness.
  - assistance with family planning and sexual health.
  - early anticipation of any surgical needs.
- Guidelines to support the development of young person clinics include *You're Welcome Quality Criteria* (Department of Health) and *Transition to Adult Care: Ready Steady Go* (University of Southampton).

# JIA subtypes and their specific features

### Oligoarticular JIA (oligo-JIA)

- Oligo-JIA is the commonest subtype, accounting for 30–40% of JIA and is characterized by the risk of uveitis. See Table 9.1
- It predominantly affects females with peak ages of onset between 2 to 4 years and 7 to 13 years.
- About 50% of cases are monoarticular in presentation.
- If >4 joints become involved after 6 months of disease activity the condition is reclassified as *extended* oligo-JIA.
- Extension to polyarticular JIA is more likely in those with uveitis and rare beyond 5 years from diagnosis.
- The commonest joints involved are elbow, knee, and ankle.
- Joint or a limb deformity is of great concern in the growing patient.
- Leg length discrepancy is more common when arthritis of the knee begins <3 years of age. To accommodate for the excess length, the child stands with the knee flexed resulting in a flexion contracture.
- Hip monoarthritis or primary coxitis can occur especially in peripubertal Asian girls, but a search to rule out other causes is essential. The following should be considered: septic arthritis, leukaemia (e.g. in an at-risk population such as Down's syndrome), psoriatic arthritis, IBD-associated arthritis, and juvenile SpA.
- Studies have shown that over 80% of patients have little or no disability or joint damage after 15 years of follow-up.
- The HLA associations with oligo-JIA include HLA-DRB1*08 with additional susceptibility haplotypes HLA-DRB*1103/1104.
- HLA-DRB1*0401, found in RA, is protective for selected subtypes of JIA.

### Polyarticular JIA (poly-JIA)

- Poly-JIA is diagnosed when >4 joints are involved within the first 6 months of disease activity (excluding psoriatic arthritis, IBD-associated arthritis, and enthesitis related arthritis).
- Pragmatically, decision-making for extended oligo-JIA is similar to that for poly-JIA and long-term data indicates a similar outcome.
- A polyarticular course occurs in 20–30% of JIA and is subdivided by the presence or absence of RF, which should be checked (on latex) on two occasions at least 3 months apart.
- RF positive JIA occurs in <5% of JIA, is most common in females and has a phenotype very similar to RA in adults.

### Rheumatoid factor-negative polyarticular JIA

- In RF-negative poly-JIA there is often incomplete control of arthritis despite major advances in treatment.
- RF-negative poly-JIA is associated with higher levels of disability especially during flares of the arthritis.
- Joint restriction often indicates disease activity and is commonly associated with muscle atrophy, disability, and joint damage.

- There is a poly-JIA phenotype with boggy synovitis that is not associated with much pain or disability and joints are commonly well preserved. Tenosynovitis can coexist with joint synovitis and can remain undisclosed unless suspected.
- Another poly-JIA subtype is characterized by predominantly foot and ankle involvement, the consequences of which can be a reduction in generalized mobility, tarsal fusion, tenosynovitis, and bursitis.
- TMJ involvement is often insidious in onset. It is unlikely to be missed if pGALS (see ➲ Chapter 1) is undertaken at each clinic visit. If left undertreated, TMJ arthritis may result in micrognathia and dental malocclusion.
- Neck involvement can cause marked irritability and be particularly disabling in the classroom. Occupational therapy assessment is advisable.

## Juvenile psoriatic arthritis (JPsA)

- JPsA is considered as one of the juvenile spondyloarthritides (JSpA; see ➲ Chapter 8; and for ILAR diagnostic criteria see ➲ Chapter 8, p. 318).
- Features of JPsA are similar to adult PsA (see ➲ Chapter 8, p. 318).
- JPsA should be considered even if there is no psoriasis but there is a history of psoriasis in a first-degree relative.
- Nail pitting, dactylitis, previous or concurrent acute panuveitis, and inflammatory back pain history may be present.
- JPsA can be oligo- or polyarticular.
- JPsA is frequently resistant to conventional treatment strategies including GC resistance.

## Juvenile spondyloarthritis (JSpA) and enthesitis-related arthritis (ERA)

- See ➲ Chapter 8 for additional detail.
- JSpA should only be considered in patients older than 6 years, especially males, and when there is asymmetric large joint involvement.
- Enthesitis is the inflammation at the sites of bony insertion of tendons and ligaments. In ERA, enthesitis can be very painful and disproportionate to examination findings.
- HLA-B27 is found in 30–50% of ERA patients and is associated with an increased risk of developing juvenile ankylosing spondylitis.
- ERA is generally associated with a low-grade grumbling disease persisting into adulthood but associated with little erosive joint disease. In a minority of patients with ERA there may be high levels of disability responsive to anti-TNFα therapy.

## Systemic-onset JIA (SoJIA)

This form of JIA, presenting with fever and rash, affects just 5–8% of the JIA population. A broad approach to diagnosis is essential—many conditions can present with MSK pains, rash, and systemic symptoms.

SoJIA is best considered as an umbrella term that covers several autoinflammatory disorders (see ➲ Chapter 18 and Table 18.1, p. 544 ) and poly-JIA triggered by or presenting with a viral infection.

Previously known as 'Still's disease', this term is now discouraged due to the confusion it may cause.

- Incidence: M = F. SoJIA occurs at any age including infants with peak onset between 2 and 3 years old.
- Typically: high levels of IL-1 and IL-6 in serum and synovial fluid.

*Diagnosis of SoJIA*
- No specific diagnostic tests exist.
- There is a broad differential diagnosis that requires assessment by a paediatric rheumatologist.
- Many of the characteristic features including fever, rash, polyarthritis, lymphadenopathy, and hepatosplenomegaly overlap with other conditions (see Table 9.4).
- Similarly, acute lymphoblastic leukaemia can present with fever, rash, and joint/limb pains (attributable to marrow invasion).
- Neuroblastoma should be considered in patients <5 years old.
- A history of travel and contact with animals or tics should be taken.
- True persistent joint inflammation may not be found at diagnosis or for many months (up to 9 years old) after diagnosis.
- The fever, of up to 39°C, is typically quotidian—occurring once or twice per day in a diurnal distribution with return to a normal baseline between fever spikes.
- Typical blood results include high ESR and CRP, neutrophilia (of the order of $20 \times 10^9$/L), thrombocytopenia (often >600 $\times 10^9$/L), and anaemia of chronic inflammation (often <80 g/L).

*Treatment of SoJIA*
The initial treatment of SoJIA focuses on the need to allow time for investigations to exclude other causes of fever and manage pain and disability.
- A trial of NSAIDs for 2 weeks is used initially, though NSAIDs may have no effect on serositis, or florid polyarthropathy.
- SoJIA is a GC-responsive condition, but there's little evidence that GCs alter the long-term outcome.
- GCs may be used once other conditions have been ruled out. A short or limited course of GCs may be used to temporize pain, fatigue, and disability to see if inflammation of a post-infectious origin settles on its own.
- GCs provide effective symptomatic relief while waiting for a sDMARD (typically MTX) response.
- Biologic DMARDs (bDMARDs) are used when:
  - unable to wean off GCs despite use of MTX.
  - MAS is persistent.
  - when a flare of joint pains/disease occurs despite MTX being taken at a therapeutic dose for >3 months.
- If SoJIA is unresponsive to anakinra (an anti-IL-1 bDMARD) after 4 weeks treatment, then treatment should be switched to tocilizumab.
- Tocilizumab is recommended in the UK by NICE.
- Anti-TNFα therapy can be used for children with a polyarticular course of SoJIA once systemic features have settled.
- Other less routine treatments for SoJIA include ciclosporin, canakinumab, IVIg, and stem cell transplantation in severe disease.

# Macrophage activation syndrome

Macrophage activation syndrome (MAS) is rare but is life-threatening (mortality is 8–22%). MAS can complicate other diseases. MAS is also termed secondary haemophagocytic lymphohistiocytosis (HLH). For a summary see http://www.the-rheumatologist.org/article/macrophage-activation- syndrome/6/)

The reader is referred to Chapter 25

## Uveitis

# Uveitis

This important association of JIA occurs in 10–20% of patients and within 7 years of arthritis onset.

- Visual loss occurs in ~25% of JIA-associated uveitis and irreversible blindness occurs without symptoms or changes in eye appearance.
- Irreversible complications may occur after only a few weeks of uncontrolled uveal inflammation.
- However, about half of children with anterior or intermediate uveitis do not experience visual loss despite prolonged inflammation.
- There are numerous causes of uveitis (Table 9.5).

## Uveitis surveillance (screening) programmes

All paediatric rheumatology units/physicians should have an agreed mechanism of systematically screening for, managing, and having emergency access to, a suitably resourced ophthalmology team skilled in examining very young children.

- Uveitis surveillance in JIA is essential because uveitis:
  - is sight-threatening.
  - is rarely apparent from routine history and examination, especially in children <8 years of age.
  - is not predictable and is unrelated to the severity of arthritis.
  - is present in 40% cases at the time of the first eye screen.
  - complications, especially cataract, occur in up to 40%.
  - is most likely to respond with aggressive treatment.
- Other major ophthalmological concerns include glaucoma, macular oedema, retinal detachment, band keratopathy, and hypotony.
- There should be immediate access to advice and assessment should eye symptoms develop.
- A uveitis screening interval schedule should be adopted (e.g. Table 9.6) to avoid irreversible eye damage.
- Uveitis surveillance schedules should be adapted to the risk of uveitis, and in the context of treatment use (e.g. when stopping MTX).

**Table 9.5** The differential diagnosis of causes of paediatric uveitis

| Infectious | Non-infectious |
| --- | --- |
| *Toxoplasma* | Trauma (sympathetic ophthalmia) |
| Varicella | Inflammatory bowel disease |
| Herpes simplex | Sarcoid |
| CMV | Tubulointerstitial nephritis |
| TB | Blau syndrome |
| *Borrelia* (Lyme disease) | Behçet's disease |
| *Bartonella* | Periodic fevers |
| Other: toxocariasis, *Ascaris*, fungal, histoplasmosis, *Syphilis* | Multiple sclerosis |
| | Vogt–Koyanagi–Harada |
| | Vasculitis (including Kawasaki disease) |

**Table 9.6** Uveitis surveillance: recommended frequency of slit lamp examination (summarised from the UK Royal College of Ophthalmology Guidelines)

| Condition | Frequency |
|---|---|
| SoJIA | Yearly |
| Onset of JIA <7 yrs old | ANA +ve: every 2 months for 6 months, then every 3 months for 3.5 yrs, then 6 monthly for 3 yrs or until aged 12 yrs, then yearly (if previous uveitis has occurred) |
| | ANA –ve: every 6 months for 7 years or until aged 12 yrs, then yearly (if previous uveitis has occurred) |
| Onset of JIA ≥7 yrs old | 6 monthly for 4 yrs then yearly (if previous uveitis has occurred) |

- Eye screening continues until 12 years of age when a patient can reliably self-report features of inflammation such as floaters and pain.
- Cessation of eye screening at 12 years old does not indicate that uveitis may not occur, but the risk beyond this age is sufficiently low to make self-report more reliable.

## Management of uveitis

Uveitis management aims to balance long-term risk of visual loss with short- and long-term risks of treatment.
- First-line treatment of anterior uveitis: topical GCs (e.g. Maxidex® or Predsol® eye drops) given up to hourly depending on the severity. Topical GCs are less effective in intermediate or posterior uveitis.
- There is a dose-dependent increase in risk of cataract formation from using steroid eye drops. The risk from one drop per day is 0.1% per year and rises with more frequent and prolonged use.
- Other topical agents include mydriatics to reduce the risk of the iris sticking to the lens (posterior synaechiae) and glaucoma agents.
- Systemic or periocular GCs are used in the presence of panuveitis and features inadequately responsive to eye drops.
- Aggressive or long-term treatment should be confined to those with a significant risk of permanent visual loss.
- sDMARDs or bDMARDs are used when recurrent courses or prolonged use of steroid eyedrops is required to maintain inflammation to less the 0.5+ activity using the SUN criteria.[3]
- Poor outcome from uveitis is associated with presence of ocular damage at presentation, when uveitis precedes arthritis, when there is delay in treatment initiation, and with failure to achieve early remission.

## Reference

3. Scottish Uveitis Network (SUN). *Guidelines.* ✍ http://www.sun.scot.nhs.uk/guidelines.html

# Systemic lupus erythematosus

# Introduction

Systemic lupus erythematosus (SLE/'lupus') is a multisystem autoimmune disorder with a broad spectrum of clinical features involving almost all organs and tissues.

- SLE is a chronic disease which remits and relapses. A preclinical phase exists characterized by autoantibodies common to other autoimmune diseases, followed by a disease-specific autoimmune phase.
- Variations exist in the incidence of clinical features between ethnic groups necessitating a keen sense of awareness of a variety of multisystem pathologies and appreciation that SLE has taken on the mantle of syphilis as the great mimic of other conditions.

## Epidemiology

- Prevalence varies worldwide, but in the UK it is 97 per 100,000.
- SLE is 10–20× more common in women than men, and most likely to develop between the ages of 15 and 40 years.
- It is more common and often more severe in certain ethnic groups such as those of African-Caribbean, India, Hispanic, and Chinese origin living in the USA and Europe than in white Caucasians.

## Classification

- The American College of Rheumatology (ACR) published its revised criteria for the classification of SLE in 1997 (Table 10.1).
- Criteria are for the classification of SLE for epidemiological and research purposes and not for diagnostic purposes. In practice, however, criteria naturally tend to form the cornerstone for clinical diagnosis. The criteria were developed and validated in patients with established, long-standing disease and therefore may exclude patients with early or limited disease.
- The Systemic Lupus International Collaborating Clinic (SLICC) classification criteria for SLE are similar to the ACR classification criteria. The main differences are that, for the SLICC classification:
  - Haematological abnormalities need be present on only one occasion.
  - There is inclusion of low C3, C4, and CH50 levels and a positive Coombs test in the absence of haemolytic anaemia.
  - The criteria also include non-scarring alopecia and a broader range of cutaneous and neurological manifestations.

**Table 10.1** 1997 update of the 1982 American College of Rheumatology revised criteria for the classification of SLE

| 1 | Malar rash | Fixed erythema flat or raised over malar eminences tending to spare the nasolabial folds |
|---|---|---|
| 2 | Discoid rash | Erythematous raised patches with adherent keratotic scaling and follicular plugging; atrophic scarring may occur in older lesions |
| 3 | Photo-sensitivity | Skin rash as a result of an unusual reaction to sunlight by patient history or physician observation |
| 4 | Oral ulcers | Oral or nasopharyngeal ulceration, usually painless observed by physician |
| 5 | Non-erosive arthritis | Involving 2 or more peripheral joints characterized by tenderness, swelling, or effusion |
| 6 | Serositis | Pleuritis (history of pleuritic pain or rub heard by physician or evidence of pleural effusion) or pericarditis (documented by ECG or rub or pericardial effusion) |
| 7 | Renal disorder | Persistent proteinuria >0.5 g/24 hrs or >3+ if quantitation not done or cellular casts (red blood cell, Hb, granular, tubular or mixed) |
| 8 | Neurological disorder | Seizures or psychosis in the absence of offending drugs or known metabolic derangements, e.g. uraemia, ketoacidosis, or electrolyte imbalance |
| 9 | Haematological disorder | Haemolytic anaemia with reticulocytosis or leucopenia $<4.0 \times 10^9$/L on ≥2 occasions or lymphopenia $<1.5 \times 10^9$/L on ≥2 occasions or thrombocytopenia <100,000/mm$^3$ in the absence of offending drugs |
| 10 | Immunological disorder | Anti-dsDNA antibody to native DNA in abnormal titre or anti-Sm antibody or antiphospholipid (APL) antibodies (abnormal level of IgM or IgG cardiolipin antibodies or positive lupus anticoagulant or 'false-positive' test result for >6 months confirmed by *T. pallidum* immobilization or fluorescent treponemal antibody absorption test) |
| 11 | Positive ANA | Abnormal ANA titre by immunofluorescence or equivalent assay (any point in time and in the absence of drugs) |

SLE may be diagnosed if 4 or more of the 11 criteria are present either serially or simultaneously

Reproduced from Hochberg 'Updating the American college of rheumatology revised criteria for the classification of systemic lupus erythematosus' (1997) *Arthritis & Rheumatology* 40(9):1725 with permission from Wiley.

# Pathophysiology

The cause of SLE is incompletely understood but genetic, immunological, and environmental factors all play an important role.

## Genetics

- There is a higher concordance in monozygotic twins and the disease is strongly associated with polymorphic variants at the HLA locus.
- In a few cases, SLE is associated with inherited mutations in complement components C1q, C2, and C4, and in the immunoglobulin receptor FcγRIIIb or in the DNA exonuclease TREX1.
- Genome-wide association studies have identified common polymorphisms near several other genes that predispose to SLE, most of which are involved in regulating immune cell function.

## Serology and immune complexes

The characteristic feature of SLE is autoantibody production.

- Autoantibodies have specificity for a wide range of targets, but many are directed against antigens in the cell or within the nucleus.
- SLE may occur because of defects in apoptosis or in the clearance of apoptotic cells, which causes inappropriate exposure of intracellular antigens on the cell surface, leading to polyclonal B- and T-cell activation and autoantibody production.
- Following autoantibody production, immune complex formation is thought to be an important mechanism of tissue damage in SLE, leading to vasculitis and organ damage.

## Environmental factors

- Environmental factors cause flares of lupus.
- UV light and infections increase oxidative stress and cause cell damage.
- Stress can aggravate SLE.

# Clinical features of systemic lupus erythematosus (SLE)

There is an extensive number of clinical features which can occur in SLE. Of the several non-specific features that are common to many chronic diseases, lethargy and fatigue are often the most disabling.

## Mucocutaneous

Approximately half of patients diagnosed with SLE will have the classic UV-sensitive 'butterfly' rash over the nasal bridge and malar bones. The cutaneous manifestations of SLE include a combination of acute, subacute, chronic, and other rashes, listed in Table 10.2.

## Musculoskeletal features

- Musculoskeletal immobility-related stiffness and polyarticular, symmetrical arthralgia or arthritis occur in 90% of cases.
- In most cases, symptoms outweigh objective clinical signs, and overt joint damage from synovitis is confined to <10% of patients.
- Reversible subluxation of joints without erosive disease (Jaccoud arthropathy) can also occur.
- Osteonecrosis occurs in 5–10% of patients; most cases are associated with previous glucocorticoid (GC/'steroid') use or secondary to antiphospholipid syndrome (APS).
- Raynaud's disease, vasculitis, fat emboli, GCs, and APS can result in bone ischaemia.
- Myalgia is common, but true myositis is seen in <5%.
- Myopathy may be a consequence of steroid treatment.

**Table 10.2** Mucocutaneous manifestations of SLE

| Frequency | Feature |
|---|---|
| Common (20–50%) | Malar rash |
| | Photosensitive rash |
| | Chronic discoid lesions |
| | Non-scarring alopecia |
| Less common (5–20%) | Mucosal ulcers |
| Occasional (5%) | Periorbital oedema |
| | Bullous lupus |
| | Severe scarring alopecia |
| | Subacute cutaneous lupus |
| | Leg ulcers |
| | Panniculitis |
| | Cutaneous vasculitis |

## Cardiovascular disease

- Pericardial disease is the most common manifestation.
- Most cases of pericardial disease are asymptomatic. A mild pericarditis is more common than a clinically significant pericardial effusion. On echocardiography, pericardial thickening is seen more frequently than pericardial effusions.
- Although SLE can lead to life-threatening pericardial effusions or constrictive pericarditis, these manifestations are quite rare.
- Myocarditis, present in 8–25% of patients, is often asymptomatic.
- Clinical myocarditis (defined by combinations of tachycardia, dysrhythmias, a prolonged PR interval on ECG, cardiomegaly, or congestive cardiac failure) is considerably less common. Blood testing often reveals a raised troponin level and N-terminal pro-BNP. Diagnosis is confirmed by cardiac MRI.
- Valvular heart disease is common. The most frequent abnormality is diffuse thickening of the mitral and aortic valves followed by vegetations, valvular regurgitation, and stenosis. Any valve vegetations identified in a patient who is febrile should raise the possibility of bacterial endocarditis. Libman-Sacks endocarditis is characterised by immune-complex dominant vegetations classically on the mitral or the aortic valves in patients with SLE. The vegetations are associated with lupus duration, disease activity and anticardiolipin antibodies, among others.
- SLE patients have increased morbidity and mortality from cardiovascular disease. Patients are 5–10× more likely to have clinically evident coronary artery disease than the general population.
- Subclinical cardiovascular disease is also seen, with increased prevalence of carotid plaque and faster progression of plaque formation. The pathogenesis of early cardiovascular disease is multifactorial including traditional risk factors (smoking, obesity, hypertension, diabetes mellitus, hyperlipidaemia, and positive family history), SLE-related risk factors (disease activity and damage, GC use, disease duration), and factors related to the inflammatory process (raised C-reactive protein and pro-inflammatory cytokine levels, elevated homocysteine levels).
- Reducing cardiovascular morbidity and mortality requires management of traditional risk factors, using antihypertensive agents and statins as appropriate, as well as minimizing GC and NSAID use and achieving early and prolonged control of disease activity.
- GCs, although indicated for inflammatory cardiac disease, are an added risk factor for atherosclerosis given its propensity to induce hypertension, hypercholesterolaemia, and obesity.

## Pulmonary disease

- Because of the tendency for disease to be subclinical, CXR and pulmonary function tests invariably indicate a greater degree of involvement than is evident clinically.
- Patients may present quite late in the disease process following a history of slow-onset non-productive cough and increased dyspnoea.
- Pulmonary function tests typically show reduced total lung capacity and peak flow rates.
- Shrinking lung is associated with unexplained dyspnoea, initially exertional, but then at rest and on lying flat, small lung volumes on CXR, diaphragmatic elevation, and restrictive pulmonary function tests in the absence of parenchymal lung disease.

- Pleuritic pain/pleuritis is present in up to 60% of cases, with a clinically apparent pleural effusion in up to 50%.
- Pleural effusions are a feature in one-third of patients, but they are usually small and clinically insignificant.
- Interstitial fibrosis, pulmonary vasculitis, and pneumonitis are found in up to 20% of patients.
- Pulmonary haemorrhage is rare but potentially a catastrophic complication of SLE.
- Pulmonary hypertension is found in ~10% of patients with SLE, and is associated with Raynaud's disease, vasculitis, and APL antibodies.
- Patients presenting with pleuritic pain and/or pulmonary hypertension should be investigated for the presence of pulmonary emboli and APS (see ➜ Chapter 11).

## Renal disease

Assessment of blood pressure for hypertension, urine for protein, blood, and casts, and the serum creatinine, urea, and albumin is an essential part of regular proactive monitoring.

- Symptoms suggesting renal failure rarely become obvious until substantial damage has occurred.
- If early disease is suspected, a spot urine protein:creatinine ratio (uPCR), is more accurate than urine dipstick and more convenient than the conventional 24-hour urine collection for protein and creatinine.
- Even low levels of proteinuria (<100 mg/mmol) may indicate renal involvement.
- The glomerular filtration rate (GFR) and renal function may also be assessed by nuclear medicine techniques.
- A uPCR of >50 mg/mmol should be investigated in a patient with SLE. A uPCR of >300 mg/mmol is suggestive of nephrotic range proteinuria.
- Renal biopsy should be considered if there is any evidence of new-onset proteinuria, increasing proteinuria, haematuria, casts, or acute kidney injury.
- Biopsy should be done in centres with a high degree of experience.
- In 2003, the International Society of Nephrology (ISN) and Renal Pathology Society (RPS) released a new classification of SLE ('lupus') nephritis designed to standardize definitions. The 2003 ISN/RPS classification of lupus nephritis replaced the 1982 modified World Health Organization (WHO) classification:
  - *Class I:* minimal mesangial lupus nephritis.
  - *Class II:* mesangial proliferative lupus nephritis.
  - *Class III:* focal lupus nephritis (< 50% of glomeruli).
  - *Class III (A):* active lesions.
  - *Class III (A/C):* active and chronic lesions.
  - *Class III (C):* chronic inactive lesions.
  - *Class IV:* diffuse lupus nephritis (50% glomeruli), divided into diffuse segmental (IV-S) or global (IV-G) lupus nephritis.
  - *Class IV-(A):* active lesions.
  - *Class IV-(A/C):* active and chronic lesions.
  - *Class IV-(C):* chronic inactive lesions.
  - *Class V:* membranous lupus nephritis.
  - *Class VI:* advanced sclerosing lupus nephritis (90% globally sclerosed glomeruli without evidence of activity).
- Chronic inactive lesions (glomerulosclerosis) are a poor prognostic feature.

- A repeat renal biopsy may be considered when there is increasing proteinuria or progressive renal failure in the absence of an alternative cause (i.e. poorly controlled blood pressure, intercurrent infection, or non-compliance with medication).
- Active lupus nephritis may be present in otherwise clinically quiescent disease.
- Patients with lupus nephritis should have good blood pressure control with a target of ≤130/80 mmHg.

## Haematological features

- A microcytic anaemia may be due to anaemia of chronic disease, NSAID-related peptic ulcer disease, dietary deficiency of iron, gastrointestinal blood loss, haemoglobinopathy, or menorrhagia.
- A normocytic anaemia can be due to myelosuppression from immunosuppressants, chronic kidney disease due to nephritis, macrophage activation syndrome (MAS), or rarely acute bleeding in alveolar haemorrhage or in the context of autoimmune thrombocytopenia.
- Macrocytosis can be caused by immunosuppression (e.g. azathioprine (AZA) or methotrexate (MTX)) or as a consequence of hypothyroidism, alcohol excess, vitamin B12, or folate deficiency or occasionally with a reticulocytosis after haemolysis.
- Autoimmune haemolytic anaemia causes fragments on blood film, an increased reticulocyte count, low haptoglobin, raised lactate dehydrogenase (LDH) and bilirubin, and a positive Coombs test (direct antiglobulin test).
- Leucopenia and lymphopenia are common abnormalities, in 50% and 80% of patients, respectively.
- A leucocytosis is rare, suggesting infection or GC therapy.
- There are several forms of clinical thrombocytopenia. Chronic, indolent, and uncomplicated thrombocytopenia ($<100 \times 10^9$/L) is present in up to 20% of patients, particularly among patients with APL antibodies. A rarer acute and life-threatening severe thrombocytopenia is also recognized, as well as thrombotic thrombocytopenic purpura (TTP).
- Some patients may also present with immune thrombocytopenia, later followed by other manifestations of SLE.
- Thrombocytopenia also occurs in the context of MAS. This 'cytokine storm' requires urgent treatment with high-dose GCs (see ➲ Chapter 9 and ➲ 25).

## Neurological disease

Features of neurological disease range from cognitive impairment (in up to 50% of patients) to psychoses and seizures (in 5–10% of patients over the course of their disease).

- About 10% of patients develop a sensory (or, less often, sensorimotor) peripheral neuropathy.
- Cranial nerve involvement is not common.
- Up to 70% prevalence of psychiatric illness has been quoted in the literature (includes anxiety and depression).
- While it is accepted that GCs can induce psychiatric symptoms, in general it is felt the drugs given in SLE are not responsible for most of the psychiatric manifestations observed.

- Examination of CSF in neuropsychiatric disease should be done as part of the initial evaluation—it may reveal a raised protein and/or white cell count, and glucose may be low. CSF can also be normal, making diagnosis challenging.
- Electroencephalography is often non-specific.
- MRI with contrast is more sensitive than CT in detecting small vessel vasculopathy associated with SLE.
- Brain biopsy can be used to exclude opportunistic infection or neoplastic disease but is often not required. The pathological findings in lupus cerebritis are of a small vessel vasculopathy.

## Other clinical features and important comorbidities

Other clinical features are listed in Table 10.3.

### Vitamin D deficiency

This may be associated with loss of immune tolerance. Most patients with SLE have insufficient levels of vitamin D, and the effect of replacement on disease activity remains uncertain.

### Osteoporosis and osteopenia

There is a high prevalence of fractures in young patients with SLE, due to a reduction in bone density.

- Factors that contribute to osteopenia and osteoporosis include GCs, renal osteodystrophy, low vitamin D levels due to sun avoidance, premature menopause, or cyclophosphamide (CYC) treatment.

### Malignancy

There is a 7× increased risk of non-Hodgkin lymphoma with SLE. There is increased incidence of cervical cancer due to human papilloma virus in SLE.

| Table 10.3 Other clinical features of SLE | |
|---|---|
| Vascular | Raynaud's disease |
| | Cutaneous vasculitis |
| | Digital ulcers and gangrene |
| Gastrointestinal | Hepatomegaly (25%) |
| | Abdominal serositis (10–20%) |
| | Splenomegaly (10%) |
| | Mesenteric vasculitis (rare) |
| | Pancreatitis (rare) |
| Immunological | Hypergammaglobulinaemia (60%) |
| Ocular | Keratoconjunctivitis sicca |
| | Episcleritis |
| | Scleritis |
| | Anterior uveitis |
| | Retinal vasculitis |
| | Retinal vessel occlusion |

# Investigations

- Important initial investigations are shown in Box 10.1.
- There are a variety of circulating autoantibodies to a range of nuclear, cytoplasmic, and plasma membrane antigens (Table 10.4).
- Most patients (≥98%) will have antinuclear antibodies (ANAs). ~60% have double-stranded DNA (dsDNA) antibodies (detected by immunofluorescence on crithidia lucillae or by ELISA or radioimmunoassay).
- Some patients have varying combinations of antibodies that may change over the course of the disease.
- SLE is associated with deficiencies of the early classical pathway of complement (e.g. C1q, C1r, C1s, and C2).
- Reduced levels of complement C3 and C4 are common in SLE, particularly at the time of a disease flare.
- A subset of patients will be 'serologically active but clinically quiescent', meaning they will have low complement levels and raised dsDNA antibody titre, but no signs of active disease.
- Patients should always be treated on the basis of symptoms rather than blood tests alone, but should be closely monitored for a flare in the context of a rising anti-dsDNA antibody level and falling C3.
- Some individuals may have high levels of RF and features of RA (thus an 'overlap' syndrome termed 'rhupus').

---

**Box 10.1 Initial investigations in patients who have, or are suspected of having, SLE**

- Full blood count
- Urea and electrolytes
- ESR and CRP
- Liver function tests
- Urinalysis
- Urine microscopy
- Blood pressure
- Urinary protein:creatinine ratio
- ANA and extractable nuclear antigens (ENAs)
- Complement C3 and C4
- Anti-dsDNA antibody titre (ELISA)
- Direct antiglobulin test (Coombs test)
- Anticardiolipin antibodies
- Lupus anticoagulant (dilute Russell viper venom test)
- Rheumatoid factor

**Table 10.4** Autoantibodies in SLE

| Autoantibody specificity | | Prevalence in SLE patients | Associations |
|---|---|---|---|
| Intracellular: | dsDNA | 40–90% | Renal disease |
| | Histone | 30–80% | Drug-induced SLE |
| | Sm | 30% (Afro-Caribbeans) 10% (Caucasians) | Renal or neurological disease |
| | U1 RNP | 20–30% | Mixed connective tissue disease |
| | Ro/SS-A | 25–40% | Sjögren's syndrome, cutaneous SLE, congenital heart block |
| | La/SS-B | 10–15% | As for Ro/SS-A (see above in table) |
| Cell membrane | Cardiolipin | 20–40% | Pregnancy loss, thrombosis |
| | Red cell | <10% | Haemolytic anaemia |
| | Platelet | <10% | Immune thrombocytopenia |
| Extracellular | RF | 25% | |
| | C1q | 50% | |

# Antiphospholipid syndrome and SLE

(See also ➲ Chapter 11.) Abnormal procoagulant factors occurring in SLE patients include a positive lupus anticoagulant test, anticardiolipin and anti-$\beta_2$ glycoprotein-1 (GP1) antibodies.

- Antiphospholipid (APL) antibodies occur in up to 33% of SLE patients.
- Although the presence of APL antibodies alone is not sufficient to make a diagnosis of APS, 50% of SLE patients with positive APL antibodies will develop hypercoagulopathy.
- The manifestations of SLE-associated APS include venous and arterial thrombosis, thrombocytopenia, cerebral disease, recurrent fetal loss, pulmonary hypertension, and livedo reticularis.
- Some patients with APL antibodies develop renal impairment (e.g. hypertension or proteinuria) due to multiple small thrombi.

# Pregnancy and SLE

- There is debate about whether pregnancy is associated with an increased risk of SLE flare. However, pregnancy does not appear to worsen the long-term outcome of SLE.
- A USA study[1] has shown that SLE patients suffer more from gestational diabetes mellitus, hypertension, pulmonary hypertension, renal failure, and thrombotic episodes in pregnancy.
- Incidence of intrauterine growth retardation, pre-term delivery, and incidence of caesarean sections are also increased.
- Active disease increases the risk of miscarriage and preterm birth.
- A major complication is pre-eclampsia—it occurs in 22.5% of women with SLE. Pre-existing renal disease is an important risk factor.
- SLE is associated with an increased rate of fetal death late in pregnancy. ~10% of SLE pregnancies result in fetal loss.
- APS-associated complications are discussed in ➜ Chapter 11.
- Anti-Ro associates with fetal heart block and neonatal lupus.
- Women who wish to conceive should receive appropriate counselling to discuss discontinuation of teratogenic drugs.
- Features of a high-risk pregnancy include increasing age, significant organ impairment/damage, lupus nephritis, active disease, high-dose GCs, and presence of APL/Ro/La antibodies.
- Women at high risk should be managed in a combined medical-obstetric clinic, and care should continue into the postpartum period, when flares and thromboembolic events can occur.

## Reference

1. Clowse MEB, Jamison M, Myers E, et al. A national study of the complications of lupus in pregnancy. *Am J Obstet Gynecol* 2008;199:127.e1–127.

## Assessment of disease activity

Assessment of changes in SLE activity is an essential part of decision-making and drug treatment.

- Several global activity indices have been produced that correlate well and are reliable.
- Global scoring systems such as the Systemic Lupus Erythematosus Disease Activity Index (SLEDAI) and the British Isles Lupus Assessment Group (BILAG) activity index are of some value, both in the context of clinical trials and long-term follow-up of patients.
- Equally constructive is the concept of an index of damage as distinct from disease activity. For example, a patient with dyspnoea may have an active but reversible pneumonitis or irreversible fibrosis.
- The distinction between disease activity and damage is important since treatments/management for each situation are different.
- The SLICC damage index has been developed as a method of recording damage in patients with SLE.[2,3]

### References

2. Gladman DD, Goldsmith CH, Urowitz MB, et al. Sensitivity to change of 3 Systemic Lupus Erythematosus Disease Activity Indices: international validation. *J Rheumatol* 1994;21:1468–71.
3. Gladman DD, Ginzler E, Goldsmith C, et al. The development and initial validation of the Systemic Lupus International Collaborating Clinics/American College of Rheumatology damage index for systemic lupus erythematosus. *Arthritis Rheum* 1996;39:363–9.

# Drug-induced SLE

Drug-induced lupus erythematosus (DILE) should be suspected in patients with no history of SLE, who develop a positive ANA and at least one clinical feature of SLE after an appropriate duration of drug exposure.

- Drugs most commonly associated with DILE are:
  - minocycline.
  - hydralazine.
  - procainamide.
  - isoniazid.
  - quinidine.
  - methyldopa.
  - chlorpromazine.
  - sulfasalazine (SSZ).
  - anti-TNFα drugs.
- Hydralazine-associated DILE is considered to be dose dependent, and procainamide, time dependent.
- Up to 90% of patients taking procainamide develop a positive ANA and 30% of these develop DILE.
- Renal, central nervous system, and skin features of SLE are rare in DILE. Other features of SLE such as musculoskeletal, pulmonary, and serosal disease are common.
- In the majority of cases, the condition subsides on withdrawing the drug.

# Management of SLE

## General measures

- It is important to avoid overexposure to UV/sunlight.
- Sunblock should be SPF30 or greater, and should protect against both UVA and UVB.
- Advice should include supplement intake of vitamin D and in some cases calcium to maintain adequate vitamin D levels (>50 nmol/L 25-hydroxyvitamin D (25OHD)).
- Postmenopausal women and men >50 years old on long-term GCs should be offered a bisphosphonate as prevention against GC-induced osteoporosis (GIO).
- In premenopausal women and men <50 years old, a DXA scan should be obtained, and FRAX assessment done, and fracture risk—and need for bisphosphonates—assessed accordingly.
- Live vaccines (e.g. yellow fever, polio) are contraindicated in patients taking immunosuppressants. Other vaccinations are not contraindicated though the degree of response to a vaccine may differ from the healthy individual.
- Oestrogen-containing contraceptives should be avoided ideally. Progesterone only contraceptives or other methods of contraception are advised in preference.
- All oral contraceptives should be avoided by women with SLE who have APL antibodies (or positive lupus anticoagulant).
- Many patients tolerate hormone replacement therapy (HRT) but use of HRT in the menopause is controversial. There is, for example, a 20% increase in SLE flares among women taking HRT.

## Reduction of cardiovascular disease risk factors

There is an excess incidence of cardiovascular disease (CVD) in SLE patients compared with non-SLE general population.

- Management of basic CVD risks is essential (smoking, hypertension, diabetes, obesity).
- Consider statins for hypercholesterolaemia.
- Aspirin or formal anticoagulation in the presence of APS or if APL antibodies are present (but see also ➜ Chapter 11).
- Tight control of SLE disease may reduce risk (see Table 10.5)

## Immunosuppression

(See Fig. 10.1.)

### Glucocorticoids (GCs)

- Prednisolone is frequently used with immunosuppressive drugs to rapidly reduce SLE disease activity.
- Dosing of GCs varies widely depending on the severity of disease activity, and is gradually tapered.
- Intravenous 'pulsed' methylprednisolone 0.25–1 g used daily for 3 consecutive days is preferred in serious organ or life-threatening disease.

**Table 10.5** Recommendations for drug use in SLE

| Symptom | Drug | Regimen |
|---|---|---|
| Arthralgia/fever | NSAIDs (caution with renal disease) | No special recommendation |
| Arthralgia/myalgia/lethargy | Hydroxychloroquine | 200–400 mg daily |
| Malar/discoid rash | Prednisolone, hydroxychloroquine, sunscreen, topical steroid, or tacrolimus | |
| Arthritis/serositis/myositis | Prednisolone, MTX, AZA | 20–40 mg of prednisolone daily for 2–4 weeks, then reducing dose in 5 mg steps each week. Requires bone prophylaxis against osteoporosis if dose treatment lasts for >3 months |
| Autoimmune anaemia or thrombocytopenia (ITP) | Prednisolone, IVIg, AZA, rituximab (RTX) | IV methylprednisolone followed by 60–80 mg prednisolone daily for 2 weeks, reducing in 10 mg steps per week, depending on response. ITP often requires immunoglobulin. Refractory cases may be treated with RTX, AZA, or splenectomy |
| Renal | Prednisolone, AZA, CYC, mycophenolate mofetil (MMF), RTX, tacrolimus | Control BP with ACE inhibitor or angiotensin receptor blocker: BP target <130/80 mmHg |
| Central nervous system | Prednisolone, AZA, MMF, CYC, RTX | |
| Raynaud's disease | Calcium channel blockers, losartan | |

*Antimalarial drugs*

- Hydroxychloroquine (HCQ) 200–400 mg/day is an initial treatment for patients with mild SLE symptoms.
- HCQ reduces the frequency of flares so is normally continued in all patients, even when they require additional immunosuppression.
- Patients should be advised about the need for annual eye testing, and after 5 years of use they should be referred to an ophthalmologist to assess for retinal toxicity.
- Eye examination should include examination of central visual field, visual and reading acuity, slit lamp of the cornea, and stereoscopic slit lamp of the retina.
- For patients intolerant of HCQ, chloroquine phosphate 250 mg daily is a useful alternative.
- Mepacrine is an antimalarial effective in treating SLE skin rashes, but does not treat other manifestations of the disease.

*Treatment with an immunosuppressive agent is recommended in class IIIA or IIIA/C (±V) and IVA or IVA/C (±V) nephritis, and also in pure class V nephritis if proteinuria exceeds 1g/24h despite the optimal use of renin-angiotensin-aldosterone system blockers. Glucocorticoids ± immunosuppressive may also be indicated in certain situations in class I or II nephritis – see full guideline for details.*

| Induction | MMF (3 g/day) or CYC (3 g total over 3 months Euro-lupus regime)<br>+<br>IV methylprednisolone 500–700 mg pulsed on 3 consecutive days then prednisolone 0.5 mg/kg/day for 4 weeks, then wean to ≤10 mg/day by 4–6 weeks<br>(AZA can be considered if no adverse features and unable to have MMF or CYC)<br><br>*Or if adverse features*<br>*(acute deterioration in renal function, substantial cellular casts or fibrinoid necrosis), consider as alternative:*<br><br>CYC 0.75–1 g/m² for 6 months or oral CYC<br>+<br>IV methylprednisolone 500–700 mg pulsed on 3 consecutive days then prednisolone 0.5 mg/kg/day for 4 weeks, then wean to ≤10 mg/day by 4–6 months |
|---|---|
| Maintenance | MMF (at least 2 g/day) or AZA 2 mg/kg/day (or calcineurin inhibitor in class V nephritis)<br>+<br>Prednisolone 5–7.5 mg /day<br>(3 years at least before consider gradual treatment withdrawal, starting with steroid first) |
| Refractory | MMF change to CYC or CYC change to MMF and/or Rituximab<br>Additional options maybe calcineurin inhibitors, IVIG, plasma exchange for rapidly progressive GN or immunoadsorption |

| *Additional treatment considerations* |
|---|
| – ACE or ARB if uPCR > 50 mg/mmol or Hypertension<br>– Statin for high LDL (>2.58 mmol/L)<br>– Hydroxychloroquine<br>– Anticoagulation if nephrotic range proteinuria and serum albumin < 20 g/L<br>– Management of CKD complications i.e. metabolic bone, anaemia<br>– Dialysis if indicated despite treatment |

**Fig. 10.1** Management of lupus nephritis. Data from Bertsias GK, Tektonidou M, Amoura Z, et al. Joint European League Against Rheumatism and European Renal Association–European Dialysis and Transplant Association (EULAR/ERA-EDTA) recommendations for the management of adult and paediatric lupus nephritis. *Ann Rheum Dis* 2012;71:1771–82.

### Azathioprine, mycophenolate mofetil (MMF), and methotrexate

- Azathioprine (AZA) 2–3 mg/kg/day or mycophenolate mofetil (MMF) 0.5–3g/day are used in moderate to severe disease.
- MMF is often preferred to AZA for lupus nephritis after the ALMS trial[4] demonstrated superiority as a maintenance treatment with significantly less time to treatment failure (and equivalence of MMF to IV CYC as an induction agent[5]).
- Trial data show MMF is useful in treating non-renal manifestations.
- MTX is used when arthritis is the main clinical manifestation of SLE, or in overlap syndromes with RA.
- A recent systematic review found MTX is also associated with a significant reduction in SLEDAI.

### Rituximab

RTX depletes circulating B cells through targeting anti-CD20. It is a monoclonal antibody that was first used effectively in 2002 in patients with active SLE which had failed, or only had partially responded to, conventional treatments.

- Open-label studies using pulse IV infusions of RTX confirmed the efficacy, with benefits extending to 6 months.
- However, a major RCT failed to demonstrate that RTX was beneficial to patients with moderate-to-severe SLE.
- In NHS England healthcare, RTX is allowed for use in SLE, as long as the patient has one BILAG A and/or 2B scores or SLEDAI-2K score >6, in addition to having failed at least two immunosuppressive drugs (at least one of these must be MMF or CYC).
- B-cell depletion can be tested by monitoring the CD19 count.
- Significant side effects include infusion-related reactions and infection. Rarely, progressive multifocal leucoencephalopathy (PML) has been reported in association with RTX, but PML is also seen in SLE patients who have never received RTX.
- Low IgG levels can occur with successive cycles, with very low levels occasionally preventing further treatment, or necessitating the use of maintenance immunoglobulin.

### Cyclophosphamide (CYC)

- IV 'pulsed' CYC is commonly used for many of the severe manifestations of SLE, and has been demonstrated to be particularly effective for renal and neurological disease.
- The 'Euro-Lupus' regimen (low-dose IV CYC) is often used with clinical outcomes similar to the higher-dose regimens.
- As an alkylating agent with a broad effect on different cells, CYC depletes both B and T cells.
- Major side effects include infection, hair fall, premature menopause, and bladder toxicity (now rare due to co-treatment with mesna).
- There is some evidence that using GnRH agonists given prior to each dose of CYC may prevent premature menopause and preserve fertility following treatment.

*Belimumab*

- Belimumab is a fully-humanized antibody that neutralizes the activity of the soluble B-lymphocyte stimulator (BLyS)/B-cell activating factor (BAFF). BLyS/BAFF is also known as TALL-1, and THANK, and is a TNF superfamily member (TNFSF13B) best known for its role in the survival and maturation of B cells.
- It is the first drug to be licensed for SLE in approximately 50 years, and is currently approved by NICE in the UK.
- Given IV, belimumab has principally demonstrated a positive effect in MSK and mucocutaneous disease, as well as reduction in disease activity and flares.
- Its efficacy in neurological and renal SLE remains uncertain.

*Plasma exchange (PE)*

- PE is a treatment option for severe manifestations of SLE such as alveolar haemorrhage, refractory nephritis, or associated catastrophic APS, though the limited trial data for its use are conflicting.

*Stem cell transplantation*

- Haemopoietic stem cell transplantation (HSCT) is used to treat haematological disease, but has also been used in patients with severe refractory SLE.
- HSCT is effective in inducing remission but is curative only in <50%.
- Mortality is high and long-term effects are unknown.
- New autoimmune conditions have been reported after HSCT.
- It is currently used only in those with life-threatening SLE.
- Mesenchymal stem cell transplantation has recently emerged as an alternative treatment. It significantly reduces SLE activity and may induce remission in up to 50% of patients.

*Other agents*

- Tocilizumab has been shown to improve disease activity scores and dsDNA antibody titres in open-label studies.
- Epratuzumab, an anti-CD22 monoclonal antibody, reduces disease activity and seems to deplete a more 'lupus-specific' set of B-cells than RTX. It is currently undergoing phase III trials.
- Ofatumumab is a fully humanized anti-CD20 monoclonal antibody that may be useful in SLE as an alternative to RTX when there has been an infusion reaction.
- Eculizumab, a fully humanized monoclonal antibody against complement C5 has passed phase I trials in SLE. There are case reports of its benefit.
- Atacicept is a recombinant fusion protein that acts on B cells inhibiting BAFF/BlyS and a proliferation-inducing ligand (APRIL). In recent studies it significantly reduced the SLE flare rate. Phase IIb trials are ongoing.
- Tacrolimus, a calcineurin inhibitor, may be used in lupus nephritis. A recent RCT suggests it may be non-inferior to MMF when used as an induction agent.

- Pooled immunoglobulin (IVIg) may be of use in severely ill patients not responding to other therapies, and especially in situations where sepsis is the trigger and life-threatening.
- IVIg may have a role in drug-resistant membranous and membranoproliferative nephritis, and has been used in severe immune thrombocytopenia and haemolytic anaemia with good effect.

For additional detail on all drug therapies used for rheumatic disease, including immunosuppressants, see Chapter 23.

### References

4. Dooley MA, Jayne D, Ginzler EM, et al. Mycophenolate versus AZA as a maintenance therapy for lupus nephritis. *N Engl J Med* 2011;365:1886–95.
5. Appel GB, Contreras G, Dooley MA, et al. Mycophenolate mofetil versus cyclophosphamide for induction treatment of lupus nephritis. *J Am Soc Nephrol* 2009;20:1103–12.

# Prognosis and survival

Many studies of the duration of disease and survival rates are confounded by inadequate attention paid to the ethnic group, age of onset, and socioeconomic status of individual patients. The number of patients lost to follow-up is also high.

- In relevant studies, with the division of patients into those with or without overt nephritis, there is a 5-year survival in SLE of 90%.
- At 15 years, only 60% of those with nephritis will be alive compared with 85% of those patients without renal disease.
- A bi-modal mortality curve is considered to exist. Patients who die within 5 years usually have very active disease, requiring high doses of immunosuppressive drugs.
- Patients dying after 5 years tend to do so from cardiovascular disease, renal disease, and possibly infection.
- The combined effect of the disease and its treatment is to increase the risk of infection markedly. The possibility of infection must always be considered and treated aggressively as outcomes from sepsis can be very poor.
- SLE increases the risk of all malignancies compared to the general population, particularly non-Hodgkin's lymphoma.
- Cervical dysplasia is increased in SLE patients and regular monitoring should be emphasized.
- The exact contribution of disease activity, duration, and immunosuppressive drug exposure to the risk of developing a malignancy requires further research. Clinicians should be aware of this increased risk and be alert to investigating worrying symptoms promptly.

# Juvenile SLE

## Epidemiology

Approximately 20% of patients with SLE present before 18 years of age, commonly between 12 and 14 years.

- Increased incidence of renal, haematological, and neuropsychiatric disease is seen in juvenile SLE (JSLE).
- The overall incidence of JSLE is 0.4–0.6 per 100,000, but is much higher in Afro-Caribbean and Asian populations.
- F:M ratio is less pronounced than in adults and is 3:1 pre puberty but increases to 9:1 post puberty.

## Clinical features

The clinical features of JSLE are extremely variable, ranging from a mild illness with rash, fatigue, and joint involvement to severe life-threatening organ involvement.

- JSLE tends to be a more severe phenotype than adult disease, accruing a greater burden of organ damage.
- JSLE has a similar presentation to adult disease and follows a relapsing/remitting course.
- Other differences from adult disease include:
  - Raynaud's disease is less common (10–20% of patients).
  - Avascular necrosis of the hip is more common in JSLE.
  - In JSLE, the disease itself and its treatments have significant consequences on growth and physical development.
- Malar rash occurs in 30% of cases at diagnosis.
- Prevalence of renal disease is high at diagnosis, up to 60% of cases.
- Neuropsychiatric disease is present in up to 40% of cases.

## Diagnosis and investigations

- Similar to adult SLE, diagnosis is based on both clinical and laboratory features.
- The ACR revised classification criteria for SLE have also been validated in JSLE.
- Of the ACR criteria features, the commonest found in JSLE include ANA positivity, arthritis, haematological disorders, malar rash, renal and neuropsychiatric involvement.
- Assessment of JSLE includes history, examination, and disease activity assessment using tools used in adult SLE, including BILAG and SLEDAI.

### Initial assessment investigations

- ANA (+ve in >95%), dsDNA (+ve in 60%), ENAs—most commonly include anti-Ro and La, anti-Sm antibodies.
- Lupus anticoagulant (LA), ACL IgG and IgM, $\beta_2$GP1 antibodies.
- Clotting screen—prolonged in APLS and MAS.
- Fibrinogen—increased in inflammation, low in MAS.
- Coombs test/DAT—positive in autoimmune haemolytic anaemia.
- Immunity status to measles and varicella IgG.

*At each review*
- FBC (Hb low in anaemia of chronic disease or autoimmune anaemia, leucocyte count increased in infection and serositis, low platelets often).
- If pancytopenia on FBC in unwell patient—consider MAS.
- ESR typically increased in flares, low in MAS.
- CRP—if increased consider infection, serositis, polyarthritis.
- Complement: low C3 and C4 levels can correlate with disease activity but with low sensitivity.
- Urinalysis for blood and protein to check for renal involvement. If protein present, quantification is needed with uPCR.

## Management of JSLE

Early and aggressive therapy is key to improve outcome and prevent organ damage. This includes induction and maintenance therapies.
- Management is similar to adult SLE (see ➲ 'Management of SLE', pp. 360–5).
- The current treatment paradigm is to treat all children with HCQ to minimize flares, skin disease, and limit atherogenic and thrombotic risks associated with JSLE.
- Provide advice regarding sun and UV avoidance and use of sunblock (SPF 50) to reduce flares and photosensitive rashes.
- Induction therapy typically includes use of IV GCs (e.g. IV methylprednisolone on 3 consecutive days), followed by a dose reduction regimen of oral prednisolone (from 1–2 mg/kg/day) together with a sDMARD.
- The role of IV CYC in induction is less clear and MMF is typically preferred in JSLE nephritis.
- CYC is still used in neurological disease, systemic vasculitis, and refractory JSLE nephritis.
- Mild to moderate disease at presentation is treated with GCs, MMF, or AZA. MTX is used when arthritis or cutaneous manifestations (including discoid lupus) predominate.
- Maintenance treatment is with AZA, MMF, or MTX—similar to adult disease.
- RTX is effective in JSLE and can be used in disease refractory to first-line induction therapy or in patients experiencing unwanted adverse effects of alternative treatments.
- Anticoagulants (heparin and/or warfarin) should be considered in APLS, and low-dose aspirin in cases of positive LA or ACL antibodies. Optimum anticoagulation regimens, are not known, however.
- Hypertension and proteinuria should be aggressively managed with ACE inhibitors and calcium channel blockers to prevent organ damage.
- Close surveillance of patients at intervals of 1–3 months is necessary to ensure there are no unexpected complications of JSLE or its treatment.

## Prognosis and survival

- The prognosis of JSLE is often determined by the severity, management, and outcome of renal disease.
- Risk factors for poor outcome include severe JSLE flares, infection, neuropsychiatric manifestations, and some features, seen notably in black and Hispanic populations, such as persistent anaemia, high creatinine, hypertension and persistently low C3.
- JSLE continues to have a 2× higher mortality than adult SLE, although outcome has improved in recent years.
- 5-year survival of JSLE now exceeds 90%.

## Further reading

Brunner HI, Huggins J, Klein-Gitelman MS. Paediatric SLE – towards a comprehensive management plan. *Nat Rev Rheumatol* 2011;7:225–33.

Midgley A, Watson L, Beresford MW. New insights into the pathogenesis and management of lupus in children. *Arch Dis Child* 2014;99:563–7.

Thorbinson C, Oni L, Smith E, Pharmacological management of childhood-onset systemic lupus erythematosus. *Pediatr Drugs* 2016;18:181–95.

# Neonatal lupus syndrome

Neonatal lupus erythematosus (NLE) is an autoimmune condition attributable to transfer of maternal autoantibodies across the placenta, such as anti-SSA/Ro and/or anti-SSB/La antibodies.

- The condition can present *in utero* or postnatally.
- ~50% of mothers of babies with NLE are healthy at childbirth with no recognized symptoms of AICTD.
- Only 1–2% of autoantibody-positive mothers will have an infant who develops NLE, although subsequent risk increases to 10–25% for future pregnancies.
- NLE is transient in cases other than those with heart block. Skin and haematological manifestations resolve as maternal antibodies disappear at 3–6 months post birth.
- Severe hepatitis can be life-threatening and mortality in cardiac NLE is 20–30%.

## Clinical features

There should be suspicion of the presence of NLE where there is a persistent bradycardia or a combination of non-scarring rash, transaminitis, and cytopenia in a baby 0–6 months old.

### Skin

- Rashes occur in 70% of NLE babies—typically present at birth.
- Typical lesions are transient and similar to subacute cutaneous LE with annular pink scaly plaques.
- Lesions may be crusted and may affect head and neck as elsewhere.
- Telangiectasia and petechiae are also common and may occur alone.

### Cardiac manifestations

- Cardiac lesions occur in 65% of NLE babies.
- A third of affected babies have congenital complete heart block, which usually develops between 18 and 20 weeks of gestation.
- Other problems include bradycardia, prolonged QT interval, ventricular tachycardias, valve disease, cardiomyopathy, and heart failure.

### Other manifestations

- Haematological effects usually appear during the second week of life and include thrombocytopenia, haemolytic anaemia, and neutropenia.
- Liver involvement includes transaminitis in half of patients and conjugated jaundice.
- Other effects of NLE can include transient neurological and lung involvement. The former may be manifest by asymptomatic neuroimaging abnormalities.

## Investigations

- All women of childbearing age with an AICTD should be tested for anti-Ro and anti-La antibodies early in their pregnancy.
- Women testing positive for anti-Ro and/or anti-La antibodies should be referred to a specialist obstetric unit for weekly fetal US-echocardiography from 16 weeks' gestation onwards.
- The frequency of US-echo may be reduced in absence of complete heart block after week 26.
- Diagnosis is made on the basis of clinical features and in the presence of positive autoantibodies in neonatal or maternal serum.

## Management of NLE

- In complete heart block, 64% of live births require a pacemaker, almost all in the first year of life. About 60% of cases require a pacemaker during the first 10 days after birth.
- GCs, HCQ, and IVIg may reduce the risk of NLE-related cardiac lesions overall.
- Skin lesions can be managed with UV avoidance, sun block, and topical steroids (± HCQ).

## Prognosis

- Affected babies may be at increased risk of future autoimmune conditions but development of JSLE is rare.
- Other inflammatory conditions in infants that may subsequently occur include autoinflammatory conditions such as CINCA/NOMID, Kawasaki disease, and systemic-onset JIA.

## Further reading

Brito-Zerón P, Izmirly PM, Ramos-Casals M, et al. The clinical spectrum of autoimmune congenital heart block. *Nat Rev Rheumatol* 2015;11:301–12.

Johnson B. Overview of neonatal lupus. *J Paediat Health Care* 2014;28:331–41

Saxena A, Izmirly PM, Mendez B, et al. Prevention and treatment in utero of autoimmune associate congenital heart block. *Cardiol Rev* 2014;22:263–7.

# Antiphospholipid syndrome

# Antiphospholipid syndrome

## Classification

Antiphospholipid syndrome (APS) is a systemic autoimmune disease characterized by recurrent arterial or venous thrombosis. APS can be primary or secondary to an underlying autoimmune disease—commonly SLE (see ⊃ Chapter 10).

- Patients may be classified in terms of the antibody present. Anticardiolipin (ACL) and anti-$\beta_2$ glycoprotein 1 ($\beta_2$GP1) are detected by quantitative enzyme-linked immunosorbent assays (ELISA). See Table 11.1.
- Lupus anticoagulant (LA) is a functional test that quantifies coagulation *in vitro*.

### Table 11.1 Classification criteria for antiphospholipid syndrome

| Clinical criteria | |
| --- | --- |
| Vascular thrombosis | One or more clinical episodes of arterial, venous, or small vessel thrombosis in any tissue or organ, confirmed by objective criteria. Histopathology should show thrombosis without significant inflammation in the vessel wall |
| Pregnancy morbidity | One or more unexplained death of a morphologically normal fetus at or beyond 10 weeks' gestation<br><br>*or*<br><br>One or more premature birth of a morphologically normal neonate at or before 34 weeks' gestation due to pre-eclampsia, eclampsia, or placental insufficiency<br><br>*or*<br><br>Three or more unexplained, consecutive, spontaneous abortions before 10 weeks' gestation, excluding maternal anatomical or hormonal abnormalities, and excluding maternal and paternal chromosomal causes |
| **Laboratory criteria** | |
| ACL antibodies | Medium/high titre of IgG and/or IgM isotype anticardiolipin antibody in blood on 2 or more occasions at least 12 weeks apart using standard assays |
| Anti-$\beta_2$ glycoprotein 1 antibodies | Anti-$\beta_2$ glycoprotein 1 IgG or IgM in blood on 2 or more occasions at least 12 weeks apart using standard assays |
| Lupus anticoagulant (LA) | LA present in plasma on ≥2 occasions >12 weeks apart |

*A diagnosis of APS requires the presence of one positive clinical criterion manifested by thrombosis or pregnancy loss, plus one positive laboratory criterion (any one of the three antibodies) on two different occasions separated by 12 weeks.*

Adapted from Miyakis S et al. International consensus statement on an update of the classification criteria for definite antiphospholipid syndrome (APS). *J Thromb Haemostasis* 2006;4:295–306 with permission from Wiley.

## Epidemiology

- Case–control studies estimate the prevalence of ACL antibodies in the normal population to be 1–4%.
- Prevalence of ACL antibodies in people >65 years increases to 12–50% depending on the study.
- Age-dependent reference ranges do not exist but have been suggested by some authors.
- Prevalence of ACL antibodies and LA in SLE patients is estimated at 20–40% and 10–20%, respectively. These differences arise due to treatment history and the lack of uniformity of assay methods.

## Pathophysiology

- APL antibodies are directed against phosphorus-fat components of cell membranes called phospholipids.
- Certain blood proteins will bind with phospholipids to form complexes to which antibodies may occur.
- ACL antibodies are a family of the immunoglobulins IgG, IgM, IgA, or a combination of these isotopes. The IgG subtypes have a stronger association with clinical complications compared with IgM.
- High levels of the IgM isotype can be associated with autoimmune haemolytic anaemia.
- The clinical consequences of IgA ACL antibodies are unclear.
- $\beta_2$GPI is a plasma glycoprotein co-factor to which ACL binds. Anti-$\beta_2$GPI is more specific than ACL antibody in predicting thrombosis, and can occur in ~10% of APS patients as the only positive test.
- LA is a functional measurement of the capacity of heterogeneous APL antibodies that interferes with phospholipid-dependent stages of blood coagulation in vitro, inhibiting both the intrinsic and extrinsic pathways.
- Hence, in vitro, LA exhibits anticoagulant properties, whereas in vivo it functions as a procoagulant. APL antibodies are therefore paradoxically associated with thrombosis, rather than haemorrhage.
- Apart from clinical suspicion, a clue to the presence of APS is prolonged clotting time in assays for the 'internal pathway' clotting cascade. Around 50% of patients with positive LA antibodies have a prolonged activated partial thromboplastin time (APTT).

## Differential diagnosis

The most characteristic feature of APS is thrombosis in the presence of thrombocytopenia.

- The main differential diagnosis to consider is thrombotic thrombocytopenic purpura (TTP).
- TTP is a microvascular disorder, often associated with neurological features of confusion, seizures, and altered consciousness.
- The differential diagnosis of unexplained thrombosis includes genetic causes (e.g. protein C and S, and antithrombin III deficiencies) and drugs (including oestrogen, thalidomide, IVIg). Therefore a full thrombophilia screen should be carried out in patients with recurrent venous thrombosis.

## Clinical features
(See also Table 11.2.)

*Thrombosis*
- Vessels of all sizes, venous or arterial, may be affected without evidence of an inflammatory infiltrate, hence the range of clinical features is wide.
- Unlike in most clotting disorders, arterial thrombosis is a major feature of APS.
- Thrombosis can be present with or without a history of relevant pathology associated with pregnancy.
- Occlusion of the intracranial arteries is the most common arterial manifestation, with the majority of patients presenting with stroke.
- APL antibodies should be sought in the younger stroke patient, where they may account for up to 20% of cases.

*Catastrophic antiphospholipid syndrome*
- Widespread thrombosis is the feature of life-threatening 'catastrophic antiphospholipid syndrome' (cAPS).
- cAPS may present with acute collapse, severe thrombocytopenia, multiorgan failure (notably cerebral and renal), and adult respiratory distress syndrome (ARDS).

**Table 11.2** Clinical features of antiphospholipid syndrome

| Feature | Subgroup | Frequency (%) |
|---|---|---|
| Thrombosis | Deep vein thrombosis | 39 |
| | Pulmonary embolism | 14 |
| | Arterial thrombosis, legs | 4 |
| | Arterial thrombosis, arms | 3 |
| | Stroke | 20 |
| | Transient ischaemic attack | 11 |
| | Valve thickening/dysfunction | 12 |
| | Livedo reticularis | 24 |
| Pregnancy manifestations | Early loss (<10 weeks) | 35 |
| | Late loss (≥10 weeks) | 17 |
| | Live birth | 48 |
| | Premature birth | 11 |
| **Thrombocytopenia** | | 30 |
| Associated features | Skin ulcers, livedo reticularis, thrombophlebitis | |
| | Heart valve lesions and myocardial infarction | |
| | Budd Chiari, transverse myelitis, chorea, cognitive deficits, pulmonary hypertension | |
| Less common features | Splinter haemorrhages, digital gangrene, amaurosis fugax, retinal artery and vein occlusion, renal artery stenosis/thrombosis, osteonecrosis, Addison's disease, ARDS | |

Reproduced from Cervera R et al. Antiphospholipid syndrome: clinical and immunologic manifestations and patterns of disease expression in a cohort of 1000 patients. *Arthritis Rheum* 2002;46: 1019–27 with permission from Wiley.

*Fetal loss*
- Recurrent spontaneous pregnancy loss is a common manifestation of APS, which occurs as either recurrent early miscarriage or intrauterine fetal demise.
- Screening for APL antibodies in the context of previous pregnancy history is of importance in determining the significance of positive APL antibodies.
- In APL antibody-positive pregnancies that do not end in miscarriage, there is a high incidence of early onset pre-eclampsia, intrauterine growth restriction, placental abruption, and premature delivery.

*Skin lesions*
- The most frequent manifestations are livedo reticularis and skin ulcers.
- Livedo reticularis is characterized by a mottled purple reticular pattern. Appearances look similar to a fishnet pattern and in APS is usually disseminated. Livedo is a marker of poor prognosis and disease severity.
- Skin ulcers can be found in the extremities, and extensive cutaneous necrosis has been reported. Digital gangrene has also been described.
- Subungual splinter haemorrhages are seen in ~5%, and may suggest the occurrence of other thrombotic events.
- Other cutaneous lesions also described include purpura, tender nodules, papules, palmar–plantar erythema, and anetoderma.

*Liver and gastrointestinal tract*
- Liver abnormalities are common in APS, possibly due to vascular sludging or small vessel thrombosis.
- Budd–Chiari syndrome was a feature of the original description of APS. It is caused by thrombosis of the hepatic veins, presenting as a triad of abdominal pain, ascites, and liver enlargement. It may be fulminant, acute, chronic, or asymptomatic.
- Intestinal ischaemia and perforation due to thrombosis and coeliac artery stenosis have also been described.

*Musculoskeletal*
- Osteonecrosis is a complication of APS. It is most commonly of the femoral head but can affect other bones such as the navicular.
- Non-specific arthralgia may occur. Joint pains and stiffness are more common in APS associated with SLE and other autoimmune rheumatic and connective tissue diseases.
- Metatarsal fractures and other spontaneous vertebral and rib fractures have also been reported.

*Endocrine*
- Adrenal insufficiency is the most common endocrinological manifestation, and can be the presenting feature of APS.
- A few cases of hypopituitarism and ovarian/testicular involvement have been reported.

### Kidney
- The kidney is a major target organ in APS.
- Renal artery occlusion and renal artery stenosis have been described in APS patients with hypertension, and may result in renal infarction.
- Thrombosis of the renal veins and thrombotic microangiography has been described.
- Distinguishing between SLE nephritis (immune complex mediated) and APS nephritis (thrombotic disease) can only be established by renal biopsy.

### Lungs
- Pulmonary embolism and infarction is the most common lung manifestation of APS.
- Pulmonary hypertension is found in around 2% of APS patients.
- ARDS is rare with high mortality of ~50%, usually seen in cAPS.

### Central nervous system
- Cerebral ischaemia associated with APL antibodies is the most common arterial thrombotic manifestation. Less commonly associated is sagittal venous sinus thrombosis.
- Migraine is a common complaint, and cognitive deficits can occur.
- APS patients may exhibit features seen with multiple sclerosis, and MRIs may fail to differentiate.
- Seizures can occur, thought to be secondary to the interaction of APL antibodies and neuronal tissue.
- Transverse myelopathy, though rare, has a strong association with APL antibodies.
- Other less frequent manifestations include chorea, Guillain–Barré syndrome, sensorineural hearing loss, and retinal ischaemia.

### Cardiac features
- APS may be associated with multiple cardiovascular complications including accelerated atherosclerosis, valvular heart disease, and intracardiac thrombi.
- Cardiac manifestations of APS result in significant morbidity in around 5% of patients.
- In a European cohort, myocardial infarction was a presenting feature of APS in 3% of patients, and was seen during follow-up in 5.5%.
- The prevalence of APL antibodies in patients with myocardial infarction is estimated at 5–15%, but screening is not indicated, except in younger patients, patients with other symptoms and signs of APS, and those with a family history of autoimmune disease.
- Mitral and aortic valve thickening and dysfunction is commonly seen on echocardiography, but significant morbidity is uncommon.
- Intracardiac thrombus is a rare manifestation of APS.

## Laboratory features

### Thrombocytopenia
- Thrombocytopenia is common, seen in ~25%. It is rarely severe enough to cause bleeding.
- ACL antibodies have been found in up to 30% of presumed cases of immune thrombocytopenic purpura.
- Haemolytic anaemia with a positive direct antiglobulin test may co-exist with thrombocytopenia (Evans syndrome).

*General aspects*

- Given an association with all AICTDs, extensive autoantibody screening should be considered: ANA, RF, anti-CCP antibodies.
- C3, C4, Coombs test/DAT, bilirubin, LFTs, FBC, ESR, CRP, and organ function tests should be checked.

## Treatment of APS

There is no evidence for the role of warfarin in primary prevention ('primary prevention' defined by prevention before diagnosed thrombosis). Modifiable risk factors for thrombosis and cardiovascular lesions should be addressed (e.g. smoking, high cholesterol, increased blood pressure, systemic inflammation, oestrogen use).

- Hydroxychloroquine has antiplatelet, anti-inflammatory, and anticoagulant properties, and is recommended in SLE patients with positive APL antibodies (Table 11.3 and Table 11.4). It has also been shown to reduce APL antibody titres.
- HMG CoA reductase inhibitors lower cholesterol levels and have anti-inflammatory, immunoregulatory, and antithrombotic effects.

**Table 11.3** The treatment of APS and clinical scenarios involving APL antibodies/positive LA: summary

| Clinical situation | | Treatment |
|---|---|---|
| Non-SLE patients with high-risk APS profile | No previous thrombosis | Low-dose aspirin 75–150 mg/day (LDA) |
| SLE patients with LA/APL antibodies at high titres | No previous thrombosis | Hydroxychloroquine 200–400 mg/day ± LDA |
| Definite APS with thrombosis | After 1st venous event | Lifelong warfarin (INR 2–3) or 3–6 months warfarin (INR 2–3) if low-risk APL profile or other transient/reversible risk factors at time of thrombosis |
| | After 1st arterial thrombosis | * Lifelong warfarin (INR 3–4) or combined warfarin (INR 2–3) with antiaggregant anticoagulant therapy  *Assess bleeding risk* |
| | After 1st non-cardio-embolic cerebral arterial event with low APL profile ± reversible factors | Consider antiplatelet agents |
| | Catastrophic APS | IV heparin  IV methylprednisolone plus plasmapheresis or IVIg |

*(Continued)*

**Table 11.3** (Contd.)

| Clinical situation | | Treatment |
|---|---|---|
| Definite APS with pregnancy | Recurrent miscarriage (<10 weeks' gestation) or late complications (>10 weeks' gestation) | Low-dose aspirin plus unfractionated LMWH at thrombo-prophylactic doses *Consider LDA alone for selected cases within 1st trimester* |
| | Pregnancy and previous thrombosis | LDA plus LMWH at therapeutic doses |
| | Repeat fetal loss despite heparin and aspirin | Unknown |
| Definite APS with thrombocytopenia | Mild (100–150 × 10⁹/L) | Observe |
| | Moderate (50–100 × 10⁹/L) | Observe |
| | Severe (<50 × 10⁹/L) | GCs (as ITP), IVIg, immunosuppression (e.g. RTX) |

**Table 11.4** Summary of the recommendations for refractory/difficult APL cases from the 14th International Congress on APS treatment task force[2]

| | |
|---|---|
| Novel oral anticoagulant (NOAC) | Consider in a first or recurrent venous thromboembolism if warfarin allergy/intolerance or poor anticoagulant control |
| Older non-heparin/warfarin anticoagulants | Danaparoid, fondaparinux, and argatroban can be used in heparin-induced thrombocytopenia |
| Hydroxychloroquine | Recommended in SLE patients with APL antibodies. Consider in refractory cases (adjuvant treatment). No evidence for use in primary APS |
| Statins | May be of benefit in patients with recurrent history of thromboembolism despite adequate anticoagulation |
| B-cell inhibition | Recommended for refractory cases of APS possibly in patients with haematological and micro-angiopathic manifestations |
| Complement inhibition monoclonal antibody therapy | Not recommended yet. Data only from animal studies. May have a role as adjuvant or main therapy for patients refractory to anticoagulation |

- Studies have shown that fluvastatin may prevent thrombosis in patients with APS by inhibiting tissue factor and other monocyte markers that contribute to activation of the coagulation pathway, in addition to reducing thrombus formation biomarkers.[1]
- Rituximab (RTX), an anti-CD20 monoclonal antibody that depletes CD20-positive B-cell populations, has been used in APS-related thrombocytopenia, haemolytic anaemia, venous and arterial thrombosis, ischaemic cardiac and bowel events, cutaneous lesions, diffuse alveolar haemorrhage, nephropathy, and cAPS.
- RTX may be used in refractory cases of APS after failure of anticoagulation.
- Glucocorticoids (GCs), immunosuppressive drugs, IVIg, or plasmapheresis have been used in the treatment of APS with thrombosis, but the latter are more justified in cAPS.
- Over the last 4 years, successful treatment with eculizumab (a complement inhibitor) has been reported in a few cases, showing benefit in preventing recurrence of APS among transplant recipients, and in refractory cAPS.

*Anticoagulation in primary thromboprophylaxis (APL antibody positive without previous thrombotic event)*

- Recommendations for primary thromboprophylaxis in APS support the use of low-dose aspirin (75–100 mg/day).

*Anticoagulation in secondary thromboprophylaxis (APS—after first venous or arterial event)*

- After the first thrombotic event (either arterial or venous), recurrence of thrombosis is common, but can be prevented by treatment with warfarin.
- Patients <50 years of age with cerebrovascular events and positive APL antibodies, have a 5× increased risk of further ischaemic stroke.
- In venous thrombosis with transient or reversible risk factors or low-risk APL antibody profile, 3–6 months of treatment may be adequate, aiming for an international normalized ratio (INR) of 2–3.
- High-intensity anticoagulation (an INR of 3–4) is associated with increased bleeding risk compared to standard intensity treatment (INR of 2–3) with no clear reduction in thrombotic events according to studies.
- Hence, high-intensity anticoagulation is not recommended, but could be considered in complicated cases where thrombosis occurs despite warfarinizing with an INR of 2–3.
- For patients with refractory thrombosis, fluctuating INR levels, or high risk of major bleeding, alternative therapeutic options to warfarin should be considered, such as long-term low-molecular-weight heparin (LMWH), hydroxychloroquine, or statins.
- Table 11.4 summarizes APS treatments in patients refractory to anticoagulation or who are unable to take warfarin.
- Mild thrombocytopenia need not be treated but severe cases (<50 × 10⁹/L) should be treated with oral GCs in the first instance. In those failing to respond, IVIg, danazol, and splenectomy have been used with varying success.

*Anticoagulation in obstetric APS*
See Table 11.5.

*Novel oral anticoagulants (NOACs)*
- Anticoagulation with warfarin is limited by drug and food interactions, teratogenicity, high variability in response and necessity of frequent blood monitoring.
- NOACs directly inhibit a single enzyme of the coagulation cascade, and seem to be promising in the prevention of thrombosis in APS (but no APS trials).
- Minimal drug and food interactions and fixed drug dosing without the need for laboratory monitoring contribute to the advantage of NOACs compared to warfarin. However, the lack of antidotes remains a limitation. Some studies report a risk of major bleeding of up to 10% of cases per year.
- NOACs include direct thrombin inhibitors such as dabigatran, and direct anti-Xa inhibitors such as rivaroxaban, apixaban, and edoxaban. The Rivaroxaban for Antiphospholipid Antibody Syndrome (RAPS) study is currently underway comparing the effects of warfarin versus rivaroxaban in thrombotic APS patients.

**Table 11.5** Summary of treatment of obstetric APL syndrome

| Recurrent early miscarriage (<10 weeks' gestation) | Late complications (>10 weeks' gestation) | Pregnant patients with previous thrombosis |
|---|---|---|
| Low-dose aspirin 0.75–150 mg/day (LDA) plus unfractionated / LMWH combination at thromboprophylactic doses | LDA plus unfractionated/LMWH combination at thromboprophylactic doses | LDA plus unfractionated/LMWH combination at therapeutic doses, then warfarin (INR 2–3) postpartum |
| LDA alone in selected cases | | |

## Catastrophic antiphospholipid syndrome

# Catastrophic antiphospholipid syndrome

## Introduction

This rare variant of APS (<1% cases) affects small vessels and visceral organs and was first described in 1992.

- Catastrophic antiphospholipid syndrome (cAPS) is an important and serious condition that can present in previously asymptomatic patients.
- The trigger is an infection in 20% of cases. Other precipitating factors include trauma/surgery, malignancy, warfarin withdrawal in a patient with APS, pregnancy, and oral contraceptives. However, it is estimated that 45% of cAPS cases have no known trigger.
- cAPS is associated with other autoimmune conditions such as SLE (see ➋ Chapter 10), RA (see ➋ Chapter 5), and SScl (see ➋ Chapter 13).
- Mortality is high at 50%, and most patients require care in an intensive care unit.

## Clinical features

- Diffuse peripheral and central thrombosis occurs leading to:
  - limb arterial and venous occlusion.
  - intra-abdominal organ infarction including renal failure.
  - pulmonary emboli and ARDS.
  - small vessel cerebrovascular disease.
  - aortic and mitral valve defects, and myocardial infarction.
  - other thrombotic complications, such as ovarian, testicular, and retinal vessel occlusion.
- Livedo reticularis, gangrene, and purpura are visible markers of the disorder on the skin.
- Bone marrow infarction has also been reported.
- Following the production of classification criteria, data from 300 patients in a cAPS registry have shown the majority are female (72%), almost half had primary APS (46%), and a precipitating factor was found in 53%.[2]
- Data from the cAPS registry also show the most common sites are renal (71%), pulmonary (64%), cerebral (62%), and cardiac (51%).
- The presence of systemic immune response syndrome, in which pro-inflammatory cytokines are released from affected tissues, is also thought to contribute to morbidity and mortality.

## Laboratory features

- Moderate-to-severe thrombocytopenia.
- Haemolysis with schistocytes.
- Disseminated intravascular coagulation.
- High levels of IgG ACL antibodies or presence of a LA.

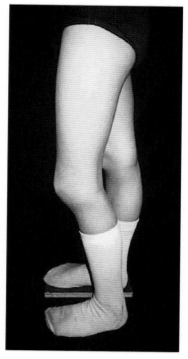

**Plate 1** Increased growth of the left lower limb due to chronic knee inflammation in (rheumatoid factor-negative) juvenile idiopathic arthritis.

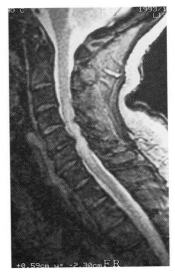

**Plate 2** Magnetic resonance scan of the neck showing loss of height and signal affecting several discs with multisegmental spondylotic bars, compression of the cord from protrusion of the C5/6 disc, and myelopathic changes (high signal) in the cord.

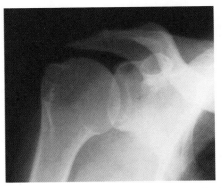

**Plate 3** Patterns of radiographic abnormality in chronic subacromial impingement: sclerosis and cystic changes in the greater tuberosity.

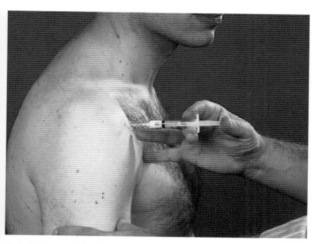

**Plate 4** Injection of the glenohumeral joint via the anterior route.

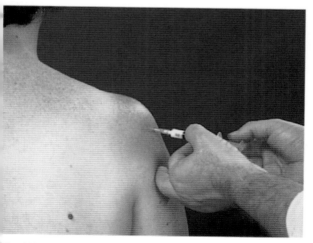

**Plate 5** Injection of the subacromial space.

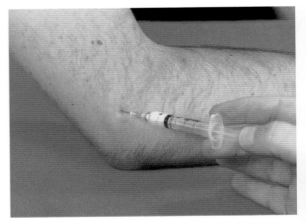

**Plate 6** Injection of tennis elbow (lateral humeral epicondylitis/enthesitis).

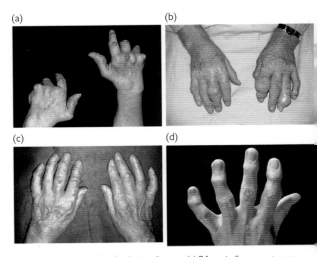

(a)

(b)

(c)

(d)

**Plate 7** Nodules associated with joint diseases. (a) RA: typically over extensor surfaces and pressure areas. (b) Chronic tophaceous gout: tophi can be indistinguishable clinically from RA nodules though may appear as eccentric swellings around joints (image provided courtesy of Dr R.A. Watts). (c) Multicentric reticulohistiocytosis: nodules are in the skin, are small, yellowish-brown, and are often around nails. (d) Nodal OA: swelling is bony, typically at PIPJs and DIPJs.

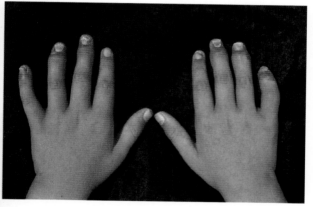

**Plate 8** Dactylitis, nail changes, and DIPJ arthritis in psoriatic arthritis.

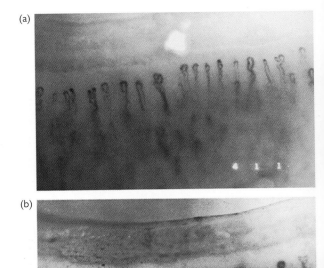

**Plate 9** (a) Normal nailfold capillaries. (b) Nailfold capillaries in scleroderma showing avascular areas and dilated capillaries in an irregular orientation (original magnification ×65).

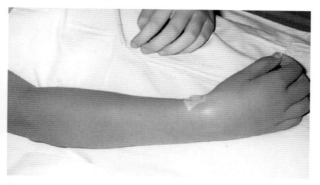

**Plate 10** Diffuse arm and hand swelling in chronic regional pain syndrome (osteodystrophy) in a 13-year-old girl.

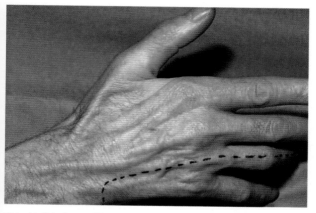

**Plate 11** Slight flexion of fourth and fifth fingers as a result of an ulnar nerve lesion at the elbow. The area of sensory loss is indicated by the dashed line.

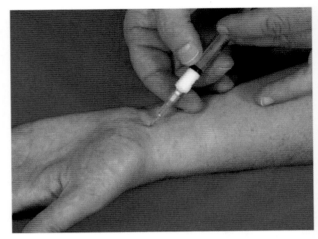

**Plate 12** Injection of the carpal tunnel to the ulnar side of palmaris longus tendon.

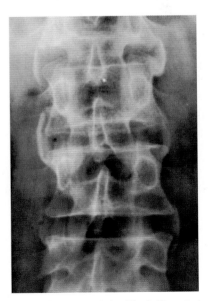

**Plate 13** Psoriatic spondylitis: non-marginal and 'floating' (non-attached) syndesmophytes.

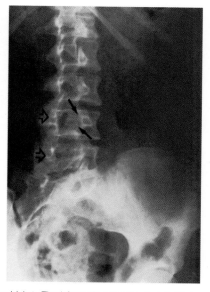

**Plate 14** Spondylolysis. The defect in the pars interarticularis (black arrows) may only be noted on an oblique view. The patient has had a spinal fusion (open arrows).

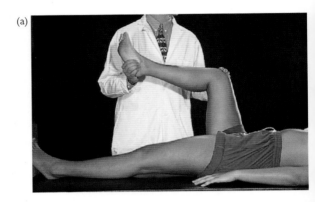

(a)

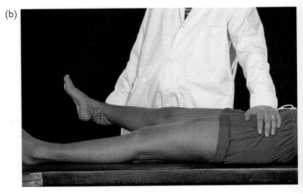

(b)

**Plate 15** Testing passive hip flexion and rotational movements (a) and hip abduction. (b) The pelvis should be fixed when testing abduction and adduction.

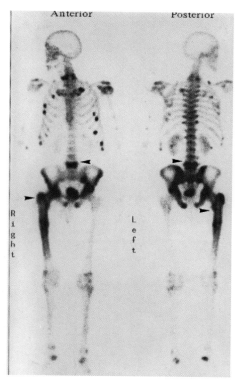

**Plate 16** Bone scintigraphy ($^{99m}$Tc-MDP) of a 65-year-old man with widespread bone pain and weakness suspected to have metastatic malignancy. Anterior view (left); posterior view (right). Undecalcified transiliac bone biopsy confirmed severe osteomalacia. There was coincidental right femoral Paget's disease (arrowed lesions).

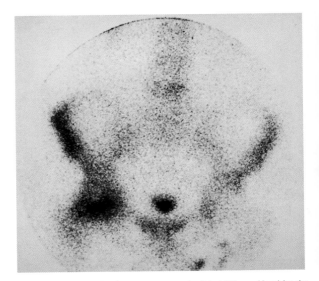

**Plate 17** Bone scintigraphy showing osteonecrosis of the left femoral head (on the right-hand side as this is an anterior view). High tracer localisation indicates increased bone turnover though in some instances there may be photopenia (an early sign) which corresponds to ischaemia.

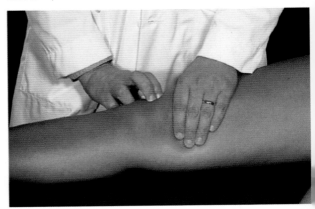

**Plate18** The 'patellar tap' test. Any fluid in the suprapatellar pouch is squeezed distally by the left hand. The patella is depressed by the right hand. It will normally tap the underlying femur immediately. Any delay in eliciting the tap or a feeling of damping as the patella is depressed suggests a joint effusion.

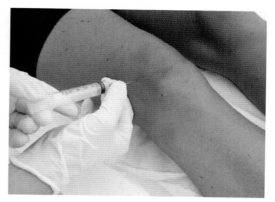

**Plate 19** Injection of the knee. Courtesy of Mrs Carey Tierney.

(a)

(b)

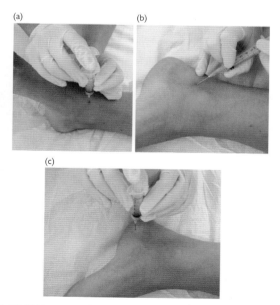

(c)

**Plate 20** (a) Injection to ankle joint, (b) tarsal tunnel, and (c) plantar fascia. Images courtesy of Mrs Carey Tierney.

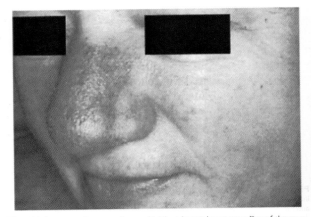

**Plate 21** Lupus pernio presenting as a bluish-red or violaceous swelling of the nose extending onto the cheek.

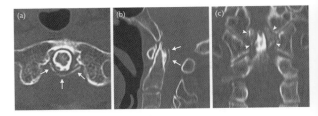

**Plate 22** Calcium pyrophosphate deposition disease (CPPD). This is a typical axial skeletal CPPD lesion: calcification of periodontoid ligaments and soft-tissue (termed 'crowned-dens syndrome') shown on CT scan: (a) axial view; (b) sagittal view; (c) coronal view.

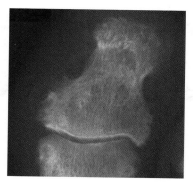

**Plate 23** Psoriatic arthritis (PsA). Lesions at/around a distal great toe interphalangeal joint. In early disease the articular surfaces often appear normal and there is 'fluffy' juxta-articular new bone. See CASPAR criteria for diagnosis and 'Investigations' for PsA in ➲ Chapter 8.

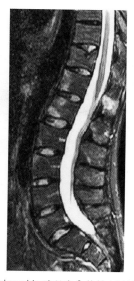

**Plaate 24** Osteitis in axial spondyloarthritis (axSpA). Vertebral (corner) osteitis is seen as high signal on this fat-suppressed sagittal spinal magnetic resonance image, indicating current inflammation on four contiguous vertebrae (T12–L3) and faintly in L5. Intervertebral discs appear normal (high signal indicating well hydrated) so not degenerate—suggesting against the vertebral high signal being 'Modic lesions' (associated with degenerate disc disease).

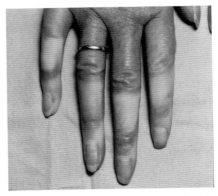

**Plate 25** Raynaud's disease (RD) in systemic sclerosis (SScl). Note clear margins to ischaemic (white) areas.

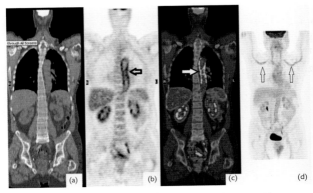

**Plate 26** Contiguous CT (a) and ¹⁸F-FDG-PET (b) images showing aortitis (arrowed in (b) and in CT-PET registered image (c)) and vasculitis of subclavian arteries (arrowed in (d) in non-contiguous ¹⁸F-FDG-PET scan image) in vasculitis (in a 75-year-old, treated as giant cell arteritis).

## Differential diagnosis

- The clinician should consider the following conditions:
  - Thrombotic thrombocytopenic purpura (red cell fragments more numerous than in cAPS).
  - HELLP syndrome (haemolysis, elevated liver enzymes and low platelets).
  - Haemolytic–uraemic syndrome.
  - Cryoglobulinaemia.
  - Vasculitis.

## Treatment and prognosis

- Apart from techniques and therapies used in the intensive support of multiple organ failure, IV heparin, GCs, plasma exchange, and IVIg (for 4–5 days at a dose of 0.4 g/kg/day) can be used.
- Case reports exist in single patients describing the use of epoprostenol, defibrotide (not licensed in the UK), and fibrinolytics.
- RTX can be used in refractory cases or in the presence of micro-angiopathic haemolytic anaemia.
- CYC has been shown to be beneficial in cAPS with the presence of secondary autoimmune disease such as SLE.
- A RCT on belimumab (a B-cell activating factor inhibitor) in SLE patients has shown a decrease in ACL IgA.
- Mortality remains >50% and 25% of survivors will develop further APS-related events.
- Recurrence of cAPS is very rare.

## References

1. Merashli M, Noureldine MH, Uthman I, et al. Antiphophopholipid syndrome: an update. *Eur J Clin Invest* 2015;45:653–62.
2. Cerevera R. Catastrophic antiphospholipid syndrome (cAPS): update from the 'cAPS Registry'. *Lupus* 2010;19:412–18.

# Sjögren's syndrome

# Epidemiology and pathophysiology

Sjögren's syndrome (SS) is a chronic autoimmune disease of unknown aetiology, characterized by lymphocyte infiltration of exocrine glands resulting in dryness of mucosal surfaces including mouth (xerostomia), eyes (xerophthalmia), nose, pharynx, larynx, and vagina.

- SS may be *primary*, associated with specific extraglandular (systemic) disease, or *secondary*, in association with a number of other autoimmune diseases including RA (see ➔ Chapter 5), SLE (see ➔ Chapter 10), thyroid disease, coeliac disease, and primary biliary cirrhosis (PBC).
- SS is (rarely) associated with progression to lymphoid malignancy.
- SS has a F:M ratio of 14–24:1 in the largest reported series, and is common between 40 and 60 years of age.
- Population prevalence is estimated at 1%, similar to that of RA.
- EBV and retroviruses have been implicated in pathogenesis.
- Antibodies to nuclear proteins Ro/SSA and La/SSB may be formed when Ro and La are exposed on the surface of apoptotic cells.
- Rheumatoid factor (RF) and a positive ANA are also common and patients may be erroneously diagnosed with RA.
- HLA-DR3 is strongly associated with SS.

**Table 12.1** Classification criteria for primary Sjögren's syndrome for use in the context of sicca symptoms

| Criteria | Comment | Score |
|---|---|---|
| Positive Schirmer test | <5 mm/5 min | 1 |
| Low unstimulated salivary flow | < 0.1 mL/min | 1 |
| Anti-Ro antibody positive | | 3 |
| Abnormal lip biopsy | ≥1 foci/4 mm$^2$ | 3 |
| Abnormal ocular staining score | ≥5 | 1 |

Individuals with signs and/or symptoms suggestive of SS who have a total score of ≥4 for the above-listed items meet the criteria for primary SS.

Data adapted from Shiboski CH, Shiboski SC, Seror R, et al. 2016 American College of Rheumatology/European League Against Rheumatism classification criteria for primary Sjögren's syndrome: a consensus and data-driven methodology involving three international patient cohorts. *Ann Rheum Dis* 2017;76:9–16.

# Clinical manifestations and classification criteria

The classification criteria for primary SS are listed in Table 12.1. These represent an update of the 1993 European Community Criteria for classifying SS and have been adopted by the scientific community worldwide. They have a sensitivity and specificity of around 94%.

- Exclusions include head and neck irradiation, hepatitis C, AIDS, pre-existing lymphoma, sarcoidosis, graft vs host disease and anticholinergic drug use.
- Extraglandular disease is seen in one-third of patients with primary SS. The main symptoms are fatigue, low-grade fever, myalgia, and arthralgia (Table 12.2).

## Glandular disease

- The initial manifestations can be non-specific and 8–10 years can elapse before the diagnosis is established.
- Typical initial features of 'sicca' syndrome include dry eyes (xerophthalmia) in >50% at presentation, dry mouth (xerostomia) in 40%, and parotid/salivary gland enlargement in 25%. The prevalence of these manifestations increase with the duration of disease.
- Concurrent corneal and conjunctival damage (keratoconjunctivitis sicca), and dental caries from poor tear and salivary flow respectively, can occur.
- Lack of secretions may also affect the respiratory tract (nasal dryness, cough, or hoarse voice), oesophagus and pharynx (dysphagia) or vagina (dyspareunia and pruritus).
- A number of conditions can cause xerostomia and other 'dryness' symptoms and also parotid/salivary gland swelling (see Table 12.3).

**Table 12.2** The frequency of extraglandular manifestations of primary Sjögren's syndrome

| Condition | Frequency (%) |
| --- | --- |
| Arthralgia/arthritis | 37 |
| Raynaud's disease | 16 |
| Cutaneous vasculitis | 12 |
| Pulmonary disease | 9 |
| Lymphadenopathy | 7 |
| Peripheral neuropathy | 7 |
| Renal disease | 6 |
| Autoimmune hepatitis | 2 |
| Lymphoproliferative disease | 2 |
| Myositis | 1 |

**Table 12.3** The differential diagnosis of the glandular features of Sjögren's syndrome

| Feature | Differential diagnosis |
|---------|------------------------|
| Parotid and other salivary gland enlargement | Neoplasia |
| | Infections (e.g. EBV, mumps, HIV, CMV) |
| | Granulomatous diseases (sarcoid, TB) |
| | Endocrine causes (diabetes, hypothyroidism, acromegaly) |
| | Chronic recurrent idiopathic parotitis |
| | Calculi |
| | Amyloidosis |
| | IgG4-related disease |
| Xerostomia and xerophthalmia ('dryness') | Age/elderly |
| | Drugs (diuretics, antihypertensive, parasympathetic, psychotropic) |
| | Dehydration |
| | Psychogenic |
| | Irradiation damage |
| | SOX syndrome |
| | Congenital |
| | Graft vs host disease |
| | Hepatitis C |
| | IgG4-related disease |

## Joints

Joint disease needs careful assessment. Associated ('overlap') RA can occur (ACPA positive and typical RA erosions on radiographs) and generalized inflammatory osteoarthritis (OA) is common in the same age/gender demography as primary SS. Whether a true SS-associated arthritis or (or) whether (there is) there is a significant association between generalized OA and PSS, is debated but essentially is not known.

- Non-erosive arthritis is more frequent in patients with Raynaud's phenomenon, and the latter can pre-date SS by many years.
- A milder form of SS has been linked to generalized OA and has been termed 'SOX syndrome' (sialadenitis, osteoarthritis, xerostomia).

## Skin

- Itchy annular erythema, alopecia, and hyper/hypopigmentation can occur. A hypersensitivity vasculitis may also develop.
- Vascular involvement in SS affects small- and medium-sized vessels. The most common manifestations are cutaneous purpura, urticaria, and skin ulceration.

- Skin vasculitis in SS is benign and treatment with glucocorticoids (GCs) not always needed.
- Cryoglobulins are present in 10–20% of patients with skin vasculitis in SS (and may be associated with hepatitis C positivity).
- In contrast to SScl (see ⊃ Chapter 13), Raynaud's disease in SS is not typically associated with digital ulceration and infarcts.

## Pulmonary disease

Pulmonary disease is common.
- Pulmonary function abnormalities are seen in 25% of patients, although they are not usually clinically significant.
- Rarely a lymphocytic interstitial pneumonitis (LIP) may occur, causing pyrexia, cough, and dyspnoea.
- In LIP, lymphocytic infiltration occurs around bronchioles, leading to cryptogenic organizing pneumonia. This responds well to GCs.

## Renal disease

Overt renal disease is found in 10% of patients with primary SS.
- A renal tubular acidosis (RTA) may occur, causing a normal anion gap metabolic acidosis, a urine pH of >5.5, and hypokalaemia.
- RTA is typically type 1 distal tubule predominant in SS.
- Long-term RTA can result in nephrocalcinosis or nephrolithiasis.
- Glomerulonephritis is rare and seen mainly in those with SS/SLE overlap. In many cases, a consistent finding is cryoglobulinaemia and hypocomplementaemia.

## Gastrointestinal and hepatobiliary disease

- Dysphagia due to dryness of the pharynx and oesophagus is common. Chronic atrophic gastritis may occur due to lymphocytic infiltration similar to that seen in the salivary glands.
- Subclinical hyperamylasaemia is a common finding in up to 25% of cases and there may be a close link between the 'autoimmune cholangitis' of SS and PBC. Sicca syndrome is found in 50% of PBC cases.
- Transaminitis may be due to hepatitis C, which can cause a Sjögren's-like disease often in association with a 'mixed' cryoglobulinaemia.

## Neuromuscular disease

- Peripheral sensory neuropathy is the most common neuromuscular feature of SS. This may be a sensory ataxic neuropathy (dorsal root ganglionopathy) or a painful small fibre neuropathy.
- Autonomic neuropathy is rarely seen.
- Mononeuritis multiplex as a consequence of vasculitis is well recognized as is the isolated involvement of cranial nerves, particularly the trigeminal and optic nerve.
- Involvement of the central nervous system remains a controversy. Demyelinating, multiple sclerosis-like syndromes may be seen.
- Myalgia is common but myositis is rare. The pattern of myositis is like polymyositis and is treated as such accordingly (see ⊃ Chapter 14).

## Lymphoproliferative disease

- Patients with SS have an ~16% increased risk of developing a lymphoma, compared to age-, gender-, and race-matched normal controls.
- The lymphomas are primarily B cell in origin, usually expressing the monoclonal IgMκ, and of two major types, either highly undifferentiated, or well-differentiated immunocytomas.
- The clinical picture is diverse. The approach to therapy should be determined by the stage and histological grade of the disease.
- The salivary glands are the main site of lymphomatous change. The presence of lymphadenopathy, organomegaly, or persistent, painful, and continuously enlarged salivary glands, in the absence of infection, should raise suspicion and warrants biopsy.
- Other organs and systems may be affected including lungs, kidneys, and GI tract.
- Risk factors include monoclonal gammopathy, cryoglobulins, hypocomplementaemia, and ganglionopathy.

## Cardiovascular system

- Anti-Ro and La antibodies cross the placenta and can cause fetal congenital heart block. Mothers with these antibodies have a 1 in 20 risk of having an affected pregnancy (see ➋ Chapter 10).
- Fetal heart rate monitoring in specialist centres is needed.
- Oral dexamethasone given to mothers early following detection of heart block may reverse the condition.
- Neonatal lupus erythematosus (NLE) is also seen (see ➋ Chapter 10).

## Fatigue

- Fatigue is often the worst symptom for many patients with SS.
- Patients often learn to cope with fatigue with the most successful adopting a frame of mind that 'accepts' the fatigue; having close relatives and family realize that fatigue is part of the disease; pacing their activities; and undertaking some regular aerobic exercise.
- Failure to cope with fatigue may lead to chronic pain.

## Other pathology in SS

- Over 50% of patients have antithyroid antibodies and altered thyroid biochemistry without necessarily overt clinical symptoms.
- Non-bacterial interstitial cystitis due to an intense inflammation of the mucosa can cause frequency, nocturia, and perineal pain.
- Mild normochromic, normocytic anaemia is common. Leucopenia is seen in 15–20% of patients with SS. The ESR is often raised (requiring a paraprotein to be excluded), but the CRP is usually normal.

## Other autoimmune diseases

In a recent retrospective case review of 114 patients with primary SS, 33% had an additional autoimmune disease, 6% two diseases, and 2% three diseases. Hypothyroidism was the most common condition seen. Coeliac disease is also commonly associated.

# Investigations

Common laboratory findings in primary SS are detailed in Table 12.4.

## Assessment of sicca symptoms

- Salivary flow rates (sialometry) can be measured for whole saliva or separate secretions from different salivary glands, with or without stimulation.
- Patients with overt SS have decreased unstimulated salivary flow rates. Measuring salivary flow rate is simple but can be confounded by concomitant use of drugs with anticholinergic properties.
- However, a simple screening test is to have a patient spit all saliva into a graded measuring sample pot for 10 min. More than 2 mL (>0.2 mL/min) makes primary SS unlikely.
- Anatomical changes in the ductal system can be assessed by radiocontrast sialography. This can, however, be painful and there is some controversy as to its sensitivity and specificity.
- Scintigraphy, with uptake of $^{99}$Tc, may provide a functional evaluation of all the salivary glands by observing the rate and density of uptake and the time for it to appear in the mouth after IV administration. Scanning has a high sensitivity albeit low specificity, but has a greater sensitivity and specificity than unstimulated sialometry.

**Table 12.4** Common laboratory findings in primary SS.

| Finding | | Frequency (%) |
|---|---|---|
| General | Anaemia | 20 |
| | Thrombocytopenia | 13 |
| | Leucopenia | 16 |
| | Raised ESR | 22 |
| | Monoclonal gammopathy | 22 |
| | Hypergammaglobulinaemia | 22 |
| Cryoglobulinaemia | | 9 |
| Autoimmune serology | ANA | 74 |
| | Rheumatoid factor | 38 |
| | Ro/SS-A | 40 |
| | La/SS-B | 26 |
| | ANCA | 6 |
| | Antimitochondrial | 5 |

Reproduced from Garcia-Carrasco M, et al. Primary Sjögren syndrome: Clinical and immunologic disease patterns in a cohort of 400 patients. *Medicine* 2002;81:270–80 with permission from Wolters Kluwer.

- The Schirmer test is used for the evaluation of tear secretion. Strips of filter paper 30 mm in length are slipped over the inferior eyelid by a fold at one end of the strip. After 5 min the length of paper that has been made wet by the tears is measured; wetting of <5 mm is a strong indication of diminished tear secretion.
- Salivary gland US is emerging as a useful non-invasive tool in the diagnosis of SS. It has a high specificity and has been shown to correlate well with labial gland biopsy findings. It is used in some centres to establish whether a labial gland biopsy is required.

## Biopsy

A labial gland biopsy is often essential to the establishment of a diagnosis of SS, particularly when the patient lacks anti-Ro or anti-La antibodies.

- Because there is a risk of sensory nerve damage, the biopsy should be done by a surgeon with experience in the technique.
- At least 4–6 glands must be biopsied, since the pathologic process is invariably focal.
- Biopsies should not be taken if there is mucosal inflammation overlying the biopsy site or there is a past history of therapeutic head and neck irradiation.
- The biopsy must be scored for the number of lymphocytic foci (i.e. aggregates of 50 or more lymphocytes) that surround ducts or blood vessels, and are adjacent to histologically normal acini.
- A score of 1 or more foci per 4 mm$^2$ is compatible with SS. However, focal lymphocytic sialadenitis can also be seen in hepatitis C, HIV, graft vs host disease, and patients with autoimmune disease in the absence of sicca symptoms.

# Treatment

Table 12.5 summarizes the general and organ-directed treatment options for SS. For more extensive detail the reader is directed to the 2017 BSR Guideline for the management of adults with primary Sjögren's syndrome.

- Dental input and close collaboration is essential.
- Patients should be encouraged not to smoke, to avoid sugar-laden foods, and to attend dental hygienist sessions regularly.
- Periodically, swabbing palate, tongue, and pharynx for oral *Candida* overgrowth is prudent, especially if dysgeusia develops.
- There is merit in patients trialling topical preparations for xerophthalmia and xerostomia as there may be personal preference to one preparation or another.
- Many patients favour the combination use of a runny eye drop for frequent use during the day and a more viscous preparation at night or in situations where frequent drop insertion is impracticable.

## Synthetic DMARDs (sDMARDs)

- Hydroxychloroquine (HCQ) is the most commonly used sDMARD though evidence for its effectivity in SS is weak.
- Significant improvements have been described in a retrospective study in terms of the sicca features, parotid gland enlargement, oral infection, myalgia, arthralgia, fatigue, and joint swelling following 12 months of treatment with HCQ.
- In a 2014 study reported in *JAMA*, HCQ was no better than placebo in improving pain, fatigue, or dryness.
- There is no evidence that other sDMARDS or anti-TNFα therapies are effective in primary SS.

## Biologic DMARDs (bDMARDs)

- Rituximab (RTX; anti-CD20/anti-B-cell monoclonal antibody) has only shown short-lasting benefit in clinical trials, but may be useful for SS-related cryoglobulinaemia or neuropathy, as well as for other coexisting immune-driven conditions, e.g. coeliac disease.
- Belimumab (anti-BAFF monoclonal antibody (B-cell activating factor, also known as BLyS, TALL-1, and THANK), is a TNF superfamily member (TNFSF13B) best known for its role in the survival and maturation of B cells) has demonstrated efficacy in open label phase II trials, but salivary flow and the Schirmer test did not improve.
- Tocilizumab (anti-IL-6 receptor monoclonal antibody) is currently undergoing phase II/III trials.
- Epratuzumab, (humanized anti-CD22 monoclonal antibody) has demonstrated response in an open label phase I/II study.

For greater detail on all drug therapies including immunosuppressants, see Chapter 23

**Table 12.5** The treatment of Sjögren's syndrome

| Condition | Treatment |
|---|---|
| Xerophthalmia | Artificial tears (preferably preservative free) |
| | Topical ciclosporin drops |
| | Punctal occlusion (plugs) |
| | Treatment of meibomian gland dysfunction (with warm compresses). In persistent inflammation and blepharitis, doxycycline 50 mg once daily for at least 3 months may be considered |
| Xerostomia | Frequent sips of water, good oral hygiene (e.g. chlorhexidine mouthwash), high-concentration fluoride toothpastes) |
| | Sugar-free gum and lozenges (e.g. Salivix® or SST® pastilles) |
| | Artificial saliva or mouth lubricating sprays |
| Sicca features | May improve with pilocarpine 5 mg up to 4 times daily (side-effects include flushing/sweating), or cevimeline, which is currently not licensed in the UK (fewer side-effects) |
| Vaginal dryness | Patients may respond to propionic acid gels. Rigorous treatment of infection. Advice on lubricants, use of pessaries, and for intercourse, the presence of dyspareunia |
| Salivary gland | Infection—tetracycline (500 mg, 4 times a day) and NSAIDs. Persistent pain and swelling—biopsy |
| Arthralgia | Hydroxychloroquine 200–400 mg/day if RA and generalized inflammatory OA have been ruled out (though hydroxychloroquine may be effective for joint symptoms associated with these diagnoses) |
| Systemic vasculitis | Necrotizing vasculitis and glomerulonephritis—prednisone and/or cyclophosphamide. Leucocytoclastic vasculitis—no specific therapy but MMF or azathioprine may have a role. |
| Liver disease | Cholestasis may respond to ursodeoxycholic acid 10–15 mg/kg/day |
| Chronic erythematosus candidiasis | Topical nystatin, miconazole, or ketoconazole |
| Interstitial lung disease (LIP) | Prednisolone, cyclophosphamide |

# Prognosis

There are few studies on the prognosis of primary SS.

- Some studies suggest the presence of vasculitis, cryoglobulins, or low complement may be adverse prognostic markers.
- Outcomes in secondary SS are likely to correlate with the associated condition.

# Systemic sclerosis and related disorders

# Introduction and definitions

Systemic sclerosis (SScl) is a generalized autoimmune connective tissue disease. Scleroderma—the cutaneous lesion which is prominent and key to a diagnosis of SScl—is epidermal-dermal tethering associated with microangiopathy and excessive collagen production and fibrosis. *Morphoea* essentially describes localized scleroderma and it can exist in a number of forms though all forms are not associated with systemic disease/internal organ lesions (unlike in SScl).

- The classification of SScl is shown in Table 13.1.
- Raynaud's disease (RD) describes (usually cold-induced) peripheral digital vasospasm and is highly associated with SScl (See ➜ Plate 25).
- The spectrum of morphoea conditions includes:
  - *Generalized morphoea* which is characterized by widespread indurated plaques and pigmentary changes.
  - *Linear scleroderma* is localized scleroderma, which is characterized by a line of thickened skin which can affect the bones and muscles underneath it. It most often occurs in the arms, legs, or forehead. It is also most likely to be on just one side of the body. Linear scleroderma generally first appears in young children.
  - *Other:* morphoea profunda, morphoea-lichen sclerosis et atrophicus, frontolinear scleroderma (morphoea en coup de sabre). (See ➜ 'Morphoea, localized scleroderma, and scleroderma-like fibrosing disorders', pp. 422–3)

**Table 13.1** ACR/EULAR classification criteria for SScl

| Feature | Details | Weight/score |
|---|---|---|
| Skin thickening of the fingers of both hands extending proximal to MCPJs *(sufficient criterion)* | | 9 |
| Skin thickening of the fingers *(only count the higher score)* | Puffy fingers | 2 |
| | Sclerodactyly of the fingers (distal to MCPJs, proximal to PIPJs) | 4 |
| Telangiectasia | | 2 |
| Abnormal nailfold capillaries | | 2 |
| Pulmonary arterial hypertension and/or interstitial lung disease | | 2 |
| Raynaud's disease | | 3 |
| SSc-related autoantibodies (anti-centromere, anti-topoisomerase I, anti-RNA polymerase III) | | 3 |

*Add to maximum weight in each category to calculate the total score*

*Patients having a total score of ≥9 are classified as having SScl*

Reproduced from van den Hoogen F et al. 2013 Classification criteria for systemic sclerosis: an American college of rheumatology/European league against rheumatism collaborative initiative. *Annals of the Rheumatic Diseases* 2013;72:1747–1755 with permission from the BMJ.

# Epidemiology and pathophysiology of systemic sclerosis (SScl)

## Epidemiology

- The incidence and prevalence of SScl varies in different populations.
- SScl appears to be less prevalent in Europe (80–150 cases per million adults) compared with the USA (276 cases per million adults).
- There is a racial difference in the prevalence of SScl—greater in Europeans than in Asians.
- Mild disease often remains undiagnosed. Therefore, the true prevalence of SScl is probably underestimated.
- Annual incidence is reported at 1–20 cases per million. Males and females are both affected.

## Pathophysiology

SScl is characterized by three main pathogenetic features: microvasculopathy, immune activation with inflammation, and increase of extracellular matrix deposition in the skin and internal organs resulting in fibrosis.

### General

(For a recent review, see reference 1). Currently, the mechanisms involved in SScl pathogenesis remain unknown and are likely to be very complex. Evidence suggests a close connection between environmental factors and SScl pathogenesis.

### Immune cell activation and cytokines

- The activation of T cells is considered to play an important role in the development of the vasculopathy and fibrosis in SScl.
- Activated oligoclonal CD8 T cells may be detected in the blood and lungs of SScl patients and effector memory CD8 T cells may be involved in the pathogenesis of organ involvement in SScl.

### Genetics/epigenetics

- The genetic heritability for SScl is <0.01; however, there is a higher incidence in patients with a family history than in the general population and a positive family history significantly increases the relative risk (RR) of SScl by 15–19-fold in siblings—indicating a genetic influence on pathogenesis.
- Epigenetic effects such as DNA methylation, histone modification, non-coding RNA effects (microRNA) are all thought to play a key role in pathogenesis. For example, hypomethylation of the gene encoding integrin-α9, a membrane glycoprotein that mediates cell–cell and cell–matrix adhesion, can produce an overexpression of integrins causing myofibroblast differentiation and increased TGFβ production promoting fibrogenesis.

*Environmental factors*

Several chemical agents have been implicated in the development of scleroderma, although exposures account for only a small fraction of patients who develop scleroderma or similar conditions.
• Possible chemical triggers of scleroderma include silica, organic chemicals, aliphatic hydrocarbons (e.g. vinyl chloride, naphtha), aromatic hydrocarbons (e.g. benzene, toluene), drugs (e.g. hydroxytryptophan, carbidopa, fenfluramine, bleomycin).

*Vasculopathy*

Vascular injury may be the primary pathophysiological event either by vasomotor instability or microvascular intimal proliferation and vessel obliteration. Intravascular pathology in the form of increased platelet activity, red cell rigidity, and thrombosis may also be a factor.

*Inflammation*

Occurs early in SScl, and may no longer be present at the time of diagnosis. Causes oedematous (not indurated) skin.

*Fibrosis*

Consequence of inflammation, widespread and non-organ-specific in SScl. Excess extracellular matrix protein in the skin and internal organs.
• TGFβ plays a crucial role particularly through the activation of collagen production that leads to fibrosis.

## Reference
1. Barsotti S, Stagnaro C, d'Ascanio A, et al. One year in review 2016: systemic sclerosis. *Clin Exp Rheumatol* 2016;(34 Suppl 100):S3–S13.

# Classification of SScl

## Classification and disease patterns

Patients with SScl have a potentially wide range of features of pathology affecting different organ systems, and can present in varied ways. The ACR/EULAR 2013 classification criteria for SScl (Table 13.1) have a sensitivity of 91% and specificity of 92%.

- Clinical features are wide ranging and their classification, in association with typical serological findings, within disease patterns is shown in Table 13.2.
- Table 13.2 highlights the two main clinical forms of SScl: limited cutaneous (lcSScl) and diffuse cutaneous (dcSScl). Over 60% of cases are in the 'limited' subset, where visceral involvement is late, and some 10–30 years after onset of Raynaud's disease (RD).
- The definition of 'limited cutaneous' subsumes the definition of CREST (Calcinosis, Raynaud's disease, (o)Esophageal dysmotility, Sclerodactyly, Telangiectasia) syndrome, although this acronym is a useful reminder of the common characteristics of lcSScl.
- SScl can develop insidiously and in early disease non-SScl scleroderma-associated disorders need to be considered (see ➔ Table 13.3, p. 409).

**Table 13.2** Patterns of clinical and serological features in the different forms of systemic sclerosis (SScl)

| | |
|---|---|
| Early SScl | Raynaud's phenomenon, nailfold capillary changes |
| | Disease-specific antinuclear antibodies (ANAs):<br>• Antitopoisomerase-1 (Scl-70)<br>• Anticentromere (ACA)<br>• Anti-RNA polymerase III<br>• Nucleolar |
| Diffuse cutaneous SScl | Skin changes within 1 year of Raynaud's. Truncal and acral (face, arms, hands, feet) skin involvement |
| | Tendon friction rubs |
| | Early, significant organ disease:<br>• Interstitial lung disease<br>• Scleroderma renal crisis<br>• Myocardial disease<br>• GI disease |
| | Nailfold capillary dilatation and/or 'drop out' |
| | Scl-70 antibodies in up to 60% of patients |
| Limited cutaneous SScl | Raynaud's phenomenon for many years |
| | Acral skin involvement |
| | Late incidence of pulmonary hypertension with or without interstitial lung disease |
| | Skin calcification and telangiectasia |
| | Nailfold capillary dilatation and/or 'drop out' |
| | ACA antibodies in 70–80% of patients |
| SScl sine scleroderma | Raynaud's |
| | No skin involvement |
| | Presentation with lung fibrosis, renal crisis, cardiac, or GI disease |
| | ANA |

# Approach to diagnosis of SScl

## Differential diagnosis

The principles that underlie diagnosis include considering first whether there is a form of systemic sclerosis (dcSScl or lcSScl; Table 13.2) or a disease that mimics SScl (Table 13.3) or a scleroderma-associated fibrosing disease (see later in this chapter, ➐ 'Morphoea, localized scleroderma, and Scleroderma-like fibrosing disorders', p. 422. Then, if SScl is likely, establish the extent of disease.

- The input of a dermatologist may be very helpful if a scleroderma-like fibrosing disorder is possible.
- Nephrology input should be considered early.
- A skin biopsy should not be taken unless discussed with a dermatologist and pathologist first and probably should only be done once the patient has seen the dermatologist.
- The extent of involvement of SScl requires a methodological approach to evaluating organs and bodily systems (see later in this topic).
- Assessment may be aided by an appreciation of how early or late the disease is likely to be (Table 13.4).

## Essential initial investigations

The extent of organ involvement disease should be assessed by baseline investigations as follows:

- Blood pressure measurement and urinalysis.
- Barium swallow/GI endoscopy depending on symptoms.
- Chest radiograph and lung function tests.
- High-resolution CT lung scan if auscultation of the lungs reveals crackles or if lung function abnormal.
- Laboratory tests: renal and liver function, paraprotein, FBC, ESR, CRP, TSH, random glucose, ANA/ENAs; RF, complement C3, immunoglobulins.
- ECG and transthoracic echocardiography (with estimate of pulmonary artery pressure).
- Nailfold capillaroscopy and distal upper limb thermography with cold stimulation challenge (in specialist centres) can highlight abnormal patterns of disease and can point to systemic disease in cases with limited early features.

**Table 13.3** The differential diagnosis of SScl

| | | |
|---|---|---|
| Metabolic and inherited conditions | Carcinoid syndrome | Scleroderma-like lesions can be found with malignant carcinoid |
| | Acromegaly | Associated with skin puffiness and increase in sebum and sweat |
| | Phenylketonuria | Phenylalanine-restricted diet may improve skin changes |
| | Amyloidosis | Plaques from direct dermal infiltration can mimic SScl; more common are alopecia, ecchymoses, and nail dystrophy |
| Immunological and inflammatory conditions | Chronic graft vs host disease | Skin changes favour the trunk, hips, and thighs, but can affect the entire body. Associated with pruritus and hypopigmentation |
| | Eosinophilic fasciitis | Associated with painful induration of the skin, hypereosinophilia, and hypergammaglobulinaemia. Early skin changes described as 'peau d'orange' |
| | Scleroedema | Occurs with diabetes, monoclonal gammopathies, and after infections (e.g. post-streptococcal throat infection). Unlike SScl, can occur without Raynaud's phenomenon |
| | Sclero-myxoedema | Waxy induration of the skin along the forehead, neck, and behind the ears. Not associated with Raynaud's phenomenon |
| | Nephrogenic fibrosing dermopathy | Rapid induration of the skin and other organs associated with exposure to gadolinium-based contrast used for MRI |
| | POEMS | Polyneuropathy, organomegaly, endocrinopathy, M-protein, and skin changes. Hyperpigmentation is most common, but acrocyanosis/skin thickening are seen |
| Acquired | Lipodermato-sclerosis | Hyperpigmentation and induration of lower legs associated with chronic venous insufficiency/stasis ('champagne bottle legs') |
| | Eosinophilic myalgia syndrome | Acute syndrome caused by exposure to L-tryptophan |
| | Bleomycin exposure | Used as a model to study scleroderma |

Table 13.4 Characteristic findings in early- and late-onset SScl

|  | Early onset (<3 yrs from disease onset) | Late onset (>3 yrs from disease onset) |
|---|---|---|
| **dcSScl** | | |
| Constitutional | Fatigue, weight loss | Minimal |
| Vascular | Raynaud's (often mild) | Severe Raynaud's. Telangiectasia |
| Cutaneous | Rapid progression involving arms, face, and trunk | Stable or some regression |
| Musculoskeletal | Arthralgia, myalgia, stiffness | Flexion contractures |
| Gastrointestinal | Dysphagia and 'heart burn' | More severe dysphagia. Midgut and anorectal disease |
| Cardiopulmonary | Myocarditis, pericarditis, lung fibrosis | Progression of established disease/pulmonary hypertension |
| Renal | Maximum risk of scleroderma renal crisis | Crisis uncommon after 4 years |
| **lcSScl** | | |
| Constitutional | None | Worsened by vasculopathy, GI symptoms. |
| Vascular | Severe Raynaud's. Telangiectasia | Digital ulceration or gangrene |
| Cutaneous | Mild sclerosis on face | Stable, calcinosis |
| Musculoskeletal | Occasional joint stiffness | Flexion contractures More severe symptoms common. |
| Gastrointestinal | Dysphagia and 'heart burn' | Midgut and anorectal disease |
| Cardiopulmonary | Rarely involved | Slow progressive lung fibrosis. Pulmonary hypertension Right-sided heart failure |
| Renal | No direct involvement | Rarely involved |

# Clinical features of SScl

### Raynaud's disease (RD)

The overall prevalence of RD is 3–10% worldwide, variation depending on climate, skin colour, and racial background.

- In SScl, RD is present in 95% of cases.
- History: classic triphasic response to cold starting with episodic pallor of the digits (due to ischaemia, see ➜ Plate 25), followed by cyanosis (due to deoxygenation), and then redness and suffusion. The last stage of redness is a reactive hyperaemia following the return of blood and is the most painful phase, also associated with tingling/numbness.
- Continuous blueness/cyanosis with pain is not characteristic of RD and the main differential diagnosis then is chilblains or vasculitis.
- Symptoms that might suggest secondary RD include an onset in men, patients >45 years, symptoms all year round, digital ulceration, and asymmetry.
- ANA should be tested and nail-fold capillaroscopy obtained (see ➜ Plate 9). Pathological changes seen on capillaroscopy include nailfold capillary dilatation, haemorrhage, and drop-out. Both have a high predictive power for detecting those patients likely to develop SScl.
- Conservative measures should be directed at keeping the core body (i.e. base of neck and upper trunk) temperature warm.
- Smoking cessation is essential.
- Severe RD can cause digital ulceration (DU). Ulcers can become infected and may lead to osteomyelitis. Treatment is usually conservative with antibiotics.
- Early finger pulp tissue threat/pathology (hardening, cracks, callus and small erythematous lesions)—can be painful. Skin infection can ensue— the process worsened by subcutaneous calcification. Regular application of fusidic acid and hydrocortisone cream can help soften the skin and lessen pain.
- Digital gangrene may occur following prolonged ischaemia, leading to auto-amputation of digits. Surgery is usually avoided due to poor wound healing.
- RD can occur in fingers, toes, ear lobes, and even genitalia in SScl.

### Skin—scleroderma

Scleroderma in dcSScl and lcSScl usually proceeds through three phases early, classic, late. In the early stage there may be non-pitting oedema of the hands and feet, marked in the mornings and associated with RD. The skin then becomes taut, the epidermis thins, hair growth ceases, and skin creases disappear—the 'classic' changes of scleroderma become pronounced. The classic changes remain static for many years.

- The late phase may evolve at any time. Truncal and limb skin softens such that it can be difficult to know that a person ever had sclerosis. However, the hand changes rarely resolve and continue to show the ravages of fibrosis and contractures.

**Table 13.5** The treatment of Raynaud's disease

| Treatment | Examples | Comments |
|---|---|---|
| Simple | Hand warmers. Protective clothing | Universally helpful |
| | Evening primrose oil | Effective in clinical trials |
| | Fish-oil capsules | |
| Parenteral vasodilator | Nifedipine or amlodipine (calcium channel blockers) | Effective, but may cause oedema, hypotension, headache, resulting in poor tolerability etc. |
| | Losartan (angiotensin II receptor blocker) | 25–50 mg once daily |
| | Fluoxetine | 20–40 mg once daily |
| | Sildenafil (phosphodiesterase inhibitor) | 25–50 mg three times daily |
| | Topical glyceryl trinitrate | High rate of discontinuation due to side effects |
| | Epoprostenol | For severe attacks with prolonged ischaemia, digital ulceration gangrene, and prior to hand surgery. Side effects include headache, nausea and hypotension |
| | Bosentan (endothelin receptor antagonist) | Endothelin receptor antagonist. In England—for use when digital ulcers are present despite treatment with sildenafil and epoprostenol |
| Surgery | Chemical or operative lumbar or digital sympathectomy with or without botulinum toxin. Debridement. Amputation | Caution prior to any surgery as wound healing is poor. |

During the late phase, digital pitting scars, loss of finger pad tissue, ulcers, telangiectasia, and calcinosis can occur.

All patients with SScl will have some involvement of the face and the digits (although this involvement may be mild). Skin thickening limited to the fingers, but sparing the proximal upper extremities is called *sclerodactyly*.

lcSScl is associated with skin involvement limited to the face and distal extremities (below the elbows and knees).

dcSScl is associated with taut hypo- or hyperpigmented skin involvement proximal to the elbow, knee, or clavicle.

**Gastrointestinal**

The GI tract is probably the most commonly involved system in SScl (Table 13.6).

- Over 90% of all patients with lcSScl and dcSScl develop oesophageal hypomotility, with >50% of patients with lcSScl having serious disease.
- The cause of GI dysfunction in SScl is not entirely clear. Possible contributing factors include neural dysfunction, tissue fibrosis, and muscle atrophy. In the earliest stages of neural dysfunction most patients are asymptomatic.
- Prokinetic drugs such as metoclopramide may help some patients with oesophageal hypomotility.
- Many patients develop reflux oesophagitis. Simple advice such as raising the head of the bed, taking frequent small meals, and avoiding late night snacks, may help. Patients often require high-dose proton-pump inhibitors.
- Small bowel disease with hypomotility can lead to weight loss and malabsorption; bacterial overgrowth may exacerbate the situation requiring rotational courses of antibiotics and the use of prokinetic drugs. Ultimately, the small bowel may fail, necessitating total parenteral nutrition.

**Table 13.6** Gastrointestinal pathology associated with SScl

| Site | Disorder | Investigation | Treatment |
|------|----------|---------------|-----------|
| Mouth | Caries, sicca syndrome | Dental radiographs | Oral hygiene. Artificial saliva |
| Oesophagus | Hypomotility | Barium swallow | Metoclopramide (dopamine receptor antagonist) |
| | Strictures | Endoscopy | Dilatation |
| Stomach | Gastroparesis | Endoscopy | Metoclopramide |
| | Gastro-oesophageal reflux disease | Barium swallow Endoscopy | Proton-pump inhibitor. Dopamine receptor antagonist |
| Small bowel | Hypomotility | Barium follow-through | Metoclopramide |
| | Malabsorption | Hydrogen breath test | Pancreatic supplements. Low-dose octreotide. Nutritional support including parental feeding if refractory, antibiotics |
| | | Jejunal aspiration/biopsy | If serologic evidence of coeliac disease is present |
| | | Stool cultures | |
| Large bowel | Hypomotility | Barium enema | Stool bulking agents |
| Anus | Incontinence | Rectal manometry | Surgery. Neurostimulator |

- Atony and hypomotility of the rectum and sigmoid colon may cause constipation and incontinence, best managed with bulking agents, although severe cases may need limited surgery or the use of implantable sacral stimulators.
- Anaemia due to vascular lesions in the GI mucosa is now widely recognized. The classic appearance in the stomach is now called gastric antrum venous ectasia (watermelon stomach), and these lesions may be treated by argon laser therapy if blood loss is significant, although this is not curative.

## Pulmonary and cardiac disease

Pulmonary disease ranks second to oesophageal disease in SScl in frequency of internal organ effects (Table 13.7).

- Pulmonary disease is now the major cause of death in SScl.
- The major lesions are parenchymal lung disease (interstitial lung disease, organizing pneumonia, and traction bronchiectasis) and pulmonary vascular disease (isolated pulmonary hypertension, pulmonary hypertension associated with interstitial lung disease, and pulmonary oedema).
- Far less common lung conditions include pleurisy, aspiration pneumonia, drug-induced pneumonitis, and spontaneous pneumothorax.
- Interstitial lung disease often develops insidiously and established fibrosis is currently untreatable. Early diagnosis is therefore vital. Most centres would now treat active disease with oral GCs and either oral or IV cyclophosphamide.
- The CXR is not a sensitive test for early fibrosis. Lung function tests can be discriminatory. The single-breath diffusion test (diffusion capacity for carbon monoxide (DLCO)) is abnormal in >70% of early cases and lung volumes are often decreased.
- Low DLCO with normal lung volumes may signify pulmonary hypertension.
- High-resolution lung CT will confirm and stage lung disease and serial imaging can be compared with changes in DLCO and functional indices (e.g. 6-min timed walking test).
- Fibrosis tends to occur mainly in dcSScl and is associated with anti-topoisomerase I antibodies; and pulmonary artery hypertension (PAH) associates with lcSScl and anti-centromere antibody.
- Heart block has been reported, but is rare.
- Severe left ventricle impairment from myocarditis is treated with cyclophosphamide and an implantable cardioverter defibrillator (ICD) may be indicated to treat ventricular arrhythmias.
- Recent studies suggest a prevalence of PAH of 12–15% in SScl.
- Right heart catheterization is the gold standard method of diagnosis, but screening using this method is not practical. Annual transthoracic echocardiography done by experienced practitioners, lung function tests, and clinical assessment are essential to help detect subclinical disease.

Table 13.7 Cardiopulmonary pathology in SScl

| Disease | Frequency | Investigation | Treatment |
|---------|-----------|---------------|-----------|
| **Pulmonary disease** | | | |
| Pulmonary fibrosis | Most common in dcSScl (Scl-70+) | Chest radiograph, lung function tests, high-resolution CT scan | Low dose GCs, mycophenolate or cyclophosphamide (alkylating agent) depending on extent of disease. Rituximab is used in refractory disease where there is extensive lung involvement |
| Pleurisy | Uncommon | Chest radiograph | NSAIDs. Low-dose oral prednisolone |
| Bronchiectasis | Rare | Chest CT scan | Antibiotics. Physiotherapy |
| Pneumothorax | Rare | Chest radiograph | Chest tube, pleurodesis |
| Pulmonary artery hypertension (PAH) | 10–15% overall | Doppler echocardiogram. Catheter studies | Endothelial 1 receptor antagonists (bosentan), epoprostenol, sildenafil, ambrisentan/tadalfil combination, macitentan or riociguat. Anticoagulation. Long-term oxygen therapy |
| **Cardiac disease** | | | |
| Dysrhythmias and conduction defects | Common, but rarely symptomatic | ECG. 24 h ambulatory cardiac monitor | Dependent on rhythm—drugs, pacemaker, ICD if indicated |
| Pericarditis | 10–15% overall | Echocardiogram | As for pleurisy (see above in table) |
| Myocarditis | Rare | | Prednisolone, cyclophosphamide. Diuretics. ICD if indicated, beta blockers maybe used but may cause worsening RD and/or digital ischaemia |
| Myocardial fibrosis | 30–50% of dcSScl | | Controversial; consider diuretics, ACE inhibitors |

- DETECT (⌘ http://detect-pah.com/home) is a composite data calculator that can be used to screen for patients with SScl who may have PAH, to identify patients who should proceed to right heart catheter. DETECT has a sensitivity of 96% and specificity of 48% and comprises:
  - FVC% predicted/DLCO% predicted.
  - current/past telangiectasia.
  - anticentromere antibody.

- serum NT pro-BNP.
- serum urate.
- right-axis deviation on ECG.
- echo findings of right atrial area and TR velocity.

## Treatment of PAH associated with SScl

- The treatment options and outcome have developed rapidly over the last 5–10 years.
- Historically continuous parenteral epoprostenol was used for moderate and severe PAH. However, the treatment improves symptoms and pulmonary artery pressures, but not mortality.
- Bosentan, an oral endothelin receptor antagonist, improves function.
- Sildenafil inhibits phosphodiesterase type 5 (PDE5), enhancing relaxation of vascular smooth muscle and also inhibits endothelial cell growth.
- A recent double-blind placebo-controlled study of patients with idiopathic or autoimmune connective tissue disease-associated PAH found that sildenafil significantly improves the 6-min walk times and mean pulmonary artery pressures.
- Combination treatment with ambrisentan (another endothelin receptor antagonist) and tadalafil (a PDE5 inhibitor) have improved functional status and haemodynamics in a recent open label trial.
- Macitentan is a dual endothelin receptor antagonist with a better side effect profile and longer duration of action, with similar outcomes in therapy studies of PAH.
- Riociguat is a soluble guanylate cyclase stimulator that has demonstrated efficacy in PAH.

## Renal disease

Renal disease has been superseded by lung disease as the main cause of death in SScl due to the impact of ACE inhibitors in the treatment of SScl hypertensive renal crisis (see also ➜ Chapter 25).

- Both epithelial and endothelial damage typically occurs before becoming clinically detectable.
- A renal crisis characteristically occurs in dcSScl within the first 5 years of disease onset. Risk factors include exposure to prednisolone at doses >20 mg, rapidly progressive skin disease, diffuse cutaneous disease, and the presence of antibodies to Scl-70 or RNA polymerase III. In high-risk patients, the incidence may be as high as 20%.
- A renal crisis presents acutely with features of hypertension, acute kidney injury (mild haemoproteinuria and sometimes casts), micro-angiopathic haemolytic anaemia often with thrombocytopenia and fragments on blood film, pulmonary oedema, hypertensive retinopathy, encephalopathy, and convulsions. Mortality may reach 10%.
- Essential basic investigations to establish any presence of renal involvement in all patients are blood pressure measurement, urea and electrolytes, NT pro-BNP, troponin, serum urate, creatinine clearance, and urinalysis for proteinuria.
- In some patients, a renal crisis can begin indolently, initially with just hypertension.

- Hypertension should be treated rapidly, even in the presence of acute kidney injury, with ACE inhibitors and titrated to aim for a target blood pressure of <150/85 mmHg.
- Continuous epoprostenol is often also given during a renal crisis. Dialysis may become necessary. It is important to know that considerable recovery of renal function can be made after an acute crisis and that decisions involving renal transplantation should be withheld for up to 2 years.
- APL antibodies or lupus anticoagulant can contribute to renal SScl disease (including a crisis).

## Other organ involvement

Table 13.8 summarizes the involvement of other organs in SScl.

**Table 13.8.** Other organ pathology associated with SScl

| Organ | Effect | Frequency |
|---|---|---|
| Thyroid | Hypothyroidism is common | 20–40% |
| Liver | Primary biliary cirrhosis | 3% of lcSScl* |
| Nervous system | Trigeminal neuralgia | 5% |
| | Carpal tunnel syndrome | 3% |
| | Sensorimotor neuropathy | |
| | Autonomic neuropathy | |
| Genital | Cavernosal artery fibrosis causing impotence | Up to 50% |

* Antimitochondrial antibodies found in up to 25% of patients with SScl and anticentromere antibodies found in 10–20% of patients with primary biliary cirrhosis.

# Treatment and prognosis of SScl

# Treatment and prognosis of SScL

## General disease treatments

Currently no treatment can induce complete remission of the disease. Some therapies can offer partial relief and control of end-organ damage, and many of these are advised by the 2016 BSR and BHPR guidelines for the treatment of SScl.

- The evaluation of treatments is extremely difficult given the complexity, heterogeneity, and episodic nature of SScl, as well as the paucity of patients for recruitment.
- Active phase skin disease is treated with methotrexate (MTX) or mycophenolate mofetil (MMF) 1g twice daily, sometimes with low-dose prednisolone (≤10 mg daily).
- MMF can be used for lung fibrosis when the disease not extensive.
- Tocilizumab improves skin scores in phase II trials and could be an important new therapy for SScl.
- Cyclophosphamide may offer benefit in cardiac or lung disease.
- Rituximab is used in refractory cases of severe pulmonary fibrosis, with trial evidence demonstrating prevention of progression of lung disease and improvement in skin score.
- IVIg is useful in SScl overlap syndromes with myositis and may have a beneficial effect on severe GI manifestations. There are ongoing trials assessing IVIg effectiveness in treating skin disease.
- Autologous stem cell transplantation has been undertaken in severe SScl disease, but has a high mortality rate.

For additional detail on all drug therapies including immunosuppressants see Chapter 23

## Prognosis

SScl has the highest case-specific mortality of any autoimmune rheumatic or connective tissue disease. However, major advances in the management of SScl have taken place over the past decade, confirming the effectiveness of treatment.

- Estimates of 5-year mortality in SScl range from 34% to 73%. Standardized mortality ratios have been estimated at 3–4× expected.
- Logistic regression modelling suggests three factors (proteinuria, elevated ESR, and low DLCO) are >80% accurate at predicting mortality >5 years.
- Patients with renal crisis had a mortality of 50%, although the use of ACE inhibitors and renal replacement therapies may have reduced this figure in recent years.
- Anti-topoisomerase I and anti-RNA polymerase antibodies have also been associated with a higher incidence of SScl-related mortality.
- Advances in the understanding of mechanisms leading to PAH has led to new therapies that, with time, may show significant impact in slowing disease progression.

# Morphoea, localized scleroderma, and scleroderma-like fibrosing disorders

## Morphoea

Morphoea may be 'circumscribed' with just one or two lesions or 'generalized'. The generalized form may be very symptomatic and distressing as it progresses.

- The rash is often itchy, violaceous or erythematous, and progresses to firm 'hide-bound' skin with hypo- or hyperpigmentation and subsequent atrophy.
- The 'circumscribed' lesion tends to resolve within 3–5 years and treatment is often unnecessary.
- The 'generalized' morphoea form can be disfiguring, leading to contractures, ulceration, and occasionally malignancy.
- Generalized morphoea may respond to PUVA, systemic/topical or intralesional GC, topical tacrolimus, MTX, ciclosporin, or MMF.
- *Guttate morphoea* is a variant with small 1 cm diameter papules and minimal sclerosis, resembling lichen *sclerosus et atrophicus*. The lesions usually occur on the neck, shoulders, and anterior chest wall.

## Linear scleroderma

This describes a band-like pattern of sclerosis, often in a dermatomal distribution. The sclerotic areas often cross over joints, and are associated with soft tissue and bone atrophy, and growth defects.

- Treatment is similar to that previously described for generalized morphoea. Physiotherapy and appropriate exercises may help to minimize growth defects in the childhood form.
- *En coup-de-sabre* is linear sclerosis involving the face or scalp, and associated with hemi-atrophy of the face on the same side. The lesion assumes a depressed appearance like a scar from a sabre.

## Eosinophilic fasciitis

(See also **➲** Chapter 18.)
- Characterized by the rapid spread of skin changes ('*peau d'orange*') over extremities. Skin becomes indurated.
- Unlike SScl, the epidermis is spared (i.e. superficial wrinkling is intact) and nail-fold capillaroscopy is normal.
- The condition may resolve spontaneously or respond to GCs.
- The condition may be a paraneoplastic phenomenon in some patients (haematological malignancy).
- MTX and MMF can be used as well as GCs (no RCTs).

## Nephrogenic systemic fibrosis

Nephrogenic systemic fibrosis (NSF)—also known as nephrogenic fibrosing dermopathy—is a systemic disease, which can lead to fibrosis in skeletal muscle, myocardium, lungs, kidneys, and testes.

- NSF is characterized by the presence of skin induration, nodular plaques, and flexion contractures in the absence of RD.

- Lesions develop over days to weeks, and initially favour the lower extremities.
- The majority of patients will have end-stage renal disease and a history of exposure to gadolinium-based contrast.
- Histologically, NSF lesions are characterized by collagen bundles surrounded by fibroblast-like epithelioid or stellate cells, and mucin deposition, which can extend into the fascia and muscles.
- Response to immunosuppressive agents is disappointing.
- Early institution of physical therapy to prevent contractures and muscle wasting is important. Pain management may be especially challenging.

## Scleromyxoedema

Is characterized by waxy induration of the skin along the forehead (glabella), the neck, and behind the ears.

- Scleromyxoedema may also affect the middle of the back, which is generally spared in SScl.
- Scleromyxoedema can be associated with oesophageal dysmotility and myopathy.
- Case reports have shown an association with severe neurological sequelae, including encephalopathy, seizures, coma, and psychosis.
- Scleromyxoedema may respond to IVIg.

## Scleroedema

Scleroedema is a fibromucinous connective tissue disease, a scleroderma-like disorder associated with doughy induration of the skin along the back, neck, face, and chest.

- Unlike in SScl, the extremities are typically spared.
- It is seen in association with poorly controlled diabetes, monoclonal gammopathy or following infections (e.g. *Streptococcus*).
- Prognosis depends on the underlying aetiology. Scleroedema that occurs after infection may resolve spontaneously. Scleroedema associated with diabetes may improve with better glucose control.
- For some patients, ultraviolet light therapy (such as UVA-1, PUVA, and photophoresis) may be beneficial.

# Idiopathic inflammatory myopathies including polymyositis and dermatomyositis

# Idiopathic inflammatory myositis

### General considerations and classification

The idiopathic inflammatory myopathies (IIMs) are a heterogeneous group of conditions characterized by varied patterns of inflammation within striated muscle and evidence of autoimmune-mediated muscle breakdown. The IIMs are believed to be autoimmune in nature. They have distinct pathological features, but the aetiopathogenesis of each subtype remains largely unknown.

- The strongest genetic association of IIMs is with HLA class II alleles. In Caucasians, HLA-DRB1*0301 and -DQA1*0501 are strongly associated, compared to HLA-B7 in Asian populations. HLA-DQA1*01 seems to be a protective factor.
- Proximal, symmetrical, and painless weakness of muscles is the hallmark of IIMs.
- Polymyositis (PM) and dermatomyositis (DM) are the most common forms of IIM, the latter distinguished by the presence of a characteristic rash.
- Overlap with other autoimmune diseases occur in 15–20% of cases.
- The classification of IIM conditions is shown in Box 14.1.
- Secondary causes of myopathies are discussed later in this chapter.
- IIM has an estimated incidence of 2–8 per million.
- PM and DM are more common in women than in men (2:1), and peak incidence is at 50–60 years old.
- The F:M ratio is lower in myositis associated with malignancy, and higher during childbearing years (5:1).
- There is a latitude gradient of prevalence of PM and DM. DM is more common closer to the equator correlating directly with UV-light irradiation, and PM is more common in northern countries.
- The criteria for PM and DM diagnosis are shown in Box 14.2.
- The principal features of PM and DM are listed in Table 14.1.

### Box 14.1 Modified Bohan and Peter's classification of PM and DM

1. Primary idiopathic polymyositis.
2. Primary idiopathic dermatomyositis.
3. 1 or 2 above in list, with malignancy.
4. Juvenile poly(dermato)myositis.
5. Overlap syndromes with other autoimmune rheumatic diseases.
6. Inclusion-body myositis.
7. Rare myositis: granulomatous, eosinophilic, focal, orbital.
8. Drug-induced.

Information from Bohan A, Peter J. Polymyositis and dematomyositis. *N Engl J Med* 1975; 292:344–7.

## Box 14.2 Diagnostic criteria for the diagnosis of PM and DM

1. Symmetrical proximal muscle weakness developing over weeks or months.
2. Elevated serum muscle enzymes: creatine kinase (CK), aldolase, AST, ALT, and lactate dehydrogenase.
3. Typical electromyographic findings: myopathic potentials (low amplitude, short duration, polyphasic) fibrillation, positive sharp waves, increased insertional activity, complex repetitive discharges.
4. Typical muscle biopsy findings.
5. Dermatological features of DM:
   * Gottron's papules, involving fingers, elbows, knees, and medial malleoli.
   * Heliotrope sign around the eyes.
   * Erythematous and/or poikilodermatous rash.

Definite PM: all of criteria 1–4; probable PM: 3 of criteria 1–4; possible PM: 2 of criteria 1–4.

Definite DM: 3 of criteria 1–4 *plus* criterion 5; probable DM: 2 of criteria 1–4 *plus* criterion 5; possible: 1 of criteria 1–4 *plus* criterion 5.

After Bohan A, Peter J. Polymyositis and dematomyositis. *N Engl J Med* 1975; 292:344–7.

**Table 14.1** Key features of PM and DM

|  | PM | DM |
|---|---|---|
| Typical patient | Any age<br>Unusual in children<br>Female and African American predominance | Any age<br>Juvenile form common<br>Female and African American predominance |
| Muscle groups affected | Proximal > distal<br>Symmetrical | Proximal > distal<br>Symmetrical |
| CK elevation | 40–50× normal not unusual | 40–50× normal not unusual<br>Weakness sometimes out of proportion to CK level |
| Myositis specific antibodies (MSAs) | Anti-aminoacyl t-RNA synthetase antibodies; anti-SRP | Anti-aminoacyl t-RNA synthetase antibodies; anti-Mi-2 |
| Histopathology | Endomysial inflammation<br>CD8+ cells invading non-necrotic muscle fibres | Perivascular<br>Interfascicular inflammation<br>CD4+ predominance; complement membrane attack complex present; capillary obliteration; endothelial damage; perifascicular atrophy |
| Malignancy association | Yes | Yes |
| Other features | Interstitial lung disease (ILD)<br>Cardiac<br>Malignancy | Skin<br>ILD<br>Cardiac<br>Intramuscular calcification<br>Vasculitis<br>Malignancy |

# Polymyositis and dermatomyositis

Application of the criteria for diagnosis of PM or DM assumes infective, toxic, metabolic, dystrophy, and endocrine myopathies are excluded.

## Pathogenesis

- DM has been conceptualized traditionally as a complement-mediated microangiopathy, but this paradigm has limitations.
- PM arises from a cytotoxic T-cell immune-mediated inflammation on muscle.
- Type I interferon signature is upregulated in DM and PM, but not in IBM.
- Aberrant expression of major histocompatibility complex (MHC) proteins contributes to muscle damage both directly and indirectly in all subtypes of IIM.
- A characteristic pattern of autoantibody production often occurs, in PM and DM and in overlap myositis disorders.
- There is evidence of inflammasome complex activity in the IIMs.
- Toll-like receptors (TLRs) are upregulated in IIMs and may link innate and adaptive immune processes.
- Autophagy is upregulated in IIM tissue, particularly within regenerating myofibres, and this may occur via activation of TLR3 and TLR4.
- Immature and regenerating muscle cells may perpetuate the immune-mediated attack in IIMs.

## Clinical features

### Myositis

- Muscle weakness is the main clinical feature in both conditions and is almost universal, tending to develop insidiously over months, but occasionally with great speed.
- Weakness is usually symmetrical and diffuse, involving the proximal muscles of the neck, shoulders, trunk, hips, and thighs. The lower limb muscles tend to be clinically symptomatic first.
- Weakness of the distal muscles is rare, but can occur late in the disease. The face and ocular muscles may also be involved.
- Myalgia occurs in about 50% of cases: it can be mild and sometimes difficult to distinguish from polymyalgia rheumatica.
- There may be muscle atrophy in chronic disease, more so in PM than DM, and contractures may occur in disease of long duration.
- Often the distinction between autoimmune rheumatic disease overlapping with PM or DM and an autoimmune rheumatic disease with myositis as a manifestation can be very difficult.

### Skin and cutaneous disease

- The rash of DM commonly precedes the weakness by weeks to months. The rash may parallel the weakness or remain independent, persisting after the myositis resolves.
- Erythematous or violaceous papules or plaques (Gottron's papules) or macular patches (Gottron's sign) may occur over the metacarpophalangeal and proximal (occasionally distal) interphalangeal joints. The rash is present in up to 80% of cases.

- Occasionally, these lesions may be found on the extensor surfaces of the knees, wrists, elbows, or medial malleoli.
- Periungual abnormalities affecting the capillary nailbeds in DM and PM with erythema and in some cases tenderness can be seen.
- Vascular changes observed at the nailbed resemble those found in other connective tissue diseases, e.g. systemic sclerosis and SLE. Abnormal capillary loops may alternate with areas of vascular dilatation and dropout.
- A macular eruption may involve the upper chest, neck, shoulders, extremities, face, and scalp. This may develop into poikiloderma, hyper- or hypopigmentation with atrophy and telangiectasia. Typical features include the 'V' sign at the base of the neck anteriorly, and the 'shawl' sign at the back of the neck and across the shoulders.
- The heliotrope rash, found in 30–60% of cases, is a purple/lilac coloured suffusion around the eyes, often associated with periorbital oedema. It is characteristic, but not pathognomonic.
- Some patients have typical cutaneous DM, but do not develop overt myositis. The term 'amyopathic DM' is applied. The same risk of malignancy and systemic complications remains.
- Calcinosis, cutaneous vasculitis, and ulceration are more common in juvenile DM.

### Joints

Coexistent polyarthralgia is quite common. It is usually non-erosive and glucocorticoid (GC) responsive.

### Cardiac disease

- Clinical features of heart involvement are rare in PM and DM.
- Asymptomatic subclinical manifestations are often reported, and can occur in up to 70% of patients. These are mainly conduction abnormalities and arrhythmias detected by ECG.
- Cardiovascular disease is a major risk factor for death in myositis, and should therefore not be overlooked. The most frequently overt manifestations are congestive heart failure, conduction abnormalities, and coronary heart disease.
- The underlying pathophysiological mechanisms responsible include myocarditis, coronary artery disease, and involvement of the small vessels of the myocardium.

### Pulmonary

- Shortness of breath may be a consequence of diaphragmatic and intercostal muscle weakness (as well as other causes that will be discussed later), and should be assessed.
- ILD is common, with a variable response to immunosuppression.

### Gastrointestinal

- Dysphagia occurs in up to 30%.
- Cricopharyngeal myotomy is occasionally needed.

*Malignancy*
- Studies suggest a modest increase in malignancies within 1–2 years of onset in DM. In the majority of cases, cancer and myositis have an independent course.
- The largest population studies suggest malignancy occurs in 15% of cases of DM (relative risk in men 2.4/in women 3.4) and 9% of cases of PM (relative risk in men 1.8/in women 1.7).
- Cancer deaths in studies suggest an increase in DM, but not PM, supporting a true association with DM, rather than a study bias due to intensive searching.
- The highest cancer risk appears to be in men >45 years with DM who lack myositis autoantibodies or overlap autoimmune connective tissue disease.
- Tumours that are frequent in the general population are frequent in PM and DM. However, there appears to be an increase in ovarian, breast, lung, stomach, colon, and bladder cancers out of proportion to that of other tumours.
- The extent of investigations required is debated. Thorough physical assessment should always include rectal, pelvic, and breast examination. Specific investigations should include a chest radiograph, urinalysis, prostate-specific antigen in men, faecal occult blood testing, mammography, and cervical smear, and probably pelvic ultrasound and CA125 levels in women.
- Further bowel investigations are open to debate and determined by individual patient symptoms. An elevated ALT may be from muscle and need not indicate liver pathology.
- Malignancy can manifest as paraneoplastic myopathy (see ➲ Chapter 4).

## Clinical assessments

*Features suggesting an alternative diagnosis to IIM*
It is important to consider whether there are features of non-inflammatory myopathy, which may point towards storage diseases, genetic myopathies and neuropathy.
- Drug history: a number of medications are associated with causing myositis (Table 14.2).
- Weakness/cramp worsened by exercise or dietary changes (e.g. fasting, carbohydrate intake), which might suggest a metabolic or mitochondrial myopathy.
- Muscle atrophy without pain or hypertrophy can suggest a muscular dystrophy.
- Fasciculation or myotonia and other neurological signs may suggest a primary neurological disease (e.g. motor neuron disease).
- Facial and shoulder girdle muscle involvement may suggest facioscapulohumeral dystrophy.
- A family history of myopathy may suggest a genetic myopathy.

**Table 14.2** Drug-induced myopathy

| Clinical picture | Examples |
|---|---|
| Myopathy with weakness, myalgia, and high CK | Penicillamine |
| | Anti-TNFα |
| | Cimetidine |
| | L-tryptophan |
| | Zidovudine |
| | Colchicine |
| | Hydroxychloroquine |
| | Lipid-lowering agents |
| | Ciclosporin |
| | Vincristine |
| | Carbimazole, propylthiouracil |
| | Alcohol |
| | NSAIDs—rare with aspirin |
| Rhabdomyolysis picture | Alcohol |
| | Recreational drugs—cocaine, heroin, ecstasy |
| | Amphetamines |
| | Barbiturates |
| | Statins (particularly high dose) |
| | Anaesthetics—malignant hyperthermia |
| | Psychotropics—neuroleptic-malignant syndrome |

*Assessment of disease impact*

See Table 14.3.

Changes in muscle strength and function may change slowly with indolent disease, or with treatment, and measures of long-term muscle and general function are important to take regularly. General (Likert scale) patient and physician global disease activity scores are easy to take and reproduce:

- HAQ or SF36 may be used.
- Muscle metrology from an experienced physiotherapist.
- The manual muscle test (MMT) is the most often used test of muscle strength, although only partly validated in adult myositis.
- Quantitative muscle atrophy (e.g. by MRI).
- Several scales of composite measures are available e.g. MYOACT (activity) and MYODAM (damage) and MDI (disease index). The latter have recently been demonstrated to have good construct and validity in adult and juvenile IIM.[1,2]

**Table 14.3** Systemic manifestations of PM and DM

| Organ/system | Features |
|---|---|
| General | Fatigue, malaise, weight loss |
| | Fevers—in 40% overall |
| | Raynaud's phenomenon |
| Pulmonary | Due to muscle weakness: aspiration pneumonia, respiratory failure (low TLC, VC, high RV) |
| | Due to local disease: interstitial fibrosis, pulmonary vasculitis, pulmonary hypertension (common) |
| | Due to treatment: hypersensitivity pneumonitis, opportunistic infection |
| Gastrointestinal | Oesophageal dysphagia—in 30% |
| | Striated muscle dysfunction |
| | Cricopharyngeal dysfunction |
| | Low oesophageal dysfunction |
| | Stomach and bowel dysmotility* |
| Cardiovascular | Cardiomyopathy—<5% |
| | Pericardial effusion—up to 20% |
| | Hypertension and ischaemic heart disease (common)[3] |
| | Heart block—rare |
| | Dysrhythmias—uncommon |
| Skeletal | Arthropathy |
| | Deformity, mild erosive arthritis |
| Renal | Very rare. Possible myoglobinuria |

RV, residual volume; TLC, total lung capacity; VC, vital capacity.

* Intestinal vasculitis, perforation, and pneumatosis cystoides intestinalis, features of juvenile DM, are very rare in the adult.

## References

1. Isenberg DA, Allen E, Farewell V, et al. International consensus outcome measures for patients with idiopathic inflammatory myopathies. Development and initial validation of myositis activity and damage indices in patients with adult onset disease. *Rheumatology* 2004;43:49–54.
2. Rider LG, Lachenbruch PA, Monroe JB, et al. Damage extent and predictors in adult and juvenile dermatomyositis and polymyositis as determined with the myositis damage index. *Arthritis Rheum* 2009;60:3425–35.
3. Bohan A, Peter JB. Polymyositis and dermatomyositis. *N Engl J Med* 1975;292:344–7.

# Investigations

# Investigations

The investigation of potential malignancy in DM/PM has been discussed earlier in this chapter.

## Muscle enzymes

- Serum levels of enzymes released from damaged muscle are helpful in the diagnosis and monitoring of the disease. Creatine kinase (CK) is most widely used. Aldolase may be more sensitive in some cases.
- There are a number of other causes for raised CK levels (Table 14.4). Muscle bulk influences the CK levels. But it is also possible, despite active myositis, for the CK levels not be elevated (i.e. relative chronic muscle atrophy). In these cases, imaging such as MRI may be a useful indicator of damage/severity.

**Table 14.4** Causes of a raised creatine kinase

| Cause | Examples |
| --- | --- |
| Strenuous prolonged exercise | Delayed-onset muscular strain (DOMS) |
| Muscle trauma | |
| Diseases affecting muscle | Myositis |
| | Metabolic (e.g. glycogen storage) |
| | Muscular dystrophy |
| | Myocardial infarction |
| | Rhabdomyolysis |
| Drugs (also see Table 14.7) | Necrotizing myopathy (statins, ciclosporin, labetalol, alcohol, anti-TNFα) |
| | Induction of myositis (L-tryptophan, L-dopa, phenytoin, lamotrigine, hydroxycarbamide) |
| | Amphiphillic ((hydroxy)chloroquine, amiodarone) |
| | Microtubule (colchicine, vincristine) |
| | Inhibition of CK excretion (morphine, diazepam) |
| Metabolic abnormalities | Hypothyroidism |
| | Hypokalaemia including drug induced (diuretics, laxatives, GCs) |
| | Ketoacidosis |
| | Renal failure |
| Normal variants | Ethnic group (often higher normal values in the black population) |
| | Increased muscle mass |
| | Technical artefact |

- The isoenzyme CK-MB can be elevated in myositis and less often in myocarditis. It is released from regenerating skeletal muscle fibres and also damaged myocardiocytes.
- As a guide, patients with myositis without cardiac involvement may have a CK-MB/total CK ratio of >3%.
- A more specific marker for myocardial damage in myositis is the cardiac isoform troponin I.
- Other cardiac troponin isoforms such as troponin C (cTnC) and troponin T (cTnT) are less specific and expressed in skeletal muscle, hence levels can be raised in various muscle disorders.

### Muscle biopsy

- All patients should have a muscle biopsy to confirm the diagnosis and to exclude conditions that may resemble IIM.
- There is an argument for not obtaining a biopsy in patients with proximal weakness, elevated enzymes, typical EMG changes, a rash of DM, confirmed myositis-specific autoantibodies, or an overlap autoimmune rheumatic disease and myositis-associated autoantibodies.
- For most patients however, it is important to remember that the mimics of IIM are more common than the IIMs themselves. Therefore, patients with a clinical diagnosis of PM/DM who do not respond to immunosuppressive treatment as expected should have a biopsy in order to confirm an alternative diagnosis.
- A negative biopsy does not exclude myositis, as inflammatory changes can be focal. Therefore the site of biopsy should be preferably from a symptomatic muscle which is not atrophic.
- Muscle biopsy samples are stained with haematoxylin and eosin.
- Further immunohistochemical staining for MHC class antigens provide additional useful information. The presence of MHC class I and II antigens in muscle fibres is a feature of inflamed muscles tissue.
- There are important histological descriptions that associate with specific diagnoses:
  - Fibre hypertrophy suggests dystrophy.
  - Inclusion bodies are seen in IBM.
  - Widespread necrosis with profuse regeneration is the typical finding in rhabdomyolysis.
- Inflammation affects striated muscle and occasionally heart muscle, but not smooth muscle.
- Histologically, the cellular infiltrates of skeletal muscle involve mainly T lymphocytes and macrophages. Dendritic cells, B cells, and plasma cells can also be found.
- IIMs often have specific biopsy features:
  - In DM, there are mainly perivascular and perimysial inflammatory infiltrates with a predominance of CD4+ T cells.
  - In PM, there is endomysial (intramuscular) inflammatory infiltrates with a predominance of CD8+ T cells causing destruction of muscle fibres and fatty replacement.
  - In IBM, the early disease may be indistinguishable from the histological appearances of PM. Characteristic findings are intracellular amyloid deposits or basophilic intracellular vacuoles ('inclusion bodies') seen on electron microscopy.

- Optimal processing, evaluation, and minimizing of artefacts require coordination with the pathologist prior to biopsy, to ensure appropriate handling of samples and maximum diagnostic information.

## Autoantibodies

- Autoantibodies are present in ~60–70% of patients with PM and DM. The main antibody is antinuclear antibody (ANA).
- Myositis-specific autoantibodies (MSAs) are associated with specific clinical phenotypes, and favour PM/DM over other myopathies.
- The most prevalent MSA is an antibody directed against histidyl transfer RNA synthetase (anti-Jo1) present in around 11–33% of patients with PM/DM.
- Histidyl is one of a number of amino-acyl transfer RNA synthetase relevant targets for antibody formation.
- The various clinical associations of the main myositis-associated (MAAs) and MSAs are shown in Table 14.5.
- Anti-signal recognition peptide (SRP) antibodies occur in ~5% of myositis patients and herald an acute-onset aggressive disease. It is not linked to skin manifestations. Muscle biopsy tends to show a necrotizing myopathy with few inflammatory cells. Treatment response is often poor.
- Anti-Mi2 and anti-CADM-140 are found in 10–20% of DM cases.
- Statin-induced myopathy is associated with anti-HMG-CoA antibodies. The presence of these antibodies is not linked to statin exposure in every case.

**Table 14.5** Antibodies in PM and DM

| Antibody class | Antibody subclass | Percentage of PM/DM | Myositis subgroup |
|---|---|---|---|
| *Myositis-specific:* | | In total 30–40 | |
| Anticytoplasmic | Anti-Jo-1 | 20 | Antisynthetase syndrome |
| | Anti-PL-7/ PL-12/OJ/EJ | <5 each | |
| | Anti-SRP | 4 | PM |
| Antinuclear | Anti-Mi-2 | 8 | DM |
| | Anti-56 kDa | 90 | All |
| *Myositis-associated* | Anti-PM-Scl | 8 | PM/DM–SScl overlap |
| | Anti-U1-RNP | 12 | PM/DM overlap syndromes |
| | Anti-U2/ U5-RNP | <2 | PM |
| | Anti-Ro and Anti-La | 5–10 | SLE. Primary Sjögren's syndrome |

- Anti-p155/p140 (anti-MJ) is found in up to 25% of cases of juvenile DM and is associated with calcinosis.
- Detailed description of all MAAs/MSAs is beyond this text. New antibodies are described regularly. It is worth noting up-to-date publications in this area given that antibody immunological tests through specialist labs can help in difficult cases where malignancy and drugs are being considered as causes.

## Electromyography

- Electromyography (EMG) cannot establish the diagnosis of PM/DM with certainty, but can demonstrate a myopathic process, and help to exclude neuropathies and distinguish some myopathies.
- 90% of patients will have abnormal EMG studies.
- Early findings include low-amplitude, short-duration, polyphasic potentials, with early recruitment and full interference patterns (i.e. more fibres are required to achieve a given force). The latter features are in contrast to neuropathies where there is decreased recruitment and interference.
- With time, re-innervation of denervated fibres leads to high-amplitude, long-duration, polyphasic potentials.
- Other features include spontaneous activity in up to 75% of cases, fibrillations, and repetitive discharges akin to myotonia, but of constant amplitude and starting and stopping abruptly.

## Imaging

- Magnetic resonance imaging (MRI), ultrasound (US), computed tomography (CT), $^{99m}$Tc, and thallium have been used to assess the distribution of disease.
- MRI with T2-weighted images and fat suppression or short tau inversion recovery (STIR) is best at identifying areas of muscle inflammation, atrophy, or fatty infiltration.
- On MRI, active myositis results in the appearance of fluid signal changes in muscle—interpreted as oedema.
- When evaluating a patient for weakness, MRI may be particularly useful in distinguishing weakness due to active inflammation from weakness due to previous damage or GC myopathy (which would not be expected to show muscle oedema).
- Because muscle involvement may be patchy, MRI can help identify an optimal site for muscle biopsy.

## Other tests

- The ESR is elevated in 50% of cases, but correlates poorly with disease activity and response to therapy.
- CRP is not specific; high levels suggest a concurrent infection.
- Complement levels in PM/DM are usually normal.
- Proteinuria may be the result of myoglobinuria.
- Serial spirometry for respiratory muscle weakness may be required.

# Treatment

Treatment should be started promptly pending completion of investigations, particularly in acute-onset weakness, dysphagia, respiratory insufficiency, and systemic complications.

- GCs have never been tested adequately in randomized, placebo-controlled trials, but are the cornerstone of therapy.
- 90% of patients will have at least a partial response to GC therapy. Most require treatment with a GC-sparing agent to maintain disease remission and to minimize GC exposure.
- An exercise programme helps improve fatigue and muscle strength. Exercise should be used with caution during periods of disease activity, but there is no evidence that it causes prolonged worsening in muscle enzyme levels or inflammation.

## Glucocorticoids. See also ⮕ p. 660

- Most clinicians use a starting oral prednisolone dose of 1–2 mg/kg until a decline in CK and/or a substantial improvement in muscle strength is seen.
- Lower GC doses of 0.5 mg/kg may be sufficient. Severe cases (or extraskeletal involvement) may be treated with IV methylprednisolone 0.5–1 g/day for 3 days before starting oral prednisolone.
- As high doses are required for several months, early vitamin D/calcium supplementation and bisphosphonates should be considered to prevent GC-induced osteoporosis.
- IIM patients are at increased risk of developing osteoporosis also due to decreased skeletal loading and immobility.
- A case–control study has also shown that most IIM patients have low serum levels of vitamin D. This may confer a risk factor for developing adult myositis, suggesting vitamin D replacement therapy is important.
- Most patients will respond to treatment, but this can be slow and partial. CK levels often improve quicker than any apparent improvement in strength.
- Failure to respond despite 4–6 months of treatment may be due to one of several reasons (especially if the ANA is negative):
  - Incorrect diagnosis.
  - Hereditary myopathy or 'inclusion-body' myositis.
  - GC myopathy.
  - Permanent loss of strength.
  - No response to GC therapy.

## Synthetic disease-modifying antirheumatic drugs (sDMARDs). See also ⮕ pp. 662–80

- Methotrexate (MTX) and azathioprine (AZA) have demonstrable efficacy; AZA may be a better option for patients with ILD or hepatitis, but may take longer to show effectiveness.
- Studies have shown a synergistic effect of MTX and AZA where a single drug has failed.

- Cyclophosphamide (CYC) has had variable results and is used in resistant cases or in those cases where there is severe extraskeletal involvement such as vasculitis or lung disease.
- Tacrolimus has been used in refractory patients with PM/DM-ILD, with improvement in muscle strength, lung function, and cutaneous manifestations.
- Ciclosporin can be a useful therapy in patients where MTX and AZA have been ineffective/not tolerated. It has been used in combination with MTX or IVIg.
- Mycophenolate mofetil (MMF) and chlorambucil have been reported to achieve disease remission in some refractory cases.

## Intravenous immunoglobulin (IVIg)

- Efficacy of IVIg has been demonstrated in small double-blind controlled trials and one open-label trial, showing significant clinical improvement in muscle strength and reduction in CK levels after 3 months of treatment, compared with placebo.
- Case reports have suggested efficacy of IVIg in the treatment of PM/DM-ILD, and it has been used in one case of refractory amyopathic DM-ILD with good response.
- High-dose regimens in the form of 2 g/kg/day for 2–5 days every month for 3–6 months have been advocated, and can be used concomitantly with other sDMARDs.
- Duration of efficacy of each treatment may be limited to a few months, but the dose or interval can be changed based on severity of disease and treatment responsiveness.
- A major advantage of IVIg is that it is safe to use in the context of active infections, but its high cost may restrict long-term use. There is also a risk of tachyphylaxis.

## Biologic therapies

There is growing interest in evaluating biologics that target various pathways involved in the pathogenesis of IIM.

- Anti-TNFα therapy has been studied in small patient series. There have been suggestions that it may trigger IIM, therefore they should be used with caution.
- In open label studies, rituximab (RTX) has been used in refractory DM with reports of clinical improvement.
- The first placebo-phase trial to assess the efficacy of RTX in refractory myositis did not show a significant difference between the two treatment groups.
- A recent summary of published evidence for RTX effect in IIM suggested a majority of patients derived benefit though markers of response varied and there was of course marked heterogeneity of disease at the outset.
- Further research is required to assess the role of biologic therapies though many treatments have been tried (Table 14.6).

**Table 14.6** Biologic therapies used for treating IIMs

| Biologic | Level of evidence |
| --- | --- |
| Adalimumab | One case report of a 'hard-to-treat' patient showing increased muscle strength and reduced CK levels |
| Etanercept | Pilot trial of 16 treatment naïve patients showed no benefits, apart from GC sparing[4] |
| Infliximab | Retrospective studies. Utility in IIMs limited due to potential for *inducing* PM and DM. Not recommended |
| Rituximab | Double-blind trial showing primary outcomes not met, but most achieved the IMACS* definition of improvement |
| Tocilizumab | 3 case reports of refractory IIM. Some clinical benefits seen with reduced enzyme levels in each case |
| Anakinra | 12-month open label trial. Improvement in 7/15 patients with refractory myositis. Inflammatory infiltrates in repeat biopsies did not resolve and IL-1 expression was not correlated to clinical response[5] |
| Alemtuzumab | 1 case report (PM/ILD) showing rapid improvement. Post infusion-related reaction/respiratory compromise. Concerns about immunosuppressive properties and infection risk |
| Abatacept | Ongoing clinical trial (ARTEMIS). Favourable outcomes in JDM with calcinosis and refractory anti- SRP myositis |
| Sifalimumab | Phase 1b trial. Suppression of genes induced by type 1 IFNγ (blood and muscle) with improved muscle strength |

* International Myositis Assessment and Clinical Studies Group (IMACS)

Adapted from Moghadam-Kia S et al. Modern Therapies for Idiopathic Inflammatory Myopathies (IIMs): Role of Biologics. *Clin Rev Allergy Immunol.* 2017 Feb; 52(1): 81–87 with permission from Springer.

## Treatment of extramuscular disease

- The rash of DM may respond to the treatment of the myositis. If lesions persist, hydroxychloroquine (HCQ) at 200–400 mg/day or topical tacrolimus may be of benefit. Photosensitivity can respond to sunscreens. Topical GCs are often not successful.
- The treatment of amyopathic DM is controversial. Sunscreens and HCQ can be used and in some severe cases, GCs or immunosuppressives are justified for the cutaneous disease. If treatment is withheld due to an absence of myositis, the patient should be followed closely, especially in the first 2 years after onset to avoid delay in treatment should myositis develop.
- Calcinosis, principally a problem in juvenile disease, is difficult to treat and does not respond to immunosuppression. Surgical resection may help for accessible deposits.

- Active exercise is discouraged during acute inflammation, but passive range of motion exercises should be commenced early to avoid joint contractures. Isometric exercise should be introduced once inflammation subsides. This must be supervised by a physiotherapist to avoid muscle overuse.
- ILD is managed as in other autoimmune connective tissue diseases with oral GCs and oral or IV CYC.
- Distal oesophageal dysmotility does not generally respond to immunosuppression, but measures similar to treatment of reflux may help.

## Prognosis in PM and DM

- PM and DM are diseases with a high mortality and morbidity. One retrospective study estimated a mortality rate of 22%, mostly due to malignancy and pulmonary disease.
- In most cases, the course of disease is either monophasic, remitting/relapsing, or chronic progressive.
- A small number (5–10%) make a full recovery following treatment.
- The use of prolonged immunosuppressive therapy increases the risk of infection, especially with unusual organisms.
- Case reports have described atypical mycobacterial infections in patients with long-standing PM/DM.
- A worse prognosis is associated with increasing age, bulbar muscle, and cardiopulmonary involvement.

## References

4. Muscle Study Group. A randomized, pilot trial of etanercept in dermatomyositis. *Ann Neurol* 2011;70;427–36.
5. Zong M, Dorph C, Dastmalchi M, et al. Anakinra treatment in patients with refractory inflammatory myopathies and possible predictive response biomarkers: a mechanistic study with 12 months follow-up. *Ann Rheum Dis* 2014; 75;913.

# Inclusion-body myositis

- Inclusion-body myositis (IBM) is a distinct disorder that comprises 20–30% of idiopathic myositis cases. IBM usually begins after the age of 50 years and is 3× more common in men. The difficulty in distinguishing it from PM and its insidious onset can lead to considerable delay in diagnosis by 3–5 years.
- Distal weakness and wasting can be as common as proximal, often involving the lower limbs before the upper, and sparing the face.
- Unlike PM or DM, IBM can present with diminished hand-grip strength, in addition to proximal muscle weakness.
- Dysphagia is a feature in 40% of cases, and myalgias in 20%.
- An open biopsy (as opposed to needle biopsy) is essential to diagnose IBM.
- A needle biopsy may not be sufficient to allow the recognition of important clues that point away from other forms of myositis.
- There is a significant inflammatory component early in the disease course, that may partially respond to GCs, though generally patients are usually non-responsive to GCs.
- There may be a period of stabilization for a few months but this may reflect the natural history of disease.
- Prolonged administration of GCs may result in worsening of disease despite improvements in CK levels.
- Treatment usually begins with high-dose GCs for 3 months, adding in MTX or AZA if clinical improvement or in patients with another autoimmune connective tissue disease. If there is continued decline in strength or function, immunosuppression should be discontinued.
- Anti-T-lymphocyte globulin, interferon-β, MMF, and anabolic GCs such as oxandrolone, may have beneficial effects as in some reports.
- Weakness will progress in most patients but this is often very slow. Patients may need assistance with daily activities within 10 years and some may be wheelchair bound within 15 years from onset of symptoms.

# Other (adult) inflammatory myopathies

## Drug-induced myopathies

- The range of myositis severity caused by different drugs varies, from asymptomatic increases in CK to necrotizing severe myopathies resulting in rhabdomyolysis.
- HMG-CoA reductase inhibitors (statins) can cause myalgia and cramps along with an elevated CK level and may be exacerbated by the use of other drugs (ciclosporin and fibrates) or other diseases (hypothyroidism).
- Patients on any drugs suspected of causing myositis, presenting with myalgia, should have their renal function and CK checked and the drug stopped.
- See ➜ Table 14.2, p. 431 for an overview.

## PM/DM with interstitial lung disease

Polymyositis or dermatomyositis occurring together with interstitial lung disease (PM/DM-ILD) may be a distinct condition.

- Characteristic features include myositis, ILD, Raynaud's disease, 'mechanic's hands' (i.e. dry, cracked skin across the digits), and small joint polyarthritis.
- Associated with a range of autoantibodies directed against aminoacyl transfer RNA synthetases including histidyl-tRNA synthetase (HRS; termed the anti-Jo1 autoantibody).
- Anti-Jo-1 is present in ~20% of PM/DM patients and titre of antibody can be associated with disease activity.
- Can be associated with fevers at onset or during flares.
- Some patients presenting with ILD or arthritis may go on to develop myositis later, so presentation of components of the disease may not be concordant.
- Patients need to be managed with a chest physician monitoring lung function tests and inflammatory disease activity.
- CYC, MMF, and RTX give alternative choices for therapies in addition to GCs.

# Juvenile idiopathic inflammatory myopathy

## Introduction

- The juvenile IIMs are heterogeneous inflammatory conditions in young people <17 years of age characterized by proximal myopathy, rashes, and other organ involvement.
- Juvenile IIMs are classified into groups that share similar clinical and laboratory features, treatment responses, and prognosis.
- The juvenile IIMs are:
  - juvenile dermatomyositis (JDM): 80%.
  - juvenile polymyositis (JPM): 5%.
  - overlap myositis: 10%.
  - rare forms: macrophagic myofasciitis, focal myositis, granulomatous, and graft-vs-host myositis.
  - inclusion body myositis and cancer associated myositis are exceptionally rare in children.
- A form of inclusion body myositis also occurs in critical illness myopathy seen in intensive care units.
- Benign acute childhood myositis is self-limiting and typically presents with calf pain, walking difficulty, and very high CK levels.
- Benign acute myositis can be misdiagnosed as something more severe or complex resulting in unnecessary tests, admission, and follow-up.
- Although the 1975 'Bohan and Peter' criteria[6] remain in principle the diagnostic criteria (see → Box 14.2, p. 427), the invasive nature of EMG and biopsy means they are rarely used and MRI and US are often substituted for confirmation of muscle involvement.

## Differential diagnosis of muscle weakness in childhood

Muscle weakness may be a sign of muscle disease or a manifestation of a muscle function-related pathology or even general pathology.

- Viral myositis or benign acute childhood myositis.
- Drug-induced myopathy.
- Critical illness myopathy (e.g. patients in intensive care units).
- Muscular dystrophy and congenital myopathy.
- Juvenile fibromyalgia.
- Other multisystem inflammatory diseases (MCTD, SLE, vasculitis).
- Skeletal dysplasias.
- Electrolyte imbalances (potassium and calcium).

## Juvenile dermatomyositis (JDM)

- JDM is by far the commonest inflammatory myopathy in children and adolescents and in typical circumstances does not require a search for neoplasia.
- The incidence is 2–4 per million (USA and UK) with a median age of onset of 7 years old (25% are <4 years old at diagnosis).
- Presentation is typically with a classical rash and insidious onset of muscle weakness.

- A facial rash is common with a photosensitive malar distribution and nasolabial-sparing characteristic of SLE.
- Distinguishing JDM from SLE is important. With JDM there are shiny raised red marks on the knuckles, elbows, knees, and ankles (Gottron's papules) and a dusky purple-red hue to the upper eyelids (heliotrope rash).
- Weakness manifests as difficulty getting upstairs or out of bed, difficulty with putting on a jumper or T-shirt, or tiring more quickly than usual during sport.
- Other features include low-grade fever, weight loss, arthralgia, abdominal pain, melaena, change in character of voice, and difficulty swallowing.
- ILD and dilated cardiomyopathy may occur in chronic disease.
- The clinical course of JDM falls into different patterns:
  - Monocyclic (lasting up to 3 years) in 25–40%.
  - Polycyclic (periods of remission and relapse relapse) or chronic, both of which can be lifelong, in 50–60%.
  - Ulcerative in 10–20%.

*Myositis-specific autoantibodies (MSAs)*
- MSAs have been identified in ~70% of JDM patients.
- All autoantibodies are seen in JDM. More common MSAs include:
  - anti-TIF1-gamma associated with classical JDM (18%), extensive skin involvement (and lipodystrophy), and chronic course.
  - anti-MJ, anti-NPX2 (15%): both associated with a monocyclic course, but more severe calcinosis, dysphonia, and joint contractures.
  - MDA5 (6%): patients are less likely to be weak, but cutaneous ulceration and arthritis are common. Associated ILD is uncommon.

## Treatment
- Managing JDM requires a multidisciplinary approach to optimize muscle strength, function, and quality of life while controlling inflammation of skin, muscle, gut, and other organs, and aiming to avoid calcinosis evolving.
- Calcinosis cutis (occurring in up to 35% of JDM cases) can be a major cause of morbidity due to pain, cosmetic problems, tethering of skin, muscles, and nerves, and as a nidus for infection.
- GCs are the mainstay of treatment and universally supplemented with synthetic DMARDs (MTX, HCQ, ciclosporin, and IVIg).
- Early aggressive treatment to rapidly and completely control inflammation is essential to fully restore muscle function and avoid damage and calcinosis.
- Consensus guidelines (CARRA 2012, USA) recommend escalating immunosuppression for the first 2 months depending on disease severity.
- The treatment regimens utilize SC MTX, and a GC tapering schedule based on weight and severity of disease (e.g. see Table 3 in reference 7).
- IV methylprednisolone is added for rapid induction especially for severe disease and to replace oral prednisolone when there is gut involvement.

- If there is initial clinical improvement, then prednisolone dose is reduced at weekly intervals initially and then monthly at lower doses with the aim of being off GCs by 10–12 months.
- CYC is typically used for ulcerative cases, severe muscle disease, and ILD.
- IVIg is used for refractory and skin-predominant disease, or when there is severe weakness.
- More recently MMF, RTX, and anti-TNFα agents have been used for refractory disease.

## Amyopathic JDM
- Has the characteristic rash but no obvious muscle disease, although typically muscle inflammation and weakness is subclinical and insidious in onset.
- Amyopathic JDM is not generally associated with calcinosis or ILD.

## Overlap myositis
- Occurs with scleroderma, SLE, JIA, Sjögren's disease, and type 1 diabetes and more often in non-Caucasian populations.
- It is often associated with Raynaud's and ILD resulting in a higher mortality.

## Juvenile polymyositis
- Is very rare and results in more clinically apparent proximal and distal muscle weakness with little skin involvement.
- It is usually severe at onset with very high CK levels, affects older children (adolescents), and frequently has cardiac involvement.
- A muscle biopsy is required to differentiate from muscular dystrophy and shows endomysial infiltrates.

## References

6. Bohan A, Peter JB. Polymyositis and dermatomyositis. *N Engl J Med* 1975;292:344–7.
7. Huber AM, Robinson AB, Reed AM, et al. Consensus treatments for moderate juvenile dermatomyositis: beyond the first two months. Results of the second Childhood Arthritis and Rheumatology Research Alliance consensus conference. *Arthritis Care Res* 2012;64:546–53.

# Primary vasculitides

# Introduction

- The vasculitides are a heterogeneous group of relatively uncommon diseases that can arise as primary conditions or secondary to an established disease such as rheumatoid arthritis (RA) (see ➲ Chapter 5) or systemic lupus erythematosus (SLE) (see ➲ Chapter 13).
- The vasculitides are linked by the presence of vascular inflammation, which can lead to one of two common outcomes:
  - Vessel wall destruction: leading to aneurysm or rupture.
  - Stenosis: leading to tissue ischaemia and necrosis.
- In 1990, the American College of Rheumatology (ACR) developed a classification system based on vessel size, with the inclusion of a division between primary and secondary vasculitis (Table 15.1).
- This classification system is not perfect. Patients with 'large vessel vasculitis' and 'small vessel vasculitis' can have disease that affects some medium-sized vessels. Moreover, not all patients with 'antineutrophil cytoplasmic antibody (ANCA)-associated vasculitis (AAV)' have detectable levels of ANCA. However, this is a useful framework for the clinician, since categorizing the patient into one of these groups can narrow the differential diagnosis considerably.
- The Chapel Hill Consensus Conference (CHCC) in 1994 had developed the most widely used nomenclature system for most forms of vasculitis. This was revised in the 2012 CHCC to include new insights gained over the past two decades, add new forms of vasculitis, and address issues surrounding eponyms. (Box 15.1).
- The notable changes of the 2012 CHCC are:
  - the adoption of new names for several conditions, consistent with the trend of replacing eponyms with disease names that reflect pathology.
  - formally adopting the term ANCA-associated vasculitis (AAV) for the major systemic small vessel vasculitis subtypes.
  - adoption of additional categories to include variable vessel vasculitis and secondary forms of vasculitis.

**Table 15.1** A classification of systemic vasculitis

| Dominant vessel | Disorders | |
|---|---|---|
| Large arteries | Giant cell arteritis. Takayasu arteritis. Isolated central nervous system angiitis | Aortitis in AS. Infection, e.g. syphilis |
| Medium arteries | Classical polyarteritis nodosa, Kawasaki disease | Infection, e.g. hepatitis B. Hairy cell leukaemia |
| Medium arteries/small vessel | AAVs (e.g. GPA, EGPA/Churg–Strauss, microscopic polyangiitis) | Vasculitis secondary to autoimmune disease. Malignancy. Drugs. Infection, e.g. HIV |
| Small vessel (leucocytoclastic) | Henoch–Schönlein purpura. Essential mixed cryoglobulinaemia. Cutaneous leucocytoclastic angiitis | Drugs. Malignancy. Infection, e.g. hepatitis B/C |

- This nomenclature does not substitute the classification criteria.
- The AAVs have a predilection for the respiratory tract and kidneys.

The AAVs are granulomatosis and polyangiitis (GPA; formerly Wegener's granulomatosis), microscopic polyangiitis (MPA), and eosinophilic granulomatosis with polyangiitis (EGPA; formerly Churg–Strauss syndrome).

## Box 15.1 The 2012 CHCC nomenclature of vasculitis

*Large vessel vasculitis*
- Takayasu arteritis (TA)
- Giant cell arteritis (GCA).

*Medium vessel vasculitis*
- Polyarteritis nodosa (PAN)
- Kawasaki disease (KD).

*Small vessel vasculitis*

*AAVs*
- Microscopic polyangiitis (MPA)
- Granulomatosis with polyangiitis (GPA)
- Eosinophilic granulomatosis with polyangiitis (EGPA).

*Immune-complex small vessel vasculitis*
- Anti-glomerular basement membrane (anti-GBM) disease
- Cryoglobulinaemic vasculitis
- IgA vasculitis (Henoch–Schönlein purpura) (IgAV)
- Hypocomplementaemic urticarial vasculitis (HUV) (anti-C1q vasculitis).

*Variable-sized vessel vasculitis*
- Behçet's disease (BD)
- Cogan's syndrome (CS).

*Single-organ vasculitis*
- Cutaneous leucocytoclastic angiitis
- Cutaneous arteritis
- Primary central nervous system vasculitis
- Isolated aortitis
- Others.

*Vasculitis associated with systemic diseases*
- Lupus vasculitis
- Rheumatoid vasculitis
- Sarcoid vasculitis
- Others.

*Vasculitis associated with probable aetiology*
- Hepatitis C virus-associated cryoglobulinaemic vasculitis
- Hepatitis B virus-associated vasculitis
- Syphilis-associated aortitis
- Drug-associated immune complex vasculitis
- Drug-associated AAV
- Cancer-associated vasculitis
- Others.

Modified from Jennette et al. '2012 Revised International Chapel Hill Consensus Conference Nomenclature of Vasculitides' *Arthritis & Rheumatism*, 65:1–11 with permission from Wiley.

### Antineutrophil cytoplasmic antibody

- ANCA exists in two main forms based on neutrophil autoantibody immunofluorescence patterns:
  - Cytoplasmic (C-ANCA; antibodies against proteinase-3 (PR3)).
  - Perinuclear (P-ANCA; antibodies against myeloperoxidase (MPO)).
- Other ANCA-staining patterns (i.e. non-cytoplasmic, non-perinuclear) can occur.
- P-ANCA pattern may be caused by antibodies against antigens other than myeloperoxidase. These are sometimes referred to as 'atypical ANCA', and do not predict the presence of vasculitis, although they can be found in inflammatory bowel disease, immune-mediated neutropenia, and other autoimmune diseases.
- C-ANCA is found in patients with GPA.
- Patients with MPA and EGPA tend to be P-ANCA positive.
- Counterintuitively, patients with AAV can be ANCA negative in up to 50% of cases.
- AAV patients with active or untreated disease are more likely to be ANCA positive.
- The role that ANCAs play in the pathogenesis of vasculitis remains controversial.

### General principles of vasculitis management

- To be complete, any evaluation of a chronic disease (such as primary systemic vasculitis) must include both an assessment of disease activity and of disease damage. The concept of damage denotes the aspects of disease that are unlikely to reverse with immunosuppression (such as pulmonary fibrosis or renal insufficiency).
- Clinical trials of vasculitis commonly use the Birmingham Vasculitis Activity Score (BVAS) and Vasculitis Damage Index (VDI) to assess activity and damage, respectively.
- Other clinical indices exist. The French Vasculitis Study Group (FVSG) has developed a prognostic Five-Factor Score (FFS). This index provides another useful method of classifying patients with vasculitis. Patients with PAN or AAV who have a FFS >0 have substantially higher mortality than patients with a FFS = 0.
- The FFS was revised in 2008, and now includes the following: age >65, renal insufficiency, cardiac involvement, and gastrointestinal (GI) manifestations. The presence of ear, nose, and throat signs was found to correlate with an improved outcome among patients with GPA.

# Large vessel vasculitis

# Large vessel vasculitis

- The 'large vessels' include the aorta and its main branches (i.e. the subclavian, carotid, and brachiocephalic arteries). Primary and secondary forms of large vessel vasculitis are shown in Table 15.2.
- The classic forms of primary large vessel vasculitis are TA (see ➔ 'Takayasu arteritis', pp. 454–5) and giant cell arteritis (GCA). GCA is associated with PMR.
- Recent studies demonstrate that many patients with polymyalgia rheumatica (PMR) have subclinical aortic inflammation, which seems to validate this classification scheme.
- The clinical manifestations of large vessel vasculitis can be predicted by the pattern of vessel involvement. Arch aortitis leads to aneurysmal dilatation and aortic regurgitation. Subclavian involvement causes arm claudication and diminished pulses on examination. Carotid involvement may lead to visual loss, jaw claudication, and stroke. Involvement of any major blood vessel may cause bruits of physical examination.

**Table 15.2** Causes of large vessel vasculitis

| Primary | Takayasu arteritis |
| --- | --- |
| | Giant cell arteritis* |
| Secondary† | Infection: bacterial, fungal, mycobacterial, spirochaete |
| | Rheumatoid arthritis |
| | Seronegative spondyloarthritis |
| | Systemic lupus erythematosus |
| | Sarcoidosis |
| | Relapsing polychondritis |
| | Juvenile arthritis |

* Giant cell arteritis is discussed in this chapter in the section on polymyalgia rheumatica.

† The secondary causes of large vessel vasculitis are discussed in their respective sections.

# Takayasu arteritis

# Takayasu arteritis

Takayasu arteritis (TA) is a chronic granulomatous arteritis that affects the aorta and the great vessels. The pulmonary arteries can also be involved, although this is relatively uncommon.

## Epidemiology

- It is most common in Japan, Southeast Asia, India, and Mexico. It is rare in the UK and in the USA, its annual incidence is estimated at 2.6 per million, where it is not limited to patients of Asian descent—the majority of patients in the USA are Caucasian.
- TA tends to affect women (90% of cases) with adolescents and young adults 20–40 years old at greatest risk.
- The hallmark of the disease is arteritic inflammatory infiltrates that cause luminal narrowing or occlusion presenting with bruits, claudication, and diminished (or asymmetric) pulses.

## Presentation

- Systemic symptoms are common in the early phase of the disease, including fever, malaise, weight loss, and fatigue.
- As the disease progresses, consequences of vascular inflammation and insufficiency can become apparent.
- Arthralgias and myalgias are common.
- Clinically evident synovitis is rare.
- Lightheadedness, visual disturbance, and strokes can occur. Subclavian steal can be an important cause of neurological symptoms.
- Hypertension may develop as a consequence of renal artery stenosis.
- Myoarthralgias are not uncommon.
- Cardiovascular complications are an important cause of morbidity, and include aortic insufficiency, congestive heart failure, systemic hypertension, and ostial involvement of the coronary arteries.

## Investigation

- Traditionally, the diagnosis of TA has depended on angiography to demonstrate the characteristic changes of arterial dilatation, thrombosis, and aneurysm formation.
- Conventional angiography has the added benefit of allowing a comparison between central and peripheral blood pressures—important because subclavian stenosis is a common consequence of this disease and a standard arm cuff blood pressure reading may underestimate hypertension. Angiography may also allow for therapeutic intervention, e.g. angioplasty or stenting of the stenotic vessels.
- Magnetic resonance imaging/angiography (MRI/MRA) have excellent resolution at the level of the large vessels. MRI can also demonstrate evidence of vessel wall inflammation, which could support a diagnosis of TA.
- High-resolution US is sensitive for detecting carotid lesions.
- [18]F-FDG PET-CT scanning is useful for identifying the presence of large vessel vasculitis, but it is not clear whether it can be used to monitor response to therapy.

## Treatment

- Initial medical treatment is with glucocorticoids (GCs) such as prednisolone 40–60 mg per day in an average-sized adult.
- Tapering GC dose is attempted when symptoms and laboratory tests of inflammation subside. About one-half of all patients have steroid-resistant disease. In this group, methotrexate (MTX), azathioprine (AZA), mycophenolate mofetil (MMF), or leflunomide (LEF) may be tried.
- In severe forms of the disease, or if there is continuing evidence of disease activity, cyclophosphamide (CYC) may be given.
- Experience with biologics is limited. Anti-TNFα agents or tocilizumab (anti-IL6r) may be tried in severe or resistant cases.
- Hypertension can be difficult to manage, and may require angioplasty or surgery to address renal artery stenosis.
- Surgical management ranges from angioplasty to bypass procedures. These are best performed during the inactive phase of disease.
- Angioplasty is often a temporizing measure, and lesions tend to restenose over time. Restenosis is less likely following bypass grafting. Operative mortality is 4%—mostly with aneurysm rupture.
- The prognosis depends mainly on the presence of hypertension and aortic incompetence. The majority of patients (75%) will have some impairment of daily living, and 50% are permanently disabled.
- Mortality is low, with 5-year and 10-year survival rates reported as 80% and 90%, respectively.
- TA is not a contraindication to pregnancy. Cytotoxic agents should be stopped and GCs kept to as low a dose as possible.
- Obstetric decisions can be made on their own merits and not because of coexistence of TA. The main complications are exacerbations of hypertension and congestive cardiac failure. The anaesthetist should be made aware of the diagnosis, as the patient may require invasive blood pressure monitoring during delivery.

# Polymyalgia rheumatica and giant cell arteritis

## Polymyalgia rheumatica

Polymyalgia rheumatica (PMR) is characterized by pain and stiffness affecting structures of the shoulder and pelvic girdle areas. Neck pain and stiffness is also a feature.

### Epidemiology

- PMR is rare in patients <50 years old. The mean age of onset is 70 years.
- Prevalence among patients older than 50 years is 1 in 133, and women are affected more than men (ratio 2:1).
- There is a higher frequency of diagnosis in northern latitudes.

### Pathology

- Parainfluenza, parvovirus B19, *Mycoplasma pneumonia*, and *Chlamydia pneumoniae* infections have been shown to have a temporal relation to incidence peaks of PMR, although other studies have found no relationship.
- HLA-DRB1*04 and -DRB*01 predict disease susceptibility.
- PMR and GCA have a close clinical relationship. One-half of patients with GCA have symptoms of PMR and up to 20% of patients with PMR have histological or clinical evidence of GCA.
- The pathogenesis of both conditions is not known.

### Presentation

- The diagnosis of PMR is based on clinical features. The criteria of Jones and Hazleman 1981[1] are succinct and practical (Box 15.2).
- The European League Against Rheumatology (EULAR) and the ACR have proposed classification criteria to be used as a research tool to identify patients with PMR.[2]

---

### Box 15.2 Criteria for the diagnosis of PMR

All the following need to be valid/relevant:

1. Shoulder and pelvic girdle pain which is primarily muscular in the absence of true muscle weakness.
2. Morning stiffness.
3. Duration of at least 2 months (unless treated).
4. ESR >30 mm/hour or CRP >6 mg/dL.
5. Absence of inflammatory arthritis or malignancy.
6. Absence of muscle disease.
7. Prompt and dramatic response to glucocorticoids.

Criteria from Jones JG, Hazleman BL. The prognosis and management of PMR. *Ann Rheum Dis* 1981;40:1–5.

- EULAR/ACR criteria include 3 required criteria and 4 points from additional criteria:
  - Required criteria include age ≥50 years, bilateral shoulder aching, and an abnormal ESR or CRP.
  - A scoring algorithm was developed for the additional criteria, which include morning stiffness ≥45 minutes (2 points); pain or limited range of motion at hip (1 point); absence of RF or anti-CCP (2 points); absence of peripheral joint pain (1 point).
- There may be apparent muscle weakness on testing, which is due to pain rather than intrinsic muscle disease.
- Symptoms may start asymmetrically, but soon become bilateral.
- Systemic features of malaise, weight loss, low-grade fever, and depression are common.
- Arthralgia and synovitis may occur. Up to 5% of patients with RA (see ⮕ Chapter 5) have an initial PMR-like presentation.

*Investigation*

- The lack of specific clinical features, a specific laboratory test, and the presence of several conditions that can present with PMR-like symptoms, makes PMR a diagnosis of exclusion (see Box 15.3).

## Giant cell arteritis (GCA)

GCA is a granulomatous arteritis of the aorta and larger vessels, including extracranial branches of the carotid artery. For diagnostic criteria, see Table 15.3.

*Epidemiology*

- GCA is the most common form of primary systemic vasculitis. In North America the annual incidence is estimated at 18 per 100,000.
- Like PMR, the female to male ratio is 2:1.

*Pathology*

- Infectious and genetic associations are also similar to PMR with evidence of disease 'clustering'.
- Increasing age and ethnicity are the major risk factors for developing GCA. GCA is rare among African Americans.

---

### Box 15.3 Conditions that can present with PMR-type symptoms

1. Rheumatoid arthritis
2. Inflammatory myopathy
3. Hypo/hyperthyroidism
4. Myeloma or other malignancy
5. Chronic sepsis
6. Bilateral shoulder capsulitis
7. Calcium pyrophosphate deposition disease
8. Spondyloarthritis/PsA
9. Inflammatory phase osteoarthritis
10. Parkinsonism.

Table 15.3 Diagnostic criteria for GCA

| | |
|---|---|
| Jones and Hazleman (1981) | All the following:<br>• Positive temporal artery biopsy or cranial artery tenderness.<br>• One or more of: visual disturbance, headache, jaw pain, cerebrovascular insufficiency; ESR >30 mm/hour or CRP >6 mg/L; response to glucocorticoids |
| ACR criteria | Three or more of:<br>• Age at onset >50 years.<br>• New headache.<br>• Temporal artery tenderness or decreased pulsation.<br>• ESR >50 mm/hour.<br>• Abnormal artery biopsies showing necrotizing arteritis with mononuclear infiltrate or granulomatous inflammation usually with multinucleated giant cells |

Information from Jones JG, Hazleman BL. The prognosis and management of PMR. *Ann Rheum Dis* 1981;40:1–5 and Hunder G et al. The American College of Rheumatology 1990 criteria for the classification of the giant cell arteritis. *Arthritis Rheum* 1990;33:1122–8.

*Presentation*
• Severe headache and scalp tenderness localized to the occiput or temporal area are common initial symptoms, and are present in 70% of cases. The critical feature of the headache is that it is new.
• Headache is often localized to the temples, but may be frontal, occipital, or generalized.
• The temporal artery can be swollen, tender, and pulseless.
• Jaw claudication is present in about half of the patients. Some patients report tongue claudication. Jaw claudication is strongly associated with a positive biopsy.
• Scalp necrosis has also been reported.
• Large arteries are affected in 15% of cases, leading to claudication, bruits, absent neck and arm pulses, and thoracic aorta aneurysm and dissection.
• Visual disturbance is usually an early finding. Patients may describe symptoms of amaurosis fugax by temporary 'curtaining' of the visual field. Visual loss due to retinal ischaemia may be irreversible within hours. A history of prior transient visual loss is the strongest predictor for subsequent permanent visual loss.
• Diplopia and ptosis may also occur.
• Fundoscopy may show optic disc pallor, haemorrhages, and exudates. Optic atrophy is a late finding.
• Arteritic anterior ischaemic optic neuropathy is the most common finding, and must be differentiated from non-arteritic anterior ischaemic optic neuropathy, a cause of visual loss that does not respond to steroids.
• Malaise, fatigue, weight loss, fever, and anaemia are common.

*Investigation*

- The ESR and CRP are characteristically elevated, but can be normal in up to 3% of cases.
- Patients suspected of having GCA should be evaluated with bilateral temporal artery biopsies, taking segments of 1.5 cm each.
- Treatment should not be delayed. Biopsies may be helpful to confirm the diagnosis up to 2 weeks after steroids are started.
- Unlike most forms of vasculitis, GCA does not cause fibrinoid necrosis and the presence of fibrinoid necrosis on a temporal artery biopsy should prompt a search for another form of vasculitis, such as GPA or cryoglobulinaemic vasculitis.
- Temporal artery biopsies may be negative in 12% of patients. A negative temporal artery biopsy does not exclude a diagnosis of GCA.
- Data regarding the usefulness of Doppler ultrasound for the diagnosis of GCA are mixed. Various abnormalities described include stenosis, occlusion and the presence of a hypoechoic 'halo' (halo sign) around the temporal arteries.
- The sensitivity and specificity of the halo sign for the diagnosis of GCA are 69% and 82%, respectively.
- MRA is useful to diagnose GCA, identify regions of temporal artery involvement, help gauge disease activity, and assess response to treatment.
- $^{18}$F-FDG-PET-CT may be useful in showing abnormal metabolic activity in the aorta of many patients with GCA (see ➲ Plate 26). Direct evaluation of the temporal arteries is not possible using $^{18}$F-FDG-PET-CT.

## Treatment of PMR and GCA

- Both conditions require GC treatment; however, the amount and duration of treatment required are quite different.[3,4]
- PMR responds dramatically to low–moderate doses of GC (i.e. prednisone 15–20 mg daily) within 24 hours.
- Some patients respond immediately to prednisolone, and the vast majority of patients have a substantial improvement within days of starting treatment.
- ACR/EULAR suggest use of the minimum effective dose of prednisolone, ranging from 12.5–25 mg prednisolone (or equivalent) per day.
- Lower doses of 7.5–10 mg prednisolone may be sufficient in those with mild symptoms.
- Persistent symptoms despite treatment mandate consideration of an alternate diagnosis.
- After treatment for 2–4 weeks, the prednisone dose may be decreased by 2.5 mg every 2 weeks until the patient reaches a maintenance dose of 10 mg/day. Prednisone may subsequently be tapered in 1 mg per month increments.
- GCA requires treatment with high-dose GCs (i.e. prednisone 40–60 mg daily) and the patient may take a week or longer to experience substantial relief.
- Treatment with GCs should be instituted once a diagnosis of GCA is suspected, even before it is confirmed.

- After treatment for 1 month, prednisone may be gradually tapered over 9–12 months.
- In patients who have GC-resistant or GC-dependent disease, or develop significant adverse effects with treatment, MTX may be added as a steroid-sparing drug.
- A meta-analysis (of 161 patients) showed that the use of MTX resulted in a cumulative reduction in the steroid dose over 48 weeks.
- Tocilizumab can be effective as GC-sparing, as demonstrated in a small trial of 30 patients with newly diagnosed or relapsing GCA.
- Small uncontrolled studies have suggested that CYC may also be considered for this indication.
- Patients with visual symptoms associated with GCA should be treated with intravenous pulse methylprednisolone therapy (1 g daily for 3 days) prior to initiating therapy with prednisone.
- Daily low-dose (e.g. 75 mg) aspirin may prevent cranial ischaemic events, such as stroke and blindness, and should be considered if there is no contraindication.
- Osteoporotic fracture protection against GC-induced osteoporosis is essential. All patients with either GCA or PMR should be commenced at the time of starting GCs, on either a weekly oral bisphosphonate or IV zoledronic acid, alongside daily calcium and vitamin D supplements.

## References

1. Jones JG, Hazleman BL. The prognosis and management of polymyalgia rheumatica. *Ann Rheum Dis* 1981;40:1–5.
2. Dasgupta B. 2012 provisional classification criteria for polymyalgia rheumatica: a European League Against Rheumatism/American College of Rheumatology collaborative initiative. *Arthritis Rheum* 2012;64:943–54.
3. Dasgupta B, Borg FA, Hassan N, et al. BSR and BHPR guidelines for the management of polymyalgia rheumatica. *Rheumatol (Oxf)* 2010;49:186–90.
4. Dasgupta B, Borg FA, Hassan N, et al. BSR and BHPR Guidelines for the management of giant cell arteritis. *Rheumatol (Oxf)* 2010;49(8):1594–s7.

# Polyarteritis nodosa

Polyarteritis nodosa (PAN) was the first form of systemic vasculitis described in the literature. It is characterized by a necrotizing vasculitis of medium-sized arteries, which can lead to cutaneous ulcers, kidney infarction, GI haemorrhage, and mononeuritis multiplex.

The CHCC created a distinction between 'classic' PAN (i.e. an ANCA-negative, medium vessel vasculitis associated with renal infarcts) and microscopic PAN (i.e. an ANCA-positive, medium vessel and small vessel vasculitis characterized by glomerulonephritis). This re-classification (and the hepatitis B vaccine) has made PAN increasingly uncommon.

## Aetiology

• Some cases of PAN have been linked to infection with hepatitis B.
• Patients with PAN should be screened for viral hepatitis, as antiviral therapy may be needed in addition to immunosuppression.

## Presentation and clinical features

• The clinical features are shown in Table 15.4.
• Patients often present with non-specific features of systemic disease including myalgias, arthralgias, weight loss, and fever.
• About 50% of cases develop a vasculitic rash, which includes purpura, nodules, livedo reticularis, bullous and vesicular lesions, ulcers, often with 'punched out' border in the lower extremities.
• GI involvement occurs in up to 50% of cases. Non-specific abdominal pain, gut/gallbladder infarction, and pancreatitis are all features.
• Renal involvement occurs in up to 50% of cases in the form of renal infarct and hypertension. Renal impairment is often mild and present in around 20% of cases.
• Mononeuritis multiplex occurs in up to 70% of patients.
• Isolated organ involvement is rare, but disease affecting the skin, testes, epididymis, breasts, uterus, appendix, and gallbladder has been reported.

## Treatment

• Treatment and prognosis in all the small vessel and medium vessel vasculitides ARE discussed at the end of this section.

**Table 15.4** Clinical features at presentation (as % of cases)

| Clinical feature | PAN | MPA | EGPA |
| --- | --- | --- | --- |
| Renal impairment | 25% | 90% | 50% |
| Pulmonary disease | 40% | 50% | General 50%, asthma 100% |
| Fever | 60% | 40% | |
| Skin vasculitis | 40% | 50% | 50% |
| Gastrointestinal disease | 45% | 20% | 60% |
| Cardiovascular | 15% | 20% | 45% |
| Peripheral neuropathy | 10% | 10% | 60% |
| Ear, nose, and throat | 10% | 20% | |
| Ocular disease | 10% | 20% | |

# ANCA-associated vasculitides

### Granulomatosis with polyangiitis (formerly Wegener's granulomatosis)

- Granulomatosis with polyangiitis (GPA) is the most prevalent of the AAVs. Renal-limited vasculitis and drug-induced AAV are less-common members of this group.
- The CHCC has defined GPA as: 'necrotizing granulomatous inflammation usually involving the upper and lower respiratory tract, and necrotizing vasculitis affecting predominantly small to medium vessels (e.g. capillaries, venules, arterioles, arteries and veins). Necrotizing glomerulonephritis is common.'

*Epidemiology*
- GPA is a worldwide disease with an incidence of 4–9 per million.
- It is slightly more common in men than women.
- It most often appears in the fourth and fifth decades.

*Presentation and clinical features*
- GPA is often a clinical triad with manifestations affecting the upper respiratory tract, lower respiratory tract, and kidneys.
- Patients can present with a wide range of clinical manifestations.
- Some patients have an indolent presentation characterized by respiratory tract involvement, such as sinusitis and pulmonary nodules.
- However, rapidly progressive glomerulonephritis and pulmonary haemorrhage can occur (Box 15.4).

*Musculoskeletal symptoms*
- Rheumatic symptoms are seen in 60% of cases.
- Symptoms can range from mild myalgias (in 50% of the cases) and arthralgias to overt arthritis. 20–30% of rheumatic symptoms may be related to a non-erosive and non-deforming polyarthropathy.
- Migratory arthralgias are a classic presentation for GPA.

---

**Box 15.4 American College of Rheumatology 1990 classification criteria of GPA\***

Diagnosis requires two or more of the following:

1. *Nasal or oral inflammation: development of painful or painless oral ulcers or purulent or bloody nasal discharge.*
2. *Abnormal chest radiograph:* the chest radiograph may show nodules, cavities, or infiltrate.
3. *Urinary sediment:* microscopic haematuria or red cell casts.
4. Histological changes of granulomatous inflammation on biopsy.
5. PR3-ANCA (C-ANCA) positivity.

\* Then known as 'Wegener's granulomatosis'.

Reproduced from Leavitt et al. (1990). The American College of Rheumatology 1990 criteria for the classification of wegener's granulomatosis. *Arthritis & Rheumatism*, 33: 1101–1107 with permission from Wiley.

*Ear, nose, and throat symptoms*
- Up to 90% of patients have ear, nose, and throat involvement.
- Chronic sinusitis is a common initial presentation for GPA and typically many patients will have been treated with several courses of antibiotics before the correct diagnosis is reached.
- Other manifestations include nasal septal perforation, bloody nasal discharge ('crusts'), and nasal bridge collapse due to erosion of underlying cartilage ('saddle nose').
- Patients may also complain of diminished hearing, either due to sensorineural hearing loss or Eustachian tube dysfunction.
- Subglottic stenosis is a classic feature of GPA and may present with hoarseness and stridor. Subglottic stenosis may worsen even when a patient is otherwise in remission, and responds better to steroid injections than systemic therapy.
- In the oral cavity and oropharynx, inflammation can lead to mucosal ulcers or gingivitis ('strawberry gums').
- It is thought that *Staphylococcus aureus* has a role in disease pathogenesis. Nasal carriage in GPA patients is 3× that of the healthy population. The exact mechanisms leading to disease are unclear, but trimethoprim/sulfamethoxazole may benefit patients with GPA by eliminating *S. aureus* colonization.

*Pulmonary disease*
- 80% of cases have pulmonary disease.
- The tracheobronchial tree may be locally involved before any signs of generalized disease.
- Subglottic pseudo-tumours and/or stenosis cause stridor or dyspnoea. Lower bronchial stenosis may cause atelectasis and obstructive pneumonia. Multiple nodules with or without cavitation are found in the lungs of asymptomatic patients.
- Severe pulmonary disease is associated with alveolar capillaritis, haemorrhage and haemoptysis, with infiltrates on CXR (typically an alveolar or mixed alveolar–interstitial pattern; the distribution is often like that of pulmonary oedema and focal infection).

*Renal disease*
- Up to 90% of patients with 'severe' GPA have renal involvement.
- Renal involvement can range from milder focal and segmental glomerulonephritis to fulminant diffuse necrotizing (rapidly progressive) and crescentic glomerulonephritis, which can rapidly lead to end-stage renal disease.
- The milder form of the condition is most common, manifesting in the asymptomatic patient as a nephritic picture of microscopic haematuria, active sediment, and mild renal impairment.

*Skin disease*
- 40% of cases have skin disease.
- Features include palpable purpura due to a leucocytoclastic vasculitis, necrotic papules ('Churg–Strauss nodules'), livedo reticularis, and pyoderma gangrenosum.

*Nervous system*
- About 30% of patients with GPA have involvement with mononeuritis multiplex and distal sensorimotor polyneuropathy the main lesions. Seizures and cerebritis are much less frequent events.
- Disseminated granulomatous lesions ('pachymeningitis') can involve the retropharyngeal area and skull base affecting cranial nerves I, II, III, VI, VII, and VIII. Pachymeningitis can also be associated with diabetes insipidus and meningitis.

*Eye disease*
- Granulomatous lesions may obstruct the nasolacrimal duct and cause orbital pseudotumour, with optic nerve compression from masses developing in the retrobulbar space.
- Rarely a purulent sinusitis may spread and cause secondary bacterial orbital infection.
- Manifestations in the generalized stage of GPA include episcleritis (red eye), vasculitis of the optic nerve, and occlusion of retinal arteries, in addition to the granulomatous lesions described earlier.

*Investigation*
(See ➔ Table 4.3, p. 214 for laboratory tests to consider.)
- A biopsy should be done in patients with suspected AAV to confirm the diagnosis. In some patients, biopsy is not feasible and so a presumptive diagnosis is made on the clinical features and ANCA.
- Laboratory investigation should include FBC with differential, routine chemistry, ESR, CRP, and urinalysis to look for active sediment.
- A positive ANCA strongly suggests the diagnosis of vasculitis; however, false-positive and false-negative results are seen.
- About 82% of patients with GPA have a positive ANCA. This is usually specific for proteinase-3.
- 10% of GPA cases are ANCA negative. A negative ANCA does not exclude the diagnosis.
- CXR and HRCT chest should be considered in all cases as the chance of pulmonary lesions is high despite sometimes few symptoms.

*Treatment*
- Treatment and prognosis of GPA is discussed later in this section with the other AAVs.

## ANCA-associated vasculitides: microscopic polyangiitis

- MPA is classified as a pulmonary-renal (haemorrhage) syndrome, a group that also includes Goodpasture's disease and SLE. GPA may also occasionally present as a pulmonary-renal syndrome.
- MPA lacks the granulomatous manifestations characteristic of GPA, such as sinus disease and pulmonary nodules.
- Unlike GPA, MPA is characterized by MPO-ANCA antibodies, which are associated with a P-ANCA immunofluorescence pattern. Up to 80% of patients with MPA will be ANCA positive.
- Like PAN, the male to female ratio is 2:1, with the majority of patients being Caucasian. The mean age of presentation is 50 years.

- Most patients with MPA will present with renal involvement in the form of a necrotizing glomerulonephritis, similar to what can be seen with GPA. Unlike most forms of vasculitis, glomerulonephritis from AAV is 'pauci-immune' (i.e. there is only minimal immunoglobulin deposition on immunofluorescence stains).
- Pulmonary haemorrhage presents as haemoptysis, and can be surprisingly subtle in some patients. Bronchoscopy with bronchoalveolar lavage will demonstrate haemosiderin-laden macrophages. Chronic pulmonary capillaritis may eventually lead to pulmonary fibrosis.
- Other clinical features of the disease are shown in Table 15.4.

## ANCA-associated vasculitides: eosinophilic granulomatosis with polyangiitis (EGPA/formerly Churg–Strauss syndrome)

- EGPA is often described as a clinical triad of adult-onset asthma, eosinophilia, and vasculitis.
- Typically, the asthma gradually worsens in intensity until the patient requires daily oral steroids for symptom control. Many of these patients will have been treated with a leukotriene inhibitor (although leukotriene inhibitors do not cause the disease).
- Peripheral blood hyper-eosinophilia is typically mild and resolves quickly upon treatment with oral steroids.
- Other manifestations of hyper-eosinophilia include 'fleeting' pulmonary infiltrates, myocarditis, and interstitial nephritis; frank glomerulonephritis is much less common in this diagnosis.
- Nerve involvement is a common manifestation of vasculitis among patients with EGPA, and patients should be examined for evidence of a sensory neuropathy or mononeuritis multiplex.
- Cutaneous granulomata that form along the elbows and fingers are called 'Churg–Strauss nodules'. Ironically, they appear more commonly in association with GPA.
- Cardiac involvement is one of the more serious manifestations of EGPA, accounting for approximately half of all deaths in patients with EGPA. Clinical manifestations include arrhythmias, pericarditis, and heart failure.
- Treatment and prognosis in all the small vessel and medium vessel vasculitides are discussed at the end of this section.

## The treatment of ANCA-associated vasculitides

- Assessment of disease activity in GPA or MPA is usually done using the BVAS.
- BVAS ranges from 0 to 68; with a score of 0 indicating remission.
- AAV are managed with treatment aiming to provide *remission induction* and then *remission maintenance*.
- Current treatment choices are based on classifying patients as having 'severe generalized disease or poor prognosis' versus 'localized, early systemic disease or good prognosis'.
- Initial immunosuppressive therapy consists of GCs in combination with either CYC or rituximab (RTX). MTX with GCs can be used in patients with mild extrarenal disease.
- In a select group, those who present with severe disease, plasma exchange may be tried.

*Severe generalized GPA and MPA*

- The National Institutes of Health regimen consisted of 1 year of oral CYC (2 mg/kg daily) with prednisolone (1 mg/kg daily tapered over 6–12 months). This has been modified in the last decade to minimize exposure to CYC and GCs.
- The induction phase consists of 3–6 months of CYC, followed by either AZA (CYCAZAREM trial)[5] or MTX (WEGENT trial)[6] to maintain remission.
- MMF was found to be inferior compared to AZA in a randomized trial (IMPROVE trial).[7]
- IVIg leflunomide and calcineurin inhibitors have been used in a small number of patients, but data to access their efficacy is insufficient.
- Etanercept was found to be ineffective in maintaining remission in a placebo-controlled trial (WGET trial).[8]
- The optimal length of maintenance therapy is unclear but continuation for 12–18 months after remission is reasonable as the majority of patients flare after therapy is discontinued.
- The CYCLOPS trial compared daily oral to IV pulse CYC.[9] Both regimens resulted in similar rates of remission. Extended follow-up for a duration of 4.3 years showed comparable survival rates of about 80%, and similar side effect profile. However, relapses were more common with pulse therapy.
- RTX has demonstrated efficacy and short-term safety comparable to CYC and AZA.
- In the RAVE trial, 64% of patients who received RTX for 6 months discontinued prednisolone compared to 53% who had CYC.[10] RTX was more efficacious compared with CYC in those who had relapsing disease at baseline.
- At 12 months, 42% of patients in the RTX arm remained in remission compared with 38% in the CYC arm.
- In the RITUXIVAS trial, about 90% of patients attained remission in both the RTX and CYC arms, and 90% and 85% respectively remained relapse free at 12 months.[11]
- RTX may be preferable to CYC for induction of remission in patients with concerns about fertility or those with a high risk of malignancy.

*Localized and early generalized GPA and MPA*

- Disease may respond to a combination of MTX and prednisolone. In the NORAM trial,[12] which compared MTX with CYC, remission at 6 months was achieved in about 90% of patients in both treatment arms. But relapses after drug discontinuation were significantly higher in those given MTX.
- Trimethoprim-sulfamethoxazole may decrease the risk of relapse in patients with localized disease.

*Other treatments*

- Plasma exchange has been used with some effect in those with severe renal disease, although the benefit is transient.
- IVIg has a short-lived benefit, but may be used in patients at high risk of systemic infection.

- Treatment of a vasculitis associated with an infectious disease (e.g. hepatitis B-associated PAN, hepatitis C-associated cryoglobulinaemic vasculitis) should include treatment of the pathogen.
- There is evidence that respiratory tract infections may trigger a relapse of GPA. Trimethoprim-sulfamethoxazole in patients with stable disease on maintenance therapy may decrease respiratory infection, and is also useful for prevention of pneumocystis among patients treated with CYC.

*EGPA*

- Patients without poor prognostic factors (FFS = 0) achieve remission with GCs alone in >90% of cases. Although about a third may relapse, the long-term prognosis is excellent.
- In patients with poor prognostic factors (FFS ≥1) IV CYC pulses are effective. Flares are frequent on CYC discontinuation. Extrapolating results from GPA/MPA trials, AZA may be used for maintaining remission.
- Successful treatment with RTX has been described in case series and case reports.
- Mepolizumab, an anti-IL5 monoclonal antibody, has demonstrated encouraging results in pilot trials.

## Prognosis of ANCA-associated vasculitides

- Prior to the introduction of CYC and GCs, mortality associated with AAV approached 100%. Modern immunosuppressive regimens have transformed these diseases into chronic conditions, characterized by cycles of relapse and remission.
- For many patients, the consequences of treatment (such as GC-associated complications) may lead to greater morbidity than the underlying disease itself.
- Mortality due to infection continues to be an important consideration for patients treated for AAV; indeed, patients with 'treatment-resistant' AAV should be carefully evaluated for the presence of *Nocardia*, *Aspergillus*, and other infections that can mimic some of the manifestations of the AAV.

## References

5. Jayne D, Rasmussen N, Andrassy K, et al. A randomized trial of maintenance therapy for vasculitis associated with antineutrophil cytoplasmic autoantibodies. *N Engl J Med* 2003;349:36–44.
6. Pagnoux C, Mahr A, Hamidou MA, et al. Azathioprine or methotrexate maintenance for ANCA-associated vasculitis. *N Engl J Med* 2008;359:2790–803.
7. Hiemstra TF, Walsh M, Mahr A, et al. Mycophenolate mofetil vs azathioprine for remission maintenance in antineutrophil cytoplasmic antibody-associated vasculitis: a randomized controlled trial. *JAMA* 2010;304:2381–8.
8. Wegener's Granulomatosis Etanercept Trial (WGET) Research Group. Etanercept plus standard therapy for Wegener's granulomatosis. *N Engl J Med* 2005;352:351–61.
9. de Groot K, Harper L, Jayne DR, et al. Pulse versus daily oral cyclophosphamide for induction of remission in antineutrophil cytoplasmic antibody-associated vasculitis: a randomized trial. *Ann Intern Med* 2009;150:670–80.
10. Stone JH, Merkel PA, Spiera R, et al. Rituximab versus cyclophosphamide for ANCA-associated vasculitis. *N Engl J Med* 2010;363:221–32.
11. Jones RB, Tervaert JW, Hauser T, et al. Rituximab versus cyclophosphamide in ANCA-associated renal vasculitis. *N Engl J Med* 2010;363:211–20.
12. De Groot K, Rasmussen N, Bacon PA, et al. Randomized trial of cyclophosphamide versus methotrexate for induction of remission in early systemic antineutrophil cytoplasmic antibody-associated vasculitis. *Rheum* 2005;52:2461–9.

# Small vessel vasculitis

The definition of small vessel vasculitis is open to different interpretations. Small vessel disease can be one feature of GPA, MPA, and EGPA. However, there are a range of clinical and pathological features that define a specific group of small vessel vasculitides outlined in Table 15.5. See also ➲ Table 4.3, p. 214 for advice on laboratory investigation.

## Leucocytoclastic vasculitis

- Histologically, leucocytoclastic vasculitis appears as a neutrophil infiltration in and around small vessels, with fragmentation of the neutrophils (leucocytoclasis), fibrin deposition, and endothelial cell necrosis. Immune complex deposition appears to be important in pathogenesis.
- Small vessel vasculitis usually presents in the skin, although the microvasculature of any tissue may be affected.
- Some forms of cutaneous vasculitis are predominantly lymphocytic, without evidence of neutrophils or leucocytoclasis. However, the division into leucocytoclastic and non-leucocytoclastic (lymphocytic) vasculitis is not absolute. Likewise, the clinical presentation of cutaneous vasculitis can vary considerably.
- The finding of leucocytoclasis should prompt a thorough review of drug treatment (e.g. sulfonamides, penicillin, thiazides), a search for infection (hepatitis B, HIV, β-haemolytic streptococcus), a screen for autoimmune rheumatic disease, malignancy (in particular myelo- and lymphoproliferative diseases), inflammatory bowel disease, chronic active hepatitis, and cryoglobulinaemia (see later).

**Table 15.5** Conditions associated with small vessel vasculitis

| Leucocytoclastic vasculitis | Allergic vasculitis (hypersensitivity angiitis): drugs, infection, inflammation, autoimmune disease, malignancy, Henoch–Schönlein purpura |
| --- | --- |
| | Urticarial vasculitis (hypocomplementaemic vasculitis) |
| | Cryoglobulinaemia |
| | Hypergammaglobulinaemia |
| | Erythema elevatum diutinum and granulomafaciale |
| Non-leucocytoclastic vasculitis (lymphocytic vasculitis) | Drugs (penicillins, thiazides) |
| | Nodular vasculitis (see ➲ 'Panniculitis', p. 473) |
| | Livedoid vasculitis |
| | Pityriasis lichenoides |

## Allergic (hypersensitivity) vasculitis

(See also ➋ Table 4.2, p. 212.)

- Allergic vasculitis is the most common pattern of presentation in adults, both sexes being affected equally.
- Non-blanching haemorrhagic papules (palpable purpura), purpuric macules, plaques, pustules, bullae, and ulcers may occur, classically distributed maximally over the lower leg.
- A low-grade fever, arthralgias, and microscopic haematuria may accompany such presentation.
- Often the condition is self-limiting and identifiable causes should be managed as appropriate. Analgesia may be needed and systemic steroids may be required for acute organ disease, especially progressive renal impairment.
- AZA may be appropriate for refractory disease but removal of the offending drug or exposure is the most effective treatment strategy.

## Henöch–Schönlein purpura (HSP; IgA vasculitis)

- HSP occurs most often in children (see ➋ 'Childhood-onset vasculitides', pp. 474–81), but can affect adults of any age. IgA is usually detected in skin, gut, or renal biopsies.
- The classic presentation is with purpura, and in adults: arthritis (50%), haemorrhagic GI disease (40%), and glomerulonephritis (50%).
- GCs given early may relieve joint and GI symptoms, but there is little evidence that they prevent progression of renal disease or influence overall outcome.
- If renal function is rapidly deteriorating, pulsed methylprednisolone and/or plasmapheresis may be of benefit.
- Patients who present with a nephritic or nephrotic syndrome have an increased lifetime prevalence of renal complications, including hypertension.
- Although most cases are self-limited, HSP can (rarely) become a chronic, relapsing disease. Such patients should be evaluated for the presence of a monoclonal IgA antibody, which may herald a pre-malignant lesion.

## Urticarial vasculitis

- Urticarial lesions with arthralgias are the most common features of this condition, with men outnumbering women by 2:1. The typical age of onset is 40–50 years.
- Morphologically, the skin lesions resemble ordinary urticaria and sometimes may be mistaken for erythema multiforme.
- Unlike ordinary urticaria, urticarial vasculitis tends to last for days (not hours) and tend to be burning and painful (not pruritic).
- Patients with hypocomplementaemic urticarial vasculitis tend to develop more systemic features such as renal, GI, and pulmonary disease. Less common manifestations include lymphadenopathy, uveitis, and benign intracranial hypertension.
- Systemic antihistamines are widely used, but their effects tend to be disappointing.

- There are anecdotal reports of success with indometacin, hydroxychloroquine (HCQ), colchicine, ciclosporin, and dapsone. AZA may be particularly effective.
- For the majority of patients, the condition is chronic and benign. For those with end-organ damage, chronic immunosuppression may be necessary.

## Cryoglobulinaemic vasculitis

- Cryoglobulins are immunoglobulins that precipitate when cold. They are divided into three types: type I (monoclonal), type II (mixed monoclonal and polyclonal), and type III (polyclonal).
- Mixed cryoglobulins are associated with autoimmune rheumatic diseases, infection, and lymphoproliferative disorders. Hepatitis B and C viral infection should always be excluded; the latter in particular is strongly associated with mixed essential cryoglobulinaemia.
- Mixed essential cryoglobulinaemia presents with purpuric skin lesions showing a leucocytoclastic vasculitis on biopsy; polyarthralgias (70%), weakness, progressive renal disease (55%), and transaminitis (70%) are common.
- Women are affected twice as frequently as men.
- Less common problems include oedema, hypertension, leg ulcers, Raynaud's disease, abdominal pain, neuropathy, and susceptibility to bacterial pneumonia.
- The prognosis is worse with renal disease.
- The main causes of death among patients with cryoglobulinaemia include renal failure and infection.
- Treatment requires management of the underlying cause; immunosuppression by itself is frequently unsatisfactory.
- Choice of immunosuppression should be dictated by the disease manifestations; the most severe forms may require treatment with CYC, pulse steroids, and plasmapheresis.

## Hypergammaglobulinaemic purpura

- This is a rare, benign IgM condition presenting as long-standing leucocytoclastic purpura similar to the cutaneous features of Sjögren's syndrome (see ➍ Chapter 12).
- It should not be confused with Waldenström's macroglobulinaemia, a monoclonal IgM paraproteinaemia associated with lymphoma.

## Erythema elevatum diutinum and granuloma faciale

- These are rare distinctive forms of chronic localized leucocytoclastic vasculitis. There are no systemic effects and the aetiology is unknown.
- Erythema elevatum diutinum (EED) is characterized by slowly enlarging oedematous purplish-brown plaques or blisters over the backs of the hands, elbows, or knees. They heal very slowly (months to years) with fibrosis. It may respond to dapsone.
- Granuloma faciale (GF) presents as single or multiple pink-brown, well-defined, smooth papules and plaques on the face. They persist for years. It is distinguished histologically from EED by the presence of eosinophils and a normal collagen beneath the epidermis. It may respond to intralesional steroids.

## Non-leucocytoclastic (lymphocytic) vasculitides

- The differential diagnosis of nodular forms of cutaneous vasculitis embraces a wide range of disorders, including the panniculitides (see ➲ Chapter 18 and Chapter 4, p. 206).
- Nodular vasculitis is regarded as a distinct group characterized by recurrent subcutaneous nodules. Patients are otherwise healthy though it may be associated with streptococcal infection.
- Bazin's disease is sometimes used to describe the nodular vasculitis that occurs in tuberculosis. The condition resolves spontaneously, but may take many years. Intralesional triamcinolone may help.
- Livedoid vasculitis is characterized histologically by endothelial cell proliferation and intraluminal thrombosis leading to ischaemia.
- Livedoid vasculitis has been attributed to defects in the tissue plasminogen activator (tPA) gene, although similar lesions can be seen in the antiphospholipid syndrome. The lesions heal with white atrophic scar ('atrophie blanche').
- Pityriasis lichenoides is an uncommon disorder of pink papules, which enlarge rapidly and may become haemorrhagic before becoming necrotic and heal with scarring. It is usually self-limiting and may respond to ultraviolet B irradiation.

# Childhood-onset vasculitides

- The primary vasculitides in children are rare but life-threatening conditions. The commonest are Kawasaki disease (KD) and the acute usually self-limiting Henoch–Schönlein purpura (HSP).
- Suspicion of the chronic vasculitides (Table 15.6) arises in the presence of fever (often low grade), weight loss, rash, and multisystem clinical features.
- As in adults, perivascular inflammation occurs and the site and size of affected vessels influences the spectrum of presentation.
- A history should be taken of infection, immunizations, family history and drug exposure.
- The first paediatric specific classification of vasculitis by EULAR and the Pediatric Rheumatology European Society (PRES) was developed in 2005 and validated in 2010.

## Epidemiology of childhood vasculitis

The incidence and prevalence of childhood-onset vasculitides are not accurately described and vary depending on the population studied.

- The prevalence of HSP is 3–20 per 100,000 of the general population, and of KD is 9–32 per 100,000 of the population in the USA and 134 per 100,000 of the population in Japan.
- The other childhood-onset vasculitides occur in 1–10 per million of the population.

**Table 15.6** Childhood-onset vasculitides

| Predominantly large vessel | Takayasu arteritis |
| --- | --- |
| Predominantly medium-sized vessel | Kawasaki disease<br>Systemic PAN<br>Cutaneous polyarteritis |
| Predominantly small vessel | *Non-granulomatous:*<br>HSP, leucocytoclastic, MPA, urticarial vasculitis |
| | *Granulomatous:*<br>GPA/Wegener's; EGPA/Churg–Strauss |
| Variable sized vessel involvement | Behçet's disease<br>Childhood primary angiitis of the CNS<br>Cogan's syndrome |
| Associated with systemic diseases or clear aetiologic factors | Relapsing polychondritis<br>Cryoglobulinaemia (/hepatitis C)<br>Malignancies<br>Autoimmune connective tissue diseases Drugs |

# Kawasaki disease

- KD is the leading cause of childhood acquired heart disease in developed countries and includes coronary artery aneurysms (in 15–25% of untreated cases) which often appear late.
- Pericarditis, myocarditis, and myocardial infarction may occur.
- With rapid detection and IVIg treatment, aneurysms occur in less than 5–10% of patients and mortality is reduced from 3–4% to <1%.
- The burden of adult cardiovascular disease and premature atherosclerosis is the subject of ongoing research.

## Epidemiology and pathogenesis

- The annual UK incidence of KD is 5–8 per 100,000 of the population, with a peak incidence in children aged 1–2 years (0–5 years typically), differing to Japan with a peak at 6–12 months of age.
- 5–10% of KD cases occur in children aged 5–10 years.
- The aetiology is unknown. Pronounced seasonality and clustering suggests an infectious or environmental trigger in genetically susceptible individuals.
- Recent epidemics have been linked to large-scale tropospheric wind currents originating in central Asia.

## Presentation

- Diagnostic criteria require a high spiking fever (usually ≥40°C) for ≥5 days; plus ≥4 of the following (*all criteria are not required at one time*):
  - Widespread polymorphic erythematous rash.
  - Bilateral conjunctival injection or congestion.
  - Reddening of the palms and soles, indurative oedema, and subsequent desquamation (Beau lines are seen in retrospect).
  - Reddening/cracking of lips, strawberry tongue, oral and pharyngeal injection.
  - Acute, usually single (>1.5 cm), non-purulent cervical lymphadenopathy.
- Fever may occur abruptly but there is a prodrome including coryza, abdominal pain, diarrhoea, vomiting, and arthralgia.
- Irritability is considered universal.
- KD is also diagnosed when there are <5 features *with* coronary aneurysm or dilatation or in an infant with pronounced irritability.
- *Incomplete* KD is diagnosed in patients with a fever and fewer than 4 additional features so that they receive IVIg before 10 days from fever onset. This is most common in infants.
- *Atypical* KD is diagnosed in children older than 9 years, younger than 6 months, and when there are additional inflammatory features.
- Other features include induration or redness at the BCG inoculation site; arthritis, uveitis, aseptic meningitis, pneumonitis, intestinal obstruction, hydrops of the gallbladder and jaundice, encephalopathy, macrophage activation syndrome, and SIADH.
- Persisting additional features should raise the possibility of alternative diagnoses. Coronary ectasia can occur in other conditions including systemic onset JIA, TA, and PAN.

*Investigations*
- Echocardiography should be done at diagnosis, 2 weeks, and 6–8 weeks after disease onset to detect myocardial inflammation and coronary aneurysmal formation.
- ECG will show conduction defects.
- There are no diagnostic blood tests but marked thrombocytosis may alert clinicians to KD.
- Viral serology (IgG and IgM) for mycoplasma pneumonia, enterovirus, adenovirus, measles, parvovirus, Epstein–Barr virus, and cytomegalovirus can be positive.

*Treatment*
The reduction in risk of long-term cardiac disease is best achieved with IVIg and aspirin started within 10 days of onset of fever.
- IVIg reduces the risk of coronary artery aneurysm formation from about 20% to 6%.
- IVIg (2 g/kg) is administered over 10–12 hours, except in infants with cardiac failure when the dose is split over 2–4 days.
- If the fever recurs or persists 36 hours after initial IVIg, a second dose is given.
- Although the evidence supports early use of IVIg, it may be given after 10 days of illness.
- Aspirin is initially given at a dose of 80–100 mg/kg/day, and reduced to 2–5 mg/kg/day when the fever has settled (low dose).
- Low-dose aspirin can be continued for a minimum of 6 weeks. It is then stopped if echocardiography is normal or when aneurysms have returned to normal.
- However, there is debate over the use of aspirin as RCT data are not available, and the positive considerations of its use must be balanced against the risk of Reye syndrome.
- Clopidogrel or dipyridamole may be temporarily substituted for aspirin in patients who develop influenza or varicella. Warfarin is substituted in the presence of giant aneurysms (>8 mm).
- Fever that recurs after two doses of IVIg is termed *IVIg resistance* and occurs in 10–20% of cases. It is associated with an increased risk of aneurysm.
- IVIg resistance is often treated with IV methylprednisolone 30 mg/kg (maximum 1 g) for 1–3 days followed by oral prednisolone (1–2 mg/kg daily) then with gradual dose reduction.
- Alternatively, infliximab (5 mg/kg) is associated with fewer days of fever and hospitalization compared to a second dose of IVIg, but a reduced rate aneurysm formation has not yet been defined.

## Henoch–Schönlein purpura
- HSP is the most common systemic vasculitis in childhood.
- HSP is a small vessel, non-granulomatous IgA leucocytoclastic vasculitis of unknown aetiology.
- HSP is generally a benign, self-limiting disease with most patients experiencing a full resolution within 8 weeks (<5% of patients develop chronic symptoms).

- One-third of children have symptoms for up to a fortnight, and another third for up to a 1 month.
- Recurrent disease occurs in 50% within 6 weeks.
- HSP nephritis accounts for up to 3% of all childhood cases of end-stage renal failure (ESRF) in the UK.

*Epidemiology*
- UK incidence is 20 per 100,000 of the general population per year (0.8/ 100,000 in adults).
- 75% occurs at the age of 2–11 years, and is rare in infancy.
- HSP is most prevalent during the winter and spring, and associations have been considered with infectious disease such as group A streptococci, hepatitis, CMV, HSV, human parvovirus B19, coxsackievirus, adenovirus, and some vaccinations.

*Presentation and clinical features*
- HSP has a characteristic purpuric rash (in 95% at presentation) affecting backs of the legs, buttocks, and arms, and in children needs to be distinguished from meningococcal septicaemia, acute haemorrhagic oedema of infancy, immune thrombocytopenic purpura, acute post-streptococcal glomerulonephritis, haemolytic-uraemic syndrome.
- Purpura rarely involves trunk or face. Urticaria, angio-oedema, deep bruising, or necrotic appearances may also occur.
- Abdominal pain may precede the rash by 2 weeks and may be associated with vomiting, haematemesis, and melena.
- GI complications are rare but include intussusception, appendicitis, cholecystitis, pancreatitis, ulceration, infarction, and perforation.
- Arthralgia or arthritis (47% of cases), typically of the knees and ankles, tends to be self-limiting.
- Nephritis affects 25–60% of patients.
- However, <5% of cases progress to CKD, and only 1–2% to ESRF (20% of children with renal disease and over 10–25 years).
- Renal prognosis is best in children <7 years.
- Renal disease occurs in 97% of children within 3 months of disease onset but generally <10% of patients require renal biopsy (usually for persisting haematuria and nephropathy).
- Rare manifestations include orchitis, pulmonary haemorrhage, and cerebral vasculitis.

*Treatment and monitoring*
- No treatment has been shown to shorten the duration of HSP or significantly improve long-term renal outcome.
- Treatment is primarily symptomatic (rest, analgesia, and hydration).
- Admission can be helpful where there is severe abdominal pain, GI haemorrhage and renal failure and occasionally for arthritis.
- Glucocorticoids (GCs) are used for symptomatic improvement and severe facial or scrotal oedema. Prednisolone dose is adjusted according to response and typically started at 1 mg/kg/day orally for 5 days. If higher doses or methylprednisolone are used, tertiary centre input is recommended.

- GCs are also used for persisting renal disease and where there are >50% crescentic glomerular involvement on renal biopsy.
- Severe renal involvement may require GC-sparing immunosuppression, antiproteinuric, and antihypertensive agents.
- Monitoring of the condition should be weekly for the first month, alternate weeks for 1 month and then monthly—the frequency increasing with renal involvement.
- Monthly urinalysis screening is recommended up to 6 months.

## Leucocytoclastic vasculitis

Leucocytoclastic vasculitis is a common small vessel vasculitis in children and presents as palpable purpura often with urticaria, vesicles, bullae, or pustules, but not itch, pain, or burning.

### Presentation and clinical features

- Internal involvement may include joints, GI system, and renal system.
- About 50% of cases may be idiopathic, 10–15% secondary to autoimmune disease (e.g. RA, SLE, IBD), about 5% are associated with malignancy and other cases attributed to medications or herbal remedies, food additives, or primarily underlying infection.
- ~10% of patients have chronic or recurrent disease.
- Erythema elevatum diutinum and granuloma faciale are rare distinctive forms of disease (with pink/purple-brown well-defined lesions).

### Investigations

(See also ➜ Table 4.2, p. 212 and Table 4.3, p. 214.)
- Investigations are for underlying infections (group A streptococci, viral hepatitis, and HIV), autoimmunity or malignancy.
- Measure total haemolytic complement (CH50 or CH100), C3, C4, anti-C1q antibodies if urticarial vasculitis is being considered and cryoglobulins if there is a suggestion of previous hepatitis C.
- Consider a skin biopsy if there is multisystem involvement and appearances are not typical of HSP.

### Treatment

- Treat underlying conditions and withdraw suspicious medications
- Treatment of primary disease includes GCs, colchicine, HCQ, dapsone, AZA, or MTX.
- RTX has been shown to be more effective than CYC for those with systemic involvement.

## Cutaneous polyarteritis nodosa

Cutaneous PAN is a paediatric condition that runs a benign course, over months to years, distinct from systemic polyarteritis nodosa.

### Presentation and clinical features

- Arthralgias, myalgias, and neuralgia may occur, but there is invariably no internal organ damage.
- Distinct from a leucocytoclastic vasculitis, cutaneous PAN results in larger inflammatory plaques, tender lumps and erythema nodosum (or other forms of panniculitis), ulceration.

- Infarcts attributable to medium vessel and pan-arteritis involvement. Post-inflammatory pigmentation may occur.
- Triggers include *Streptococcus* A, hepatitis B and C, HIV, and parvovirus B19.

*Investigations*

- Skin biopsy should confirm the diagnosis. See also ➔ Table 4.3, pp. 213–14.

*Treatment*

- Prednisolone is considered the mainstay of treatment, although there are no RCTs for glucocorticoids, colchicine, IVIg, or MTX.
- Penicillin is given for Strep A infection.
- Symptomatic treatment is often required for pain and ulcers.

## (Systemic) Polyarteritis nodosa

- PAN is the third most common vasculitis in children and adolescents.
- Childhood PAN is now more common than PAN in adults since the introduction of hepatitis B vaccine.
- PAN has an incidence of 3–7 per 100,000 per year.
- PAN characterized by a necrotizing vasculitis of medium-sized arteries, aneurysmal formation, thrombi, ischaemia, and infarction. It spares the smallest vessels and venules.

*Presentation and clinical features*

- PAN should be considered in patients with malaise, fever, weight loss (>5%), myalgia, arthropathy, and:
  - vasculitic rash (especially on the legs, palms, or soles).
  - mono/poly neuropathy (pure sensory or motor or mixed).
  - testicular tenderness or pain.
  - muscle tenderness or focal weakness.
- PAN is usually idiopathic, but may be secondary to viral hepatitis.
- Permanent morbidity is relatively rare but relapses occur in 35–50% over a mean of 6 years.
- Mortality is 4% over 5 years improved from 87% without treatment.
- Complications can include:
  - ulcerations and gangrene.
  - stroke, encephalopathy, myelopathy, and neuropathy.
  - pericarditis, coronary aneurysms, MI, and heart failure.
  - GI bleeding and infarction.
  - renal failure.
  - However, lungs are rarely affected.

*Investigations*

- Routine haematology, ESR, CRP, liver and renal biochemistry, CK, and hepatitis serology should be checked. See also ➔ Table 4.3, p. 214.
- Conventional renal and mesenteric angiography shows aneurysms and stenoses (not generally shown by CT or MRI angiography).
- Consider EMG, sural nerve, and muscle (e.g. vastus lateralis) biopsy.
- Biopsy of nodules and deep dermal ulcer margins may be helpful; however, renal biopsy is unhelpful and often associated with postoperative bleeding and fistulae.
- Other features include hypertension, retinal vasculitis, unexplained tachycardia, psychiatric symptoms, polymyositis, livedo reticularis, and Raynaud's disease.

*Treatment and prognosis*
- Active or latent hepatitis B may require concurrent antiviral therapy (e.g. lamivudine) in addition to immunosuppression.
- GC therapy should be combined with either MMF, MTX, or AZA.
- CYC is used for serious organ involvement or steroid-refractory disease.
- The role of plasmapheresis remains to be determined.
- Prognostic scoring, using the FFS may be useful (FFS =1 has a mortality of 25%; FFS = 2 has a mortality of 45%; etc.). The five factors—each scoring one—are.
  - Renal failure.
  - Proteinuria (>1 g/dL).
  - GI bleed or perforation or infarction or pancreatitis.
  - Cardiomyopathy.
  - CNS involvement (<10%).

## Primary angiitis of central nervous system in children (cPACNS)
- CNS vasculitis is increasingly recognized in children but presents a diagnostic challenge. A lack of consensus on disease classification has made it difficult to establish the true incidence of the disease.
- Brainworks (ℜ http//www.sickkids.ca/research/brainworks/) is helping to better clarify this condition and provides support when there is diagnostic uncertainty.
- Secondary CNS vasculitis occurs in a broad set of systemic conditions, including neurosarcoidosis, which is a differential diagnosis.

*Presentation and clinical features*
- Clinical presentation is typically with non-focal symptoms including headaches and altered mental state (in 50% of cases).
- Alternatively, children present with localizing symptoms include lateralized weakness (30%), aphasia, ataxia, visual symptoms, and seizures (each ~15%).
- The spinal cord is involved in 5–15% of cases.
- Systemic features are rare.
- Mimics of CNS vasculitis should be considered, and include:
  - Moyamoya disease.
  - Thrombophilic conditions (e.g. antiphospholipid syndrome).
  - Neurological conditions (e.g. multiple sclerosis, Devic's disease).
  - Metabolic conditions.
  - Sarcoidosis.
  - Malignancy.

*Investigations*
- Diagnostic criteria[13] require:
  - An acquired neurological deficit.
  - Angiographic and/or histopathological features of CNS angiitis.
  - Absence of a systemic condition.
- Catheter arteriography is the gold standard diagnostic test due to an ability to detect distal lesions affecting smaller vessels and identify lesion in the posterior part of the brain.

- MRI of brain and/or spine and MRA may demonstrate acute ischaemia of varying patterns dependent on size of vessel involve and use of diffusion-weighted imaging (for large vessel disease).
- Meningeal enhancement may be seen with MRA which can reveal beading, tortuosity, stenosis, and occlusion of the vessels.
- Brain biopsy should be considered for difficult cases when arteriography is negative or in cases with a poor response to therapy.

*Treatment and prognosis*
- Current therapeutic recommendations are similar to those for systemic vasculitis:
  - Induction with IV CYC, GCs and low-dose aspirin.
  - 1–2-year maintenance therapy with MMF or AZA, simultaneously reducing the dose of prednisolone but continuing aspirin.
  - Full anticoagulation may need to be considered.
- A poor prognosis is suggested by presentation with neurocognitive dysfunction, seizures, multifocal parenchymal lesions on MRI, or distal stenosis on arteriography.

## ANCA-associated vasculitides (AAVs)
- Using internationally recognized diagnostic criteria and algorithms, 80% of paediatric AAV patients are GPA, 15% are MPA, and 5% are EGPA. Cases of renal-limited vasculitis (crescentic glomerulonephritis) are also included.
- The Paediatric Vasculitis Activity Score, PVAS (modified from BVAS), has been validated for objective assessment of childhood vasculitis.
- Of all AAV childhood cases, 55% are cANCA positive (almost consistently PR3 positive), 30% are pANCA positive (90% MPO positive), and 3% are mixed cytoplasmic and perinuclear.
- Median age at diagnosis is 14 years with a relatively high burden of disease (median PVAS of 19).
- Time from symptom onset to diagnosis is now quick, averaging 2.5 months, but rates of organ damage at this time are still high.
- 80% of patients have pulmonary or renal disease; 60% have both.
- Pulmonary presentations include alveolar haemorrhage and massive haemoptysis.
- 10–20% of cases present in renal failure which requires dialysis and 5% have end-stage renal disease.
- ENT involvement occurs in 60% and MSK in 50%.
- CYC and GCs have been used most commonly to induce disease remission but in keeping with practice with adult cases, RTX is increasingly used.
- The choice of maintenance therapy after induction of remission includes MTX, AZA, and MMF.
- Plasmapheresis is usually for pulmonary-renal syndrome and alveolar haemorrhage.
- Low-dose aspirin is used to decrease thrombosis risk.
- Co-trimoxazole use for nasal *Staphylococcus* carriage is controversial.
- High levels of organ damage still occur. In one large study of GPA in children, 40% had chronic renal impairment at 3 years of disease duration.

## Reference
3. Calabrese LH, Furlan AJ, Gragg LA, et al. Primary angiitis of the central nervous system: diagnostic criteria and clinical approach. *Cleve Clin J Med* 1992;59:293–306.

# Metabolic bone diseases

Osteogenesis imperfecta is included in ➲ Chapter 19

# Osteoporosis

Osteoporosis can be defined as a decrease in bone mass and strength resulting in an increased risk of fracture with minimal or no trauma ('fragility fracture').

- Osteoporosis can be defined using dual X-ray absorptiometry (DXA) to derive an estimate of bone mineral density (BMD).
- The clinical consequence of osteoporosis is fragility fracture and its consequences, which include pain, skeletal deformity, functional loss (including loss of mobility and independence in the elderly), and reduced life expectancy (e.g. hip fracture in the elderly).
- The risk of osteoporotic fracture is greater in women than in men and varies with site (Table 16.1).

## Pathogenesis and classification

- During childhood and adolescence, growth and skeletal modelling lead to an increase in the size, shape, strength, and composition of bone. Growth ceases with the closure of the growth plates (epiphyseal cartilage). However, remodelling and mineral homeostasis continue throughout life with bone resorption and deposition coupled by the interaction between osteoclasts and osteoblasts, respectively.
- Peak bone mass/BMD or maximal bone density is usually achieved in the third decade. Peak bone mass is determined by both genetic and environmental factors.
- After about the age of 35 years, the amount of bone produced is less than that resorbed during each remodelling cycle. The net effect is an age-related decrease in bone mass. Trabecular and cortical BMD decline by ~6% and 3% respectively per decade.
- Accelerated bone loss occurs at the time of menopause with declining ovarian function and circulating oestrogen. Up to 15% of bone mass can be lost over the 5-year period immediately after menopause. The andropause (decreased circulating bioavailable testosterone, so decreased aromatization to oestrogen) occurs for many men over many years through late-middle and advanced age. There is a moderate correlation between serum testosterone and BMD.

**Table 16.1** Risk of osteoporotic fracture with site

| Fracture site | Overall lifetime risk of fracture (%) | |
| --- | --- | --- |
| | Men | Women |
| Hip | 6 | 18 |
| Vertebral | 5 | 16 |
| Distal forearm | 2–3 | 16 |
| Any of above | 13 | 40 |

- The mechanism of age-related bone loss is multifactorial and is a consequence of genetic, environmental, and comorbid influences:
  - decreased intestinal calcium absorption.
  - decreased synthesis of vitamin D.
  - hyperparathyroidism (caused by the above).
  - factors increasing osteoclast function (e.g. oestrogen lack).
  - reduced osteoblast development (e.g. ageing-related stem cell fate—away from osteoblast in favour of adipocyte).
  - increasing immobility reducing the physical stress on bone leading to activation of bone resorption.
- Risk factors for osteoporosis (see also Table 16.2) include:
  - race (Caucasian or Asian > Afro Caribbean).
  - increasing age and female gender.
  - positive family history (especially parental hip fracture).
  - previous 'fragility' fracture.
  - drugs (e.g. glucocorticoid (GC) therapy).
  - chronic inflammatory diseases (e.g. RA, Crohn's disease, AS)
  - malabsorption (e.g. coeliac disease)
  - endocrinopathies (e.g. hyperparathyroidism, Cushing's syndrome)
  - low body mass index (BMI <18).
  - short fertile period (late menarche, early menopause).
  - diseases of bone marrow (e.g. mastocytosis, Gaucher disease)
  - immobility, sedentary lifestyle.
  - low intake of calcium (<240 mg daily).
  - excessive alcohol intake.
  - smoking.
- The World Health Organization has developed a Fracture Assessment Tool (FRAX; ℘ htpp://www.shef.ac.uk/FRAX) to identify patients at risk of fragility fracture. BMD measurement is incorporated into FRAX. Assessing BMD alone to predict fragility fracture may lead to an incomplete fragility fracture risk profile. FRAX takes account of many of the major BMD-independent fragility fracture risk factors (with the exception of falls risk) and allows a calculation of a 10-year risk of fragility fracture:
  - age, low BMI, and gender.
  - prior fragility fracture.
  - GC use.
  - parental history of hip fracture.
  - rheumatoid arthritis.
  - secondary osteoporosis (selected causes).
  - current smoker and daily alcohol >3 units.

## Idiopathic juvenile osteoporosis

- Idiopathic juvenile osteoporosis (IJO) is uncommon. It occurs before or at onset of puberty. It affects the sexes equally. The cause is unknown and there are no consistent biochemical abnormalities.
- IJO should be discriminated from osteogenesis imperfecta (OI; see ⊃ Chapter 19) and osteoporosis from secondary causes (e.g. see Table 16.2).

**Table 16.2** Diseases that cause, or are associated with, osteoporosis (incomplete)

| | |
|---|---|
| Malignancies | Multiple myeloma |
| | Leukaemia |
| | Lymphoma |
| Endocrine | Hyperparathyroidism |
| | Hypopituitarism |
| | Thyrotoxicosis |
| | Hypogonadism |
| | Cushing's syndrome |
| | Diabetes (T1DM/T2DM) |
| | Turner's syndrome |
| Chronic inflammatory diseases | Rheumatoid arthritis |
| | Ankylosing spondylitis |
| | Crohn's disease |
| | Cystic fibrosis |
| Metabolic diseases | Gaucher disease |
| | Chronic kidney diseases 3b–5 |
| | Alcoholism |
| Skeletal diseases | Osteogenesis imperfecta |
| | Mastocytosis |
| Diseases and conditions associated with immobilization | Multiple sclerosis |
| | Paraplegia |
| | Space flight |
| Drugs | Glucocorticoids (GCs) |
| | Anticonvulsants |
| | Calcineurin inhibitors |
| | Levothyroxine (in excess) |
| | Heparin |

- The child presents with pain, non-traumatic fractures around the weight-bearing joints, and collapsed vertebrae. No specific treatment is available and for most, bone mass increases to normal values as puberty progresses; however, in some cases fractures may lead to deformity. Supportive physical therapy should be made available.
- Children with IJO and all forms of osteoporosis have low BMD for their age and skeletal development. It is essential that DXA scan-derived BMD data are adjusted for skeletal development if growth deviates from average velocity significantly (see ISCD position statements online: ℘ https://www.iscd.org/official-positions/) using skeletal growth adjustment algorithms (for UK data, using bone mineral apparent density (BMAD)).

*Glucocorticoid-induced osteoporosis (GIO)*

- GIO is a common and (as published audits continually suggest) a poorly managed condition.
- Numerous guidelines for managing GIO risk exist (e.g. ACR, EULAR, American Society of Bone Mineral Research (USA), National Osteoporosis Foundation (USA), National Osteoporosis Society (UK))
- The effects of GIO are greatest in the older patient given the additional osteoporosis risk factors and comorbidities likely.
- The effect of GCs on the skeleton is most profound with early GC treatment, so preventive osteoporosis strategies need considering at the beginning of GC use, particularly in the elderly.
- Any vitamin D deficiency and secondary hyperparathyroidism requires correcting at the outset of any GC treatment.
- GP patient databases suggest patients on long-term inhaled GCs may be at increased of osteoporosis defined by DXA, but there is no overall evidence that there is an increased risk of fracture compared to control patients with underlying lung diseases.
- The pathogenesis of GIO is complex. There are direct effects of GCs on bone cells and indirect effects through an influence of metabolic and endocrine factors though convincing data in humans for all these effects being systematic are lacking (Table 16.3).
- A bisphosphonate should be recommended, to patients ≥65 years and 50–65 years old with multiple risk factors for osteoporosis, who will take GCs ≥3 months and should be started simultaneously with the GCs.
- For younger patients FRAX (⅍ http://www.shef.ac.uk/FRAX) is useful to predict major fragility fracture risk or very low risk in patients before starting GCs. FRAX can be used without DXA scan data and can be adjusted depending on GC dose.

Table 16.3 Pathogenesis of glucocorticoid-induced osteoporosis (GIO)

| Mechanism | Effect |
|---|---|
| Direct effects on bone cells | Reduced recruitment of osteoblasts from bone marrow precursors |
| | Induce apoptosis of osteocytes |
| Possible contributing indirect effects | Reduce production of sex hormones |
| | Increased PTH production and PTH sensitivity |
| | Reduced GI calcium absorption |
| | Decreased calcium reabsorption from kidney |
| | Decreased efficiency of vitamin D activation |
| | Sarcopenic effect of steroids (falls risk etc.) |

## Clinical features

- Osteoporosis frequently presents with low-trauma fracture.
- Other presentations include back pain (vertebral fracture due to osteoporosis), loss of height evident in the spine by 'xmas-tree' folds of skin of the back or the lower rib cage margin approximating to the iliac crests, thoracic spine kyphosis (multiple vertebral fractures can cause this though this is not the commonest cause for kyphosis).
- Features of the cause of osteoporosis may be obvious or not. For example, immobility due to spinal cord injury and paraplegia (potent cause of bone loss) but hypogonadism in men, though detectable to an experienced clinician, may be subtle and relatively 'invisible'.
- Obvious and/or important clinical features that might be detected to indicate conditions highly associated with osteoporosis include stigmata for chronic alcohol excess, hypogonadism features in men, Cushing's disease appearance, etc.
- High falls risk is an important clinical feature. Though high falls risk does not define osteoporosis, it is arguably the main risk factor for fracture in the elderly, and it can be detected systematically using guidelines (see UK advice in NICE Clinical Guideline 161).[1]

## Investigations

- People aged >50 years old who have a fragility fracture should be investigated to exclude secondary causes of osteoporosis (e.g. hyperparathyroidism, CKD3b–5, myeloma, etc.).
- Any fracture in a person >75 years suggests some degree of skeletal fragility, regardless of DXA scan-derived BMD; tests for underlying disease is advisable.
- Plain radiographs are an insensitive method of assessing bone mass but lateral spinal images are useful for staging previous vertebral fractures, which may have occurred with minimal symptomology.
- The standard technique for measuring BMD is DXA. It is quick, accurate, low in radiation dose, and is fairly precise. Sites measurable include lumbar spine, femoral neck, forearm, and whole body.
- DXA is typically interpreted in terms of the T-score or Z-score. The T-score (used only by convention for postmenopausal women and men >50 years of age) is the SD multiple difference between the individual's BMD compared with the mean peak BMD achieved in the third decade matched for gender and ethnicity. The Z score (used by convention in premenopausal women and children and all men <50 years of age) is the standard deviation (SD) multiple difference between the individual's BMD and the age/gender/ethnicity-matched average. T- and Z-scores can be minus values. In postmenopausal women, for every SD decrease in BMD there is a twofold increase in the risk of fracture.
- Quantitative CT allows volume measurements and can distinguish between cortical and trabecular bone in vertebrae. It is, however, costly and entails a high radiation exposure.
- Bone ultrasound (US) of the os calcis has been used to predict fracture. Both the attenuation and speed of US in bone may relate to material properties of bone relevant to fragility and fracture.

- Bone biopsy (undecalcified transiliac) may be useful in cases of multiple comorbidity to discriminate high and low turnover disease and whether there is demineralization but is not routinely in the assessment of osteoporosis.
- Routine biochemical and haematological tests are usually normal in osteoporosis. High bone turnover disease may be indicated by high bone turnover markers (e.g. collagen crosslinks (CTX)).
- Reduction of CTX has been linked with bisphosphonate response and may be an indicator of drug adherence.

## Prevention of osteoporosis and fragility fractures

- The prevention of a first fragility (osteoporotic) fracture is termed 'primary prevention' and prevention of second and subsequent fragility fractures—'secondary prevention' (/treatment of osteoporosis).
- All people who have a fragility fracture after the age of 50 years (or for women, if post-menopausal) should be assessed for their risk of further fragility fracture and osteoporosis. Typically, this will be done by a Fracture Liaison Service (FLS) linked to the Orthopaedic Unit (secondary prevention assessment).
- Underlying diseases (known or unknown) and modifiable clinical or lifestyle issues relevant to skeletal health will be identified in many patients by such an assessment. FLSs will triage patients for specialist assessment or secondary fracture prevention management including DXA scanning and considering osteoporosis medications.
- Primary prevention is best undertaken by case-finding based on the presence of osteoporosis risk factors, utilizing the FRAX risk factor tool (% http://www.shef.ac.uk/FRAX) then obtaining DXA in people with multiple risk factors or high scores on FRAX. Osteoporosis treatment can be considered based on BMD and fracture risk.

### Calcium

- Calcium intake, either increased by dietary intake or supplements, has not been shown to prevent osteoporotic fractures.
- However, chronic calcium lack leads to secondary hyperparathyroidism which can cause accelerated bone loss and this may contribute to osteoporosis and bone fragility.
- Providing calcium supplements is wise if there is a low-calcium diet (e.g. poor in dairy products) and/or secondary hyperparathyroidism.
- Calcium supplementation in pre-pubertal children enhances the rate of increase in BMD with age but whether this translates into higher peak BMD is unknown.
- At present the use of calcium supplements is recommended for:
  - calcium deficiency indicated by secondary hyperparathyroidism if vitamin D levels are replete (but reasonable then to rule out coeliac disease/poor GI absorption).
  - poor calcium diet particularly in children (<400 mg/day).
  - to optimize the effect of bisphosphonate therapy.
- There has been considerable debate as to whether calcium supplementation is associated with an increased risk of cardio/cerebrovascular disease.

*Exercise*
- There is some evidence to suggest that weight-bearing activity decreases the rate of bone loss around the menopause, although the level and type of activity remains unclear.
- There is little impact of exercise in improving bone mass once osteoporotic, although it may aid in preventing further loss.
- Profound losses of hip BMD in the elderly may be highly and predominantly influenced by reduction of mobility/weight-bearing.

*Hormone replacement*
- Oestrogen replacement therapy is an effective way of preventing post-menopausal bone loss. The addition of a progestogen allows endometrial shedding and minimizes risk of neoplasia.
- The minimum oral dose of estradiol required is 1 mg/day, and conjugated oestrogen 0.3 mg/day. Estradiol gels and transdermal treatments should be started at 1 mg/day or 25 micrograms/day, respectively.
- Evidence suggests that the use of HRT increases risk of DVT, coronary artery disease, breast cancer, and stroke. HRT should therefore be used with caution, should be time limited, and used when the risks of these diseases otherwise is lowest.

*Bisphosphonates*
- Weekly oral bisphosphonates (risedronate or alendronic acid) reduce fragility fractures by 35–50% at the spine and by less at the hip in women who have had a fragility fracture or osteoporosis-range BMD.
- Monthly ibandronic acid 150 mg is also licensed for postmenopausal osteoporosis. Cyclical etidronate is nowadays seldom used.
- Fracture prevention data with oral bisphosphonates is not as extensive for men as for women but treatment is considered effective for men with fragility fracture and with DXA-defined osteoporosis.
- IV zoledronic acid 5 mg given yearly (×3 years original RCT data), is available if oral therapies fail, are not tolerated or contraindicated. Fracture prevention is as much as 70% for vertebral fractures in 3 years.
- Ibandronic acid 3 mg IV ('push' injection taking just a few seconds) once every 3 months is licensed also for postmenopausal women and some bone physicians considered it relatively safe in mild renal impairment, where zoledronic acid is not used (i.e. estimated GFR 25–35 mL/min/1.73 m²) and denosumab is contraindicated.
- Currently most physicians will review the balance of risks and benefits of long-term bisphosphonate therapy after 5-year oral, and 3-year parenteral, bisphosphonate use. For those patients still at high fracture risk though, treatment can be continued for a further 3–5 years accordingly.
- The emerging concern about the incidence of atypical femoral fractures (AFFs) in long-term bisphosphonate users has prompted changes in strategic long-term planning of medications for osteoporosis. AFFs can present with proximal femoral bone pain for many months before (somewhat catastrophic) subtrochanteric fracture, and can be bilateral. Cause is unknown but thought to be a combination of low bone turnover/bone replacement at a site of critical weight-bearing stress on the femoral bone.

- In general, bisphosphates are well tolerated, but should be used with caution in renal impairment (estimated GFR <30 mL/min/1.73 m²), history of oesophageal reflux/hiatus hernia, or poor dentition requiring dental work (risk of mandibular osteonecrosis).
- Oral medications should be taken fasting. Absorption may be optimum if food intake is avoided for 60 minutes following taking the tablet. Symptoms of nausea and reflux can be lessened by taking with plenty of water and avoid lying down after taking the tablet.
- Adherence with oral therapy is variable with reports from the USA of <30%, but reports in the UK of >80% at 2–4 years' therapy. Adherence is best when treatment is started by a FLS following fragility fracture in comparison to starting as part of primary fragility fracture prevention treatment plan.
- The effects of bisphosphonates are optimized if vitamin D remains replete and there is sufficient calcium intake to prevent deficiency (e.g. no secondary hyperparathyroidism).
- The therapeutic effect of bisphosphonates can be predicted to a degree by demonstration of a reduction in bone resorption biomarkers (e.g. CTX) measured on serum or plasma before and 2 months after treatment is started.

*Strontium ranelate*

- Strontium ranelate 2 g daily was shown to decrease fracture risk over 3 years in men and postmenopausal women (by about 40%), but its use has been considerably restricted in recent years because it increases vascular disease risk (e.g. CVD, IHD, and thrombosis). Strontium has now been withdrawn from use.
- Strontium is similar to calcium chemically but much 'heavier'. It is incorporated into the hydroxyapatite bone matrix and naturally leads to large increases in BMD, though the relationship of change in BMD to change in fracture risk is neither linear nor proportional to BMD changes associated with fracture risk reduction seen in other therapies, for example.
- The association with markedly increased BMD is important to note when reviewing serial DXA scan data on patients previously treated with strontium.

*Teriparatide*

- Teriparatide is a parathyroid hormone analogue given as a SC injection daily for 2 years.
- Licensed for use in postmenopausal osteoporosis, though not in men, it reduced vertebral fracture risk by about 70%.
- Teriparatide initially triggers osteoblast-mediated bone matrix production then an increase in bone turnover. It may achieve therefore a gain in bone ('anabolic') unlike anti-resorption therapies.
- In the UK, teriparatide is heavily restricted for use for NHS postmenopausal osteoporosis by NICE and cannot be used without specialist application for individual funding for men with osteoporosis.

*Denosumab*
- Denosumab is a fully human monoclonal antibody that inhibits the RANK ligand, and is a potent inhibitor of bone resorption.
- Denosumab is licensed in Europe for a range of bone loss conditions including post-menopausal osteoporosis and bone loss in patients being treated with hormone ablation for prostate and breast cancer.
- Denosumab 60 mg SC injection once every 6 months reduces vertebral fracture rate by about 70% in postmenopausal women with osteoporosis over 3 years (FREEDOM trial).
- The FREEDOM trial extension now shows fracture prevention, BMD accrual, and no major safety issues for up to 8 years' continuous use.

*Odanacatib*
- Odanacatib was developed a cathepsin K inhibitor to inhibit osteoclastic bone resorption, then slowing bone loss.
- Phase II data indicate that 50 mg once weekly inhibits bone resorption and increases BMD, with only a transient decrease in bone formation.
- In a phase III RCT, fracture reduction was shown but subsequently the drug was withdrawn due to an unacceptably high number of cerebrovascular events in patients in the treatment arm.

*Romosozumab*
- The monoclonal antibody romosozumab binds to sclerostin thus inhibiting the effect of sclerostin, which is an osteocyte-derived inhibitor of osteoblast activity, thus increasing bone formation.
- In the phase III FRAME (FRActure study in postmenopausal woMen with ostEoporosis) study, which enrolled 7180 women, SC 210 mg dose of romosozumab resulted in a statistically significant 73% reduction in the relative risk of a new vertebral fracture at 12 months compared to those receiving placebo (fracture incidence 0.5% vs 1.8%, respectively ($p$ <0.001).
- At time of going to press the licensing for romosozumab is on hold pending further investigation into cardiovascular adverse events in clinical trials.

*Abaloparatide*
- Abaloparatide is a novel synthetic analogue of human PTHrP (1–34).
- It can stimulate bone formation with less accompanying bone resorption and hypercalcaemic effects that can occur with PTH (1–34).
- In postmenopausal osteoporosis, weekly SC abaloparatide, compared with placebo, reduced the risk of new vertebral and non-vertebral fractures over 18 months (ACTIVE study).
- Treatment with a bisphosphonate after an 18-month course of abaloparatide may consolidate BMD and fracture risk reduction gains.

*Other therapies*
- Vertebroplasty is the percutaneous injection of bone cement into painful fractured vertebrae. It can be used to treat osseous haemangiomas and fractures caused by malignancy.
- Initially vertebroplasty was reported to reduce the pain of vertebral fractures though RCTs then showed conflicting results. Currently a large RCT (vs sham procedure) is in process (VERTOS IV).

- Kyphoplasty (balloon inflation in the vertebral body then balloon injected with bone cement as for vertebroplasty) is unproven by robust study as to whether there is cost-effectivity of the procedure vs conservative fracture pain management or vs vertebroplasty.

*Guidelines for managing osteoporosis*

- In the UK, Europe and North America, numerous societies have generated guidelines for managing osteoporosis.
- In the UK, NICE guidelines operate to control funding treatments in the NHS. Guidelines are based on economic models of disease and treatment effects, not on clinical factors alone. The reader is advised to consult the NICE Technology Appraisal Guidance (TA204 and TA464) and Clinical Guideline 146.[2]
- In the UK the National Osteoporosis Guideline Group regularly posts consensus guidelines (e.g. see: ℘ https://www.shef.ac.uk/NOGG/).

### References

1. NICE. *Falls in Older People: Assessing Risk and Prevention* (CG161). London: NICE, 2017. ℘ https://www.nice.org.uk/guidance/cg161
2. NICE CG146. ℘ https://www.nice.org.uk/guidance/cg146

# Vitamin D deficiency, osteomalacia, and rickets

- Osteomalacia (adults) and rickets (children) are characterized by defective mineralization of bone and cartilage and the accumulation of unmineralized bone matrix (osteoid).
- Rickets is the term used for this defect in growing children before the closure of the epiphyses.
- There is considerable debate over the level of 25-hydroxyvitamin D (25(OH)D) that constitutes 'repletion' and 'deficiency'. For the majority of the UK population a reasonable 'repletion' level is >50 nmol/L and deficiency level <30 nmol/L. In the elderly, levels of 'insufficiency' (30– 50 nmol/L) may be pathologically relevant and a better 'repletion' level taken as >75 nmol/L.
- There are many causes of osteomalacia, but essentially they all occur due to either a deficiency (low sunlight exposure, dietary lack, or suboptimal metabolism) or resistance to vitamin D, or a non-PTH related defect in renal handling of phosphate (Table 16.4).
- In both osteomalacia and rickets, PTH is invariably raised due to vitamin D-associated calcium lack. High PTH can increase bone turnover/bone loss and amplify bone loss in osteoporosis.
- Both vitamin $D_2$ (ergocalciferol) from vegetables in the diet, and vitamin $D_3$ (cholecalciferol) from animal tissues and *de novo* synthesis in skin, are metabolized in the liver to 25(OH)D (25(OH)$D_2$/25(OH)$D_3$) and then in the kidney to 1,25-dihydroxyvitamin $D_2$/$D_3$ respectively: the active forms of vitamin D.

**Table 16.4** A simple classification of osteomalacia

| Low 25(OH)D | Reduced availability | Poor diet, UV skin exposure or malabsorption |
| --- | --- | --- |
| | Metabolic | Chronic renal failure |
| | | Anticonvulsant drugs |
| | | Hepatobiliary disease |
| Normal 25(OH)D | 1α-hydroxylase mutations | Vitamin D-dependent rickets type I |
| | Vitamin D receptor mutations | Vitamin D-dependent rickets type II |
| Phosphate loss | FGF23 excess | X-linked hypophosphataemia |
| | | Oncogenic—hypophosphataemia |
| | Tubular dysfunction | Fanconi syndrome |
| Skeletal toxicity | Defective mineralization | Aluminium, fluoride |

- 1,25-dihydroxyvitamin $D_3$ is considered more biologically potent than 1,25-dihydroxyvitamin $D_2$ and negatively affects both 1$\alpha$-hydroxylase (its own activating enzyme), and transcription of the PTH gene, but increases the capacity of GI calcium absorption by enhancing the transcription and therefore effect of calcium sensing receptors (CaSRs).
- 1,25-dihydroxyvitamin $D_3$ stimulates bone formation through stimulating osteoblast differentiation and activity thereby increasing coupled bone turnover.
- 25(OH)$D_3$ can be also be converted into 24,25-dihydroxyvitamin $D_3$, which is biologically inactive and destined for excretion.

## Clinical and laboratory findings

- Classical symptoms of osteomalacia are bone pain and tenderness, bone deformity (depending on age of onset), and proximal muscle weakness (waddling gait); muscle enzymes and biopsy are normal.
- The hypocalcaemia of osteomalacia usually does not cause symptoms but can cause paraesthesia and tetany. Rarely, it is severe enough to cause cardiac dysrhythmia, convulsions, or psychosis.
- Children with rickets may be hypotonic and apathetic with growth retardation and delayed walking. On weight-bearing, bones become bowed, and there is irregularity of the metaphyseal–epiphyseal junction, usually at the wrist and costochondral junctions. The latter gives rise to the feature 'rachitic rosary'. An indentation may also arise along the attachment of the diaphragm to the softened ribs (Harrison's groove). Rapid growth of the softened skull leads to craniotabes, parietal bone flattening, and frontal bossing. Dentition is delayed and poor.
- In rickets, many bony deformities persist despite treatment (unless due to simple dietary deficiency and treated early) and may require surgery, e.g. tibial osteotomy to correct lower limb alignment.
- The classical radiographic change of osteomalacia is the pseudo-fracture (Looser's zone). These are incomplete radiolucent fracture lines perpendicular to the cortex, with poor callus formation and found most often at ribs, clavicles, pubic rami, femoral neck, metatarsals, and outer border of scapulae.
- Laboratory investigations show low 25(OH)D, a low or low reference range serum calcium and phosphate, elevated ALP, low urinary calcium excretion, and secondary hyperparathyroidism.
- Osteomalacia may exist with reference range levels of calcium, phosphate, and ALP; thus only raised PTH, reduced 25(OH)D, and low urinary calcium (24 hour), tested simultaneously, disclose the diagnosis.
- Levels of 1,25-dihydroxyvitamin D may be in the reference range and are therefore not routinely tested.
- Vitamin D deficiency through poor diet intake is rare unless combined with exposure to sunlight. It is a phenomenon seen most often in the housebound elderly, and in immigrant Asian populations.
- Intestinal disorders that lead to fat malabsorption can cause vitamin D deficiency, as vitamin D is fat soluble.

## Management of hypovitaminosis D, rickets, and osteomalacia

- The strategy should be to replace 25(OH)D to target repletion level, provide enough calcium to mineralize bone normalizing any secondary hyperparathyroidism, control skeletal pain, pursue a physio-led muscle rehabilitation regimen if there is any myopathy, and finally prevent the condition from recurring.
- Quite commonly there may be two lesions in the elderly: osteomalacia and osteoporosis. It is unknown to what degree bisphosphonate therapy for osteoporosis will impair mineralization/osteomalacia recovery if treatment for both conditions is given simultaneously. Delaying osteoporosis treatment for 4–6 weeks is unlikely to harm and may give valuable time for osteomalacia healing based on necessary higher bone turnover (can be indicated by an 'ALP flare').
- Bone pain and muscle weakness respond quickly to successful replacement therapy though laboratory and radiological features may take longer to return to normal.
- In adults, various regimens for cholecalciferol replacement might be recommended (e.g. 20,000 IU cholecalciferol weekly for 5 weeks), though caution has been advised in regard of 'over-replacement regimens', which have been associated with an increased falls and fracture risk.
- An alternative (and potentially well-adhered-to regimen) is 3200 IU colecalciferol daily in twice-daily doses for a calendar month. Repletion status should then be tested with repeat 25(OH)D check and repeat course of treatment given if required.
- Vitamin-D (and calcium) lack may be habitual as it depends on UV-skin exposure and dietary preferences. Identification of repeat deficiency then in future is facilitated by periodic 25(OH)D testing.
- Co-treatment with calcium supplements isn't necessary in all cases but is usually safe at daily supplement doses of 500–1000 mg without causing hypercalcaemia.

## Vitamin D-dependent rickets

- Type I vitamin D-dependent rickets is a rare autosomal recessive disease caused by inactivating mutations in the 1α-hydroxylase gene. Low levels of 1,25-dihydroxyvitamin D result. Children are often affected with rickets before the age of 2 years, and fail to respond to normal levels of vitamin D replacement. Treatment is most effective with physiological doses of 1,25-dihydroxyvitamin D (e.g. calcitriol).
- Type II vitamin D-dependent rickets is an autosomal recessive disorder caused by loss of function mutations in the vitamin D receptor (VDR). About 70% of patients will have alopecia—an important prognostic feature when discussing likely outcome of treatment. In patients with normal hair, remission can be achieved with high levels of 1,25-dihydroxyvitamin D. Only about 50% of patients with alopecia will respond to a similar therapeutic approach.

## Osteomalacia from altered phosphate homeostasis

- Osteomalacia from phosphate depletion is histologically the same in the skeleton as 25(OH)D deficiency, although serum calcium and 25(OH)D are/can be normal.
- X-linked (AD) hypophosphataemic rickets (XLHR) is a disorder of vitamin D resistance. It is important to diagnose early in young children as treatment prevents bone deformity.
- XLHR manifests as delayed growth, short stature, lower limb skeletal deformity, and rickets.
- In XLHR, dental development can be delayed but dentition is usually normal. Proximal myopathy is not a feature. Laboratory tests show a low serum phosphate, normal serum calcium and PTH, and low/normal 1,25-dihydroxyvitamin D with high FGF23. The renal tubular maximum reabsorption of phosphate for GFR is low for the degree of hypophosphataemia (TMP-GFR).
- The treatment of XLHR is a combination of calcitriol (0.125–1.5 micrograms/day) and phosphate (25 mg/kg/day in infants, and 1–3 g elemental phosphorus in adults).
- Complications of long-term treatment include hypercalcaemia, hypercalciuria/renal lesions, and hyperparathyroidism.
- The requirements for calcitriol and phosphorus therapy in adults with XLHR is generally reduced and management of the condition refocuses on the need to address tertiary hyperparathyroidism, address osteoarthritis, and MSK symptoms caused by or associated with the enthesopathy which evolves over time.
- Renal tubular acidosis (RTA) and Fanconi syndrome may be associated with osteomalacia and rickets.
- In RTA, there is a disorder of bicarbonate handling leading to low plasma bicarbonate, metabolic acidosis, and an inappropriate urine pH. Type I distal tubular RTA occurs as a result of failure to secrete hydrogen ions.
- Type II proximal RTA is a consequence of bicarbonate wasting and is often associated with Fanconi syndrome. The development of rickets in both forms of RTA is due to hypophosphataemia. The acidosis should be treated and vitamin D supplements given.
- Fanconi syndrome is associated with a number of acquired or inherited disorders including multiple myeloma, amyloidosis, heavy metal toxicity, and disorders of carbohydrate metabolism.
- The net effect of proximal renal tubular defects is glycosuria, aminoaciduria, phosphaturia, and hypophosphataemia. Treatment is with phosphate and calcitriol supplements.

## Oncogenic hypophosphataemic osteomalacia

Also known as *tumour-induced osteomalacia*, this is caused by (usually small) benign mesenchymal tumours, which secrete FGF23. See ➲ Plate 16.

- The condition is cured after removal of the tumour though detection of the tumour can be difficult.
- Tumours can be anywhere including in bone. Many anecdotal reports of tumours existing in odd positions exist (e.g. sinuses, in skin, deep fat tissue, labia, etc.).
- Functional imaging with somatostatin receptor or PET scintigraphy (e.g. gallium-67 gadopentetate) is often used as first-line imaging with CT or MRI then used to precisely locate the lesions.
- A milder form of the condition occurs in fibrous dysplasia and neurofibromatosis.
- In the absence of curative surgery, treatment involves long-term phosphate and calcitriol supplements and careful monitoring for phosphate-induced hyperparathyroid disease and effects of hypercalciuria.

# Hypercalcaemia, parathyroid disease, and related disorders

## Hypercalcaemia

- The clinical picture of hypercalcaemia can range from the asymptomatic to an acute medical emergency.
- Serum calcium is normally balanced between homeostatic mechanisms in the gut, skeleton, kidneys, and extracellular fluids.
- Hypercalcaemia arises most often from excessive mobilization of calcium from bone by osteoclastic resorption, but may also occur due to excessive gut absorption (Table 16.5).
- The excessive bone loss, a failure of the kidneys to handle high loads of calcium, and a failure of bone to reclaim minerals quickly enough, leads to the imbalance.
- Accelerated osteoclast activity may be driven by several causes including excess parathyroid hormone (PTH) or PTH-related protein (PTHrp) and cytokines (e.g. IL-6, IL-1, TNFα, and TGF-β).
- Clinical presentation of moderate to severe hypercalcaemia includes:
  - joint, bone, muscle pain.
  - muscle weakness.
  - dehydration and polyuria.
  - lethargy.
  - fatigue.
  - acute confusional state—unconsciousness.
  - abdominal pains and vomiting.
  - renal colic pains.
  - ECG findings—short QT interval, etc.
- Primary hyperparathyroidism (PHPT) and malignancy are the most common causes of hypercalcaemia (90% of cases). Other causes include sarcoid, lymphoma, and granulomatous inflammatory conditions.
- Active vitamin $D_3$ (calcitriol/1,25-dihydroxyvitamin $D_3$) can be produced by tissue macrophages which generate 1α-hydroxylase. Macrophage/inflammatory cell calcitriol production (e.g. in sarcoid) is not regulated as occurs in renal vitamin $D_3$ activation as there is no feedback inhibition of 1α-hydroxylase nor diversion of its substrate (25-hydroxyvitamin $D_3$) to an inactive form (24,25-dihydroxyvitamin $D_3$) by increasing amounts of calcitriol, which happens in normal renal calcitriol production.
- Treatment of hypercalcaemia (Table 16.7) depends on the level of serum calcium, the presence of symptoms, renal impairment, and the underlying cause. For example, borderline high serum calcium in an asymptomatic individual with a mildly elevated PTH may simply warrant observation in the absence of renal impairment or vitamin D deficiency. On the other hand, an individual with severe hypercalcaemia, dehydration, and renal impairment due to a treatable malignancy would require urgent aggressive management.
- With acute hypercalcaemia, dehydration is very common. Early rehydration is very important and often given for 24–48 hours prior to review of serum calcium levels and the instigation of further therapies such as bisphosphonates and loop diuretics (Table 16.6).

**Table 16.5** Some causes of hypercalcaemia

| Common | Primary hyperparathyroidism | |
|---|---|---|
| | Malignancy | Lytic metastases to bone |
| | | Ectopic PTH (PTHrp) |
| | | Tumour-derived 1,25 dihydroxyvitamin D |
| Uncommon/rare | Drugs | Thiazide diuretics |
| | | Lithium |
| | | Aminophylline |
| | Granulomatous disease (tissue macrophage production of 1α-hydroxylase) | Sarcoidosis |
| | | Tuberculosis |
| | | Histoplasmosis |
| | Endocrine/metabolic | Thyrotoxicosis |
| | | Phaeochromocytoma |
| | | Excess vitamin A or D |
| | | Renal failure |
| | | Paget's disease of bone |
| | Other | Immobility ± calcium supplementation |

**Table 16.6** Treatment of hypercalcaemia

| General principles | Rehydrate with normal saline 4 L in 24 hrs if needed |
|---|---|
| | Correct hypokalaemia and hypomagnesaemia |
| | Mild metabolic acidosis need not be treated |
| Specific treatment | Loop diuretics when hydrated |
| | Bisphosphonates |
| | Calcitonin |
| | Glucocorticoids (haematological malignancies and granulomatous diseases) |

### Hypercalcaemia in infancy and childhood

- Chronic hypercalcaemia of infancy may not be associated with the more common clinical features mentioned previously. More often there is a failure to thrive, abdominal pain, and irritability. Acute hypercalcaemia is very rare in children.
- Conditions to consider are listed in Table 16.7.

**Table 16.7** Conditions that may be responsible for hypercalcaemia in infancy and childhood

| | |
|---|---|
| Williams' syndrome | A spectrum of aortic valve stenosis and facial dysmorphism ('elfin' facies) |
| Idiopathic infantile hypercalcaemia | Similar milder appearance to Williams' syndrome can be seen. There are also features of inguinal hernias, hypertension, strabismus, and kyphosis |
| Familial hypocalciuric hypercalcaemia | See later in this section |
| Neonatal primary hyperparathyroidism | |
| Other | Fat necrosis, sarcoidosis, Jansen syndrome (metaphyseal dysplasia), overdosing of milk/vitamin D |

## Parathyroid disorders

### Primary hyperparathyroidism

- Primary hyperparathyroidism (PHPT) is a relatively common condition; incidence 1 in 1000. It occurs at all ages, although is much more common after the age of 60 with a female to male ratio of 3:1. It is unusual in childhood—when it should raise the possibility of familial multiple endocrine neoplasia (MEN) type I or type II.
- A single benign adenoma accounts for 80% of cases of PHPT.
- Generalized four-gland hyperplasia accounts for 15–20% of cases.
- Parathyroid carcinoma is very rare.
- PHPT is associated with bone, renal, GI, and neuromuscular complications. Bony problems can be seen on plain radiographs and range from low BMD on DXA scanning and mild sub-periosteal bone resorption to osteitis fibrosa cystica, bone resorption of the distal phalanges and clavicles, patchy osteosclerosis (classic 'rugger jersey' spine), and multiple lytic lesions of the skull.
- General symptoms include fatigue and myalgias (myopathy is rare).
- CPPD disease is a relatively under-recognized association (look for joint chondrocalcinosis, crowned dens syndrome See ➲ Plate 22, typical features in OA joints ('OA-plus')). Kidney stones are uncommon. GI manifestations include peptic ulceration and pancreatitis.
- PHPT is easily diagnosed with raised PTH in the context of replete level 25(OH)D, and high (or high reference range) serum calcium and low (or low-reference range) phosphate. Often 24-hour urinary calcium levels are uninformative.
- Medical management includes adequate rehydration and avoidance of high calcium intake and calcium supplements, gentle correction of 25(OH)D deficiency and a bisphosphonate to limit bone loss.
- Successful parathyroidectomy from minimally invasive targeted surgery is feasible in the majority of cases for single adenomas identified by imaging (e.g. [99m]Tc-MIBI scintigraphy and US though (contrast-enhanced, delayed phase) CT is also used in equivocal cases).

- Neck exploration surgery is required if imaging fails to identify an adenoma. Surgery should only be done by experienced surgeons.
- Conservative management is acceptable if patients are asymptomatic, and do not have osteoporosis though also may be necessary if surgery is not feasible. Bisphosphonates do stabilize BMD loss as indicated by DXA and can be used long-term.
- Clinical trials with calcimimetic agents (stimulates the PTH gland Calcium sensing receptors with consequent inhibition of PTH secretion) such as cinacalcet, can be used in cases where parathyroidectomy is not feasible/failed and there are hypercalcaemic symptoms.

### Secondary and tertiary hyperparathyroidism

- Secondary HPT (SHPT) occurs as a consequence of low serum calcium and PTH gland CaSR 'sensing' of calcium levels.
- Calcium lack and thus SHPT are often due to vitamin D deficiency.
- SHPT from calcium lack alone (where there is replete 25(OH)D) is unusual though may point to a severe GI absorption problem.
- With time, persistent SHPT can lead to autonomous PTH release (tertiary HPT). This is most often seen in severe or prolonged renal bone disease or from long-term calcitriol use (e.g. XLHR).
- Calcimimetics may have an important role to play in controlling tertiary HPT but at present parathyroidectomy is the best option.

### Familial hypocalciuric hypercalcaemia (FHH)

- FHH is extremely rare. It is inherited as autosomal dominant with high penetrance. Radiographs, PTH, and renal function are normal in uncomplicated cases. Although parathyroid gland hyperplasia occurs, parathyroidectomy is invariably unsuccessful at lowering serum calcium levels.
- The two indications for parathyroidectomy in FHH are neonatal severe HPT and adult relapsing pancreatitis.
  Use of diuretics, oestrogens, or phosphate to regulate serum calcium has been unsuccessful. Patients should therefore be followed without intervention unless complications arise.
  FHH needs to be considered when diagnosing PHPT (where hypercalcaemia and elevated PTH levels are modest). First discrimination is made by repleting 25(OH)D to 100 nmol/L then retesting all biochemistry. PTH usually normalizes in FHH, unless there is tertiary HPT, but won't in PHPT. Also if the calcium:creatinine clearance ratio is <0.02 then FHH is 98% likely (CCCR = uCa/(uCr × sCr)).
  In pregnancy the three situations to be aware of are:
  - asymptomatic hypercalcaemia in an affected baby of a carrier.
  - neonatal hypercalcaemia in an affected baby of an unaffected mother (intrauterine SHPT, which resolves spontaneously).
  - hypocalcaemia in an unaffected baby of an affected mother (fetal parathyroid suppression).

### Familial primary hyperparathyroid syndromes

Up to 10% of cases of PHPT may have a hereditary syndrome. The most common of these is MEN.
MEN1 is autosomal dominant (M = F), is associated with pancreatic, thymic, gastric, and pituitary adenomas, and adrenal hyperplasia.

- Pancreatic, thymic, and bronchial neuroendocrine tumours are the leading cause of death in patients with MEN-1 and should be regularly monitored for (e.g. biannual computed tomography imaging).
- The MEN1 gene consists of ten exons, spanning 10 kb, and encodes a 610-amino acid protein ('menin'—its function as yet not fully known but may play a role in tumour suppression).
- MEN2A (Sipple syndrome) is autosomal dominant and is characterized by phaeochromocytomas and medullary thyroid carcinoma and is highly associated with the RET proto-oncogene.

*Parathyroid hormone resistant syndromes*
- Pseudohypoparathyroidism (PHP) is a term applied to a heterogeneous group of disorders whose common feature is end-organ resistance to PTH. PHP type 1A (PHP1A) is characterized by resistance to other hormones, including TSH and gonadotropins.
- PHP1A is associated with clinical features referred to as Albright hereditary osteodystrophy (AHO; includes short stature, obesity, round facies, subcutaneous ossifications, brachydactyly, other skeletal anomalies, and some patients have mental retardation).
- In PHP1A, there is decreased cellular cAMP response to PTH infusion, decreased erythrocyte Gs activity, and a GNAS1 mutation in the maternally derived allele.
- In PHP1B, there is renal PTH resistance, decreased cAMP response to PTH infusion, normal erythrocyte Gs activity, and imprinting/methylation defects at the GNAS locus resulting in lack of expression of the maternal allele in renal tissue. Classically, patients do not have features of AHO.
- PHP1B is not associated with generalized hormone resistance, although resistance to thyroid-stimulating hormone has been reported.
- Individuals with AHO without endocrine abnormalities, a normal cellular cAMP response to PTH infusion, decreased erythrocyte Gs activity and a GNAS1 mutation in the paternally-inherited allele have pseudopseudohypoparathyroidism (PPHP).

## CKD-mineral and bone disorders (CKD-MBD) incorporating renal osteodystrophy (ROD)

- The kidneys are key in regulating calcium and phosphate, are a target organ for PTH and FGF23, and are the primary source for 1α-hydroxylation mediated activation of 25(OH)D.
- CKD-MBD (the term was first proposed by Kidney Disease: Improving Global Outcomes (KDIGO) in 2005) describes a broad clinical syndrome which includes skeletal, soft tissue, and vascular abnormalities that develop as a result of CKD. Renal *skeletal* disease alone is termed 'renal osteodystrophy (ROD; Table 16.8).
- ROD can be a spectrum of bone disease from 'high turnover' (due to primary or tertiary hyperparathyroidism) to 'low turnover' (termed adynamic) bone disease where PTH levels are generally low (reference range or modest elevation).
- Phosphate retention (secondary), FGF23 elevation, hypovitaminosis D, hypocalcaemia, impaired calcitriol production, and skeletal resistance to PTH all contribute to secondary HPT in CKD with relevant effects beginning in CKD3 (estimated GFR 30–60 mL/min/1.73 m²).

**Table 16.8** The clinical manifestations of renal osteodystrophy

| Clinical feature | Comment |
|---|---|
| Bone pain | Common |
| Skeletal deformity | Common. Affects appendicular and axial skeleton |
| | *Children*: onset <3 yrs, rachitic; onset <10 yrs, bowing of long bones, widened metaphyses, pseudoclubbing, slipped epiphyses |
| | *Adults:* lumbar scoliosis, kyphosis, distorted thorax |
| Growth retardation | |
| Proximal muscle weakness | |
| Ectopic calcification | Soft-tissues. Visceral. Vascular—if severe, individuals may develop ischaemic necrosis |

- Historically low turnover, adynamic ROD has been related to excess aluminium deposition in bone in dialysis patients—thus more prevalent in peritoneal dialysis patients compared with haemodialysis.
- Bone fragility and increased fracture risk is a consequence of all types of ROD. Clinical manifestations of ROD are in Table 16.8.

*General management of ROD*

- Early dietary restriction of phosphate can maintain normal calcium levels, but low-phosphate diets are often unacceptable and normal phosphate levels are best achieved with binding agents (some contain calcium).
- Small doses of calcitriol (vitamin D) may help to lower serum PTH levels. Some individuals may be sensitive to calcitriol and serum calcium levels may increase. Most patients require doses of 0.25–0.5 micrograms daily; children may require higher doses.
- Parathyroidectomy is indicated in persistent symptomatic hypercalcaemia, ectopic calcification, and severe bone pain.

*Ectopic calcification and ossification*

- Ectopic calcification can arise from any one of a number of causes of hypercalcaemia or hyperphosphataemia. These include renal failure, hyperparathyroidism, familial hyperphosphataemia tumoural calcinosis (OMIM 211900) and sarcoidosis. Dystrophic calcification is also a feature of systemic sclerosis (see ➔ Chapter 13), dermatomyositis (see ➔ Chapter 14), and primary calcinosis.
- Ectopic ossification can be seen post trauma and following myositis. It is also a feature of several rare conditions including PHP and myositis ossificans progressiva. Early signs of muscle ossification are best detected with MRI scanning. Later ossification is easily visible on plain radiographs. Treatment is difficult, but includes physiotherapy to maintain suppleness and possibly heparins or bisphosphonates to halt bone formation.

# Paget's disease of bone

- Paget's disease of bone (PDB) is a localized disorder of bone remodelling resulting in expansion and deformity of bone.
- PDB is common (about 5% of the population >55 years) in the UK, North America, Australia, and New Zealand, with a male to female ratio of 3:2. It's uncommon in Asia, Africa, Scandinavia, and South America.
- The 'lesion' in PDB is substantially increased (coupled) bone remodelling, driven by an excess number of multinucleated, highly active osteoclasts, producing excessive woven bone (immature bone characterized by erratic collagen orientation).
- Theories of PDB being caused by viruses have largely been disproved.
- PDB has a genetic basis; 15–30% PDB patients have a positive family history; there is a 7× risk of developing PDB if your first-degree relative has it and 30% of familial cases have gene mutations at 5q35 (the gene encodes for an ubiquitin-binding protein sequestasome-1 (SQSTM1/p62)).
- SQSTM1 mutations indicate severity of PDB, the protein playing an important role in NFKβ signalling.
- PDB patients with SQSTM1 mutations can have a variable clinical phenotype however, indicating modifying gene or environmental effects also are relevant.
- The clinical features of PDB are shown in Table 16.9.

**Table 16.9** Clinical features of Paget's disease of bone

| Clinical feature | Details |
|---|---|
| Pain | Deep unremitting pain, possibly correlated to blood flow (e.g. headache from skull involvement) |
| Bone involvement | Pelvis 75%, skull 35%, femur 35%, sacrum 35%, tibia 30%, radius 15%, hands or feet 10% of cases |
| Fractures | Vertebral fractures, 'fissure' fractures at site of convexity of long bone |
| Neurological sequelae | Spinal cord compression, radiculopathy, deafness, |
| High-output cardiac failure | Rare but can occur if >40% of the skeleton is involved |
| Osteosarcoma | 0.1% of cases |
| Hypercalcaemia and hypercalciuria | Unusual. Linked to polyostotic disease and immobility. Can, if severe, lead to kidney stone disease |
| Osteoarthritis | PDB in bone adjacent to joint, can accelerate joint degeneration |
| Retinal angioid streaks | Cause unknown |

## Investigation and treatment

- Serum alkaline phosphatase (ALP), a measure of osteoblast-derived bone formation, is the most useful marker of high bone remodelling and may be elevated as much as 30× above normal.
- Reference range ALP can mean bone turnover is low ('inactive PDB') but is not specific. The degree of abnormality of ALP often associates with the number of bones affected, polyostotic disease being associated with higher ALP values.
- The differential diagnosis of increased (bone) ALP includes metastatic bone disease, osteomalacia, hyperparathyroidism, and osteomyelitis or inflammation.
- Because of the increased bone turnover, other biomarkers will be abnormal: e.g. increased urine hydroxyproline, serum/plasma CTX, P1NP.
- There is a wide variation in radiographic appearance of the condition but the main features are localized sclerosis, coarse and irregular trabecular patterning, and bone expansion.
- $^{99m}$TC methylene diphosphonate (MDP) bone scintigraphy is a sensitive investigation for defining the extent of lesions. See ➲ Plate 22.
- There are several indications for treatment of Paget's disease:
  - Pain arising from affected sites.
  - Deforming disease.
  - Fissure fractures.
  - Skull disease.
  - Reduction of vascularity in bone next to a joint planned for surgery.
  - Complications—progressive neurology, hypercalcaemia, high-output cardiac failure.
- PDB and related osteoarthritic pain may be reduced by simple analgesics, but pure pagetic bone pain responds poorly to this.
- Full biomechanical assessment, particularly looking for correctable deformities with judicious orthosis use, is invariably helpful.
- First-line treatment of PDB is a single dose of zoledronic acid 5 mg IV.
- An alternative is risedronate 30 mg daily for 2 months. The relapse rate with risedronate is significantly higher than with zoledronic acid.
- Historically, etidronate (e.g. 6 months at a dose of 5 mg/kg/day), pamidronate (e.g. 90 mg IV ×2 doses fortnight apart) and calcitonin (50–100 IU SC injection daily, reducing to 50 IU 2 or 3 times per week once a symptomatic response is achieved (usually after 4–8 weeks) have shown benefit in reducing PDB pain and ALP. However, relapse risk is moderately high compared with zoledronic acid. Calcitonin often causes nausea, flushing, and diarrhoea.
- Many PDB patients achieve long-term biochemical remission with just a single treatment of zoledronic acid 5 mg.
- Typical side effects of zoledronic acid, as with pamidronate, includes transient 'flu-like' symptoms of fever, myalgia, and arthralgia.

- Zoledronic acid 5 mg IV used for ALP rise alone does not appear to benefit PDB patients compared with patients treated on the basis of PDB symptoms alone (PRISM-EZ); indeed, it may be associated with a greater risk of fractures (in non-pagetoid bone).
- Zoledronic acid is currently being studied for its role in PDB development in high-risk (SQSTM-1 mutation-positive) patients.
- Typical surgical interventions include arthroplasty—where accelerated OA has evolved in joints adjacent to pagetoid bone, fixation of fractures, and realignment osteotomies where there is significant deformity amenable to surgical correction.
- Vitamin D deficiency is increased in frequency in PDB patients compared to expected, thus it should be sought and corrected.
- Denosumab is predicted to be effective at reducing bone turnover, pain, and ALP in PDB but treatment will be relatively expensive, relapse of PDB is likely to occur on treatment cessation, and the rebound increase in bone turnover at that time, is likely to preclude its adoption as a routine treatment for PDB.

# Childhood autoinflammatory bone diseases

## Introduction

Autoinflammatory bone diseases are disorders primarily driven by abnormalities of the innate immune system.[3]

- The most common disorders include chronic non-bacterial osteomyelitis (CNO); synovitis, acne, pustulosis, hyperostosis, and osteitis (SAPHO) syndrome; Majeed syndrome; deficiency of interleukin-1 receptor antagonist (DIRA); cherubism; and juvenile mandibular chronic osteomyelitis (JMCO).
- Bone inflammation is typically characterized by a subacute or chronic inflammation that is bacterial culture negative and with no demonstrable organism on histopathology.
- NSAIDs are typically used as first-line therapies in CNO. Bisphosphonates and anti-TNFα drugs have been used for second-line therapies to prevent pathologic fractures, pain, and disease relapse.
- CNO and SAPHO are discussed in greater detail later in this section and for the rarer autoinflammatory bone diseases see Table 16.10.

## CNO

The terminology for CNO has changed over the last 40 years. The most commonly used term is chronic recurrent multifocal osteomyelitis (CRMO); however, not all patients have multifocal bone lesions or numerous recurrences, hence the term chronic non-bacterial osteomyelitis (CNO) encompasses all possible disease presentations.

- CNO is a systemic disease that predominantly occurs in childhood. It has many similarities to SAPHO syndrome, a disorder primarily seen in adults.
- The incidence and prevalence of CNO is unknown, but the majority of reports are from Scandinavia, Europe, Australia and North America. Female predominance/mean age of onset about 10 years of age.
- CNO is a diagnosis of exclusion established by clinical presentation, imaging studies, and a culture-negative bone biopsy.
- Pain occurs with or without swelling at the site of a bony lesion. Inflammatory markers are normal or moderately raised.
- Bone lesions tend to cluster around metaphysis, but can occur at sites such as the clavicle (commonly the medial third).
- The most common CNO sites include the femur, pelvis, calcaneus, ankle, vertebrae, and clavicle. Multifocal lesions tend to have a symmetrical distribution. Unifocal disease occurs in 10–20%.
- CNO patients frequently have other coexisting chronic inflammatory diseases such as psoriasis, arthritis, inflammatory bowel disease, vasculitis, myositis/fasciitis, and parotitis.
- Imaging to clarify diagnosis: radiographs and MRI. CT can be used, but exposes children to high radiation, so is not recommended.
- Whole-body MRI can assess for asymptomatic (polyostotic) lesions, and should be considered for indeterminate CNO cases.
- Typical radiographic findings include a lytic lesion at or around the metaphysis, which may progress to sclerosis or hyperostosis.
- Bone biopsy is often required to confirm the diagnosis—important in isolated bone lesions, as malignancy can mimic CNO.

**Table 16.10** Features of the rarest autoinflammatory bone conditions

| Features | DIRA | Cherubism | Majeed syndrome |
|---|---|---|---|
| Fever | Uncommon | No | High fevers |
| Common CNO sites | Long bones especially proximal femur, vertebral bodies, ribs, clavicles | Maxilla and mandible | Femur, tibia, pelvis, calcaneus, ankle, vertebrae, and clavicle |
| Area of long bones affected | Metaphyses predominantly | Long bones rarely affected | Metaphyses predominantly |
| Extraosseous features | Skin pustulosis, systemic organ involvement | Cervical lymphadenopathy | Congenital dyserythropoietic anaemia, dermatitis, growth failure, hepatomegaly, joint contractures |
| Inflammatory markers | Elevated | Normal to mildly elevated | Elevated |
| Inheritance | AR | AD | AR |
| Gene defect | IL-1RN | SH3BP2 | LPIN2 |
| Ethnic distribution | Puerto Rican, European, Lebanese | Worldwide | Arabic, Turkish |

*Treatment*

- NSAIDs are the gold standard initial therapy.
- Case reports suggest GCs, methotrexate (MTX), and sulfasalazine (SZP) may be beneficial, but results are inconclusive.
- Reports on use of anti-TNFα are inconclusive: some responses are unsustained.
- IV bisphosphonate (e.g. pamidronate) has been used due to its effect on reducing osteoclast-driven osteitis pathophysiology.
- Several studies have demonstrated high efficacy rates and good clinical response occurring in the first 3 days, and inducing remission for 12–18 months.
- However, there are concerns regarding the use of bisphosphonates in children given the lack of long-term safety data.
- The most common adverse event of pamidronate is minor flu-like symptoms. Osteonecrosis of the jaw is a rare but serious complication and to date unreported in paediatric use.
- CNO can be a difficult condition to treat, with high rates of non-responders. If untreated, there is increased risk of pathological fractures, in addition to other possible morbidities such as generalized growth failure, scoliosis, and hyperostosis.

**Reference**

3. Stern SM, Ferguson PJ. Autoinflammatory bone diseases. *Rheum Dis Clin North Am* 2013;39:735–49.

# SAPHO syndrome

SAPHO syndrome was originally an acronym from the French term: le Syndrome Acne, Pustulose, Hyperostose et Osteite but later changed and terminology anglicized in terminology to Syndrome of Synovitis, Acne, Pustulosis, Hyperostosis and Osteitis. However, the original description is notable for the absence of synovitis, which probably is quite an uncommon lesion of the condition.

- SAPHO syndrome has similarity to CNO but can also be classified as an osteosclerotic bone disease. Furthermore, there may be overlap with the SpA diseases—some features exist in both SAPHO and some forms of psoriatic arthritis though SAPHO is not B27 related.[4]

## Patterns and spectrum of disease

- Typical presentation age 30–50 years old though childhood forms exist.
- Pathogenesis may derive from an amplified abnormal innate immune response to pathogens, with the most likely triggering pathogen being *Propionibacterium acnes*.
- A patient's disease phenotype can be indistinguishable also from axial skeletal sarcoid.
- There are similarities to and overlap with forms of psoriatic arthritis.
- CRMO has been described as the paediatric presentation of SAPHO. However, the localization of inflammation is different between the two conditions with the extremities more often affected in CRMO than SAPHO whereas for the latter, axial skeleton with costo-sternoclavicular region is the focus.
- Both enthesitis and spondylodiscitis are likely to be associated SAPHO lesions.

## Clinical features

- Painful osteitis lesions, enthesitis, and spondylodiscitis are likely to all occur in SAPHO lesions.
- Palmoplantar pustulosis (PPP) and severe acne (acne conglobata, acne fulminans, hidradenitis suppurativa) are among the typical lesions seen in SAPHO.
- PPP is more often seen in women and severe acne in men.
- Other skin lesions described in SAPHO include various types of psoriasis; pyoderma gangrenosum; Sweet's syndrome; Sneddon–Wilkinson disease.
- Systemic symptoms of fever and fatigue frequently occur.

## Differential diagnosis

- Psoriatic arthritis. This can pose diagnostic dilemma since psoriatic arthritis manifest by spondylodiscitis, osteitis, entheseal/juxta-articular hyperostosis and pustular psoriasis can mimic SAPHO.
- Infection (osteomyelitis) and neoplasia should be considered though MRI is usually discriminatory.
- In children, the following should also be considered: Ewing sarcoma, Majeed syndrome, histiocytosis, and DIRA.

## Investigations

- $^{99m}$TC MDP (bone) scintigraphy is characteristic in most cases showing marked tracer accumulation at sternoclavicular area lesions (e.g. Bull's head sign).
- On radiographs lesions are often primarily expanded and sclerotic.
- MRI discriminates osteitis from infection and malignancy.
- Laboratory tests are not specific and features of inflammation may be seen: raised CRP, ESR, platelets, C3, ACE. Immunoglobulins are usually normal and autoantibodies not detected.
- Bone should be cultured for TB, *Propionibacterium*, and general pathogens.
- Histology of bone often shows dense disorganized sclerosis with features of increased bone turnover.
- Histology of skin lesions can show neutrophilic infiltration and pseudo-abscesses (differential diagnosis—Sweet's syndrome).

## Treatment

- NSAIDs are used for pain.
- Appropriate antibiotics for culture-positive bone biopsy.
- Colchicine, GCs, oral and IV bisphosphonates, and sDMARDs (e.g. MTX) have all been used with variable effects.
- Anti-TNFα and anti-IL-1 receptor antagonist (anakinra) have shown good effect persistent disease.
- For skin manifestations, topical steroids, PUVA, and retinoids have been used.

## Reference

4. Rukavina I. SAPHO syndrome: a review. *J Child Orthop* 2015;9:19–27.

# The osteochondroses

Osteochondrosis is a trauma-induced focal disturbance of cartilage in a joint (articular), at a periarticular epiphyseal plate or tendon or ligament insertion (apophysis/enthesis).

- Lesions typically occur in active children and adolescents.
- Osteochondritis may be associated with a delay in growth-associated endochondral ossification, with a potential consequence of joint or other biomechanical deformity (see ➜ Table 16.11).
- Where the lesion is associated with cleft formation through articular cartilage, then the lesion is termed 'dissecans'.

## Scheuermann's disease

Although not consistently defined, Scheuermann's disease is a vertebral epiphyseal osteochondritis that occurs in adolescence. See also ➜ p. 620

- Although an incidental radiographic finding, Scheuermann's is also associated with diffuse spinal pain which is more likely to be present if the osteochondritis is thoracolumbar (25%), rather than thoracic (75%) and if the child is an athlete or very active.
- It can present with painless dorsal kyphosis with compensatory lumbar lordosis and lateral spine radiographs show irregularity of vertebral end-plates, anterior vertebral wedging, and kyphosis—the latter can develop in late adolescence or gradually over years.
- In adults who present late, the vertebral deformities may be mistaken for grade 1 vertebral fractures.
- Management is with physiotherapy—working on extensor spinal muscular strength, and judicious use of analgesics.

## Legg–Calvé–Perthes disease

Perthes disease is an osteonecrosis of the femoral epiphysis and occurs in the age range 3–8 years, most frequently in boys (ratio 4:1).

- Perthes disease is bilateral in 10–20% of cases.
- Symptoms include an insidious onset of limp and pain in the groin or referred to the knee/thigh that is relieved by rest.
- There may be limitation of hip internal rotation and abduction (due to adductor spasm).
- Leg length inequality suggests femoral head collapse. There may be spontaneous resolution, especially in younger patients, in whom conservative management is indicated.

## Osgood–Schlatter disease

This osteochondrosis is probably due to repetitive trauma at the site of patellar tendon insertion into the tibial tubercle.

- It typically occurs in athletic adolescents, especially young males aged 14–16 years.
- Pain is usually on exercise and eases with rest.
- The diagnosis is made clinically and on demonstrating an enlarged fragmented tibial tubercle on a lateral view radiograph.
- Bilateral knee views help to distinguish normal from abnormal.
- Differential diagnosis includes SpA-related enthesis.

**Table 16.11** Osteochondritis conditions

| Type | Site | Details |
|------|------|---------|
| Articular | Metatarsal head (Freiberg's) | Typically, 2nd metatarsal head; bilateral in 10% |
| | Hip (Legg–Calvé–Perthes) | Slipped capital femoral epiphysis; 4–10 years of age; more complications if >8 years of age; is bilateral in 10% |
| | Navicular (Kohler's) | 3–7 years of age; male to female ratio 5:1; occasionally bilateral |
| | Talus | Lateral lesions most likely to be associated with single trauma trigger |
| | Lunate (Kienbock's) | Rare <15 yrs old; commonly males; may be associated with short ulna relative to radius |
| Non-articular -at an enthesis | Vertebral end-plate (Scheuermann's) | 13–17 yrs; male:female ratio equal; usually lower thoracic > than upper lumbar; often several vertebrae affected (3–5) |
| | Tibial tubercle (Osgood–Schlatter) | Enthesitis of insertion of patellar ligament; typically 10–15 yrs of age; more often males than females; bilateral in 25% |
| | Inferior patella pole | 'Jumper's knee'; typically male adolescents involved in sports and exercise; |
| | 5th metatarsal base (Iselin's) | 9–15 yrs old; typically sports-related trauma |
| | Calcaneus (Sever's) | 'Traction enthesitis at Achilles' tendon insertion; incidence 4/1000 children 6–17 yrs |
| Epiphyseal plate | Ulna medial epiphyseal at elbow (Panner's) | Avulsion enthesitis from pitching in Little League baseball termed 'Little League elbow'; males <16 yrs old; associated with increased height velocity; extensively reported in the sports medicine literature |
| | Medial/proximal tibia (Blount's) | 'Tibia vara'; infantile <3 yrs old or late onset |
| | Slipped upper (capital) femoral epiphysis (SUFE) | Commonest adolescent hip disorder; 20% bilateral; risks: obesity, coxa profunda, femoral or acetabular retroversion, hypothyroidism, ROD, hypopituitarism; 25% risk of progression to osteonecrosis; almost all cases need surgery |

### Sinding–Larsen–Johansson disease

This osteochondrosis occurs as a consequence of overloading of the patella at its secondary centre of ossification producing a traction apophysitis at the patella lower pole.

- Although not exclusive to the group, it is a typical sports-related injury in adolescent athletes who jump, e.g. high-jump, basketball.
- Treatment is with simple analgesia or NSAIDs, and rest.

### Köhler disease

This osteochondrosis is essentially an osteonecrosis lesion of the tarsal navicular. Changes may represent a developmental variation in ossification and it presents with a painful limp. Weight-bearing is more comfortable on the outside of the foot and the navicular is tender.

### Freiberg disease

An osteonecrosis of the metatarsal (usually the second) head following trauma, is most common in adolescent females. Pain is localized and worse on weight-bearing with swelling sometimes detectable.

### An osteochondritis 'dissecans' lesion

An articular osteochondritis lesion can become a 'dissecans' lesion when a fragment of articular cartilage and subchondral bone becomes demarcated and may form an intra-articular loose body.

- Symptoms of a dissecans lesion are mainly acute-onset pain, an effusion, and limited movement of the joint.
- Plain radiographs will show a well-circumscribed, sclerotic lesion.
- In young patients before skeletal maturity there is a good chance of dissecans healing.
- After the epiphysis has closed, however, there is more risk of a loose body and secondary osteoarthritis if a dissecans lesion persists.
- Arthroscopy can assist in assessing the degree of damage and removing loose bodies.
- Surgery ranges from drilling the lesion *in situ* to encourage healing, to bone osteochondral allografts.

# Osteonecrosis

Osteonecrosis is regional ischaemic skeletal injury, which can be caused by trauma, drugs (e.g. GCs), or systemic conditions—metabolic, haematological, or endocrine (e.g. sickle cell disease, antiphospholipid syndrome).

- If severe and/or prolonged, ischaemia can cause skeletal cell death leading to necrotic bone, which can compromise regional skeletal integrity and strength and lead to fracture, damage to adjacent cartilage, and deformity.
- Osteonecrosis can be symptomatically silent and persist, with no or minimal symptoms, for years in some cases.
- Ischaemia occurs after mechanical interruption of blood delivery, non-traumatic intravascular occlusion, thrombosis, cholesterol, expanding nitrogen bubbles or other mechanisms that lead to critical ischaemia; then deposition of vascularized connective tissue can accumulate at the interface of necrotic and normal bone. Calcification can follow and necrotic tissue remains as an 'island' of inviable bone.
- Local skeletal features include pain or discomfort. Pain evolution may denote the onset of subchondral bone collapse. If secondary adjacent joint damage evolves and progresses then features of mechanical joint disease will evolve—pain and discomfort on movement, stiffness, swelling, and a functional impact accordingly.
- There may be tenderness on palpating over osteonecrotic bone and signs of joint effusion if the lesion has affected the adjacent joint causing cartilage loss or microfracture.
- MRI signs are characteristic and can contribute to grading (e.g. femoral head after Ficat). See also ➲ bone scintigraphy Plate 17.
- Practical radiographic-based osteonecrosis grading can be done using Steinberg (2001) or even ARCO (1992) grading systems.
- Laboratory testing should focus on systemic causes (Table 16.12).
- Initial management: pain control, addressing remediable underlying systemic causes/associated disease, agreeing and planning what amount of weight- or load-bearing of the affected bone is permissible.
- In the absence of data from controlled studies of treatment, management is based on stage of the lesion and degree of effect on the adjacent joint, thus for early disease with reversible cause, or repair or revascularization possible before any collapse of the subchondral bone, conservative measures are appropriate. But in late disease with subchondral bone collapse, arthroplasty is considered.
- For osteonecrosis of the femoral head (ONFH) consider an 8-week period of non-weight-bearing.
- Evidence for bisphosphonate use and its effect is anecdotal only.
- Core decompression for ONFH involves removing bone from the medullary cavity or multiple smaller holes through the bone surface. The cavity may be then filled with a vascularized fibular graft or by non-vascularized cortical bone.
- Osteotomy attempts to shift the weight from the necrotic segment but subsequent joint replacement is technically more difficult. Hemi-resurfacing preserves the bone for later arthroplasty and is an option for femoral head collapse in younger patients.
- Skeletal stem cells combined with impaction bone grafting is a novel treatment translated to the treatment of ONFH.

**Table 16.12** Conditions causing, or associated with, osteonecrosis

| Condition | Notes |
| --- | --- |
| Trauma | Fractures and fracture-dislocations, Legg–Calvé–Perthes disease, orthopaedic procedures |
| Glucocorticoids (GCs) or Cushing's disease | Associated with acute repeated high-dose GCs or high cumulative GC doses. GCs cause hypertrophy and hyperplasia of marrow fat cells. GCs divert mesenchymal cells toward an adipocyte lineage as opposed to osteoblast-osteocyte one |
| Alcohol | Risk increases >3-fold in those consuming 40 units per week or more. |
| Drugs | Cocaine; bisphosphonates and denosumab (monoclonal antibody to RANKL) both causing ONJ; oral contraceptives (rare); protease inhibitors; thalidomide |
| Gaucher disease | In the total population of 5894 ICGG Gaucher Disease Registry patients, 544 experienced at least one episode of osteonecrosis; associated with anaemia |
| SLE | Osteonecrosis reported in up to 27% of patients taking GCs, often multifocal; risk higher if there is hypertriglyceridemia |
| Transplantation | Likely multifactorial risks. Mainly associated with GCs |
| Sickle cell disease | Prevalence very high. Most commonly humeral head (28–48% prevalence); ONFH most prevalent in patients with SCD-SS α-thalassemia |
| Prothrombotic risks | Up to 50% of cases of multifocal osteonecrosis associate with pro-thrombotic conditions (e.g. antiphospholipid syndrome) |
| Dysbaria | Predominantly affects femoral head and proximal humerus in divers, caisson and tunnel workers. |
| HIV | Protease inhibitor-induced hyperlipidaemia and HIV-associated antiphospholipid syndrome |
| Malignancy | All; notably childhood leukaemia |
| Other probable associations | Pancreatitis, hyperlipidaemia, diabetes, pregnancy, hyperuricaemia/gout |

# Fibrous dysplasia

Fibrous dysplasia (FD) manifests as either an isolated (monostotic) or polyostotic condition as fibrous bone cysts.

- FD presents most often in the second to third decade of life as monostotic disease, or usually <10 years of age in polyostotic disease.
- FD is manifest by cystic expansion of bones. Lesions can cause pain and local mechanical effects due to their site and proximity to critical structures (e.g. nerve foramen in the skeleton).
- FD is due to activating or gain-of-function GNAS1 mutations.
- *McCune–Albright syndrome* is a triad of polyostotic fibrous dysplasia, hyper pigmented 'café-au-lait' patches, and endocrine abnormalities (Cushing's, thyroid, precocious puberty).
- There is genetic mosaicism given the mutation in FD and McCune–Albright syndrome is somatic in origin. The degree of extent of pathology and severity therefore depends on the stage of development at which the postzygotic somatic mutation occurred.
- When the mutation occurs at an early post-zygotic development stage, the condition is more severe (a germline GNAS1 mutation would be lethal).
- FD bone lesions grow under the influence of growth hormone (/IGF-1) and may stop growing at skeletal maturity, but need monitoring.
- Any FD bone lesion can produce FGF23 and mild hypophosphataemia is not uncommon and additional osteomalacia can result.
- Bone pain is common and difficult to treat.
- Bone pain is sometimes severe and its cause unexplained.
- Pain can be treated with serial IV pamidronate infusions. Dose regimens vary and options have not been systematically studied.
- Some FD lesions do not cause symptoms though can cause complications such as fracture, neural compromise (expansion of bone adjacent to a nerve canal), or bone collapse depending on their site. Fracture healing does not appear to be compromised however.
- Patient information is available at: ℘ http://www.gosh.nhs.uk/fibrous-dysplasia and support at: ℘ http://www.fibrousdysplasia.org and also at: ℘ http://www.fdssuk.org.uk

## Sclerosing bone disorders

# Sclerosing bone disorders

Sclerosing bone disorders comprise those affecting cortical bone (hyperostotic) and those affecting trabecular bone (osteosclerotic).

- There are many sclerosing bone disorders.[5] The most common are dealt with here but see also Table 16.13.

## Osteopetrosis

Is a term that defines a range of osteoscleroses ('the osteopetroses').

- The osteopetroses are caused by one of a number of genetic abnormalities which result in functional deficit (mostly regulation of acidification) in osteoclastic bone resorption (e.g. CLCN7, GL, CA II (causes carbonic anhydrase II deficiency)).
- AD and AR forms exist—the former lethal in childhood unless treated—the latter often benign and presents later in life. (See ⅏ http://www.omim.org for a comprehensive review of genetics.)
- Diagnosis is made on radiographs where the effects of osteoclast failure during endochondral bone formation result in 'islands' or 'bars' of calcified cartilage within trabecular bone.
- HLA identical bone marrow transplant has been very effective for some infantile forms of osteopetrosis.

## Camurati–Engelmann disease (CED) and Ribbing disease (RD)

- CED and RD are manifest by slowly evolving long bone hyperostosis in children and adolescents (CED) and in adolescents and young adults (RD).
- Bone sclerosis may be driven by release of active TGF-β from bone matrix which drives the development and activity of osteoblasts.
- CED is likely a consequence of one or a number of germline mutation in the TGF-β gene or peptides which regulate TGF-β activation.
- It is unclear whether RD is similar but with variable penetrance or whether there are acquired systemic factors that can, similar to the functional effect in CED, 'switch on' TGF-β activity.

## Primary hypertrophic osteoarthropathy (HOA)

- HOA is a familial disorder characterized by digital clubbing, hyperhidrosis, facial skin thickening, and long bone hyperostosis.
- There are variable features of pachydermia, delayed closure of the fontanelles, and congenital heart disease.
- The AD form (pachydermoperiostosis) is very rare and the genetic cause unknown. AR primary hypertrophic osteoathropathy-1 (PHOAR1) is caused by a homozygous mutation in the HPGD gene on chromosome 4q34.1.

## Pulmonary (secondary) hypertrophic osteoarthropathy (HPOA)

- HPOA differs from HOA and is characterized by digital clubbing secondary to acquired diseases, most commonly intrathoracic neoplasm.

## Endosteal hyperostosis

The process of sclerosis characterizes two conditions: *Van Buchem disease* and *sclerosteosis*.

- Both diseases are autosomal recessive and are caused by mutations in the SOST gene, which encodes for sclerostin.

Table 16.13 The spectrum of sclerosing bone disorders

| Type | Conditions |
|------|-----------|
| Dysplasias and dysostoses | Autosomal dominant osteosclerosis; central osteosclerosis with ectodermal dysplasia; craniodiaphyseal dysplasia, craniometaphyseal dysplasia; dysosteosclerosis; endosteal hyperostosis (Van Buchem disease and sclerosteosis); frontometaphyseal dysplasia; infantile cortical hyperostosis (Caffey disease); juvenile PDB; melorheostosis; metaphyseal dysplasia (Pyle's disease); mixed sclerosing bone dystrophy; oculodentoosseous dysplasia; osteopathia striata; osteopetrosis; osteopoikilosis; progressive diaphyseal dysplasia; Ribbing disease; pycnodysostosis; tubular stenosis (Kenny–Caffey syndrome) |
| Metabolic | Carbonic anhydrase II deficiency; fluorosis; heavy metal poisoning; hepatitis C associated; hypervitaminosis D/A; primary hyperparathyroidism; hypoparathyroidism, pseudohypoparathyroidism; LRP5 gain-of-function (high bone mass); milk-alkali syndrome; renal osteodystrophy; X-linked hypophosphataemic rickets |
| Other | Axial osteomalacia; DISH; Erdheim–Chester disease; fibrogenesis imperfecta ossium; pachydermoperiostosis; hypertrophic osteoarthropathy; ionizing radiation; leukaemias; lymphoma; mastocytosis; multiple myeloma; myelofibrosis; osteomyelitis; osteonecrosis; Paget's; sarcoidosis; sickle cell disease; sclerotic tumour metastases (e.g. prostate); tuberous sclerosis |

- A loss of function in sclerostin results in de-suppression of osteoblast differentiation and function thus causing generalized bone sclerosis and hyperostosis.
- The diseases have informed the development of a therapeutic inhibitor of sclerostin to treat osteoporosis.

## Osteopoikilosis

Is a benign condition often disclosed incidentally on radiographs ('spotted bones').

- Occasionally the condition is associated with the occurrence of connective tissue nevi and dermatofibrosis (Buschke–Ollendorf syndrome) and melorheostosis.

## Hepatitis C osteosclerosis

Hepatitis C can be associated with severe generalized osteosclerosis (cranium-sparing).

- Remodelling of good quality excessive bone seems accelerated during active disease, though it will respond to anti-resorption treatment and gradual spontaneous remission can occur.
- The condition may be caused by effects of IGF as there are increases in IGF binding protein ('big IGF2').

## Reference

5. Whyte MP. Sclerosing bone disorders. In: Rosen CJ (ed) *Primer on the Metabolic Bone Diseases and Disorders of Mineral Metabolism* (8th edn), pp.767–85. New York: Wiley-Blackwell, 2013.

# Bone tumours

Primary tumours of bones and joints are rare, have a peak incidence in childhood and adolescence, and can be benign or malignant. Paget's disease accounts for most cases of osteosarcoma occurring >40 years of age.

## Osteoid osteoma

An osteoid osteoma (OO) is a benign osteoid-forming tumour that can be an elusive cause of intense focal bone pain in children or adults.

- OOs are uncommon and accounts for 10% of benign bone neoplasia.
- OOs are 2–3× more common in men than women and the incidence is highest in the second and third decades of life; >66% occur in long bones and especially the femur and tibia.
- OO lesions are identified on radiographs (or more commonly CT) as a well-defined area of sclerosis with radiolucent nidus often containing speckles of calcium.
- $^{99m}$Tc MDP scintigraphy is a sensitive method of isolating a lesion and CT is valuable for localizing the nidus before surgical resection.
- Pain will respond, in part, to aspirin or NSAIDs. Provided the nidus is completely resected, surgery is curative.

## Osteosarcoma

This is a rare tumour with an incidence of 0.6–0.9 per 100,000 population. It is the commonest primary bone tumour.

- Most patients present at <30 years of age.
- The presentation is with local pain and swelling.
- Radiographs show expansion of the bone with a surrounding soft tissue mass, often containing islands of calcification.
- MRI or CT should be arranged to determine the extent of tumour.
- Patients suspected to have osteosarcoma should be referred to a specialist team for biopsy.
- Treatment depends on histology but generally involves surgical removal of the tumour (and often radical field surgery including amputation), followed by chemotherapy and radiotherapy.
- The prognosis is generally good in cases that present in childhood and adolescence, but poor in elderly patients with osteosarcoma related to Paget's disease of bone.

## Chondrosarcoma

- This is the second most common primary bone tumour. Presentation is similar to osteosarcoma. Treatment choice is between surgical resection and radiotherapy. Chondrosarcomas are relatively resistant to chemotherapy. The prognosis is good for low-grade tumours but poor for anaplastic tumours.

# Infection and rheumatic disease

# Introduction

Microorganisms have been linked directly and indirectly (through organism-specific and autoimmune responses) to a number of acute and chronic inflammatory rheumatic diseases. This chapter will introduce some examples of the inflammatory mechanisms (summarized in Table 17.1) and microorganisms (summarized in Table 17.2) linked to rheumatic disease, and then discuss septic arthritis, *Mycobacterium tuberculosis*, osteomyelitis, Lyme disease, and rheumatic fever.

**Table 17.1** Pathogenesis of rheumatic disease associated with infection

| Inflammatory process | Basic process | Example | Susceptibility |
|---|---|---|---|
| Local infection at MSK sites | Infection. Tissue inflammation and direct tissue damage | Pyogenic septic arthritis | Diabetes, complement and immunoglobulin deficiencies |
| Pathogen and pathogen-specific immune response | Infection and organism-specific response. Immune response to intact organism or fragments, probable immune complex-mediated tissue injury | Syndromes associated with viral hepatitis, e.g. Sjögren's syndrome | Not generally established |
| Pathogens, immune response and autoimmunity | i. Cross-reactive immune response. ii. Infection inferred, but not established, autoreactivity | Rheumatic fever, RA, JIA SLE | HLA class I and II genes, T-cell receptor genes |

**Table 17.2.** Examples of microorganisms associated with arthritis

| Class | Examples | Disorder |
|---|---|---|
| Bacteria | *Staphylococcus* and *Streptococcus* | Septic arthritis, osteomyelitis |
| | *Neisseria* spp. | Gonococcal arthritis |
| | *Brucella* | Septic monoarthritis |
| | *Klebsiella* | Spondyloarthritis |
| | *Chlamydia* | Reactive arthritis |
| Mycobacteria | *Mycobacterium tuberculosis* | Osteomyelitis, oligoarthritis |
| Atypical mycobacteria | *M. avium* complex *M. malmoense* | Septic arthritis in immunosuppressed patients |
| Spirochaete | *Borrelia burgdorferi* | Lyme disease |
| Viruses | Parvovirus B19 | Fifth disease |
| | Rubella | Polyarthropathy |
| | Hepatitis B | Polyarteritis nodosa |
| | Hepatitis C | Cryoglobulinaemia, Sjögren's syndrome |
| | HIV | Polyarthralgia, myopathy, vasculitis, Sicca syndrome |
| Protozoa | *Toxoplasma* | Polyarthritis |
| | *Giardia* | Oligoarthritis |
| | *Trypanosoma* | Myopathy |
| Helminths | *Toxocara* | All cause myositis and arthritis |
| | *Schistosoma* | |
| Fungi | *Histoplasma* | Monoarthropathy |
| | *Cryptococcus* | |

# Septic arthritis

Septic arthritis caused by a bacterium is a medical emergency. See also Chapter 25, p. 708 for management in adults and children.

## Epidemiology
Incidence in the general population is 2–10 per 100,000 and rising to 30–70 per 100,000 in those with autoimmune rheumatic disease or prosthetic joint replacements.

## Pathology
- Most cases are due to haematogenous seeding during transient bacteraemia, but septic arthritis can also be caused by direct penetration through the skin, or by local spread from a contiguous infected site.
- Joints damaged by chronic arthritis (e.g. RA and OA) and prosthetic joints are at increased risk of infection.
- Risk factors include advancing age (>80 years), recent joint surgery, IV drug use, alcoholism, previous intra-articular steroid injection, immunodeficiency states, CKD3b-5, and diabetes.
- The most common pathogens are *Staphylococcus aureus* (including MRSA), *Streptococcus* spp., and *Neisseria gonorrhoeae* in adults.
- The clinical features and natural history of gonococcal and non-gonococcal arthritis are sufficiently distinct to discuss them separately (Table 17.3).
- Gram-negative bacilli may be involved in patients with a current history of IV drug abuse, or those who are immunosuppressed.
- Salmonella is a common cause of septic arthritis among patients with sickle cell disease, although *Staph. aureus* remains the most common organism in this group.

## Presentation
- The most commonly affected joint is the knee (>50%).
- Wrists, ankles, and hips are also commonly involved.
- Intravenous drug users (IVDUs) are predisposed to septic arthritis involving the axial joints, e.g. sternoclavicular joint.
- Transient synovitis, particularly of the hip, is not uncommon in children, and generally occurs in the setting after upper respiratory tract infection
- Patients with septic arthritis usually present with joint pain, swelling, and restricted range of movement of the affected joint(s). Most patients are febrile; however, the elderly do not always show a systemic response.

## Investigation
Every attempt should be made to undertake joint aspiration prior to starting antibiotics.
- The aspirate should be sent for Gram stain, cell count and differential, microscopy, culture, and sensitivity, and blood cultures.
- A fluid sample should be analysed with polarized light microscopy for crystals.
- Depending on likely source of infection, skin, oral, and genital swabs should be considered.
- For a septic joint, the leucocyte count (predominantly neutrophils) in the aspirate is usually > 50,000 cells/mm$^3$.

**Table 17.3** Comparison of clinical features of gonococcal and non-gonococcal septic arthritis

| Gonococcal arthritis | Non-gonococcal septic arthritis |
|---|---|
| *Causative agent:* Neisseria gonorrhoeae | *Causative agents:* Staph. aureus (50% of cases) Staph. epidermis (15% of cases) Strep. pyogenes/pneumonia (20% of cases) Gram-negative bacteria (10% of cases) Anaerobes (5% of cases) |
| Most often in young adults | Most common in the elderly, or underlying joint or medical condition |
| Women > men | Men > women |
| Hip disease uncommon | Hip disease common (20% of cases) |
| Migratory polyarthritis common | Polyarthritis uncommon |
| | Monoarthritis very common |
| Rash, skin blisters/pustules, tenosynovitis common | Extra-articular manifestations uncommon |
| *Synovial fluid analysis:* Gram stain-positive in 25%, culture positive in 50%, lactate normal | *Synovial fluid analysis:* Gram stain-positive in 60%, culture positive in 90%, lactate raised |
| Rapid response to therapy | Often slow response to therapy. May require surgery |
| Full recovery in most cases | 10% mortality; one-third have residual joint damage |

- Routine blood tests should be done: FBC, ESR, CRP, renal function, and liver function tests.
- Plain radiographs are a useful baseline investigation for assessing for osteomyelitis or alternative pathology. In untreated septic arthritis, patchy lucencies in periarticular bone and evidence of articular cartilage loss (joint space narrowing) can be seen.
- US can confirm a joint effusion and aid diagnostic aspiration of small joints.
- If osteomyelitis is suspected, MRI is the investigation of choice.

## Management

See also ➜ Chapter 25.

Three principles determine outcome: (i) prompt diagnosis; (ii) immediate institution of appropriate antibiotics; and (iii) adequate joint drainage.
- The joint should be aspirated to dryness.
- Surgical drainage/washout, or daily arthrocentesis may be required.
- An affected joint should be rested and non-weight-bearing until the inflammation and pain have subsided enough to allow passive mobilization. Mobilization should be encouraged as soon as possible.

- Empiric therapy should be started while awaiting culture results. See local guidelines, but common regimens include flucloxacillin 2 g IV four times a day ± gentamicin IV, or an oral third-generation cephalosporin.
- In cases of suspected MRSA infection, discussion with a microbiologist and consideration of vancomycin is advised.
- *Pseudomonas* spp. should be suspected in IVDUs.
- IV antibiotics are usually continued for 2 weeks followed by 4 weeks of oral antibiotics. Prolonged courses of up to 6 weeks of IV antibiotics may be required in severe cases until swelling subsides, inflammatory markers normalize, and cultures become negative.
- There are no studies comparing long and short courses of antibiotics.
- Infection of a prosthetic joint is a challenging surgical problem, and the management should only be undertaken by specialist arthroplasty surgeons, ideally as part of a prosthetic joint infection MDT.
- Infection of a prosthesis soon after surgery or within a short period following a bacteraemic episode can sometimes be managed with prosthesis retention, but often revision of the prosthesis is required.
- Prosthesis revision is either a single operation or done in a staged manner, with an interval period during which an antibiotic impregnated cement spacer replaces the prosthesis.
- A joint should not be injected with glucocorticoid (GC) if intra-articular infection is suspected, or if there is superficial infection over the skin covering a joint (e.g. cellulitis or psoriasis).
- There is no benefit from intra-articular antibiotics. Indeed, antibiotics can cause a chemical synovitis.

## Septic bursitis

The two most common sites are the olecranon and prepatellar bursae.

- Septic bursitis should be managed with serial fluid aspiration and oral antibiotics.
- Non-responders will need IV antibiotics, and will probably need surgical incision and drainage.
- Chronically infected bursitis can lead to osteomyelitis.

## Gonococcal arthritis

Gonococcal arthritis is caused by *Neisseria gonorrhoea*.

- May present as an acute monoarthritis but is more commonly a migratory polyarthritis with tenosynovitis and dermatitis.
- The polyarthritis is usually asymmetric.
- Patients are usually afebrile.
- Investigations should include synovial fluid analysis, blood cultures, skin/ urethral/rectal/pharyngeal cultures.
- If patients are found to have gonococcal infection they should be tested for other sexually transmitted infections.
- There is increasing resistance, including multidrug resistance, of *N. gonorrhoea* to a wide range of antibiotics.
- Treatment should be guided by local policies but a common regimen is ceftriaxone 1 g IM or IV every 24 hours, with a single dose of azithromycin 1 g orally for potential *Chlamydia trachomatis* co-infection. An oral switch can be considered after 24–48 hours when clinical improvement is seen. Treatment should continue for 7 days.

# Mycobacterium tuberculosis

# *Mycobacterium tuberculosis*

## Epidemiology
- Until 1985, the number of tuberculosis (TB) cases in the USA and Europe declined. More recently, the recurrence of TB has become an important complication of new biologic DMARDs.
- It is thought that 30% of the world's population is infected with TB.
- In industrialized countries, <5% of cases of TB develop infection of bone or joints.

## Pathology
- TB can affect any MSK structure.
- Predisposing factors for MSK TB infection include pre-existing arthritis, alcoholism, use of GCs, and immunosuppression.

## Presentation
- TB of bone is usually a low-grade and slowly progressive infection associated with a variable degree of local and systemic symptoms, such as fatigue, weight loss, or night sweats.
- Onset is insidious and usually mono-articular or monostotic.
- The spine is the commonest site, whether within a vertebral body (Pott's disease), disc, or a paravertebral abscess.
- Spinal cord compression due to vertebral destruction and/or soft tissue swelling due to an abscess is a serious complication and must be treated urgently.
- Spinal stabilization procedures carry a good prognosis in preventing neurological sequelae.
- Monoarticular disease is seen most often in weight-bearing joints (hip, knee, ankle, sacroiliac joint—in order). The wrist and shoulder are less commonly affected.
- Osteomyelitis may affect any long bone and is associated with either solitary or multifocal cysts.
- In TB arthritis, typical features of septic arthritis (e.g. warmth and erythema) are often absent.

## Investigation
- The diagnosis of TB is made by identifying acid-fast bacilli from a lesion or by histopathological changes in excised tissue.
- Synovial fluid analysis is not usually diagnostic and a synovial tissue biopsy may be required.
- A high level of clinical suspicion, in the absence of other identified pathology, might lead the clinician to treat empirically.

## Management

- Standard anti-TB regimens should be used for prophylaxis or treatment, and surveillance for 1 year after treatment is recommended.
- Treatment is usually continued for 6–9 months, or 9–12 months for more advanced disease.
- Surgical intervention may be necessary—tissue biopsy, debridement of necrotic tissue, or stabilization of a joint or long bone.
- Owing to an association between biologics therapy (particularly anti-TNFα) and disseminated TB, the identification of latent TB has become increasingly important in patients being treated for chronic arthritis.
- In such patients, a tuberculin skin test (PPD) is useful. Induration of >5 mm should be considered positive in patients who are immunosuppressed.
- Quantiferon-TB gold, which is a blood-based IFNγ release assay, is also useful for the diagnosis of latent TB.

## Atypical mycobacterial infections

- Patients with autoimmune rheumatic or connective tissue diseases who are taking immunosuppressant medications are at risk of developing atypical infections.
- These infections are usually chronic in nature and can mimic an inflammatory flare of rheumatic disease, thus making a diagnosis can be difficult.
- Atypical infections should be considered in patients with autoimmune diseases who present with MSK symptoms that do not respond to conservative treatment.
- *Mycobacterium malmoense* has been described causing tenosynovitis and septic arthritis of the knee.
- *M. avium* complex and *M. chelonae* osteoarticular infections have also been described.

# Osteomyelitis

Osteomyelitis refers to any infection involving bone or bone marrow.

## Pathology

- *Staphylococcus aureus* is the most common cause of osteomyelitis. Other important pathogens to consider, particularly in the immunosuppressed patient, are TB, *Pseudomonas*, and *Salmonella*.
- The long bones are most commonly affected in children, and the vertebrae in adults.

## Investigations

- No single laboratory investigation is reliable enough to be used routinely for the diagnosis of osteomyelitis. An elevated white cell count and ESR may not be seen.
- Imaging is important in establishing the diagnosis. Which imaging technique is successful at identifying osteomyelitis depends partly on the stage of the infective process.
- Once the pathogen has reached bone, a suppurative reaction and marrow oedema occurs. This can be seen using MRI.
- The next stage—vascular congestion, ischaemia, thrombosis, and soft tissue swelling—is readily detected by CT. After 2–3 weeks, bone reaction including new periosteal bone formation and decalcification can be seen on radiographs.
- Radiographs should be requested as routine as they provide a point of reference, and assess for other disease.
- Vertebral osteomyelitis is often seen early on radiographs. There may be erosion of the vertebral body or disc, and paravertebral abscesses and vertebral collapse are common complications.
- Bone scintigraphy can help localize an area of abnormality. $^{99m}$Tc-bisphosphonate scans, however, are not specific and the negative predictive value is often greater than the positive predictive value.
- $^{111}$In-labelled leucocyte scintigraphy is an alternative.
- Bone biopsy is the gold standard investigation to confirm location of infection, identify specific organisms, to inform treatment choices.

## Management

Several general, local, and systemic factors need to be considered in the management of osteomyelitis (Table 17.4).

- Initial treatment in the acute phase is the same as that for septic monoarthritis. In general, antibiotics are needed for 6 weeks, although chronic infection may require long-term (>3 months) low-dose treatment.
- Antibiotic choice should be guided by tissue microscopy and culture results and local antibiotic therapy policy.
- Surgery may be required early in the acute phase especially if there is an abscess or spinal involvement with neurological compromise.
- Chronic osteomyelitis implies that dead bone is present, and will require surgical debridement.
- Hyperbaric oxygen has also been used successfully in the treatment of air embolism, osteonecrosis, myonecrosis, and burns patients with infection.

**Table 17.4** Factors relevant to the management of osteomyelitis

| Factors | Examples |
|---------|----------|
| General | *Age*: neonates tend to harbour *S. aureus*, Enterobacteriaceae, and β-haemolytic streptococci. In children >4 yrs, *H. influenzae* is common, and in adults *S. aureus*. |
|  | *Bone*: long bones (especially lower limb) are more susceptible than short bones to infection. Pelvic and cranial bones are infrequently involved |
| Local | Chronic lymphoedema |
|  | Venous stasis |
|  | Arterial disease with poor flow |
|  | Scars |
|  | Sensory neuropathy |
|  | Prosthetic material |
| Systemic | Malnutrition |
|  | Renal and liver failure |
|  | Immunodeficiency |
|  | Diabetes |
|  | Malignancy |
|  | Extremes of age |
|  | Chronic hypoxia |
|  | Parenteral drug use |

# Lyme disease

Lyme disease is a tick-borne infection caused by the spirochaetes *Borrelia burgdorferi*, *B. afzeli*, and *B. garinii*.

## Epidemiology

- All three spirochaetes are found in Europe but *Borrelia burgdorferi* is the only species identified in cases of Lyme disease in the USA.
- Cases of Lyme disease have been reported from most states in the USA, as well as throughout Europe, China, and Japan.
- Highest incidence is in children <15 years and middle-aged adults.
- Seasonal variation: common in the summer months of June and July.
- The tick vector *Ixodes* is found on rodents, boar or deer—animals inhabiting wooded, brush, or grassy areas.
- A history of potential exposure in an endemic country within the last 30 days is an important fact to establish in considering the diagnosis.

## Presentation

- The diagnosis is made on epidemiological history and presenting features (Table 17.5), and is confirmed with laboratory tests.
- A clear history of a tick bite is not necessary to make the diagnosis.

## Investigations

- Diagnosis is made by either isolation of the spirochaete from tissue or body fluid or detection of diagnostic levels of IgM or IgG antibodies in the serum or cerebrospinal fluid (CSF) and changes in antibody levels between acute-phase and convalescent paired sera.
- False-positive results occur in other infections (e.g. syphilis), RA, and SLE.
- Western blotting is available as a confirmatory test, distinguishing between true seroreactivity and false-positive serology.
- If the serological status is negative, then the diagnosis is unlikely and an alternative diagnosis should be sought.

## Management

The management of Lyme disease is primarily with antibiotics with choice of therapy varying depending on organ affected.

- Erythema migrans is treated with doxycycline 100 mg twice daily for 3 weeks, or with cefuroxime 500 mg twice daily for 3 weeks.
- Septic arthritis is treated similarly but antibiotic treatment may need to be continued for 30 days.
- The choice of antibiotics for neurological or cardiac disease includes IV penicillin, cefotaxime, or ceftriaxone/imipenem.
- Lyme disease can cause a post-infective inflammatory ('reactive') arthritis which is typical migratory (differential: sarcoid, post-streptococcal, palindromic RA).

**Table 17.5** The presentation of Lyme diseases

| Organ affected | Symptoms |
| --- | --- |
| Skin | *Erythema migrans (EM):* begins as a red macule/papule expanding, over days or weeks, to become a large round lesion often with partial central clearing. The lesion usually measures 5 cm or more. There may be smaller secondary lesions* |
| | An expanding lesion is often accompanied by general symptoms: fever, fatigue, arthralgia, myalgia, headache |
| | Months later a chronic lesion, acrodermatitis chronicum atrophicans (AChA), can appear. It is a violaceous infiltrative rash forming plaques or nodules) |
| MSK | Recurrent, brief attacks of joint swelling in one or a few joints (may become chronic in 60% of untreated cases weeks to years after infection). |
| | A post-Lyme syndrome of fatigue, arthralgia, and myalgia has been reported. Ongoing infection has been difficult to prove. It may be fibromyalgia syndrome |
| Neurological (may occur weeks to months after tick bite) | Lymphocytic meningitis |
| | Cranial neuritis (especially facial nerve palsy) |
| | Radiculoneuropathy (differential Guillain–Barré syndrome) |
| | Encephalomyelitis |
| Cardiovascular (may occur weeks to months after tick bite) | Acute second- or third-degree atrioventricular conduction defects often associated with myocarditis. Resolves in days to weeks. |
| | Carditis—rare and remits spontaneously |

* A similar lesion occurring within hours of a tick bite is usually a hypersensitivity reaction and does not qualify as EM.

# Rheumatic fever

Rheumatic fever is a delayed, non-suppurative sequelae to a pharyngeal infection with Lancefield group A β-haemolytic *Streptococcus*.

## Epidemiology

- Although there has been a dramatic decline in incidence in Europe and the USA, rheumatic fever still occurs, and remains common in developing countries.
- There are an estimated 10–20 million cases per year worldwide, with an annual incidence of 100–200 per 100,000 of the population.

## Pathology

- Associations have been described with HLA-DR2, -DR3, and -DR4.

## Presentation

- There is a latent period of 2–3 weeks after transmission before the appearance of the illness.
- A symptomatic pharyngitis is seen in 60% of cases.
- Patients can present with migratory arthritis (typically of the large joints), myocarditis, or valvulitis, though with chorea is unlikely.
- Diagnosis follows the revised 'Jones' criteria (Table 17.6)
- Patients who have had previous acute rheumatic fever are at risk of repeat episodes following reinfection with group A β-haemolytic streptococci. In repeat episodes, 2 major, or 1 major and 2 minor or 3 minor criteria are sufficient for diagnosis.

**Table 17.6** The revised Jones criteria for the diagnosis of acute rheumatic fever

*The diagnosis requires 2 major; or 1 major and 2 minor criteria*

| Major criteria | Carditis |
|---|---|
| | Arthritis |
| | Chorea |
| | Erythema marginatum |
| | Subcutaneous nodules |
| Minor criteria | Fever (≥38.5°C) |
| | Arthralgia |
| | Previous rheumatic fever or rheumatic heart disease |
| | Raised ESR or CRP |
| | Prolonged PR interval on ECG |
| Supporting evidence | Raised ASO titre* |
| | Positive throat cultures for group A streptococci |
| | Recent scarlet fever |
| | Normochromic normocytic anaemia |

* ASO, anti-streptolysin O antibodies. Titres peak at about 4 weeks, which is about 2 weeks into the clinical illness then titres fall rapidly over the following 2–3 months.

*Arthritis*

Joint involvement is more common and often more severe in teenagers and young adults.

- Arthritis tends to start in the large weight-bearing joints and tends to occur early. The pain can be severe. Often there is an absence of objective signs of inflammation. It lasts 2–3 weeks and is self-limiting.
- NSAIDs are the recommended first-line treatment.
- Discriminating post-streptococcal reactive arthritis (seen in the absence of carditis) from rheumatic fever can be difficult. Most patients will fulfil the Jones criteria and, therefore, should be considered as having rheumatic fever.

*Cardiac disease*

- Rheumatic heart disease is the most severe outcome of acute rheumatic fever. It remains the major cause of acquired valvular heart disease in the world.
- Rheumatic heart disease usually occurs 10–20 years after the initial infection. The mitral valve (stenosis) is most frequently involved.
- When left untreated, cardiomegaly and cardiac failure secondary to valvular disease may ensue.
- Carditis may also occur and is associated with cardiomyopathy and conduction defects including second- or third-degree heart block.

*Chorea*

- Sydenham's chorea (St Vitus' dance) consists of abrupt, purposeless movements, muscle weakness, and emotional disturbance.
- The hands and face are usually the most obviously affected parts. The movements are not present during sleep, but do occur at rest and may be more marked on one side of the body.
- Chorea may be the sole feature suggesting rheumatic fever (beyond observing new cardiac murmurs) and may occur weeks to months after onset of an arthropathy.

*Skin*

- Subcutaneous nodules of rheumatic fever are firm and painless. They range from a few mm to 2 cm in size. They are located over bony surfaces or near tendons. Lesions are present for 2–4 weeks only, and more often in patients with carditis.
- Erythema marginatum is an evanescent, non-purpuric rash, usually affecting the trunk and proximal part of the limbs, but sparing the face. Because the rash often appears to make a ring, it is also called 'erythema annulare'. The lesions come and go in a matter of hours, heat can make them appear worse, and they are more common in association with carditis. They resolve spontaneously.
- Erythema nodosum is rare.

### Investigation

- There is no diagnostic test.
- Diagnosis is based on detection of group A streptococcal infection followed by the typical clinical manifestations.
- Raised inflammatory markers and mild anaemia are often seen.
- Serial rises in ASO antibody (or anti-DNAaseB) titres may be seen if measured every 14 days.
- CXR and ECG to look for conduction defects/cardiomegaly.

### Management

- The three goals of management include symptomatic relief, eradication of group A β-haemolytic streptococci, and prophylaxis against future infection with group A β-haemolytic streptococci.
- NSAIDs should be given until all symptoms have resolved.
- Heart failure should be treated with conventional medications.
- Penicillin is given for 10 days, even in the absence of pharyngitis.
- Chorea is treated with haloperidol 1–2 mg/kg/day. GCs are sometimes also given, though there is little evidence of added benefit.
- Recurrence can occur within the first 2 years. However, recurrence rates are low, and the risk of recurrence declines with age of first attack. Recurrence is associated with increased risk of cardiac disease.
- Prophylaxis should be started as soon as antibiotic treatment has finished with oral phenoxymethylpenicillin or benzylpenicillin 1.2 million units IM every 3–4 weeks. Duration of prophylaxis depends on severity of disease. Erythromycin 250 mg daily can be used in patients allergic to penicillin.

# Rare autoinflammatory and miscellaneous diseases

# Rare autoinflammatory diseases

## Introduction

Rare autoinflammatory diseases (RAIDs) are mostly rare monogenic immunological disorders that typically present in childhood with recurrent fevers, high inflammatory markers, and systemic features.

- The typical presentation is with bouts of fever, and associated symptoms between which the patient is well ('periodic' fever).
- The term 'autoinflammatory' arose from the understanding that gene mutations result in switching on of innate immunity that has a secondary effect on adaptive immunity. This differs from autoimmunity where failure of recognition between self and non-self is caused by self-reactive T cells, involves MHC class II and leads to circulating antibodies.
- Since the discovery of the gene for familial Mediterranean fever (FMF), MEFV (pyrin innate immunity regulator), the genes of many other RAIDs have been identified and collectively have proven extremely valuable in understanding inflammatory pathways.
- Although RAIDs are not generally life-threatening, early diagnosis may avoid repeated hospital visits, unnecessary investigations and treatment, reduced quality of life, and morbidity from AA amyloid.

## Pathogenesis

- RAIDs are disorders of the innate immune system. Innate immunity is the first line of defence against pathogenic microbes and mediates host responses against cellular stress (e.g. against lipopolysaccharide or peptidoglycan constituents).
- Highly conserved molecular processes, known as pathogen-associated molecular patterns (PAMPs), are detected by intracellular pattern-recognition receptors (PRRs) such as Toll-like (TLRs) and nucleotide-binding oligomerization domain (NOD)-like receptors (NLRs), which are expressed by macrophages, monocytes, neutrophils, and lymphocytes.
- PRR signalling drives (the 'inflammasome') cytokine production such as interleukin-1β (IL-1β).
- Genotype-influenced inflammasome function can cause RAIDs and contribute to other diseases (e.g. NOD2 mutations can causes Blau syndrome and contribute to IBD phenotype also).

## Epidemiology

- FMF, the commonest RAID, has a carrier frequency in Middle Eastern populations of 30–50%.
- Fewer than 200 families have been reported with tumour necrosis factor (TNF) receptor-associated periodic syndrome (TRAPS) and there are 100 reported cases of familial cold autoinflammatory syndrome (FCAS) and Muckle–Wells syndrome (MWS).
- As an example of other RAIDs, there are fewer than 10 families reported to have Majeed syndrome, mostly arising from Jordan.

## Approach to diagnosis

Diagnosis is based on clinical suspicion, mostly in children, at times of recurrent fevers or multisystem inflammation of unknown aetiology.

- Treatable causes of fever such as infection, neoplasia, and autoimmune diseases should be excluded.
- Family history, ethnicity, age of onset of fever, especially within first year of life, characterization of the fever, and rash and manifestations are important clues to diagnosis with RAIDs.
- Characterization of the fever includes its duration and periodicity. This also helps to understand the burden of disease on quality of life.
- High inflammatory markers and a neutrophilia are typical during febrile episodes and normalize during disease-free intervals.
- Associated features also include abdominal or limb pain and:
  - Diarrhoea—present in 75% of cases with MVK deficiency.
  - Uveitis.
  - Sensorineural hearing loss.
  - Inflammatory episodes provoked by vaccination.
  - Arthritis.
- Confirmation of a RAID can be sought with genetic testing; however, >50% of RAID patients have negative genetic results.
- In the UK, genetic testing is undertaken by the National Amyloidosis centre at University College Hospital, London (℗ http://www.ucl. ac.uk/amyloidosis).
- Information about the latest genetic abnormalities is available on the In-Fever website at ℗ http://http://fmf.igh.cnrs.fr/ISSAID/infevers/.
- Urinalysis should be requested to screen for proteinuria which raises the possibility of secondary AA amyloidosis.

## Cutaneous manifestations of RAIDs

- Urticarial eruptions—typical of patients with the cryopyrinopathies— are often indistinguishable from the more common mast cell-mediated chronic urticaria. The latter is usually asymmetric with itchy recurrent wheal and flare and angio-oedema.
- Urticarial vasculitis, which is fixed in shape for >24 hours and also seen in cryopyrinopathies.
- Multiple sterile abscesses—seen in pyoderma gangrenosum, acne and pyogenic arthritis (PAPA) syndrome, SAPHO syndrome, Majeed syndrome, DIRA, early-onset IBD, and several other RAIDs.
- Psoriaform rashes: seen in congenital forms of psoriasis (e.g. CAMPS) and pustular skin lesions as in SAPHO syndrome.
- Ichthyosiform rash: tan-coloured and scaly is seen in ~90% of patients with Blau syndrome.

## RAID presentations

RAIDs might be considered in a differential diagnosis on the basis of age of presentation, familial inheritance (see Table 18.1), and typical clinical features common to certain groupings of RAIDs.

**Table 18.1** The spectrum of rare autoinflammatory diseases

| Main features | Diagnosis; molecular defect | Inheritance; gene; gene location |
|---|---|---|
| Periodic fever, macular or papular rash, abdominal pain | MKD (MVA and hyper IgD syndrome (HIDS)); MVK deficiency | AR; MVK; 12q24.11 |
| | FMF; pyrin deficiency | AR; MEFV (pyrin innate immunity regulator); 16p33.3 |
| | TRAPS; TNF receptor signalling | AD; TNFRSF1A; 12p13.31 |
| Fever and urticarial rash | CINCA, MWS, and FCAS; aberrant cryopyrin production and inflammasome responses | AD; NLRP3; 1q44 |
| Granulomatous disease with low-grade fever | Blau syndrome | AD; CARD15; 16q12.1 |
| | Early-onset IBD | AR; IL-10R |
| Pyogenic rash | PAPA | AD; PSTPIP1; 15q24.3 |
| | Majeed syndrome | AR; LPIN2; 18p11 |
| | CAMPS; abnormal activation of NFκB | AD; CARD14; 17q25 |
| | DIRA; unchecked IL-1α activation | AR; IL-1RN; 2q14.1 |
| | DITRA; as for DIRA | AR; IL-36RN; 2q14.1 |
| | CANDLE; defect in IFN signalling | AR; PSMB8; 6p21.3 |
| Skeletal disorders | Majeed syndrome/DIRA | See above |
| | CNO | Not known |
| | Caffey's disease | AD; COL1A1; 17q21.33 |
| | Cherubism | AD; SH3BP2; 4p16.3 |
| Multisystem RAID | Behçet's disease | Not known |
| | Systemic-onset JIA | Various genes |

AD, autosomal dominant; AR, autosomal recessive; CANDLE, Chronic atypical neutrophilic dermatosis with lipodystrophy and elevated temperature CAMPS, CARD14-mediated psoriasis; CINCA, chronic infantile neurological cutaneous and articular syndrome; CNO, chronic nonbacterial osteomyelitis; DIRA, deficiency of IL-1 receptor antagonist; DITRA, deficiency of interleukin 36 receptor antagonist; FCAS, familial cold autoinflammatory syndrome; FMF, Familial Mediterranean fever; IBD, inflammatory bowel disease; MKD, mevalonate kinase deficiency; MVA, mevalonic aciduria; MVK, melavonate kinase; MWS, Muckle–Wells syndrome; PAPA, pyogenic arthritis, pyoderma gangrenosum and acne; SAPHO, synovitis, acne, pustulosis, hyperostosis, osteitis; TRAPS, tumour necrosis factor-associated periodic syndrome; TNFRSF, tumour necrosis factor receptor superfamily.

*Neonatal and infantile periodic fevers*

- A RAID is considered in infancy when a fever is unresponsive to antibiotics or recurrent, when an associated rash is persistent or unusual, and there are atypical features, such as bone oedema.
- Alternative diagnoses for consideration include neonatal lupus (NLE; see ⟳ Chapter 10), Kawasaki disease, Behçet's disease, and systemic-onset JIA.
- A RAID in the first year of life includes:
  - chronic infantile neurological cutaneous and articular syndrome (CINCA), a cryopyrinopathy also known in the USA as NOMID (neonatal-onset multisystem inflammatory disease).
  - FCAS.
  - Majeed syndrome.
  - deficiency of IL-1 receptor antagonist (DIRA).
  - Blau syndrome.
  - chronic atypical neutrophilic dermatosis with lipodystrophy and elevated temperature (CANDLE).

*Childhood periodic fevers (cryopyrin-associated periodic syndromes)*

CAPS are a group of autosomal dominant RAIDs that share the same gene mutation (NLRP3) but present at different ages with variations of phenotype that includes an urticarial rash.

- NLRP3 gene encodes the protein cryopyrin. Cryopyrin is a key component of the inflammasome (an intracellular multi-protein complex), which regulates the processing of IL-1β.
- CAPS result in excess IL-1β and respond to anti-IL-1 therapy (anakinra, canakinumab, and rilonacept).
- AA amyloidosis occurs in ~25% generally in all CAPS.
- In *CINCA*, fevers are usually short lived, low grade, or absent.
- Typical features in CINCA are frontal bossing, saddle nose, midface hypoplasia; arthritis and bony overgrowth of knees, hands and feet, clubbing, CNS and ophthalmic involvement.
- Radiographs in CINCA may show irregular ossification of metaphyses and epiphyses.
- *FCAS* is also known as familial cold urticaria and associated with low-grade fever and arthralgia. It presents within the first 6 months of life.
- Typically in FCAS, cold precipitates symptoms within 1–2 hours and attacks last <24 hours.
- *MWS* typically presents in an older child with high fever, typically in the afternoon.
- In MWS, fever attacks last 1–2 days although the rash can be persistent and sensorineural deafness is common usually appearing in childhood or even early adulthood.

*Familial Mediterranean fever (FMF)*

FMF is most common in non-Ashkenazi Jews, Arabs, Turks, and Armenians as a result of a mutation in the gene which encodes pyrin. Pyrin is expressed in myeloid cells and regulates the inflammasome.

- Diagnosis is based on the presence of:
  - short, intense, self-limiting episodes of fever (1–3 days) with a leucocytosis and high ESR.
  - serositis (peritonitis and less commonly pericarditis or pleuritis).
  - comprehensive response to oral colchicine, which achieves remission in 65% of patients and 20–30% experience a reduction in the severity and number of fever attacks.
- Less common features include large joint lower limb arthritis, meningitis headache, orchitis, vasculitic rash, and myalgia.
- Genetic analysis is not always helpful.
- The recommended dose of colchicine is 0.5 mg/day for children <5 years of age, 1 mg/day for children 5–10 years, and 1.5 mg/day for children >10 years. Doses are titrated upwards for lack of efficacy and downwards for abdominal pain/diarrhoea in 0.25 mg steps (max. 2 mg/day). Colchicine virtually eliminates the risk of AA amyloid.
- Anti-IL-1 (e.g. anakinra) may be effective in colchicine-resistant FMF patients.

*TNF receptor-associated periodic syndromes (TRAPS)*

Previously known as Hibernian fever, TRAPS affects 1 per million in Europe and is caused by mutations in the p55 TNF receptor 1 (TNFR1). 50% have no family history.

- Presentation is often by 4 years with prolonged, although milder, periodic fevers, lasting 1–3 weeks. In 30%, symptoms are almost continuous. Fever is always associated with high ESR.
- Common features are myoarthralgia, tender macular rash on the extremes and/or torso, and abdominal pain, headache, pleuritic pain, conjunctivitis, periorbital oedema, and lymphadenopathy.
- Genotyping is helpful but two polymorphisms are present in 4% of the normal population (and may be associated with mild symptoms).
- Acute flares are treated with glucocorticoids (GCs) and flares best prevented with anakinra or canakinumab. Etanercept (not infliximab) may be effective.
- Without effective long-term treatment 25% develop AA amyloid.

*Mevalonate kinase deficiency (MKD; mevalonic aciduria (MVA) / hyper-IgD syndrome (HIDS))*

- The condition(s) was first identified in 1984 in six patients of Dutch ancestry with a long history of recurrent attacks of fever and high serum IgD levels.
- An AR condition, mutations in the mevalonate kinase (MVK) gene result in a deficiency of mevalonate kinase, essential in cholesterol biosynthesis. Complete absence of MVK activity results in mevalonic aciduria (MVA) associated with developmental delay, progressive ataxia, visual loss, and failure to thrive.
- MKD starts in early childhood and presents with fevers lasting 3–7 days.

- Characteristically the condition is precipitated by vaccination.
- Other features include abdominal pain, diarrhoea, lymphadenopathy, arthralgia, aphthous ulcers, and polymorphic rash.
- Diagnosis is supported by an IgD concentration >100 IU/mL during/ between attacks and increased urine mevalonic acid during fever.
- MVK gene molecular analysis is used to confirm the diagnosis.
- Treatment is symptomatic during a flare which may also respond favourably to GCs. There may be a role in treatment for inhibitors of IL-1 or TNFα.
- Symptoms improve with age and AA amyloidosis is rare.

*Periodic fever, aphthous stomatitis, pharyngitis, adenitis (PFAPA) syndrome*

PFAPA syndrome is included here as it is the commonest syndrome associated with recurrent fever, although it is not a RAID.

- It is defined by debilitating episodes of abrupt onset of fever lasting 3–6 days with recurrence every 2–6 weeks.
- Other features include sore throat, small mouth or lip ulcers, tender swelling of the cervical lymph nodes.
- The syndrome usually presents before the age of 5 years and spontaneously resolves during the second decade of life.
- CRP/ESR and neutrophils are elevated during attacks and normal (or settle) between them.
- 1–2 days of prednisolone (1–2 mg/kg) may be given at the start of an attack, which may be prevented by colchicine, anti-IL-1 therapy, or even cimetidine in some cases.

*Late-onset FMF*

This form of FMF is a milder variant of the condition in children.

- It occurs typically in men and with abdominal attacks.
- Chronic manifestations (e.g. amyloid) rarely occur.

*Late-onset TRAPS*

Of all patients with TRAPS, 9% present in adulthood with mean age of onset of 35 years and a similar phenotype to paediatric onset.

*Schnitzler's syndrome*

Very rare and usually from 50 years of age with urticarial rash and fatigue.

## When diagnosis is unclear

There is considerable overlap in features of the inherited periodic fevers making diagnosis challenging.

- In some cases genetic analysis is inconclusive. This may be because of a single mutation in an AR disorder or identification of variants of unknown significance (e.g. low-penetrance mutations, functional polymorphisms, and novel variants of unknown functional impact).
- As a guide to diagnosis in general, the Eurofever Project has produced a validated evidence-based tool (Table 18.2).

## RAIDs with prominent skin manifestations

*Pyoderma gangrenosum, acne, and pyogenic arthritis (PAPA) syndrome*

PAPA syndrome is characterized by multiple sterile abscesses or pyoderma with severe cystic acne and painful hot arthritis.

**Table 18.2** The Eurofever tool for indication for molecular analysis or clinical classification* of patients with suspected RAIDs after careful exclusion of other causes.

| FMF | | MKS | | CAPS | | TRAPS | |
|---|---|---|---|---|---|---|---|
| **Presence** | **Score** | **Presence** | **Score** | **Presence** | **Score** | **Presence** | **Score** |
| Duration of episodes <2 days | 9 | Age of onset <2 years | 9 | Urticarial rash | 25 | Periorbital oedema | 21 |
| Chest pain | 13 | Aphthous stomatitis | 13 | Neurosensorial hearing loss | 25 | Duration of episodes >6 days | 19 |
| Abdominal pain | 9 | Generalized enlargement of lymph nodes or splenomegaly | 9 | Conjunctivitis | 10 | Migratory rash† | 18 |
| Eastern Mediterranean‡ ethnicity | 22 | Painful lymph nodes | 13 | | | Myalgia | 6 |
| North Mediterranean‡ ethnicity | 7 | Diarrhoea (sometimes / often) | 20 | | | Relatives affected | 7 |
| | | Diarrhoea (always) | 37 | | | | |
| **Absence** | | **Absence** | | **Absence** | | **Absence** | |
| Aphthous stomatitis | 9 | Chest pain | 11 | Exudative pharyngitis | 11 | Vomiting | 14 |
| Urticarial rash | 15 | | | Abdominal pain | 15 | Aphthous stomatitis | 15 |
| Enlarged cervical lymph nodes | 10 | | | | | | |
| Duration of episodes >6 days | 13 | | | | | | |
| **Cut-off** | **≥60** | **Cut-off** | **≥42** | **Cut-off** | **≥52** | **Cut-off** | **≥43** |

* The clinical features should be related to the typical fever episodes (i.e. exclusion of intercurrent infection or other comorbidities).

† Centrifugal migratory, erythematous patches most typically overlying a local area of myalgia, usually on the limbs or trunk.

‡ Eastern Mediterranean: Turkish, Armenian, non-Ashkenazi Jewish, Arab. North Mediterranean: Italian, Spanish, Greek.

CAPS, cryopyrin-associated periodic syndromes; FMF, familial Mediterranean fever; MKD, mevalonate kinase deficiency; TRAPS, receptor-associated periodic fever syndrome. Reproduced from Federici, Silvia et al. Evidence-based provisional clinical classification criteria for autoinflammatory periodic fevers, *Ann Rheum Dis* 2015;74:799–805, with permission

- PAPA is attributable to mutations of the PTSTPIP1 gene that encodes a protein which interacts with pyrin.
- PAPA may be responsive to anti-TNFα or IL-1 blockade.

### Deficiency of IL-1 receptor antagonist (DIRA)

DIRA presents in the neonatal period with a pustular rash, arthritis, periostitis, and osteolytic lesions of ribs and long bones. An excellent response to IL-1 inhibition (e.g. anakinra) is seen.

### Chronic atypical neutrophilic dermatosis with lipodystrophy and elevated temperature (CANDLE) syndrome

CANDLE syndrome is AR with increased IFN-γ expression. It appears to be responsive to drugs inhibiting Janus kinases (JAKs), which mediate IFN-γ signalling.

### Blau syndrome

Blau syndrome is an AD RAID characterized by a tan-coloured ichthyosiform rash (90%) and non-caseating granulomas. Blau syndrome is indistinguishable from sarcoid, similarly affecting the joints, skin, and uveal tract.

### CARD14-mediated psoriasis (CAMPS)

In CAMPs, severe generalized pustular psoriasis presents before 3 years of age. Fevers are uncommon however.

### Further reading

Gattorno M, Federici S, Pelagatti MA, et al. Diagnosis and management of autoinflammatory diseases in childhood. *J Clin Immunol* 2008;28:S73–S83.

Koné-Paut I, Piram M. Targeting interleukin-1β in CAPS syndromes. What did we learn? *Autoimmun Rev* 2012;11:77–80.

Lachmann HJ, Kone-Paut I, Kuemmerle-Deschner JB, et al. Use of canakinumab in the cryopyrin-associated periodic syndrome. *N Engl J Med* 2009;360:2416–25.

# Behçet's disease

## Epidemiology and pathophysiology

Behçet's disease (BD) is a systemic inflammatory disorder of unknown aetiology. It is most common in the Mediterranean basin, the Middle East, and Asia.

- Prevalence is estimated at 80–370 cases/100,000 in Turkey.
- The usual onset of the disorder is in the third to fourth decades. Onset is rare before puberty or after the sixth decade.
- The M:F ratio is equal, but the disease tends to run a more severe course in men and the young.
- Patients from Eastern Asia, Middle East, and Mediterranean countries show a higher prevalence of HLA-B51; In Israelis there is an association with HLA-B52, and in the UK HLA-B57.
- BD is considered to have a strong angiopathic basis and considerable morbidity overall is caused by thrombosis in addition to inflammation.
- Mild anaemia of chronic disease and neutrophilia is seen in 15% of patients. ESR and CRP are often only moderately raised with episodes of arthritis, erythema nodosum (EN) and thrombophlebitis.
- Autoantibodies are characteristically absent (i.e. ANCA negative).

## Clinical features and their management

Full-blown BD might be easy to identify, but there are conditions that mimic the incomplete picture, including reactive arthritis, antiphospho-lipid syndrome (APS), multiple sclerosis, IBD, erythema multiforme, and neutrophilic dermatoses. The International Study Group (ISG) criteria published in 1990 are the most widely accepted diagnostic and classification criteria (see ➜ Table 18.3). For clinical manifestation frequencies, see ➜ Table 18.4.

*Skin and mucosal involvement*

- Skin lesions may be nodular (like EN), acneiform, or vasculitic.
- The pathergy reaction, a hyper-reactivity of the skin to a needle prick, is a nonspecific phenomenon, but may be helpful in diagnosis of BD (note: also positive in IBD and Sweet's Syndrome). After skin puncture with a needle, a papule or pustule forms in 24–72 hours. The reaction is thought to be unusual in patients from Northern Europe or the United States, but is positive between 60–70% of patients from Japan and Turkey.
- Painful oral aphthous ulcers may precede other features by several years. Idiopathic oral aphthous ulcers are common, and alone do not imply BD. The ulcers may resemble ordinary aphthae, but tend to be more frequent and multiple, and may heal with scarring.
- Genital ulceration in men is most prominent over the scrotum (90%). Urethritis is not seen unless there is a meatal ulcer. In women, the labia are commonly affected.

**Table 18.3** International Study Group criteria for the diagnosis of Behçet's disease

| Clinical feature required for diagnosis | Defined as: |
|---|---|
| Recurrent oral ulceration | Minor aphthous, major aphthous or herpetiform ulcers, observed by a physician or reported reliably by the patient, recurrent at least 3 times in one 12-month period |
| **Plus, any 2 of the following:** | |
| Recurrent genital ulceration | Recurrent genital aphthous ulceration or scarring, observed by a physician or reported reliably by the patient |
| Eye lesions | Anterior uveitis, posterior uveitis, or cells in vitreous on slit lamp examination; or retinal vasculitis observed by an ophthalmologist |
| Skin lesions | Erythema nodosum-like lesions, observed by a physician or reported reliably by the patient, pseudofolliculitis or papulopustular lesions; or acneiform nodules observed by a physician in post-adolescent patients not receiving GCs |
| Positive pathergy test | Test interpreted as positive by a physician at 24–48 hrs, done with an oblique insertion of a 20-gauge or smaller needle under sterile conditions |

**Table 18.4** Frequency of clinical manifestations in Behçet's disease

| Lesion | Prevalence (%) |
|---|---|
| Aphthous ulcers | 97–100 |
| Genital ulcers | ~85 |
| Skin lesions | ~80 |
| Papulopustular lesions | 85 |
| Erythema nodosum | 50 |
| Pathergy reaction | ~60% (Mediterranean countries, Japan) |
| Eye lesions/uveitis | 50 |
| Arthritis | 30–50 |
| Subcutaneous thrombophlebitis | 25 |
| Arterial occlusion/aneurysm | ~4 |
| Gastrointestinal lesions | 1–30 (more prevalent in Japan) |
| Epididymitis | ~5 |
| Deep vein thrombosis | 5–20 |
| Neurological disease | ~5 |
| Secondary amyloidosis | 0.04–3 |

*Skin and mucosal involvement treatment*

- Mild oral and genital ulceration may respond to topical GC preparations or GC inhalers.
- Colchicine 1.5 mg/day (0.5mg tds) can be used to treat frequent attacks of aphthous ulceration.
- More resistant cases may respond to azathioprine (AZA) 2.5 mg/kg/day, mycophenolate mofetil (MMF) and/or brief courses of prednisolone 20 mg/day.
- Anti-TNFα (etanercept and infliximab) have been shown to be beneficial for mucocutaneous disease.
- Ciclosporin and interferon alfa have been shown to be effective in RCTs. NSAIDs are frequently used for pain control.
- Thalidomide has modest benefits in mucocutaneous BD, but it is difficult to obtain and carries a significant risk of peripheral neuropathy and teratogenicity. It is generally reserved for highly resistant disease in patients who will follow strict contraception.

*Eye disease*

- Eye disease is a serious complication and a poor prognostic factor.
- It is more common in men, in the <25 years age group, is usually seen during the first 2 years of having BD, and is bilateral in 70–80%.
- The most frequent eye involvement is chronic relapsing panuveitis. The presence of a hypopyon occurs in ~20% of patients and is almost always associated with severe posterior retinal vasculitis. Recurrent bouts of inflammation result in structural change, and total loss of vision occurs in 20% of cases despite treatment.

*Eye involvement treatment*

Topical GC and mydriatics with close supervision may be sufficient in mild disease, but severe disease requires AZA 2.5 mg/kg/day, ciclosporin, up to 5 mg/kg/day, anti-TNFα therapy (especially infliximab), and cyclophosphamide (CYC) for refractory cases.

*Musculoskeletal involvement*

Arthritis or arthralgia is seen in about 50% of patients.

- MSK symptoms may precede the other findings by months or years.
- Arthritis might commonly involve knees, ankles, hands, and wrists, or occasionally symmetrical. It is usually a self-limiting synovitis, and tends to be non-erosive and non-deforming.
- Back pain is rare. However, a subgroup of patients have a reactive arthritis-like features, presenting with acne, arthritis and enthesopathy (see main differential: SAPHO syndrome, ➜ Chapter 16).

*Musculoskeletal involvement treatment*

Pain may respond to NSAIDs and colchicine (e.g. 0.5 mg three times a day)

- Inflammatory disease often requires the introduction of AZA 2.5 mg/kg/day. Other therapies include SSZ 2–3 g/day or MTX 10–20 mg weekly. Infliximab could also be considered.

*Cardiovascular and pulmonary involvement*

- BD can affect both arteries and veins. In spite of the thrombotic episodes, there is a relative absence of embolic phenomena.
- The heart is rarely involved in BD, but may manifest as endocarditis, myocarditis, pericarditis, coronary vasculitis, and ventricular aneurysms. Right-sided endomyocardial fibrosis with intracardiac thrombi is an unusual manifestation that has been observed in young males with widespread vascular disease.
- Thrombophlebitis occurs in 25% of patients. Lower limb venous thrombosis of the deep veins is often seen. Occlusion of suprahepatic veins (Budd–Chiari syndrome) is a rare complication of BD that carries a high death rate.
- Artery involvement (1.5–7.5%) carries significant associated mortality. Lesions are typically aneurysmal with a risk of rupture, or uncommonly, occlusive. The abdominal aorta is the most frequently affected resulting in abdominal pain. Peripheral arterial involvement may result in reduced/absent pulses with intermittent claudication, cold extremities, or even gangrene.
- The pulmonary pathology of BD is related to arterial vasculitis. Aneurysms, thromboses, and infarcts are found. Pulmonary embolism is rare despite high rates of thrombophlebitis.

*Cardiovascular and pulmonary involvement treatment*

- Aspirin and NSAIDs can be used for phlebitis.
- Aneurysms and arterial occlusion can be treated with endovascular surgery including intra-arterial embolization if combination immunosuppressants fail or are considered inappropriate.
- There remains debate as to whether to use heparin or oral anticoagulants for BD thrombophlebitis. Most physicians will choose to treat with anticoagulation in addition to immunosuppression. If patients have BD-associated aneurysms, anticoagulation increases the risks of haemorrhage.

*Neurological involvement*

Neurological involvement is seen in 5% of patients with BD. It usually occurs after the first 5 years of the disease, and is almost never a presenting feature. Patterns of involvement are either vascular or parenchymal.

- Parenchymal disease is usually manifested by bilateral pyramidal signs, unilateral hemiparesis, behavioural changes, and headaches.
- The most commonly affected site is the brainstem and basal ganglia. Cerebral cortices seem to be spared. Meningeal irritation and dementia may also occur. As is the case with eye disease, central nervous involvement is often more severe in men.
- Cerebrospinal fluid (CSF) changes such as pleocytosis and increased cellularity occur in 60% of patients with parenchymal involvement.
- MRI is more sensitive than CT for imaging. Signal changes, with contrast enhancement in the brainstem and basal ganglia regions, occur but are not specific (consider MS, sarcoid, APS).

- Dural sinus thrombosis is a feature characterized by headache, sixth nerve palsy, papilloedema, and raised CSF pressure. It has a better prognosis than parenchymal involvement. An association between dural sinus thrombosis and deep vein thrombosis exists.
- In contrast to other vasculitides, peripheral neuropathy is unusual.

*Neurological involvement treatment*
- Thrombosis of the dural sinuses and increased intracranial pressure should be treated with IV methylprednisolone 1 g for 3–5 days.
- Parenchymal involvement is usually treated with CYC or AZA combined with GCs.
- A small trial has found MTX may stop the progression of chronic neurological involvement, but larger studies are needed.
- A few case reports suggest infliximab may be beneficial in refractory parenchymal disease.

*Gastrointestinal involvement and its treatment*
- While seen in up to one-third of patients in Japan, gastrointestinal (GI) disease is rare in patients from the Mediterranean basin.
- The pathology is mucosal ulceration, mostly in ileum and caecum.
- The course is one of relapse and remission, and a tendency for bowel perforation. It can be difficult to distinguish the findings of GI BD from those of Crohn's disease.
- In treating GI BD, ulceration may respond to prednisolone 0.5–1 mg/ kg/day, SSZ 2–3 g/day, or infliximab. AZA is an alternative.
- Surgical evaluation may be necessary to manage severe sequelae.
- Large ulcers, high CRP and perforation are predictors of recurrence.

*Renal involvement and its treatment*
Renal disease is seen much less than might be expected with systemic vasculitis.
- There are occasional reports of glomerulonephritis, ranging from IgA nephropathy to rapidly progressive glomerulonephritis.
- Secondary amyloidosis AA usually presents with nephrotic disease, and has been reported in about 1% of patients.
- Epididymitis is seen in up to 20% of males. Other urological problems include cystitis and erectile dysfunction.
- Treatment focuses on symptom control. Patients with AA amyloidosis require therapy for BD.
- Colchicine can be used to treat both BD and amyloidosis.

# Sarcoidosis

Sarcoidosis is a multisystem disease of unknown aetiology, characterized by the presence of multiple, non-caseating granulomas.

## Epidemiology and pathophysiology

- Sarcoidosis is found worldwide but the prevalence, clinical features, and outcome varies considerably.
- It may present at any age, but prevalence peaks in the 20–40 years age group with a second peak in women >50 years old.
- It is seen more often in developed vs underdeveloped, Western vs Eastern, and in Northern vs Southern European countries.
- Sweden and Denmark have prevalence rates of 60 per 100,000, The UK 20 per 100,000. In the USA, sarcoidosis is 10–15× more prevalent in African American people than in Caucasians, and in this ethnicity, disease is often severe. Studies have suggested a link between HLA-B8, HLA-DR3, acute sarcoidosis, and arthritis.
- Granuloma and associated tissue inflammation can occur in virtually any tissue in the body and can manifest local symptoms alone. Systemic effects are not always present.

## General patterns of disease

### Acute sarcoidosis (Lofgren's syndrome)

- This presents with rapid-onset fever, acute arthritis/arthralgias, EN, and hilar lymphadenopathy.
- Löfgren's syndrome has a high rate of remission and a good prognosis.
- Treatment usually requires NSAIDs only.
- It has been reported to occur in seasonal clusters, especially winter and early spring, suggesting environmental/infectious triggers.
- The chest radiograph clears within 1 year in 60% of cases.
- Around 15% of patients with Löfgren's syndrome have a raised angiotensin converting enzyme (ACE) level at presentation.

### Chronic sarcoidosis

- Chronic sarcoid is less common than Löfgren's syndrome and has an often subtle, insidious, progressive, and highly variable clinical course. Clinical manifestations can be extensive (Table 18.5).
- Granulomata can occur in virtually any tissue in the body and can manifest local symptoms. Systemic effects are not always present.

### Early-onset (childhood) sarcoidosis

EOS refers to disease onset in the first 5 years of life and has a clinical phenotype distinct from adult-onset disease and very similar to Blau syndrome (see earlier in this chapter).

- A typical presentation is with rash, polyarthritis (typically a 'boggy' tenosynovitis), and uveitis (little pulmonary involvement).
- The rash occurs in 77% and is often unusual including a soft yellow-brown papillomatous lesion, hypopigmentation, and ulceration.
- Eye disease is often asymptomatic and uveitis requires screening with a slit lamp. Lacrimal hypertrophy and conjunctival granuloma may be found.

**Table 18.5** Clinical manifestations in chronic sarcoidosis

| Organ/system | Clinical features |
|---|---|
| Lung | Parenchymal disease in >90% of cases |
| Skin | Lupus pernio, plaques, nodules, vascular purpura |
| Ocular | Uveitis, conjunctivitis, xerophthalmia |
| Lymphatics | Lymphadenopathy, splenomegaly |
| Bone marrow | Infiltration |
| Hepatic | Failure, granulomas, portal hypertension |
| Renal | Nephrocalcinosis, granuloma, glomerular disease |
| Gastrointestinal | Granulomas (also in salivary, lacrimal glands, nose, tonsils and larynx), xerostomia |
| Cardiac | Arteritis, cardiomyopathy, conduction abnormalities |
| Nervous system | Central and peripheral neuropathy. Intracerebral lesions. Meningeal inflammation. Seizures |
| Endocrine/ reproductive organs | Granulomas |

- Other organ involvement is rare but may include parotids glands, testes, vasculitis, lungs, and renal involvement from hypercalciuria.
- Treatment is as described later in this section. There is a guarded prognosis for EOS as nearly all develop long-term morbidity despite intervention.
- Older children have a clinical phenotype similar to adult-onset disease.

## Musculoskeletal manifestations of sarcoid
### Joints
- Distinctive patterns of arthropathy are seen in both acute and chronic sarcoidosis. In acute disease, migratory arthralgias may precede other symptoms.
- Acute sarcoid arthritis is mainly oligoarticular, occasionally polyarticular, but rarely monoarticular. It commonly involves the lower limb joints, often resulting in symmetrical effusions affecting the knees and ankle joints. After recovery, recurrence rates are low.
- Chronic polyarthritis is uncommon. It is more frequent in women and in association with pulmonary disease.
- Different forms of chronic arthritis can occur: non-deforming with granulomatous synovitis, non-erosive deformity (Jaccoud's), dactylitis, and tenosynovitis. Knees and ankles are often involved.
- Rheumatoid factor is positive in 10–47% of chronic arthritis.

*Bone*
- Bone involvement is estimated to occur in up to 15% of all patients with sarcoidosis, and is usually accompanied by skin disease.
- Approximately 50% of affected patients are asymptomatic.
- Different types of bone involvement are seen: cystic (most common), lytic, sclerotic focal lesions, and osteopenia/osteoporosis.
- Bone cysts are often found incidentally on plain films, and seen most often in phalanges but may also occur in the skull, facial bones, ribs, spine, pelvis and long bones.
- Bone cysts are frequently seen with persistent disease and/or lupus pernio (i.e. erythematous induration of the skin across the face).
- Dactylitis appears as 'sausage-like' swollen digits.
- Other radiological features include thickening of cortical bone, acrosclerosis, and joint destruction.
- Lytic lesions which appear in vertebral bodies can lead to back pain, and be a cause of vertebral fractures.

*Muscles*
- Skeletal muscle involvement occurs in ~50–80% of patients with sarcoidosis, but is often asymptomatic. It may present as proximal pain, tenderness, and weakness.
- Myopathy may be focal with painful nodular granulomatous masses, insidious with a symmetrical diffuse pattern, or acute with elevated muscle enzymes.
- Muscle weakness is often more pronounced than either the symptoms of pain or the level of raised CK.
- Acute sarcoid myopathy may involve the respiratory muscles.
- Electromyography is abnormal as for polymyositis.

## Diagnosis and investigations

Diagnosis relies on the combination of clinical and radiographic findings, histological proof of non-caseating granulomas, and exclusion of other diseases with similar presentation.
- All patients with suspected sarcoidosis should undergo the following investigations: electrocardiogram (ECG), pulmonary function tests, PA chest radiograph, slit-lamp examination, tuberculin skin test, urinalysis, 24-hour urinary calcium and blood tests (urea, electrolytes, creatinine, FBC, ESR, bone profile, vitamin D, PTH, LFTs, CRP, ACE, CK) in addition to a thorough physical examination and symptom-driven evaluation.
- A CT chest will also be necessary to assess the degree of parenchymal lung involvement.
- Leucopenia can be seen in around 30% of cases, and eosinophilia in 25%. Thrombocytopenia is also relatively common.
- The ESR may be elevated in the acute phase, particularly if EN is present (see later in chapter for EN/panniculitis).

- Hypercalciuria and/or hypercalcaemia is seen in 10–20%, secondary to increased $1\alpha$-hydroxylation of 25-hydroxyvitamin D to active 1,25-dihydroxyvitamin D $(1,25(OH)_2D)$ by inflammatory cell-derived $1\alpha$-hydroxylase. Hypercalciuria can exist without there being (supra-reference range) hypercalcaemia (but PTH will be suppressed).
- Liver function tests may be deranged and a third of patients have significant proteinuria.
- Granuloma epithelial cells produce ACE. Serial measurements of ACE may be useful in monitoring the course of the disease.
- The distribution of inflammatory tissue in sarcoid and guidance to site of potential biopsy can be identified using either Ga-67 or somatostatin receptor scintigraphy.
- Other causes of granulomatous disease include tuberculosis and other viral, parasitic, bacterial, or fungal infections, lymphomas, Crohn's disease, granulomatosis with polyangiitis, and drug reactions.
- Since sarcoidosis can resemble other diseases, the diagnosis should ideally be confirmed by histology.
- Bronchoalveolar lavage (BAL) may demonstrate lymphocytosis and is useful in excluding other diagnoses. Transbronchial lung biopsy or mediastinal lymph node biopsy may also be required.

## Treatment  (see also pp. 662–80)

- Acute, transient disease may resolve spontaneously, and require only supportive care. NSAIDs alone may be effective, and should be used in conjunction with proton pump inhibitors.
- More severe disease may require treatment with GCs, either alone or in combination with MTX.
- Addition of HCQ may also help the skin and joint manifestations. Several reports also describe its use in pulmonary and neurological disease, and in hypercalcaemia.
- AZA is most often used as second-line drug therapy in patients with progressive disease despite GCs.
- CYC has been used in neuro- and cardiac sarcoidosis.
- Infliximab may be effective for refractory forms of this disease, including lupus pernio; however, relapse of sarcoidosis has been observed upon discontinuation.
- Colchicine has been used in patients with sarcoid arthritis at doses similar to those used in gout.
- No therapy is required for asymptomatic osseous or cystic bone disease, or asymptomatic muscle disease. The place for GCs in chronic sarcoid myopathy remains uncertain.
- Mortality is <5% and mainly results from respiratory failure secondary to pulmonary fibrosis and refractory neurological or cardiac disease.

# Miscellaneous skin conditions associated with arthritis

## Panniculitis

Panniculitis is inflammation in fat tissue. It is an inflammatory process involving neutrophils, leucocytes, and histiocytes that causes fibrosis and granulomas.

- The categories of panniculitis, based on histopathology are septal, lobular, mixed type septal and lobular, panniculitis with vasculitis.

### Septal panniculitis

- This includes erythema nodosum (EN) and Vilanova's disease (subacute nodular migratory panniculitis). EN is a common, acute, and self-limiting condition (typically in lower legs). It usually heals in 4–6 weeks without scarring. A rare form can cause ulceration and a migratory form can occur for several years (women 40–50 years old).
- Associations of EN are numerous (see Table 18.6).

### Lobular panniculitis

Numerous syndromes have been defined:

- *Weber–Christian disease:* a relapsing, febrile, nodular non-suppurative disorder. Multiple recurrent nodules and fever, arthralgia, myalgia, and abdominal pain. Any area of the body containing fat can be involved, e.g. mesentery, heart, lung, liver, kidney. There is a 10–15% mortality. Investigations may show typical histological features on biopsy, elevated ESR, anaemia, leucopenia, or leucocytosis.
- *Lipogranulomatosis:* this group of conditions tends to occur in children. Multiple lesions, often on the extremities, resolve with subcutaneous atrophy.
- *Post-GC use:* the pathogenesis of this rare condition is not understood. It seems to be limited to children. It occurs on withdrawal of GCs, and may clear up on GC re-administration.
- α1-antitrypsin deficiency: may predispose to panniculitis in many types—worth checking genetic status if severe, recurrent, or family history of panniculitis.

**Table 18.6** Causes/associations of erythema nodosum

| Cause | Examples |
|---|---|
| Infections | Streptococcal, TB/leprosy, *Yersinia*, *Salmonella*, histoplasmosis, blastomycosis, psittacosis |
| Drugs | Penicillin, sulfonamides |
| Pregnancy | |
| Diseases | Sarcoidosis, IBD, SLE, SScl, dermatomyositis, malignancy, Sweet's syndrome |

- *Calcifying panniculitis:* a feature of chronic renal failure. It is not the same as metastatic calcification. The prognosis is poor even with good calcium–phosphate balance. Parathyroidectomy may help.
- *Lipodermatosclerosis:* may be a result of venous insufficiency and thrombophlebitis. It should be treated with compression stockings. Intralesional GCs or low-dose aspirin may also help.
- *Lupus profundus* is a rare manifestation of chronic cutaneous SLE, occurring in <3% of cases. The lesions are usually tender and may ulcerate and calcify, commonly occur on the face, upper arms, and buttocks, and may underlie an area of discoid lupus. The lesions do not seem to follow the course of the systemic disease. It may respond to GCs.
- Associated with acute pancreatitis and acute vasculitis.

## Neutrophilic dermatoses

- The neutrophilic dermatoses are a group of non-infectious disorders characterized by the presence of an angiocentric, primary neutrophilic inflammatory cell infiltrate (Table 18.7).
- The disorders can be divided into those that cause vessel wall destruction (vasculitis) and those that do not.

### Sweet's syndrome

- This condition is rare and occurs more in women than men (4:1), between 30 and 70 years. It has occasionally been reported in children.
- It is otherwise known as acute febrile neutrophilic dermatosis and was originally described following respiratory infection, but is more commonly seen in patients with malignancy. It is also caused by drugs, especially granulocyte-colony stimulating factor.
- The characteristic features are fever, neutrophilia, and tender erythematous cutaneous lesions (plaques, nodules, and papules).
- Lesions can resemble vasculitis, especially in a febrile ill patient.
- Skin biopsy shows intense infiltrate of mature neutrophils, typically in the upper dermis.
- Untreated, the lesions resolve over 6–8 weeks, but new lesions will continue to appear.

**Table 18.7** Non-infectious neutrophilic dermatoses

| Group | Examples |
|---|---|
| Non-angiocentric | Psoriasis, reactive arthritis, acne fulminans |
| Angiocentric and vessel destruction | Leucocytoclastic vasculitis, polyarteritis nodosa |
| Angiocentric, no vessel destruction | Sweet's syndrome, pyoderma gangrenosum, bowel-associated dermatosis–arthritis, Behçet's disease, rheumatoid arthritis, ulcerative colitis, familial Mediterranean fever |

- The condition is usually an acute, GC-responsive self-limiting disorder. If longer-term treatment is required, GC dosage may be reduced by the addition of an NSAID, dapsone, colchicine, or possibly MTX.
- A secondary cause for the condition should be sought (Table 18.8).

## Pyoderma gangrenosum

- This is an uncommon, ulcerative, cutaneous lesion associated with AAVs, SLE, severe RA, and IBDs and rarely spondyloarthritis.
- The lesion is characterized by an erythematous, violaceous border overhanging a central area of ulceration and necrosis.
- The lesions start as discrete pustules, most often on the legs, and are often extremely painful, healing with scars.
- There is no specific treatment. An underlying disease should be excluded. Treatments include topical sodium cromoglicate or 5-amino salicylic acid, oral sulfonamides, dapsone, and GCs.

## Multicentric reticulohistiocytosis

- This is a rare systemic disease, occurring in adults in their 50s. Its recognized clinically by the combination of papular and nodular skin lesions and a severe destructive polyarthritis.
- It is associated with malignancy (25%).
- The arthritis mimics RA but notably involves DIPJs. The destruction may give a picture similar to arthritis mutilans. See ➋ Plate 7c.
- The skin lesions occur in ~90% of cases. Histologically, the infiltrate consists of multicentric giant cells and histiocytes from the monocyte-macrophage lineage. The lesions are often numerous, non-pruritic, skin coloured (or yellow/brown), size mm–cm in diameter, and occur most on the dorsum of the hands and face (nose, corner of the mouth, and ears). Extensive facial involvement may lead to a 'leonine' facies.
- About 25% of cases have xanthelasma.
- The differential diagnosis includes RA, PsA, sarcoid dactylitis, xanthoma, histiocytosis X, histiocytoma or tendon sheath giant-cell tumour—usually solitary.
- The condition waxes and wanes. Spontaneous remissions can occur.
- For patients with mild disease, MTX may be sufficient, but the condition can be aggressive so many patients require treatment with CYC or chlorambucil to prevent progressive damage.

**Table 18.8** Associations of Sweet's syndrome

| Associations | Examples |
| --- | --- |
| Haematological malignancy | Leukaemia, lymphoma, myelodysplastic disorders |
| Solid tumours | Breast, gastric, bladder, colon |
| Infectious diseases | HIV, hepatitis B/C, TB, salmonella |
| Inflammatory bowel disease | Ulcerative colitis, Crohn's disease |
| Autoimmune diseases | Rheumatoid arthritis, SLE, Sjögren's syndrome, Behçet's disease |

# Relapsing polychondritis

Relapsing polychondritis (RP) is a rare multisystem disorder of unknown aetiology, characterized by episodic and sometimes progressive inflammation of cartilage leading to destruction and fibrosis.

- Common sites of involvement include the ear, nose, larynx, joints, heart, and eyes. Characteristically, the cartilaginous part of the pinna is involved, sparing the non-cartilaginous lobe.
- Arthralgia involves large and small joints.
- Similar patterns of disease may be seen in PR3-positive AAV. Some patients with relapsing polychondritis are ANCA positive.
- The disease predominantly affects Caucasians, with peak incidence in the fifth decade (M=F).
- 50 paediatric cases have been reported worldwide and there appears to be an association with (monogenetic) autoinflammation.
- There is also an association with HLA-DR4.
- Approximately 30% of cases are associated with other inflammatory or autoimmune diseases, such as systemic vasculitis, RA, SLE, Sjögren's syndrome, thyroiditis, and IBD.
- There are no specific laboratory tests. Diagnosis is made on clinical grounds. The course of the disease is generally not life-threatening unless it involves the laryngotracheal cartilage or major artery roots.
- MAGIC syndrome (Mouth And Genital ulcers with Inflamed Cartilage) might represent a distinct condition but is exceptionally similar to BD with secondary RP.

## Treatment

- Treatment is based on anecdote and consensus. There are no RCTs.
- If involvement is limited to external ear and nasal cartilage with no apparent destruction or arthritis, symptoms may be controlled with NSAIDs alone.
- Dapsone (50–200 mg/day) may also be of value and some prefer small doses of GCs (10–20 mg/day) for mild disease also.
- For destructive disease in the cartilage or laryngotracheal, vestibuloneural, lung, eye, heart, kidney involvement, or systemic vasculitis—high dose GCs are used (prednisolone ~60 mg/day).
- CYC at 1–2 mg/kg/day has been considered in severe life-threatening lung, heart, or renal disease.
- Persistent or severe cases may also be treated with AZA, MTX, or ciclosporin (with due attention to renal function).
- Patients should be assessed for tracheal involvement (e.g. stridor). Some cases may require temporary or permanent tracheostomy and stents if laryngeal involvement is severe. Other measures may include continuous positive airway pressure at night.
- There have been a few case reports regarding the use of biologic therapies including anti-TNFα, and both IL-6 and IL-1 inhibitors, but clinical outcomes have been variable.

**Table 18.9** Features of relapsing polychondritis

| Organ | Clinical features | Prevalence (%) |
|---|---|---|
| External ear | | 95 |
| Arthritis | Non-deforming and non-erosive | 85 |
| Nose | Cartilage destruction, saddle-nose | 48 |
| Eye | Episcleritis, uveitis, retinal vasculitis | 57 |
| Respiratory tract | Dysphonia, dyspnoea, stridor | 67 |
| Inner ear | | 53 |
| Skin | Erythema nodosum, vasculitis, Behçet's-like ulceration | 38 |
| Kidney | Glomerulonephritis (poor prognosis) | 8 |
| Heart | Pericarditis, aortic valve incompetence, heart block | 8 |
| Blood vessels | Aneurysms (aortic root and abdominal aorta). | 12 |

Reproduced from Trentham DE, Le CH. Relapsing Polychondritis. *Ann Intern Med* 1998;129: 114–22 with permission from Wolters Kluwer.

# Amyloidosis

Amyloid—a proteinaceous, fibrillar material—is associated with many conditions. The low solubility of amyloid and its relative resistance to proteolytic enzymes contributes to the irreversible and often progressive course of amyloidosis.

- Despite morphological similarities (including the formation of a β-pleated sheet), amyloid is a heterogeneous group of proteins (at least 20). All types of amyloid fibrils have a carbohydrate moiety in the form of glycosaminoglycans and proteoglycans. Most forms of amyloid also contain the extrafibrillar protein, amyloid-P.
- Two forms are important as manifestations of a response to chronic systemic inflammation: amyloid-L (AL) and amyloid-A (AA).
- AL consists of monoclonal immunoglobulin light chains and is seen in idiopathic and myeloma-associated amyloidosis. It is the commonest systemic amyloidosis in Western countries.
- AA is derived from serum amyloid A (SAA), an acute phase apolipoprotein, and is secondary 'reactive' amyloidosis.
- It is unclear why not all chronic inflammatory disorders are associated with amyloidosis and how various precursor proteins are converted to insoluble amyloid fibrils.
- In the context of rheumatic disorders, AA amyloidosis is mainly seen in adult RA and AS.
- Several conditions are rarely associated with AA amyloidosis due to relatively low levels of acute-phase SAA protein. These include SLE SScl, and Sjögren's syndrome (SS).
- Other conditions associated with AA include chronic infections, periodic fevers, IBD, and less frequently malignancies.

## Investigations

The diagnosis of amyloidosis is made by tissue biopsy.
- Although specimens can be obtained from the liver, heart or kidneys, increased blood vessel fragility associated with amyloid deposition carries an increased bleeding risk. Therefore readily accessible abdominal subcutaneous fat is the standard aspiration (ASFA), with a sensitivity of 57–88%, and specificity of 100%.
- If the ASFA is negative, or contraindicated, biopsy of the salivary gland or rectal mucosa may be useful. Peripheral nerve biopsies vary in their diagnostic value and can cause residual dysaesthesia.
- Alkaline Congo red stain shows amyloid deposits as apple green/yellow under the polarizing microscope.
- Immunofixation of serum and urine, as well as an Ig free light chain assay should be done to confirm AL amyloidosis. If the diagnosis is uncertain, a bone marrow biopsy could be considered.
- If AL and AA amyloidoses are excluded on immunofixation, further genetic testing may help identify other weakly amyloidogenic proteins known to make up the hereditary amyloidoses.
- In patients with chronic inflammatory disease and proteinuria and/or chronic renal failure, increased SAA confirms AA amyloidosis.

**Table 18.10** The clinical features of AL and AA amyloidosis

|  | Organ/condition | Comment |
|---|---|---|
| AL | Heart | Death occurs in 50% of cases from restrictive cardiomyopathy, congestive heart failure, conduction disturbances |
|  | Lungs | 90% develop cough and dyspnoea |
|  | Skin | 40% of cases: papules, nodules, tumours |
|  | Neuropathy | 10% of cases develop carpal tunnel syndrome |
|  | Macroglossia |  |
|  | Vasculopathy |  |
|  | Amyloid arthropathy |  |
|  | Autonomic disturbance |  |
| AL and AA | Weakness |  |
|  | Fatigue |  |
|  | Weight loss |  |
|  | Renal | Nephrotic syndrome/renal failure—major cause of death in AA*, cause of death in one-third of AL patients |
|  | Gastrointestinal tract | Malabsorption, obstruction, diarrhoea, hepatosplenomegaly |

* In AA amyloid the spleen, liver, and kidneys are often involved first.

- Echocardiogram is the gold standard for diagnosing cardiac amyloid. Cardiac MRI is also highly sensitive for heart involvement.
- The serum amyloid protein contributes to stability of amyloid deposits *in vivo*. This property is used diagnostically in radiolabelled serum amyloid protein scintigraphy to detect amyloid in the body and is of value in assessing response to treatment.

### Treatment

- The condition is progressive and there is no cure. Marked heterogeneity of the hereditary amyloidoses makes counselling difficult.
- The processes by which the disorder may be controlled include liver transplantation for lysosomal amyloidosis and bone marrow transplantation.
- In the rheumatic diseases, the main goal is to control underlying disease to suppress SAA production. Various immunosuppressive agents including MTX, chlorambucil, LEF, and CYC (often in combination with GCs) have improved the prognosis in RA and JIA patients.

# Adult-onset Still's disease

## Epidemiology and pathogenesis

- Adult-onset Still's disease (AOSD) is a rare systemic inflammatory disorder of unknown aetiology, characterized by daily spiking of high fevers accompanied by a fleeting rash, arthritis, and systemic manifestations.
- Men and women are equally affected with bimodal peaks at ages 15–25 and 36–46 years though case series have suggested an association with pregnancy and in the post-partum period.
- There may be a genetic predisposition. A Canadian study found a possible link with HLA-B17, -B18, -B35, and -DR2, but this has not been confirmed in other studies. Genetic polymorphisms of the IL-18 gene may also be linked to AOSD susceptibility and/or severity.
- Various infectious triggers have been postulated, suggesting AOSD may be a reactive syndrome. These include EBV, echovirus, CMV, parvovirus 19, coxsackievirus, influenza, and bacteria including *Mycoplasma pneumoniae, Chlamydia pneumonia, Brucella abortus,* and *Borrelia burgdorferi.*
- T helper1 (Th1) cytokines present in blood and tissues are thought to play a role in the pathogenesis of AOSD in addition to IL-1, IL-6, IL-18, TNFα, and IFN-γ.

## Clinical features

Several sets of classification criteria have been proposed and are well developed from retrospective data. The Yamaguchi criteria (Box 18.1) provide the highest sensitivity (93.5%).

- Fever: acute onset of daily spiking high fever exceeding 40°C is often the first symptom. Typically peaks once daily in late afternoon or early evening (quotidian), lasting <4 hours, and normalizing in 80% without antipyretics. There may be a double quotidian pattern, with highest spikes occurring in late afternoon.
- Rash: evanescent salmon-pink, macular or macular papular eruption, predominantly involving proximal limbs and trunk. The overall incidence of the rash in AOSD is ~70%. The rash usually appears in conjunction with fever, and may exhibit Koebner phenomenon. There may be pruritus and appearances confused with drug allergy.
- Musculocutaneous disease: arthritis may initially be mild, oligoarticular, and transient, and may evolve gradually into a more severe, destructive, and symmetrical polyarthropathy—affecting mainly knees, wrists, and ankles. Elbows, shoulders, hips interphalangeal joints, and temporomandibular joints may also be involved. Generalized myalgias with fever spikes are seen in the majority of patients, but inflammatory myopathy is rare.
- Pharyngitis: estimated to occur in ~70% of AOSD cases.
- Liver: hepatomegaly occurs in 50–70%, partly influenced by NSAID use. Cases of fulminant liver failure have been described.
- Tender cervical lymphadenopathy and splenomegaly occur in 50%. Lymph node biopsy may resemble lymphoma on light microscopy, but immunohistochemistry demonstrates benign polyclonal B-cell hyperplasia.

## Box 18.1 The Yamaguchi criteria for AOSD

Diagnosis requires the presence of ≥5 criteria, including at least 2 major criteria, without the presence of any exclusion criteria.

*Major criteria*
- Fever of >39°C, intermittent, ≥1 week.
- Arthralgias or arthritis, ≥2 weeks.
- Typical rash.
- Leucocytosis (>10 ×10⁹/L) with ≥80% granulocytes.

*Minor criteria*
- Sore throat.
- Recent significant lymphadenopathy.
- Hepatomegaly or splenomegaly.
- Abnormal LFTs (including lactate dehydrogenase).
- Negative tests for ANA and RF.

*Exclusion criteria*
- Infections.
- Malignancies.
- Other rheumatic disease, i.e. vasculitis.

Information from Yamaguchi M et al. Preliminary criteria for classification of adult Still's disease. *J Rheumatol* 1992;19:424–30.

- Cardiopulmonary disease: serositis occurs in 30–40% (pleuritis, pericarditis), transient pulmonary infiltrates. ILD progressing to ARDS, cardiac tamponade, and myocarditis have been described.
- Haematological disease: is rare, but pancytopenia secondary to macrophage activation syndrome (MAS) may occur (~40% of patients), which can be life-threatening (see ➲ Chapter 25). There have been reports of pure red cell aplasia, thrombotic thrombocytopenic purpura (TTP), and haemolytic uraemic syndrome (HUS).

## Laboratory and radiographic findings

- There is no specific diagnostic test in AOSD, and no association with RF or positive ANA.
- ESR is raised in virtually all cases, and CRP may be elevated.
- Marked elevations in serum ferritin occur in ~70%, correlating with disease activity. A threshold of greater than fivefold the upper limit of normal is thought to have a diagnostic tool for AOSD is thought to have a sensitivity of 80%, but a specificity of 45%. Levels of 3000–30,000 ng/mL are not uncommon, normalizing with disease remission.
- A ferritin level of >1000 ng/mL with a glycosylated fraction of 20% or less, has diagnostic specificity of >90%.
- There is leucocytosis (>10 × 10⁹/L), with a granulocyte predominance. Normocytic normochromic anaemia and reactive thrombocytosis is common, especially during active disease.

- There is increased risk of elevated intravascular coagulation in AOSD, and this may be associated with haemophagocytosis (macrophage activation syndrome) resulting in pancytopenia, requiring prompt immunosuppression.
- Elevated liver transaminases, lactate dehydrogenase, and bilirubin levels are seen in 75% of cases, ranging from mild to fulminant. Liver biopsy changes are non-specific.
- Very high levels of IL-18 have been demonstrated in a number of studies of AOSD.
- Pregnancy and the post-partum period may be facilitative on the development of AOSD (high IL-18 responses can occur in association with pregnancy).
- Secondary haemophagocytic syndrome (HS) can occur: diffuse intravascular coagulation (DIC), hepatosplenomegaly, pancytopenia, a decrease in ESR, hypofibrinogenaemia, marked hyperferritinaemia, and raised triglycerides and liver enzymes.
- Early suspicion of HS is crucial as there is high morbidity and mortality. The gold standard diagnostic test is bone marrow aspirate to identify the presence of haemophagocytosis, but appearances may be visible on a blood film, in addition to features of haemolysis.
- There are no specific radiographic findings. Classically, there is bilateral non-erosive intercarpal and carpometacarpal joint space narrowing on radiographs, which may progress to ankylosis over several months. Rapid destruction of the hip and knee joints can occur in some cases, requiring total joint arthroplasty.

## Treatment

Treatment strategies are based on organ involvement and disease severity, aiming to control fever, arthritis, and systemic disease.

- NSAIDs can be used first line, and often a high dose of aspirin is required. Although effective for MSK symptoms and fever, efficacy rates are low, ~20% in AOSD patients
- GCs remain first-line treatment, regardless of presentation. The usual dose is 0.5–1 mg/kg/day of prednisolone. Pulsed methylprednisolone is helpful in severe disease refractory to oral GCs. GCs control disease activity in ~60%, but efficacy seems higher for systemic rather than articular symptoms.
- For refractory AOSD, MTX is a commonly used GC-sparing agent, inducing remission in ~70%.
- There is also reported efficacy of AZA, HCQ, D-penicillamine, ciclosporin, and tacrolimus.
- Intravenous immunoglobulin (IVIg) seems to have a suspensive effect, but is well tolerated and safe to use if concomitant infection. Usual dose is 2 g/kg over 2–5 days. Two randomized open label trials have demonstrated efficacy of IVIg if used early in the course of AOSD. It should also be considered in the context of macrophage activation syndrome, life-threatening complications, and in the case of AOSD flare during pregnancy.

- Biologic DMARDs used include anakinra (IL-1 antagonist), tocilizumab (IL-6 inhibitor) with beneficial effects on systemic and articular features, and anti-TNFα especially in chronic polyarticular disease.
- Adalimumab and etanercept may have led to macrophage activation in two reported cases of AOSD, and have been associated with paradoxical disease flares. Further prospective evidence is required on their use.

## Course of disease and prognosis

There are three main patterns of disease, with ~1/3 of patients falling into each category.

- *Self-limiting or monophasic pattern* characterized by a single disease episode. Most achieve complete remission within 1 year.
- *Intermittent or polycyclic systemic pattern* consisting of recurrent attacks, with remission between flares. Subsequent disease flares are often less severe, of shorter duration and may be years apart.
- *Chronic articular pattern* associated with poor prognosis. Disease is persistent with predominant articular symptoms resulting in severe destructive arthritis and arthroplasty frequent within 2 years.
- Predictors of a chronic disease course include rash, polyarthritis, and involvement of shoulders and hips. Patients with systemic disease generally have a favourable diagnosis. Serious complications from disease or treatment are rare, but amyloidosis is thought to be a common cause of death.

## Further reading

Jamilloux Y, Gerfaud-Valentin M, Henry T, et al. Treatment of adult-onset Still's disease: a review. *Ther Clin Risk Manag* 2015;11:33–43.

# Eosinophilic fasciitis

Eosinophilic fasciitis is an uncommon idiopathic condition that is characterized by the rapid spread of skin changes over the extremities.

- Skin—usually in the limbs—initially takes on a 'peau d'orange' appearance, which is replaced by induration.
- Like SScl (see ➔ Chapter 13), flexion contractures and Raynaud's disease may be present. Unlike SScl, the epidermis is spared (i.e. superficial wrinkling is intact) and nailfold capillaroscopy is normal.
- Other localized scleroderma conditions (see ➔ Chapter 13) will be in the differential diagnosis in early disease.
- The condition may resolve spontaneously. Otherwise, 70% of cases respond to GCs.
- The condition may be a paraneoplastic phenomenon.
- It is over-represented in women and in the haematological malignancies in this respect. The paraneoplastic condition often fails to respond to GCs and resolves on successful treatment of the underlying malignancy.
- MTX and MMF may be effective and are used as GC-sparing immunosuppressants.

# Immunoglobulin G4-related disease

### Epidemiology and pathophysiology

Immunoglobulin G4-related disease (IgG4-RD) is a rare systemic fibro-inflammatory disorder of unknown aetiology.

- The pathophysiology and role of the immune system in IgG4-RD is not well understood. There is Th2 cell involvement with numerous Th2 cytokines (IL-4, IL-5, and IL-13) present alongside T-regs (IL-10 and TGF-β). Circulating plasmablast levels correlate with disease activity, suggesting the importance of B cells in pathogenesis.
- Characteristic histopathological findings are a lymphoplasmacytic infiltration with IgG4-positive plasma cells, storiform fibrosis (irregularly whorled pattern of fibrosis), and obliterative phlebitis.
- It can affect multiple organ sites (see later in section) and may be localized or systemic, but most commonly affects the extra-pancreatic bile ducts, lacrimal or salivary glands, or pancreas.
- IgG4-RD often presents with a tissue mass and so may mimic a solid malignancy or lymphoma.
- It is more common in males and appears to predominantly affect patients between the age of 50–70 years.

### Clinical manifestations

- Multiple organs can be affected: extra-pancreatic bile ducts, lacrimal or salivary glands, or pancreas (Table 18.11).
- Disease is often incidentally identified on imaging or histopathology examination of a tissue specimen.

### Investigations

- Tissue biopsy is diagnostic.
- Serum IgG4 levels may be raised, although these can be normal.
- ESR and CRP may be elevated.
- Hypergammaglobulinaemia is often seen.
- Low serum complement levels occur in around one-third of patients with renal involvement.

### Treatment and prognosis

- There are no RCTs to guide treatment. GCs are effective, particularly in the inflammatory phase but less so in the fibrotic phase.
- Though frequently used, there is a lack of consensus as to whether a GC-sparing agent should be used.
- RTX has been shown to be effective in a case series and a recent prospective open-label trial.
- MMF, MTX, and AZA are suggested as treatment options, but there is little evidence base for their use.
- The natural history and prognosis are poorly described. Significant organ dysfunction may result from uncontrolled and progressive inflammation and fibrosis in involved tissues. Relapses are common on weaning GCs, particularly in systemic disease.

**Table 18.11** Organ involvement in IgG4-related disease

| Organ/system | Pathologies |
| --- | --- |
| Hepatobiliary | Pancreatitis, sclerosing cholangitis, and cholecystitis |
| Salivary and lacrimal glands | Sialadenitis, submandibular gland disease, dacryoadenitis, parotitis |
| Endocrine glands | Thyroid (Riedel's thyroiditis) |
| Ophthalmic | Orbital myositis, pan-orbital inflammation, orbital pseudo-tumour |
| Vascular and cardiac | Aortitis and periaortitis (retroperitoneal fibrosis), pericarditis |
| Pulmonary | Pleuritis, lung mass/nodules, mediastinitis |
| Lymphatic system | Lymphadenopathy |
| Neurological | Pachymeningitis, hypophysitis |
| Renal and genitourinary | Membranous glomerulonephritis, tubulointerstitial nephritis, renal pyelitis, prostatitis |
| Skin and cutaneous | Papulo-nodules, plaques, maculopapular rash, purpura, urticarial, psoriatic-like lesions |

# Rare disorders of synovium

## Pigmented villonodular synovitis (PVNS)

- PVNS is a rare non-malignant condition (2 per million) characterized by an uncontrolled proliferation of synoviocytes.
- It is associated with iron and fat deposition.
- Repeated small haemorrhages and lipid deposits stain the synovium red-brown and yellow, respectively.
- The cause of the condition is unknown, although some studies have proposed a link with chronic repetitive trauma or haemarthroses.
- Any age may be affected (mainly third to fourth decade; both sexes).
- The classic presentation is with monoarthritis.
- The knee is the most commonly affected joint and 'diffuse' disease is more aggressive and more likely to recur.
- PVNS causes an insidious onset of pain and swelling, blood-stained synovial fluid aspirate, with characteristic synovial biopsy findings.
- Differential diagnosis: malignant synovioma, TB arthritis, synovial haemangioma, synovial chondromatosis, amyloidosis, haemophilia.
- Radiographs are often normal. Calcification is not a feature of PVNS and might suggest another cause (e.g. malignant lesion, chondromatosis, gout, CPPD, trauma, etc.).
- Erosions and subchondral cysts (also on non-articular surfaces) can occur. Loss of joint space occurs late. MRI is diagnostic.

### Treatment

- Monoarticular PVNS is treated by excision of the lesion with or without preceding Yttrium-90 (Y-90) radiation synovectomy (RS).
- Y-90 RS is essentially only suitable for the knee.
- Y-90 RS can be coadministered with intra-articular steroid.
- Re-186 HEDP RS can be given for mid-size joints (e.g. elbow, ankle).
- Diffuse forms of PVNS tend to be progressive and recurrent.
- There are no robust treatment trials of PVNS. Treatment is based on radiological staging and technical feasibility.

## Synovial chondromatosis

- Synovial chondromatosis is a chondrometaplasia of the sub-synovial connective tissue. The joint contains thickened, white-blue nodular synovium.
- The cause is unknown, the disorder uncommon, and the process non-malignant. It tends to occur more often in middle-aged men and has never been reported in prepubertal childhood.
- Clinically the condition resembles PVNS but tends to be slowly progressive and sometimes can be self-limiting.
- Radiographs may show punctate calcification at the joint margin.
- The diagnosis should be confirmed on synovial biopsy. In rare cases, there may be transformation to a chondrosarcoma.
- Treatment is surgical and usually managed with arthroscopy, removing loose bodies and/or the synovial membrane.

# Hereditary disorders of connective tissue

# Background: molecular abnormalities of collagen and fibrillin

Collagen and fibrillin are major connective tissue proteins with important mechanical functions particularly in tissues relevant to MSK integrity, strength, and flexibility in tendons, ligaments, and bone. In this chapter, we outline the conditions manifest by abnormalities in collagen and fibrillin: osteogenesis imperfecta (OI), Marfan syndrome (MFS), Ehlers–Danlos syndrome (EDS), and hypermobility spectrum disorder (HSD)—the most common hereditary disorders of connective tissue (HDCT).

# Osteogenesis imperfecta

Osteogenic imperfecta (OI) is a collection of genetic disorders caused by a lack, or deficiency, of type I collagen historically known as brittle bone disease. Varied genotypes can result in related bone phenotypes.

## Epidemiology

- OI is uncommon—about 1:20,000 live births.

## Genetics

- OI occurs, in >90% of cases, because of mutations in the COL1A1 or COL1A2 gene.
- In most cases of OI type I there is a 'functional null' allele of COL1A1 on chromosome 17 or COL1A2 on chromosome 7 leading to reduced amounts of normal collagen I.
- Historically four main types have been defined on clinical criteria (Table 19.1) though at least 17 distinct genotypes are now recognized.
- OI may exhibit considerable interfamilial and intrafamilial variability in the number of fractures and degree of disability.

## Pathophysiology

- Pathology arises as a result of defects in structure or quantity of type I collagen found in bone, ligaments, teeth, sclerae, and skin.

## Clinical features

Fractures, bone deformity, ligament laxity, joint hypermobility, easy bruising, poor dentition, and hearing deficit are common features.

- Generalized osteopenia and fractures early in childhood are common. Fractures are rare in the neonatal period; fracture tendency is constant from childhood to puberty, decreases thereafter, and often increases following menopause in women and >60 years in men.

Table 19.1 The clinical and collagen abnormalities in the (historically clinically defined) four main osteogenesis imperfecta (OI) phenotypes (Sillence classification)

| Type | Clinical features | Inheritance | Defect |
|------|-------------------|-------------|--------|
| I | Normal bone growth. Normal dentition. Hearing loss in 50%. Blue sclera | AD | Decreased production of type I procollagen (null allele) |
| II | Lethal. Stillbirths | AD AR(rare) | Rearrangement of collagen IA/2A genes |
| III | Often deformed growth at birth and worsens. Poor dentition common. Hearing loss common. May have blue sclera | AD or AR | Mutations in α1 and α2 collagen chains |
| IV | Often bone deformity and short stature. Poor dentition common. Hearing loss uncommon. | AD | Mutations in the α2 chains |

AD, autosomal dominant; AR, autosomal recessive.

- OI can present in young adults with low BMD or fragility fractures including recurrent insufficiency fractures.
- Fractures in OI are treated with standard orthopaedic procedures appropriate for the type of fracture and the age, and heal rapidly with evidence of good callus formation (sometimes with hypertrophic callus formation) and without deformity.
- Using clinical, radiographic, and genetic criteria, Sillence developed the classification currently in use into OI types I to IV: a dominant form with blue sclerae, type I; a dominant form with normal sclerae, type IV; a perinatally lethal OI syndrome, type II; and a progressively deforming form with normal sclerae, type III.
- Hearing loss of conductive or mixed type occurs in about 50% of families, beginning in the late teens and leading, gradually, to profound deafness, tinnitus, and vertigo by the end of the fourth to fifth decade.
- Individuals with OI type I have blue sclerae which remain intensely blue throughout life, in contrast to the sclerae in OI type III and OI type IV which may also be blue at birth and during infancy.
- The intensity of blue sclerae fades with time such that these individuals may have sclerae of normal hue by adolescence and adult life.
- A differential diagnosis to consider in young children is non-accidental injury (NAI) and depending on the time of presentation, idiopathic juvenile osteoporosis, Cushing's, and homocystinuria.

## Management

- Fractures heal rapidly with evidence of a good callus formation, and, with good orthopaedic care, without deformity.
- Short-term use of bisphosphonates in children and adults with type I OI is associated with BMD gains and fracture risk reduction.
- In children, IV bisphosphonate is favoured over oral treatment—mostly pamidronate historically but now zoledronic acid is being increasingly used.
- Treatment with bisphosphonates can reduce bone pain and fractures, increases BMD, results in more normal skeletal growth, and is well tolerated. Greatest gains are probably in the first 2–4 years of treatment.
- In children, pamidronate is given at 1 mg/kg body weight over 4 hours on 3 successive days; infusion cycles are repeated every 4 months.
- Some evidence for a positive effect on BMD, bone pain, and fracture prevention from teriparatide exists anecdotally. Intuitively teriparatide may offer a better 'treatment fit' for OI compared with bisphosphonate in low collagen production OI.
- The long-term skeletal effects of anti-resorption therapy in adults with OI are unknown.
- There are anecdotal reports of the use of teriparatide in adults with OI where gains in BMD are documented.
- RCTs of teriparatide and abaloparatide are in planning.
- Regular hearing evaluations after adolescence and early stapedectomy or stapedotomy are recommended.
- Patient information is available at: ℘ http://www.brittlebone.org and ℘ http://www.oif.org.

## Distal arthrogryposes

Case reports of congenital contractural arachnodactyly (CCA; Beal's syndrome/distal arthrogryposis type IX) highlight the wide variation in clinical features representing variable genetic expressivity in the distal arthrogryposes (DAs).

- In the DAs, the MSK features of joint contractures, arachnodactyly, camptodactyly, and kyphoscoliosis predominate in CCA.
- The DAs types 1–10 are a group of disorders that mainly involve the distal parts of the limbs manifest by congenital contractures of two or more different body areas without primary neurologic or muscle disease. The prototypic distal arthrogryposis is type 1 (DA1)— characterized largely by camptodactyly, clubfoot, and heterozygous mutation in the TPM2 gene on chromosome 9p13 (the gene encoding beta-tropomyosin).

# Marfan syndrome and related disorders

Marfan syndrome (MFS) is due to heterozygous mutations (numerous) in the fibrillin 1 gene (FBN1) on chromosome 15q21.1.

- MFS is an autosomal dominant condition with complete penetrance and prevalence of 1 in 25,000; criteria for diagnosis are shown in Table 19.2.
- MFS is characterized by long extremities (span/height ratio >1.05), long fingers and feet (arachnodactyly) with a hand/height ratio >11% and foot/height ratio >15%, tall stature (with upper segment/lower segment ratio <0.89), pectus deformity of the chest wall, high-arched palate, mandibular hypoplasia, lens dislocations and myopia, and joint laxity.
- Other common or peculiar manifestations include striae distensae, pulmonary blebs (which predispose to spontaneous pneumothorax), and spinal arachnoid cysts or diverticula.
- All features are listed in Table 19.2.
- Mitral valve prolapse, mitral regurgitation, dilatation of the aortic root, and aortic regurgitation are cardiovascular features. Aneurysm of the aorta and aortic dissection are life-threatening.
- About 35% of affected persons have MV prolapse, aortic root enlargement or both on echocardiography, despite normal auscultatory findings on cardiac examination, thus all MFS patients should have an echocardiogram and thoracic CT/MR to assess the aortic valve and arch.
- Beta blockade has been used on the premise it will decrease the rate of aortic dilatation and improve survival.
- In comparing MFS with non-MFS children, height is a discriminant criterion when >3.3 standard deviations above the mean for age.

## Beal's syndrome

- MFS shows pleiotropism and clinical variability. It shares overlapping features with congenital contractural arachnodactyly (also termed Beal's syndrome and distal arthrogryposis type IX), which is caused by a mutation in the FBN2 gene (chromosome 5q23–q31).

## Loeys–Dietz syndrome (LDS)

LDS has similarities to MFS.
- LDS characteristics include craniofacial dysmorphism (craniosynostosis, cleft palate, hypertelorism), arachnodactyly, camptodactyly, scoliosis, joint laxity, talipes equinovarus, translucent and hyperelastic skin, umbilical hernia, and vascular lesions, e.g. dilatation of the ascending aorta.
- LDS1 is caused by a mutation in the TGF-βR1 gene.
- LDS2 is caused by a by mutation in the TGF-βR2 gene.
- LDS3, which is associated with early-onset osteoarthritis, is caused by a mutation in the SMAD3 gene.
- LDS4 is caused by a mutation in the TGF-β2 gene.
- LDS5 is caused by a mutation in the TGF-β3 gene.

**Table 19.2** The Ghent 1996 criteria for Marfan syndrome (MFS)

| Major criteria | |
| --- | --- |
| 1. Skeletal—four or more of: | Pectus carinatum |
| | Pectus excavatum (requiring surgery) |
| | Marfanoid habitus |
| | Arachnodactyly |
| | Scoliosis >20° |
| | Reduced extension at the elbow (to <170°) |
| | Pes planus |
| | Protrusio acetabulae |
| 2. Cardiovascular: dilation of the ascending aorta involving at least the sinuses of Valsalva or dissection of the ascending aorta | |
| 3. Ocular | Ectopia lentis |
| 4. Dura | Lumbosacral dural ectasia on CT or MRI |
| 5. Genetic | Parent, child, or sibling meeting the criteria or presence of a mutation in fibrillin gene known to cause MFS |
| **Minor criteria** | |
| 1. Skeletal | Mild–moderate pectus excavatum |
| | Joint hypermobility |
| | High-arched palate |
| | Facies: dolichocephaly, malar hypoplasia, enophthalmos, retrognathia |
| 2. Cardiovascular | Mitral valve prolapse |
| | Dilatation of pulmonary artery below age 40 years |
| | Dilatation or dissection of the descending thoracic or abdominal aorta below age 50 years |
| | Calcification of the mitral annulus below age 40 years |
| 3. Ocular | Flat cornea, myopia |
| 4. Skin | Striae; recurrent incisional hernia |
| 5. Pulmonary | Spontaneous pneumothorax; apical blebs |

In the absence of genetic confirmation, 2 major criteria and 1 other system involvement are required for the diagnosis. In a case where genetic mutations are known in the family, 1 other major criterion is required with involvement of one other organ system.

# Ehlers–Danlos syndrome

Ehlers–Danlos syndrome (EDS) is a clinically heterogeneous condition characterized by skin fragility, ligament laxity, short stature, spinal deformity, vascular fragility, and (rarely) retinal detachment.

## Classification

The Villefranche nosology for EDS has been updated. Villefranche recognized nine subtypes based on the severity of the clinical features, the underlying biochemical and genetic defect, and the pattern of inheritance. The 2017 updated classification (Table 19.3) lists 13 subtypes and is available online at: ℔ https://ehlers-danlos.com/wp-content/uploads/2017-EDS-Classification_March_2017.pdf

## Genotyping and clinical diagnosis

- There is considerable overlap between subtypes.
- Diagnosis is increasingly though genotyping—available on blood or saliva DNA sequencing analysis.
- For those who meet the minimal clinical requirements for an EDS subtype, but who have no access to molecular confirmation; or whose genetic testing shows one (or more) gene variants of uncertain significance in the genes identified for one of the EDS subtypes; or in whom no causative variants are identified in any of the EDS-subtype specific genes, then a 'provisional clinical diagnosis' of an EDS subtype can be made.

**Table 19.3** The 2017 classification of EDS

| Name of EDS subtype | Inheritance | Genetic basis |
|---|---|---|
| Classical (cEDS) | AR | COL5A1, COL5A2 |
| Classical-like EDS (clEDS) | AR | TNXB |
| Cardiac-valvular EDS (cvEDS) | AR | COL1A2 |
| Vascular EDS (vEDS) | AD | COL3A1 (rarely COL1A1) |
| Hypermobility EDS (hEDS) | ?? | Unknown |
| Arthrochalasia EDS (aEDS) | AD | COL1A1, COL1A2 |
| Dermatosparaxis EDS | AR | ADAMTS2 |
| Kyphoscoliotic EDS | AR | PLOD1, FKBP14 |
| Brittle cornea syndrome (BCS) | AR | ZNF469, PRDM6 |
| Spondylodysplastic EDS (spEDS) | AR | B4GALT7, B3GALT6, SLC39A13 |
| Musculocontractual EDS (mcEDS) | AR | CHST14, DSE |
| Myopathic EDS (mEDS) | AD or AR | COL12A1 |
| Periodontal EDS (pEDS) | AD | C1R |

AD, autosomal dominant; AR, autosomal recessive.

- If no diagnosis is made by genotyping and if there is an extreme clinical phenotype, then expanded molecular testing can be considered.
- Embryonic testing can be done either by pre-implantation genetic diagnosis (PGD) and pre-natal testing *in utero*. PGD is only approved for use in the vascular and classical EDS types.

## Classical EDS (cEDS)

- cEDS is often predominantly initially manifest by disability. It affects skin, wound healing, and joints. The effects often worsen over time as hypermobile joints can be unstable, causing painful dislocations, subluxations, arthritis, bursitis, tendonitis, and (later-adult) painful OA.
- Hyperextensible skin is easily torn and doesn't repair itself well, causing pain and disfiguring scarring.
- Difficulties may arise during pregnancy: joint pain from increased body weight, early rupture of membranes and premature birth, cervical incompetence and spontaneous abortion, excessive tissue trauma during delivery, and MSK complications in the post-natal period due to lifting and caring for the newborn.
- Patients are often partly resistant to local anaesthetic—cause unclear.
- Physical therapy for EDS should focus on graded exercise and joint and skin protection. Some individuals require joint splints. Spinal deformity may need bracing or surgery, and retinal disease requires ophthalmic expertise.

## Hypermobile EDS (hEDS)

The 1997 criteria for diagnosing hEDS were updated in 2017. Formerly, criteria for diagnosis were met if there was either hyperextensibility (and/or smooth velvety skin) and/or generalized joint hypermobility and the presence of ≥1 minor criteria (recurring joint dislocations, chronic joint/lib pain, positive family history).

- The 2017 criteria supercede the Brighton criteria. See are Table 19.4.
- hEDS evolves over time. Contortionism and propensity for sprains and dislocations occurs in hEDS but is not specific to the diagnosis.
- Pain initially is often limited to lower limbs.
- There may be easy fatiguability and voiding dysfunction.
- The 'pain' phase (which starts in the second to fourth decade of life) includes more widespread and progressively worsening MSK pain, pelvic pain in women, and headache.
- The 'stiffness' phase (observed in a few adults and elderly only) results in general reduction of joint mobility, significant reduction in function due to disabling pain and fatigue, and limitations from reduced muscle mass and weakness, prior injuries and arthritis.
- Patients with all types of EDS, may be at risk of developing postural orthostatic tachycardia syndrome (PoTS)—an abnormal increase in heart rate that occurs after sitting up or standing, causing dizziness, fainting, and other symptoms.
- However, the EDS-PoTS association is disputed as PoTS can be a benign condition affecting most commonly girls and women aged 15–50 years.
- PoTS can be treated with salt and fluid supplementation.

**Table 19.4** The 2017 criteria for diagnosing hypermobile EDS (hEDS)

**Criteria 1**

There is generalized joint hypermobility based on a 'positive' Beighton score (see Table 19.6) of:

- ≥6 in prepubertal children and adolescents.
- ≥5 in men and women, post-puberty up to age of 50 years.
- ≥4 in men and women older than 50 years.

**Criteria 2**

Two or more of the following features apply. There is/are:

A. At least 5 systemic manifestations of a more generalized connective tissue disorder are present (from following list).

B. A positive family history (≥1 first-degree relatives independently meeting criteria for hEDS).

C. Musculoskeletal complications (≥1 from following list)

A: *an unusually soft or velvety skin, mild skin hyperextensibility, unexplained striae without a history of significant weight change, bilateral piezogenic papules of the heel, recurrent or multiple abdominal hernias, atrophic scarring involving at least 2 sites and without the formation of truly papyraceous and/or haemosideric scars as seen in cEDS, dental crowding and high or narrow palate, pelvic floor, rectal and/or uterine prolapse in children men or nulliparous women without a history of morbid obesity or other predisposing condition, arachnodactyly defined by bilateral Steinberg and/or Walker signs, arm span to height ratio ≥1.05, mitral valve prolapse, aortic root dilatation with Z-score >+2.*

C: *MSK pain in ≥2 limbs, recurring daily for at least 3 months, chronic widespread pain for ≥3 months, recurrent joint dislocations or frank instability, in the absence of trauma (requiring both ≥3 atraumatic dislocations in same joint or more atraumatic dislocations in 2 different joints occurring at different times and medical confirmation of joint instability at ≥2 sites, unrelated to trauma.*

**Criteria 3**

*All the following are required:*

- Absence of skin fragility, which should prompt consideration of other types of EDS.
- Exclusion of other heritable and acquired connective tissue disorders including autoimmune rheumatic conditions.
- In patients with an acquired/autoimmune connective tissue disorder additional diagnosis of hEDS requires meeting both features A and B of criterion 2. Feature C of criterion 2 cannot be counted towards a diagnosis of hEDS.
- Exclusion of other diagnoses that may also include joint hypermobility by means of hypotonia and/or connective tissue laxity.

*A diagnosis of hEDS is made when all three criteria are met.*

*Vascular EDS (vEDS)*

Uterine, arterial, or visceral rupture and a history of spontaneous bleeding raises the possibility of vascular (type IV) EDS.

- There is an expected shortened lifespan (median 49 years for men and 53 years for women). Acrogeria is common.
- Appearance is often characteristic: translucent skin, increased visibility of veins, thin lips, small chin, thin nose, large eyes, receding gums. Also often seen: receding gums, easy bruising, congenital club foot.
- vEDS can cause massive bleeding (e.g. intracranial aneurysm, arterial dissection, uterine and GI bleeding).
- In vEDS, operative therapy is reserved for compelling indications in which benefit clearly warrants risk because of bleeding risk.

# Hypermobility spectrum disorder in adults

Hypermobility is now characterized through the term 'hypermobility spectrum disorder' (HSD). Generalized and localized forms are recognized (Table 19.5). Notably, having an HSD can be an advantage if it is not severe; for example, flexibility/hypermobility may present greater opportunity for enhanced motor competence and sporting prowess through increased agility, as with gymnasts and some dancers.

- Associated features of HSD include chronic widespread pain, fatigue, cardiovascular autonomic dysfunction, bowel dysfunction, pelvic organ prolapse.
- In adults, the diagnosis of both hEDS and an HSD requires knowledge of the Beighton hypermobility scale (Table 19.6). The scale has been validated across some but not all ethnic groups where the range of connective tissue laxity may vary.
- The genetics of the HSDs is poorly understood.
- Although hypermobility diminishes with age, the symptoms tend to continue and may worsen.
- It is important to remember that older patients may have been previously more mobile and that the Beighton score may not be an appropriate measure. A history of joint laxity should be sought.

## Treatment of joint hypermobility syndrome in adults

- It is important to de-medicalize simple situations of flexible joints and mild hypermobility where possible.
- Patients should be reassured that unlike other forms of heritable connective tissue disease, there are often no serious long-term complications of most HSDs and the mainstay of treatment is a combination of conservative measures such as physiotherapy and pain relief.

Table 19.5 The spectrum of joint hypermobility (JH) in addition to hEDS

| Type | Beighton score | MSK involvement | Notes |
|---|---|---|---|
| Asymptomatic generalized JH | Positive | Absent | |
| Asymptomatic peripheral JH | Usually negative | Absent | JH typically limited to hands and feet |
| Asymptomatic localized JH | Negative | Absent | JH limited to single joints or parts |
| Generalized-HSD | Positive | Present | |
| Peripheral-HSD | Usually negative | Present | JH typically limited to hands and feet |
| Localized-HSD | Negative | Present | JH limited to single joints or parts |
| Historical-HSD | Negative | Present | Historical presence of JH |

**Table 19.6** Beighton ('*Bye-ton*') adult hypermobility score

| | Subject has the ability to: | Right | Left |
|---|---|---|---|
| 1 | Passively dorsiflex the fifth metacarpophalangeal joint to 90° | 1 | 1 |
| 2 | Oppose the thumb to the volar aspect of the ipsilateral forearm | 1 | 1 |
| 3 | Hyperextend the elbow 10° | 1 | 1 |
| 4 | Hyperextend the knee 10° | 1 | 1 |
| 5 | Place hands flat on the floor without bending the knees | 1 | |
| Possible total score | | 9 | |

- Analgesics are often unhelpful for chronic pain, but have their place in acute symptoms. Pain and fatigue cause significant morbidity.
- Joint stabilizing exercises with particular reference to core stability, posture, and proprioception are beneficial, as may be advice on avoiding overuse injuries and practical ways of managing day-to-day activities. A global approach to joint stability and function, as opposed to just treating regional symptoms, is effective.
- 'Pain management' should be considered in chronic pain cases. This might include for example, cognitive behavioural therapy and management plans similar to those used in fibromyalgia.
- The role of serotonergic/noradrenergic agents in these patients is unclear. In part there may be effective control of depression; however, there may also be direct analgesic properties to these agents.
- Neuroleptic agents for neuropathic pain have not been studied in this group of patients. However, gabapentin or pregabalin and other similar agents may have a role.
- Cardiovascular autonomic dysfunction requires specialist assessment and advice.
- Pregnancy is often a concern. Unlike the rarer forms of EDS, hEDS and the HSDs are not associated with any major vascular hazard during pregnancy and labour. However, in hEDS, and generalized HSD there are a number of considerations:
  - Joint pain/dislocation may increase during pregnancy.
  - Positioning during delivery should be careful to avoid excessive strain on joints.
  - Labour may be rapid.
  - Membranes may rupture prematurely.
  - There is an apparent resistance to the effects of local anaesthetics.
  - Healing may be impaired and surgical technique may need to be modified accordingly.
  - There is no absolute indication for caesarean section.
  - Severe pelvic floor problems (uterine prolapse, etc.) May occur than otherwise anticipated.

# Hypermobility in children and adolescents

A robust definition of the HSDs in children and/or adolescents has not been established, so distinguishing 'the more hypermobile of the range of normal' (i.e. familial connective tissue laxity) from 'pathological' is challenging if based on hypermobility alone.

- Historically, use of the diagnostic terms 'benign joint hypermobility syndrome' and Ehlers–Danlos syndrome hypermobility type (EDS type 3) had a tendency to draw attention to a heterogeneous population of children and adolescents with widespread pain and other clinical features whose level of stress and disability was poorly served.
- In considering making a diagnosis of hEDS or an HSD in a child or adolescent it is important to consider that:
  - Beighton criteria have never been validated in children.
  - in the past, diagnostic labels such as EDS type 3 have been over- and misused without reference to validated criteria.
  - that joint hypermobility and connective tissue laxity is a manifestation of a number of disorders—see ➲ Box 19.1, p. 592.

## Epidemiology (of asymptomatic hypermobility)

- Hypermobility is present at high levels in the normal paediatric population. There are racial variations and a Beighton score of ≥4 is especially common in preschool children.
- In teenage girls and boys (mean 14 years), a large UK study found generalized joint laxity in 27.5% and 10.6%, respectively, using a cut-off of four hypermobile joints.
- Hyperextensibility at the little finger has been found in >40% girls and >30% scored positively for thumb apposition. One explanation of this is that hypermobility may be normal in a teenage population.

---

**Box 19.1 Childhood conditions associated with joint hypermobility**

- Osteogenesis imperfecta.
- Ehlers–Danlos syndrome (e.g. classical, vascular).
- Marfan syndrome.
- Loeys–Dietz syndrome.[1]
- Stickler syndrome.
- Distal arthrogryposis/Beal's syndrome.
- Trichorhinophalangeal syndrome (TRPS).
- Meier–Gorlin syndrome (OMIM 613805).

## The relationship of hypermobility and chronic pain in children

- A theoretical basis for problems with hypermobility is that individuals with hypermobility require greater muscular control to avoid stress, and possible damage, of the joint capsule or associated ligaments. As a result, it has been inferred that hypermobility may be a risk factor for chronic MSK pain.
- However, although there is some, if inconsistent evidence, that hypermobility in children and adolescents is associated with an increased risk of MSK pain, the true value of a diagnostic label of HSD as the cause of pain is unclear and may even be harmful in asserting a life-long condition when this is unproven.
- Pain associated with hypermobility should also be seen in the context of the general prevalence of MSK pain. Several studies have shown MSK pain can occur in a third of people from the general population.
- It is prudent to consider that if there is long-term pain in a child who has some features of hypermobility, the pain and hypermobility may not necessarily be linked through a causal mechanism:
  - A prospective study of the relationship between hypermobility (Beighton score ≥6) and MSK pain in the same population found a twofold increased risk of pain in shoulders, knees, feet, and ankles, but not other joints.
  - In the same study, the impact of pain on daily activities was found to be unrelated to hypermobility.
  - The lack of association between chronic widespread pain, hypermobility, and pain intensity is consistent across studies.
  - In a study of juvenile fibromyalgia, pain scores were similar in those with and those without hypermobility.
- As a result of the above-listed points, in a child with chronic pain where there is some evidence for hypermobility, rehabilitation and functional restoration is best achieved by a 'needs' rather than 'diagnostic' focus.

## Reference

1. Van Laer L, Dietz H, Loeys B. Loeys-Dietz syndrome. *Adv Exp Med Biol* 2014;802:95–105.

# Stickler syndrome

Stickler syndrome is a clinically variable and genetically heterogeneous disorder characterized by ocular, auditory, skeletal, and orofacial abnormalities.

Most forms of Stickler syndrome are characterized by the eye findings of high myopia, vitreoretinal degeneration, retinal detachment, and cataracts. Additional findings may include midline clefting (cleft palate or bifid uvula), Pierre Robin sequence, flat midface, sensorineural or conductive hearing loss, mild spondyloepiphyseal dysplasia, and early-onset osteoarthritis.

There are five genetic subtypes of Sticker syndrome:

- Type I is caused by heterozygous mutation in the COL2A1 gene on chromosome 12q13.
- Stickler syndrome type II (STL2), sometimes called the beaded vitreous type, is caused by mutation in the COL11A1 gene on chromosome 1p21.
- Stickler syndrome type III (STL3), sometimes called the non-ocular form, is caused by mutation in the COL11A2 gene on chromosome 6p21. STL1–3 are AD inherited.
- AR forms include Stickler syndrome type IV (STL4), caused by mutation in the COL9A1 gene on chromosome 6q12–q14, and type V (STL5), caused by mutation in the COL9A2 gene on chromosome 1p33–p32.2.

# Common upper limb musculoskeletal lesions

*For a detailed view on the differential diagnosis of the entire range of upper limb lesions, see ➔ Chapter 3*
*For steroid injection of upper limb lesions, see ➔ Chapter 24*

# Subacromial impingement

Subacromial impingement (SAI) is impingement of tissues between the humeral head (often the greater tuberosity) and an arch of overlying tissues formed by the acromion, coracoacromial ligament, and coracoid. The tissue most frequently affected is part of the rotator cuff tendon, the supraspinatus tendon.

## Clinical features

Impingement causes shoulder pain when the patient reaches up or behind their back, or rolls over on the shoulder at night.

- SAI is the most common type of presentation of shoulder pain in adults.
- Pain is often referred to the upper arm.
- Causes are acute rotator cuff tendonitis (which may be calcific), subacromial bursitis, rotator cuff tear with cuff instability and impingement, and glenohumeral (GH) instability due to a number of different lesions (e.g. labral tear, synovitis due to crystal arthritis).
- Inferior acromial osteophytes/acromioclavicular joint (ACJ) osteoarthritis (OA) can accompany any subacromial lesion, and often precede them and thus are risk factors for recurrent rotator cuff disease.
- Weakness and loss of range of motion occur particularly if the tendon tears.
- Long-term rotator cuff disease can lead to 'cuff arthropathy', with OA of the GH joint (GHJ) and significant chronic morbidity.
- In children or young adults with SAI, consideration of an underlying GH (instability) lesion is mandatory.

## Making a diagnosis

- Exclude alternative causes of shoulder pain, including rotator cuff tear, adhesive capsulitis, and referred pain from the neck or abdomen (e.g. cholecystitis with pain referred to the shoulder).
- Signs: painful arc on active arm elevation, pain on active reach behind back, positive Neer or Kennedy–Hawkins test (see ➲ Fig. 3.5 p. 91; Table 20.1).
- An AP radiograph can show changes identifying GH or bony pathology, calcific tendonitis, and chronic changes at supraspinatus insertion on humeral head.
- Consider requesting an AP view with 30° external rotation at the arm, an outlet Y view, and an axillary view.
- In many cases, US is the mainstay of further clarifying the nature of rotator cuff pathology, detecting structural damage, and identifying alternative explanations for shoulder pain.
- MRI also characterizes sites of cuff inflammation and is more sensitive than US in identifying cuff tears and can provide more information about the whole shoulder complex including GHJ lesions, deeper lying enthesitis, the ACJ, and bone lesions.
- The gold standard for diagnosing cuff tears is direct vision at arthroscopy.

**Table 20.1** The range of disorders presenting with subacromial impingement pain. Clinical testing, though it can be elaborate, has been shown repeatedly in studies not to be as specific as the original literature appeared to suggest

| Condition | Diagnosis made by |
|---|---|
| Supraspinatus/cuff tendonitis | MRI or US or arthroscopy |
| Subacromial bursitis (e.g. trauma, gout, CPPD) | US/MRI |
| Rotator cuff tear (partial or full) | MRI |
| Long head of biceps tendonitis | Clinical, US/MRI |
| OA ACJ (impingement of osteophytes on cuff) | Clinical, radiographs, MRI |
| GH instability due to labral trauma (e.g. SLAP lesion), arthritis GHJ | MRI |
| Enthesitis (e.g. deltoid origin at acromion) in SpAs (see ➔ Chapter 8) | Clinical, US, MRI |
| Lesion at suprascapular notch (e.g. cyst, tophus) | MRI |

## Management

- Avoid overhead arm activities.
- Trial a full-dose regular NSAID for 2 weeks.
- If the rotator cuff is convincingly not torn (feasible to tell only for supraspinatus by testing shoulder abduction against submaximal resistance at position of downward vertically held arm), consider steroid (e.g. methylprednisolone 40 mg; see ➔ Plate 5) with local anaesthetic injection (e.g. 5 mL 1% lidocaine). Approach laterally or posteriorly under acromion—see also ➔ Chapter 24.
- Follow-up injection with cuff physiotherapy 2 weeks later. Physiotherapy can address rotator cuff muscle(s) weakness and imbalance and abnormal posture.
- Patients should be given realistic expectations that physiotherapy may take several months to provide relief, and much self-motivation is needed.
- Consider a second injection not before 6 weeks after the first (Fig. 20.1; see also ➔ Chapter 24 for injection procedure/technique).
- Refer for surgical opinion if symptoms persist, as some are amenable to arthroscopic debridement of impinging acromial osteophytes.
- A full-thickness tear that is identified early and not fully retracted, can be amenable to surgical repair.

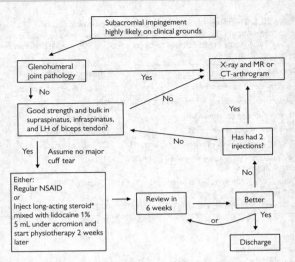

**Fig. 20.1** Pragmatic algorithm for managing subacromial impingement.

* Use 20–40 mg triamcinolone acetonide or methylprednisolone acetate. LH, long head.

# Adhesive capsulitis

Adhesive capsulitis (AC)—aetiology unknown, though it involves capsular and coracohumeral ligament contractures—is suggested by a gradual, painful loss of both active and passive range of movement of the GHJ (see also ➲ Chapter 3 for clinical assessment and differential diagnosis on presentation).

## Epidemiology

- AC is more common in females than males, and is four times more common in diabetics than the general population.
- Females are typically affected between the ages of 40 and 60 years.
- AC occurs bilaterally in 15% of patients.
- Recurrence is unusual.
- Without intervention, the pain usually resolves in <2 years, but the patient may be left with long-term restriction of shoulder movement.

## Presentation and investigations

- AC should not be confused with SAI, though the two lesions can co-exist. With SAI, passively induced GHJ movements remain intact and are less painful than active movements. With AC, passive and active movements are equally impaired.
- Clues to the diagnosis from examination include marked restriction of external rotation, early scapular abduction (normally the scapula doesn't move until 30° of abduction has been completed).
- If the presentation is delayed (e.g. >6 months), a secondary SAI may have evolved and is exposed as some range of motion begins to return.

## Management

- Rule out associated conditions: diabetes, hypothyroidism, lung carcinoma, myocardial infarction, stroke, and protease inhibitor use for human immunodeficiency virus (HIV) infection.
- Control pain during the initial painful/stiff phase of the condition. Consider NSAIDs, IA steroid injection (e.g. 40 mg methylprednisolone with 5 mL 1% lidocaine), suprascapular nerve block, or a short course of prednisone 30 mg/day for 3 weeks.
- If rotator cuff intact (confirm with US), consider image-guided hydrodilatation or manipulation under anaesthesia (MUA), early.
- Hydrodilatation improves pain and function to a greater degree than MUA when compared in RCTs.
- Mobilize with physical therapy early, but be aware this may be limited by poor pain control.

## Lateral humeral epicondylitis

# Lateral humeral epicondylitis

Lateral humeral epicondylitis (LHE)—often called tennis elbow or apophysitis of the common extensor tendon origin—is essentially an enthesitis. It is common, and affects 1–3% of the adult population, typically age 40–60 years. The dominant arm is most affected. It is rare in elite tennis players, but up to 40% of social players get it at some time. Enthesitis at the site is common and is typically associated with the SpA conditions (see ❸ Chapter 8). For clinical assessment and differential diagnosis, see ❸ Chapter 3.

## Pathophysiology

LHE is thought to be due to either cumulative trauma overuse disorder from mechanical overloading or typical SpA-related pathophysiology if an inflammatory cause.

- If chronic, it can lead to tendon degeneration and bone changes.
- True inflammation of the enthesis can occur but pain can exist without there being any identifiable inflammation.
- Poor prognosis is associated with manual work, high level physical strain at work, and high baseline pain and distress.
- Consider that the lesion may be part of SpA if bilateral, recurrent without trauma or associated with other SpA features.

## Presentation and diagnosis

(See also ❸ Chapter 3.)

- Pain is elicited by resisted force in forearm/wrist pronation (e.g. handshakes, turning doorknobs, carrying bags) or resistance of finger or wrist extension.
- Pain often extends from the LHE down the extensor compartment to the forearm.
- Enthesitis, tendon tears, and joint lesions may be diagnosed by an experienced MSK ultrasonographer.
- MRI may miss mild LHE/enthesitis and appearances are not specific. MRI is more useful for ruling out tendon tears and joint lesions.
- If lesions are bilateral then specifically consider SpA.
- The main differential diagnoses are elbow joint lesions, referred neck pain, and enthesitis (e.g. DISH or enthesitis linked to SpA, particularly PsA; see ❸ Chapter 8).

## Management

(See also ❸ Chapter 24.)

- During the acute phase, LHE can be treated with activity restriction, pain control, an elbow clasp, and immobilization.
- NSAIDs and gabapentin/pregabalin may help in some cases. Employ a treatment trial for a limited period of time and review.
- Injection around the epicondyle with methylprednisolone 20 mg should be considered if conservative therapy fails—see ❸ Chapter 3 for details (see ❸ Plate 6).
- Isometric grip exercises and stretching forearm extensor tissues (graded wrist flexion mobilisations) may also help with recovery.

- If other inflammatory MSK lesions are evident then examining for widespread enthesitis lesions and other features of SpA is indicated. With substantial SpA-related enthesopathic disease then DMARDs may be considered (e.g. sulfasalazine or methotrexate).
- Surgery is rarely indicated, and should be considered for patients with persistent symptoms despite other therapies (Fig. 20.2).
- Unproven therapies include autologous blood injection of tendon origin, lithotripsy, and therapeutic US.

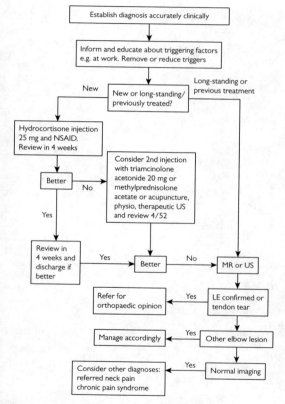

Fig. 20.2 Pragmatic algorithm for managing lateral epicondylitis (LHE).

Fig. 30.2 ...

# Spinal disorders and back pain

## Introduction

For a review of spinal anatomy and functional anatomy, see ➋ Chapter 3 under relevant sections for thoracic or lumbar spine in adults.

- The differential diagnosis of symptoms located to the neck and back is included in the relevant part of ➋ Chapter 3.
- Relevant review of issues and tables on spinal conditions include the following:
  - Painful neurological and MSK conditions of the thoracic spine and chest wall. See ➋ Table 3.12, p. 132.
  - Common and/or serious causes of neck pain in adults. See ➋ Table 3.1, p. 75.
  - Testing nerve root tension in patients with low back pain and associated leg pain. See ➋ 'Testing nerve root tension', p. 146.
  - Testing muscle strength in the lower limbs (in patients with neurogenic leg pain associated with low back pain). See ➋ Table 3.15, p. 147.
  - Principal combinations of signs used for identifying lumbar nerve root lesions. See ➋ Table 3.16, p. 148.
  - Commonly reported patterns of radiographic abnormality in adults with spinal symptoms: the interpretation, and suggested reaction. See ➋ Table 3.17, p. 149.
  - Review of choice of imaging: radiographs and CT or MRI? See ➋ Chapter 3, p. 150)

# A categorization of back pain

### Non-spinal back pain

Pain may radiate to the back from lesions in other structures, e.g. renal, aortic aneurysmal, pleuritic or pancreatic disorders, and periaortitis. For summary of conditions causing spinal pain see ⊃ 'Thoracic back and chest pain in adults', p. 132 and 'Low back pain: adults', p. 140).

### Acute non-specific back pain

- This accounts for 80–85% of all acute back pain.
- Typically, 90% of cases will recover in <6 weeks (the threshold for reassurance).
- Most causes will be 'mechanical' in origin but some causes will be neuropathic and others inflammatory in nature.

### Chronic back pain

- Describes pain that has been present for >12 weeks.
- Some causes will be neuropathic, others inflammatory in nature, but the majority can be categorized as 'mechanical'.

### Neuropathic pain

- This type of pain accounts for approximately one-third of acute and chronic low back pain.
- The painDetect® questionnaire is a useful assessment tool, as well as an aide memoire for the typical symptoms of neuropathic pain: burning, prickling, hot/cold dysaesthesia, sensitivity to touch and pressure, numbness, and sudden 'electric shock'-like symptoms.

### 'Red flags' and 'yellow flags'

This terminology is used to identify potentially serious secondary physical (red) and psychosocial (yellow) pathologies (Table 21.1).

**Table 21.1** Warning signs for sinister pathology causing back pain

| 'Red flags' | 'Yellow flags' |
| --- | --- |
| • Age of onset <20 years | • Belief that pain and activity are harmful |
| • Age of onset >55 years | • Abnormal 'sickness behaviour', e.g. extended rest |
| • Recent trauma | |
| • Pain constant, progressive, and no relief with rest | • Low/negative mood |
| • Intense night-time pain | • Work environment (low support/satisfaction conflicting evidence for high pace/demand) |
| • Thoracic pain | |
| • Past history of malignancy | • Seeking treatments that seem excessive or inappropriate |
| • Osteoporosis risk | |
| • Infection risk (immunosuppressed) | • Inappropriate expectations |
| • Systemically unwell—weight loss/fever, etc. | • Lack of social support in private life (moderate evidence) |
| • Progressive neurological signs including bladder dysfunction | • Compensation claims |
| • Structural deformity | |

# Acute and subacute back pain (adults)

## Acute mechanical back pain

- Most cases in a primary care setting are due to lumbar muscle strain or sprain presenting with diffuse pain in the lower back to buttocks, which resolves spontaneously.
- If pain is related to posture or movement, especially of the thoracic cage, and local tenderness is felt at the lumbosacral junction then the pain is highly likely to be MSK in origin.
- Within the gravid population, two-thirds of the pregnant women suffer from low back pain, typically increasing with gestational stage, impacting on sleep, work, and day-to-day function.
- 'Red flags' merit more thorough investigation. Although far less common (<15% of all cases), the following should be considered (% of cases in back pain population):
  - Fracture.
  - Symptomatic herniated disc (4%).
  - Spinal stenosis (3%).
  - Malignancy (0.7%).
  - Axial spondyloarthritis (axSpA)/ankylosing spondylitis (0.3%).
  - Cauda equina syndrome (0.04%) causing saddle anaesthesia, leg weakness, bilateral sciatica, and bladder dysfunction.
  - Spinal infection or inflammatory radiculopathy (0.01%).
- Herniated discs account for 4% of lower back pain. Disc herniation presents with leg pain radiating past the knee, and is most common in patients between 20 and 50 years of age.
- Degenerative causes of back pain, including degenerative disc disease, facet joint OA, and lumbar canal spinal stenosis, are more common in older patients.
- The immediate management is a combination of adequate and regular analgesia, titrating as per patient response, as well as encouraging gentle mobilization and normalization of activities.
- In the short term, as diazepam may be considered to decrease muscle spasm and aid sleep.
- The clinician should explore patient fears ('yellow flags') and, where appropriate, reassure that serious illness is unlikely, that tests are not usually needed, and severe pain is often short-lived.
- Radiographs are likely to be unhelpful for management in most cases unless red flag signs are present.
- MRI of the lumbar spine, for example, frequently demonstrates abnormal findings in asymptomatic patients; the relationship between such findings and clinical symptoms is not always clear.
- A rehabilitation approach should be considered (Table 21.2). The evidence for therapies is variable. Adherence may be augmented by providing patient education literature.

**Table 21.2** Therapies used in facilitating rehabilitation after acute mechanical low back pain

| | |
|---|---|
| Manipulation | Either done by an osteopath, chiropractor, or physiotherapist. Cochrane review (2012) demonstrated lack of efficacy compared to inert treatment or sham manipulation. Smaller studies since 2015 demonstrate a slight benefit, however |
| McKenzie exercises | Passive extension exercises designed to improve pain and stiffness associated with disc and anterior spinal structure pathology. May aggravate pain from posterior spine structures, e.g. facet joints, spinous processes. <br> A systematic review in 2011 has demonstrated a modest benefit in patients undertaking directional preference exercise within the McKenzie framework |
| Hydrotherapy or balneotherapy | Poorly studied, but warmth can ease movement and augment land-based exercises. Might be considered after initial painful phase to regain normal movements and mobility. May only suit a few patients and resources may be limited |
| Graded activity programmes | Useful for patients who require guidance and would be unable to gain optimally from home exercise regimen. A plan for rehabilitation with milestones is useful for some patients |
| Behavioural programmes | Focuses on psychological aspects of pain, involves moderate supervision and planned withdrawal of treatment. Differs from some other approaches in that the therapist takes over the 'control' of the back pain. Limited resources may restrict provision of this approach |

## Back pain and nerve root lesions

See also ➲ 'Low back pain: adults', pp. 144–7 for review of anatomy and functional anatomy.

- Nerve root compression occurs mostly because of acute or subacute disc prolapse or foraminal stenosis. The peak incidence is age 30–50 years. 70% resolve within 3 months and 90% within 6 months.
- Nerve root compression should be suspected if acute or subacute back pain is associated with segmental nerve or sciatic leg pain.
- Acute sciatic pain ('sciatica' affecting the outer and posterior leg) is often sharp or burning in nature, and most frequently arises from acute disc prolapse of either L4/5 or L5/S1 (>90% of cases).
- Sciatica is characterized by leg pain projecting past the knee, which may be more severe than the associated back pain.
- A patient with a herniated disc may present with sciatica.
- Evidence of disc herniation may be elicited by straight leg raise or crossed straight leg raise (i.e. elevation of unaffected leg). These tests are positive if pain is felt in the buttock or in the back at a leg angle of 30–60°. Pain elicited at a leg angle <10° is consistent with MSK back pain.
- L5 nerve root lesions give decreased strength of the foot and great toe dorsiflexion, standing on heel, and decreased ankle reflex and sensation over great toe.
- S1 root lesions give decreased strength in plantar foot flexion, difficulty in weight-bearing on toes, and decreased ankle reflex and sensation on the sole or outer part of foot.

*Principles of management*
- The natural history: 30–60% of patients recover in 1 week.
- Analgesia such as paracetamol (acetaminophen) and NSAIDs should be considered first.
- Use of diazepam may be of benefit in the short term to lessen muscle spasm. Some patients may need opiate therapy for pain control, e.g. codeine phosphate, tramadol, buprenorphine, and short- or long-acting morphine sulfate.
- Bed rest should be discouraged: prolonged bed rest leads to worse outcomes. Gentle mobilization should be encouraged.
- An epidural steroid injection can improve pain in the short term, but data from RCTs does not show better long-term outcome at 3 months or longer compared with controls.
- A meta-analysis showed that 1 in 7 patients having a steroid epidural experienced >75% improvement in pain in the short term, and 1 in 13 experienced >50% symptom improvement in the long term.
- Physical therapy and supervised rehabilitation using lumbar extensor exercise regimens may be of benefit.
- MRI can characterize lesions, but 25% of asymptomatic people have frank disc protrusions; so MRI gives poor specificity. MRI should be used to confirm a diagnosis, not to reach for one.
- The absolute indications for surgery (Table 21.3) are cauda equina syndrome, progressive muscle weakness, and neuropathy causing functional disability.

## Facet joint arthritis/syndrome

- Lumbar spine facet joint (FJ) osteoarthritis (OA) is common in middle aged/elderly adults, and can be part of generalized OA.
- FJOA is associated with degenerative and spondylolytic spondylolistheses—forward slippage of a vertebrae on the vertebrae below it.
- Psoriatic arthritis (see ➔ Chapter 8) and calcium pyrophosphate disease (CPPD; see ➔ Chapter 7) can also affect FJs and are under-recognized as causes of low back pain.
- Typical symptoms include pain on extension or rotation of the lower back. The pain is often referred to the upper buttocks, is worse while standing still, and eased by forward lumbar flexion.
- Facet hypertrophy itself cannot be felt, but true FJ syndrome is accompanied by muscle spasm and superficial soft tissue tenderness.
- Arthritic FJs may be seen on oblique spinal radiographs; however, imaging in general cannot reliably identify symptomatic FJs. FJ injection with anaesthetic may confirm the diagnosis if this results in significant pain relief.

*Management of FJ arthritis/syndrome*
- Patients can be treated according to principles applied for all patients with acute mechanical back pain except that extensor exercises are contraindicated as they will aggravate symptoms.
- Short courses of analgesics and/or NSAIDs as for OA.
- Generally, advise minimal bed rest.

**Table 21.3** Surgical approaches for lumbar disc prolapse

| | |
|---|---|
| Discectomy | Essential for discs causing cauda equina syndrome and progressive neurological deficits. Excluding above indications, compared with conservative therapy, in a randomized control trial (RCT) 66% vs 33% patients were satisfied following surgery at 1 year, and 66% vs 51% were satisfied at 4 years; thus, benefit of surgery in the long term is small. Adverse events with surgery include mortality (<0.2%), dural tears (4%), and permanent nerve root injuries (<1%). 70% success rate in short term. Risk of failure from surgery relates to hysteria or hypochondriasis scores on MMPI* and presence of litigation claims |
| Microdiscectomy | Smaller surgical field results in earlier mobilization and less postoperative disability. Outcomes similar to those of conventional discectomy from Cochrane review, 2014 |
| Percutaneous discectomy | Suctioning of central disc material causing disc decompression and relieving nerve root pressure. Associated with low complication rate and rapid rehabilitation. Small RCT studies suggest similar efficacy to discectomy and microdiscectomy |
| Chemonucleolysis | Injection of proteolytic enzyme into disc. RCTs suggest standard discectomy is superior. Rare, but devastating neurological complications; risk of anaphylaxis (0.3%) |
| Laser lumbar discectomy | Vaporizing of part of disc by laser through a needle probe. Efficacy similar to discectomy. No RCT data |
| Prosthetic intervertebral disc replacement | Also, indicated for degenerative disc disease, post-laminectomy syndrome and non-specific persistent low back pain. Artificial discs consist of two end-plates separated by pliable inner core. RCT comparative studies have shown a short-term benefit in ameliorating back pain and long-term benefit in reducing leg pain, compared with discectomy. Complication rate may be high (up to 45%) and serious: discitis, re-herniation, haematoma |

* MMPI = Minnesota Multiphasic Personality Inventory.

- Steroid injection of FJs is frequently used, although studies have failed to demonstrate benefit over placebo injection.
- Radiofrequency denervation of medial branches of dorsal rami supplying FJs can help, but the procedure should only be considered if local anaesthetic block works first.

## Lumbar canal spinal stenosis

- The diagnosis is frequently missed in the elderly.
- It presents mainly with achy, stiff pains in the legs increased on walking and easing if the patient stops walking, sits, or leans forward (neurogenic or pseudo-claudication).
- Pain, numbness/tingling, and weakness are the most common symptoms. Neurological leg signs can be accentuated after exercise.
- The diagnosis is made using MRI of the lumbar spine.

- Non-surgical management (including pain control and physical therapy) is often adequate.
- Decompressive laminectomy is required for progressive neurological symptoms, bladder dysfunction, or cauda equina syndrome.

## Non-traumatic vertebral fracture

- A fragility (minimal or not) trauma vertebral fracture is usually due to osteoporosis, collapse of an abnormal vertebra (e.g. vertebral haemangioma), or secondary to malignancy or infection.
- The history should focus on identifying risk factors for these conditions. Post-menopause or hypogonadism, previous fracture history, steroid use, and alcoholism may all contribute to osteoporosis.
- Weight loss or B-type symptoms may indicate the presence of malignancy or infection.
- Kyphosis and loss of height can occur after vertebral fracture.
- A full examination should be done to evaluate the possibility of cord compression or malignancy.
- Investigate with anteroposterior and lateral spinal radiographs, MRI, bone biochemistry (bone profile, PTH), morning luteinizing hormone (LH) and free testosterone, 25-OH vitamin D, CRP, thyroid function tests (TFTs), serum and urine electrophoresis.
- MRI is good at discriminating infection and tumours from osteoporosis, and can date fractures, but biopsy for histology and culture is essential if tumour or infection has not been ruled out by MRI.

### Management of non-traumatic vertebral fracture

- The patient should be carefully monitored for evolving neurological deficits with a low threshold for MRI whole spine.
- Pain control often requires long-acting narcotics, with short-acting narcotics for breakthrough pain as paracetamol (acetaminophen) and NSAIDs alone are unlikely to be sufficient.
- Calcitonin 100–200 IU twice-daily SC or 200 IU/day by nasal spray has an analgesic effect and reduces bone turnover in osteoporosis.
- Osteoporosis should be treated aggressively in due course (see ➲ Chapter 16) but bisphosphonates should not be regarded to have/relied on to provide an analgesic effect.
- Discuss any pathological malignancy-related fracture with a clinical oncologist.
- Consider vertebroplasty or balloon kyphoplasty where pain is uncontrolled by analgesia.

## Post-surgical back pain

- There are numerous causes and no single entity (Table 21.4).
- Post-surgical back pain presents a management challenge. A multi-disciplinary approach is often need in providing optimization of analgesia, physical therapy, behavioural modification via psychotherapy, use of nerve blocks, epidurals, and spinal cord stimulators, radio-frequency ablation as well as considering the need for re-operation.
- Some preoperative factors such as nerve root exit foraminal stenosis, smoking, obesity, and pre-morbid psychiatric conditions can lead to higher prevalence of post-surgical back pain.

**Table 21.4** Implicated causes of post-surgical back pain

| | |
|---|---|
| Recurrent disease | Example: further disc protrusion and radicular features. If re-operation not appropriate consider nerve root block, steroid epidural, etc. |
| Operation for wrong lesion | MRI can show lesions, which may not be relevant to clinical features. More than 1 or 2 lesions can coexist. Detailed clinical assessment *prior* to imaging is essential |
| Misdiagnosis originally | A structural lesion treated when an inflammatory disease, typically SpA-related disease, was present and causing ongoing symptoms |
| Altered biomechanics | Increased load burden over the adjacent structures, leading to accelerated degenerative changes in areas both above and below the surgery. Also, altered biomechanics may potentially result in increased tension over the pre-vertebral and post-vertebral muscles, leading to stiffness, spasm, and pain |
| Adverse rehabilitation conditions | Resolution of symptoms and regaining functional capacity if slow has been associated with significant psychological and social factors. Poor result of surgery also associated with an outstanding insurance claim or litigation |
| Arachnoiditis | Thought to be a direct effect of surgery. Dural tissue becomes inflamed. In nerve root/disc surgery often associated with sensory root symptoms for some months afterwards. Diagnosis with contrast-enhanced MRI. Where associated with sensory radicular symptoms, may respond to steroid root block, epidural. If radicular symptoms chronic and disabling consider spinal cord (implanted) stimulator |

- Imaging with gadolinium-enhanced MRI may be helpful to delineate inflammatory tissue around the surgical site.
- Persistent pain after surgery may be associated with adverse psychological and social factors, outstanding litigation, or insurance claims.

## Non-septic discitis

- Inflammation of the intervertebral disc is often associated with annulus enthesitis at the vertebral end-plates and vertebral osteitis.
- The causes include disc degeneration, CPPD disease, axSpA/ankylosing spondylitis ('romanus' lesions) and other SpAs; also, SAPHO (see ➲ Chapter 16.
- The lesion should be identified with MRI and treatment should include aggressive analgesia adjusted as tolerated.
- In RCTs, intradiscal steroid injections have been shown to be little help overall. IV bisphosphonate (e.g. pamidronate 60–90 mg) has anecdotally been shown to help the symptoms of axSpA and SAPHO discitis ('spondylodiscitis').

# Chronic back pain (adults)

The Global Burden of Disease Study 2010 published in *The Lancet* delineated how MSK disorders are the second main cause of disability worldwide measured by years lived with disability (YLDs). Low back pain was the leading contributor to the YLDs attributable from MSK disorders.

- Further analysis demonstrated how low back pain was the sixth out of 291 causes of global burden of disease measured by disability-adjusted life years (DALYs). In Western Europe, it is the first cause.
- In 2010, the global age-standardized prevalence of chronic back pain was 9.4%, with a higher rate in men (10.1%) than in women (8.7%).
- In Western Europe, the prevalence of low back pain was 15.5% in men and 14.5% in women.
- Managing chronic back pain requires an emphasis on psychological and social management.
- Patients with chronic back pain are likely to have set beliefs about their problem, the ability of healthcare systems to help them, and are more likely to have developed coping strategies than patients with acute or subacute back pain.
- People with chronic back pain who continually seek further and different healthcare options are likely to have less successful coping strategies.

## Initial approach to managing chronic low back pain

(See Table 21.5.)
- Be confident that there is no undiagnosed condition affecting back pain and that no new neurological lesions have evolved. If examination raises concern, use MRI to rule out lesions.
- Establish empathy and trust, taking time to get information about patients':
  - social situation.
  - health and illness beliefs.
  - intra-family dynamics.
  - work and home role.
  - perception of their role at work.
  - view on conventional and complementary therapies.
  - view on what does and doesn't work.
  - specific view of exercise therapy.
- Plan the management approach with the patient and establish short- to mid-term goals, including whether, and what type of, supervision is required (e.g. graded programme of exercise) and how often a review is needed.
- Consider 'domains' of therapy under the following headings:
  - Physical therapy.
  - Work/life commitments.
  - Psychological and social support.
  - Painkillers and medications.
  - Education (insight and coping strategies).

**Table 21.5** Management options for chronic low back pain: adults

| | |
|---|---|
| Exercises | RCT evidence supports use. Greater evidence of effect when combined with behavioural methods. Aerobic exercises augment effect of 'back school'. Should be essential part of outpatient physical retraining programme. No difference in efficacy between individual or group programmes |
| Manipulation | Trials show efficacy on pain in the long term |
| Transcutaneous electric nerve stimulation (TENS) | Disappointing results from RCTs in chronic back pain, although efficacy for other specific diagnoses are unknown |
| Posture training | May be more appropriate than corset use and easy to combine training with supervised exercise therapy |
| Pilates | Low-level evidence for short-term benefit |
| Medications | Paracetamol, especially used in conjunction with opiates to obtain a synergistic effect. |
| | NSAIDs best for acute-on-chronic pain flares, for regulating pain intensity, as shown by current RCTs. COX2-selective NSAIDs may have better GI side effect profile. |
| | Systemic review and meta-analysis has demonstrated efficacy of opiates in terms of pain reduction in the short term. The medications can be delivered in a variety of ways: oral, trans-dermal, and buccal. Chronic opiate use for chronic low back pain has not been extensively studied. A mental health evaluation before long-term prescribing is essential to avoid triggering dependency (see text); short courses, initially for a trial period, are sensible. Best supervised by a specialist with experience in pain management. |
| | Low-dose tricyclics (e.g. amitriptyline, nortriptyline) are useful particularly if chronic neuropathic pain is present. |
| | Other neuropathic agents such as gabapentin, pregabalin, and duloxetine can be used. |
| | Muscle relaxants: diazepam has been shown to have short-term benefits in acute-on-chronic exacerbations of back pain. Evidence for eperisone is currently limited. |
| | Topical lidocaine can be used as adjunctive treatment for neuropathic pain, though as yet no clear evidence base. |
| | Systemic anti-nerve growth factor agents: limited evidence, experimental phase |
| Back school | Regular programme carrying an educational component. Programmes vary from one to many sessions. May be more effective in occupational setting. Non-compliance and relapse are problems. Recent meta-analyses show inconsistent results with regard to efficacy |

(Continued)

**Table 21.5** (Contd.)

| | |
|---|---|
| Psychology-orientated rehabilitation programmes | Intensive courses often run by psychologists and 'hands-off' physical therapists can help (highly) selected patients. Focus is on learning to cope with pain and increased control of effects of pain on functioning and psyche. Not suitable for many patients. Courses few and far between. Cost-effectiveness of courses not proved. Good efficacy compared to standard care, especially with work outcomes |
| Complementary therapies | Increasingly used. By consensus, chiropractic has been shown to be helpful for chronic low back pain. Acupuncture has yet to be proved successful in robust studies. Poor evidence base otherwise |
| Epidural steroid injections | Good level of evidence for short- and medium-term efficacy in reducing back and radicular leg pain. Greater benefit established with regimen consisting of local anaesthetic and steroid |
| Epidural etanercept therapy | Does not seem to have adverse events compared to placebo but further studies needed to establish robust efficacy |
| Intrathecal opiates | Conflicting results from (only) non-controlled studies. Generally, results show overall short-term improvements regarding pain perception, but not function. Best reserved for patients where all else has failed |
| Spinal cord stimulator (SCS) | A number of good studies show that a SCS is effective for neuropathic including radicular pain. Technique is relatively safe. Careful patient selection is important. Studies show 50% reduction in pain in the long term |
| Percutaneous adhesiolysis | Robust evidence from RCTs demonstrating short- and long-term efficacy in diminishing chronic back pain and improving functional impairment |

- Plan to review progress at regular intervals.
- Evaluate patients carefully at baseline if considering long-term opiate use. There may be an increased risk of dependency if the patient currently or previously abused drugs, there is a high level of psychological distress, if short-acting opiates are used, or drugs are prescribed 'as needed'.
- Although many strategies, especially those that combine techniques, can be costly, these costs to healthcare are likely to be offset by the saving in lost wages.

### Additional sources of references on the value of interventions

Chou R, Huffman LH; American Pain Society, et al. Nonpharmacologic therapies for acute and chronic low back pain: a review of the evidence for an American Pain Society/American College of Physicians clinical practice guideline. *Ann Intern Med.* 2007;147:492–504.

Van Tulder MW, Becker A, Bekkering T, et al. Chapter 3 European guidelines for the management of acute nonspecific low back pain in primary care. *Eur Spine J* 2006;3(Suppl 2):161–191.

## Relevant Cochrane database evaluations

2003: Multidisciplinary Bio-psychosocial, Rehabilitation, Muscle relaxants.
2004: Back schools.
2005: Bed rest, Exercise therapy, Behavioural therapy, Acupuncture.
2007: Herbal medicine, Traction, Insoles, Opioids, Injection therapy, Prolotherapy and Laser therapy.

# Back pain in children and adolescents

Children with spinal problems present with deformity, back pain, limping, systemic or neurological features, or a combination of effects.

- Back pain in adolescents is common— by 20y of age, occurs in up to 80%, but is rare in children <8 years. Pain in a child <4y and pain requiring hospital admission typically predict underlying pathology.
- Age determines the likelihood of cause, with infection and tumours being more common in young children compared with adolescents (Table 21.6).
- The principles of history taking and examination in children are discussed in ⊃ Chapter 3, See pp. 154–5.

### Non-specific low back pain

- The annual incidence is 13–24% in school children.
- Adolescent back pain is linked with familial clustering, physical inactivity, sports injuries, and psychosocial factors.
- Particular risk factors from a recent birth cohort studies include female sex, muscle deconditioning previous sports injuries, sleeping problems, and persistent fatigue.
- Most children and adolescents have self-limiting symptoms.
- Management should focus on an explanation of the short natural history, reassurance, addressing predisposing factors that remain a trigger for recurrence and increasing exercise to improve muscle strength.
- Back pain associated with hyperlordosis and pain on lumbar extension of is commonly associated with tight hamstrings or hip flexors, weak core and tense paraspinal muscles with reduced forward flexion.
- A thorough assessment of gait, posture, core stability, limb strength and muscle tightness will help direct physiotherapy-led home exercise plan.

**Table 21.6** Causes of back pain in children

| | |
|---|---|
| Developmental | Painful scoliosis, Spondylolysis and spondylolisthesis, Scheuermann's disease |
| Infection | Discitis, Vertebral osteomyelitis, Spinal epidural abscess |
| Inflammation | Juvenile arthritis, Osteoporosis |
| Mechanical | Herniated disc, Muscle strain, Fractures |
| Neoplasms | Benign (osteoid osteomas, osteoblastoma, aneurysmal bone cyst), Malignant (leukaemia, lymphoma, sarcoma) |
| Visceral | Pyelonephritis, appendicitis, retroperitoneal abscess |
| Non-accidental | Fractures—ribs, spinous processes, Soft tissue injuries, burns |

## Idiopathic scoliosis

The major form of idiopathic scoliosis is vertebral malalignment in the coronal plane associated with spinal rotation accentuated on spinal flexion.

- Overall prevalence is reported to range from 0.5% to 5%, with the highest prevalence within the 12–14 years age groups.
- About 70% are asymptomatic. The incidence of back pain is probably higher than in the background population. Progression is more likely in the presence of pain or thoracic curve convex to the left—conditions that should be investigated for serious underlying spinal pathology.
- Potential interventions include scoliosis specific exercises, bracing, and surgery. There is poor quality evidence for scoliosis-specific exercises as an adjunctive treatment alongside other interventions.
- Progressive scoliosis (Fig. 21.1) requires bracing or surgery. Usually curves of 25–45° are braced; rigid bracing seems to be superior compared to elastic bracing.
- A child with a curve >40° would be considered for surgical intervention. Similar outcomes are achieved at short term follow up for both traditionally open surgery versus minimally invasive procedures.
- An MRI to look for tumour, syrinx, neural tethering or infection should be done if there is a curve concave to the left and pain.
- It's important to differentiate the cause of scoliosis (e.g. biomechanical, post-traumatic, neuromuscular, metabolic, congenital, idiopathic).

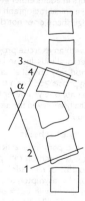

**Fig. 21.1** Measurement of the degree of scoliosis by the Cobb method: 1, the lowest vertebra whose bottom tilts to the concavity of curve; 2, the erect perpendicular to line 1; 3, the highest vertebra whose top tilts to the concavity of curve; 4, the drop perpendicular to line 3; α, the intersecting angle. Curves less than 20° are considered to be mild, 20–40° are moderate, and above 40° are severe.

## Congenital and neuromuscular scoliosis

Congenital scoliosis (CS) is associated with genitourinary malformations (20%) and, rarely, congenital heart disease. It is a rare condition, occurring in about 1 in 10,000 newborns. Neuromuscular scoliosis (NMS) is associated with cerebral palsy, muscular dystrophy, spinomuscular atrophy, and myelodysplasia.

- CS is associated with spinal dysraphism (20%), myelodysplasia, and Klippel–Fiel syndrome.
- To avoid rapid progression and increased long-term morbidity and disability, refer for prompt correction of progressive curves.

## Scheuermann's osteochondritis

- This is perhaps the most common cause of spinal deformity in children and adolescents (1–8% of all adolescents usually 13–17 years).
- The aetiology is unknown.
- Most cases are asymptomatic and present with concerns about the kyphosis. Pain occurs over the apex of the deformity often related to activity or prolonged sitting. Lumbar pain occurs with a compensatory hyperlordosis. Tightness occurs in anterior shoulder muscles, hip flexors and hamstrings.
- The typical radiographic pattern is of mild wedge vertebral deformities (<10°) of thoracic vertebrae and irregular end-plates.
- Delayed presentation occurs in adults either with (degenerative) back pains or disclosed on a spinal radiograph as 'vertebral fractures' (erroneously—as the wedge shape does not denote fracture).

*Management*
- Minor kyphosis is treated with an exercise program to increase flexibility of trunk, hamstring and pectoral muscles, and is monitored with radiographs, obtained periodically until skeletal maturity.
- Bracing is indicated for a kyphosis >55° or a thoracolumbar scoliosis >40° and should continue until one year after fusion of the iliac apophyses. Surgery is typically reserved for a thoracic kyphosis >70° or thoracolumbar scoliosis >60°.

## Spondylolysis and spondylolisthesis

Spondylolysis is a defect in the pars inter-articularis, most commonly at L4 or L5. Alone as a lesion it is common (4% preschool children and 6% <18 years). It occurs in up to 15% of elite adolescent athletes.

- Spondylolysis is a risk factor for asymptomatic and symptomatic spondylolisthesis (forward slip of a vertebra on the one below facilitated by the bilateral spondylolysis. (Fig. 21.2)).
- Progressive slippage may occur during the adolescent growth spurt.

*Management*
- If the slip is >25% (grade II, III, or IV), then effective physical therapy is important, to stabilise the spine (which is at risk of lumbar hyperextension) before a return to sports.
- Advice should be given on regular abdominal muscle exercises, avoiding gaining abdominal obesity, and consider regular bracing.
- Surgery is considered for progressive vertebral slippage or grade III/IV slip.

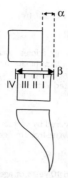

**Fig. 21.2** Spondylolisthesis measured as a % slip of L4 on L5 ($\alpha/\beta$). Grade I <25%, grade II 25–50%, grade III 50–75%, and grade IV >75%.

## Herniated disc

Herniated discs are infrequent in children <11y, but disc protrusion affects up to 20% by 18y of age.

- How much pain can be attributed to the disc protrusion is often unclear. Buttock or hip pain exacerbated by forward bend, cough or sneeze, or positive leg raise, suggests pain is due to the disc protrusion.

### Management

- Without nerve root impingement, management is conservative and includes a short period of bed rest, adequate analgesics, and NSAIDs with early exercise-based rehabilitation regimen.
- Over 50% improve with conservative treatment, but reported results from surgery for significant nerve root lesions, are very good.

## Spinal tumours

- Although rare in children, spinal tumours present with night pain increasing in intensity over time and associated with weight loss, radicular features, and focal tenderness.
- Other typical (though not specific) features include painful scoliosis and effectiveness of NSAIDs.

### Management

- Radiographs (may be negative in early disease) and MRI are essential with bone scintigraphy (+ SPECT) or CT to identify posterior element tumours (e.g. osteoid osteoma).
- Adequate analgesia is required. NSAIDs: ibuprofen in recommended but doses for weight may not be sufficient. Consider naproxen 15 mg/kg/day for adolescents.
- Bed rest is not essential, although wise if scans suggest risk of vertebral collapse or cord compression. If the latter, discuss urgently with a paediatric spinal surgeon and radiotherapist-oncologist.
- Initiate a search for other tumours known to metastasize to spine (Box 21.1). Investigation within an adolescent unit is advisable given the specific multidisciplinary input often needed.

## Box 21.1 Primary spinal tumours in children and adolescents

### Osteoid osteoma

Benign. Not uncommon. Mainly adolescents. Posterior vertebral bone usually. Pain can be severe. Discriminate from osteoblastomas by size (osteomas are <1.5 cm, osteoblastomas >1.5 cm) as histology is often identical. Lesions are associated with scoliosis (63%). Surgical excision is treatment of choice.

### Aneurysmal bone cyst

Benign. Symptoms often triggered by vertebral collapse. Take care when considering biopsy to discriminate from malignant lesions. Discuss in detail with MSK radiologist.

### Eosinophilic granuloma

Benign—often occurs around 10 years of age. Rare. Lytic. May occasionally be multiple/disseminated—staging important. Symptoms often triggered by vertebral collapse. Cord and radicular compression can occur. Biopsy essential to discriminate from malignant lesions. Surgical excision or internal spine fixation not usually needed. Consider radiotherapy if cord compression threatened. Consider external brace fixation in all and monitor for spontaneous resolution. Disseminated lesions can be treated with chemotherapy.

### Ewing sarcoma

Overall rarely affects spine (~10% cases). Can affect any part of spine including sacrum (latter cases often delayed diagnosis). Suspicion of it requires biopsy. Treat with combination chemotherapy and local radiotherapy. 5-year survival ~50%. Outcome better for tumour sizes <8 cm or localized disease.

### Leukaemia

Consider in all cases of spinal osteopenia or single/multiple vertebral collapse. May be referred pain from hip and or pelvic lesions.

Notorious association with delayed diagnosis. Associated systemic symptoms may not necessarily be present, but normal FBC at presentation unlikely (~10% cases only). Also look for eosinophilia and hypercalcaemia, and consider bone marrow aspirate.

### Lymphoma

Rarely presents with back pain; however, known cause of persistent back pain. MRI is imaging of choice: can show vertebral collapse and soft tissue paraspinal mass. Biopsy is diagnostic. Case reports of plasmacytomas presenting similarly.

### Secondary malignant tumour

Neuroblastoma, rhabdomyosarcoma, Wilms tumour, retinoblastoma, and teratoblastoma are known to present with back pain. Positive biopsy should trigger a search for the underlying primary neoplasm.

# Chronic pain syndromes

# Pain

### Introduction

Acute pain is a danger signal. Pain signals a 'threat' and stimulates a behavioural response and memory to enable avoiding future 'threat'. By nuanced contrast, chronic pain is typically a maladaptive process of reporting such a 'threat'.

- Pain is defined by the International Association for the Study of Pain as 'an unpleasant sensory and emotional experience associated with actual or potential tissue damage or described in terms of such damage'.
- The pain neuropathway can be modified—either by amplification or damped at various levels including peripherally—at the spinal cord and centrally. Modifications may occur in response to a vast array of interpretive senses such as beliefs, earlier life experiences, emotions, and emotional responses.
- The physiology and pathophysiology of pain is thus complex and it is best viewed in the context of a neuromatrix rather than a pain nerve or a simple gate theory.
- Chronic pain is considered a maladaptive sensation that both over-reports the peripheral threat signals so typical of acute pain, and directly contributes to, or may be the principal explanation for, the patient's distress.
- Viewed another way, tissue damage or inflammation cannot explain the presence or level of distress and effective pain management requires an understanding of all factors that influence pain perception.
- It is now widely recognized that effective explanation of pain processing that integrates the patient's own experiences is in itself therapeutic and allows the patient to build on the pain management strategies recommended.
- Chronic pain management strategies recognize the biopsychosocial model of pain interpretation and are most effective when they integrate a multidisciplinary approach targeting specific needs.

*For ease of explanation, chronic pain syndromes have been sub-divided into chronic widespread (or diffuse) pain (CWP) and regional (or focal) pain syndromes. Pragmatically this helps with considerations of differential diagnoses and targeting investigations effectively. Management strategies often overlap.*

### Pain neurophysiology: peripheries

Noxious painful stimuli are detected in the periphery by nociceptors on primary afferent neurons and transmitted to the dorsal horn of the spinal cord

- Nociceptive primary afferents are specialized sensory neurons: either small myelinated Aδ fibres or unmyelinated C fibres.
- These synapse mainly in lamina I and II of the spinal dorsal horn with spinal second-order interneurons. This is also one of the principal sites of pain amplification.
- It is possible that during inflammation, nociceptors may become activated at lower thresholds than usual, thus giving a degree of peripheral sensitization.

## Pain neurophysiology: central

The brain and spinal cord are responsible for central pain processing of noxious stimuli transmitted from the periphery. Numerous areas (upwards of 700 centres) within the brain influence pain perception.

• Nociceptive impulses ascend by two main spinal pathways.
• Information from Aδ fibres encodes 'fast pain' through the anterolateral neospinothalamic tract (ALNT), which transmits pain and temperature and discriminative qualities of pain: location, quality, and intensity of pain.
• This ALNT projects to the lateral thalamus with further connections to the sensory cortex allowing pain localization.
• Information from C fibres encodes 'slow pain' transmitted through the more primitive-origin spino-reticulo-diencephalic tract in the posterolateral cord. This projects to the reticular system of the brainstem, thalamus, and hypothalamus and onwards to the limbic system. These connections are responsible for the affective, emotional aspects of pain.
• Connections to the sympathetic nervous system mediate arousal.

## Theories of pain pathophysiology

Over the years, various theories have been proposed to try and explain the complex nature of pain sensation and how this is modulated.

• René Descartes first postulated the existence of pain nerves which directly transmit peripheral painful stimuli to the brain.
• The gate control theory of pain was put forward by Melzack and Wall. This states that there is a gate in the spinal cord that influences pain transmission. Non-noxious stimulation inhibits upward transmission of pain (closes the gate), hence other stimuli affecting the same peripheral nerve distribution (e.g. rubbing) reduces acute pain.
• Dissociation between peripheral stimuli and activation of the pain neuromatrix, a process known as central sensitization, is thought to underlie chronic pain that persists in the absence of tissue damage.

## Further reading

We direct those serious in their intention to help patients with chronic pain to other texts and to 'Explain Pain' delivered by the Neuro-orthopaedic Institute (ℛ http://www.noigroup.com/en/Category/EP) or similar courses.

# Generalized pain syndromes

## Chronic widespread pain

Chronic widespread pain (CWP) is a common finding present in 5–10% of the general population. In the absence of diffuse degenerative or inflammatory/autoimmune rheumatic MSK, fibromyalgia (FM) is the commonest manifestation.

- CWP affects women more than men with a ratio of 1.5:1 and is defined as pain for >6 months in two or more sites both above and below the pelvis.
- CWP may present alone, may be misinterpreted as another condition, or may be associated or complicate another condition.
- Conditions that can be associated with CWP or give rise to CWP as a secondary effect are shown in Box 22.1.
- CWP is often associated with disturbed and unrefreshed sleep.
- People with CWP often have fatigue and many may ultimately be diagnosed with chronic fatigue syndrome.
- Peripheral threat (/pain) signals will often be amplified by other threats including anxiety, depression, and any other persistent or unresolved psychological conflict. Assessment of these should be considered a normal part of the history and should be considered sympathetically as contributory but not the sole cause.

## Fibromyalgia and 'syndromic' fibromyalgia

Fibromyalgia (FM) is the term given to patients who have CWP that satisfies classification criteria: either ACR 1990 criteria for FM or ACR 2010 criteria for FM which expands the earlier criteria to include a wider spectrum of symptoms and their severity ('syndromic' FM or FM syndrome).

> **Box 22.1 Some (of the most common) conditions in adults that can either cause CWP or may be associated with it**
>
> - SLE.
> - Primary Sjögren's syndrome.
> - SOX syndrome and early generalized OA.
> - Undifferentiated AICTD.
> - Chronic sarcoidosis.
> - Antiphospholipid syndrome.
> - Psoriatic-related MSK disease.
> - SAPHO syndrome.
> - Axial or peripheral SpA.
> - Thyroid disease.
> - Primary hyperparathyroid disease.
> - Osteomalacia.
> - Large vessel arteritis.

*History of use of the term fibromyalgia*

FM is a type of CWP that has the cardinal feature of sleep disturbance. Historically this was previously labelled as muscular rheumatism or fibrositis to describe a condition with pain, fatigue, and psychological involvement.

- Both FM and CWP are often associated with other somatic symptoms, such as chronic fatigue, IBS, multiple chemical sensitivities, and headache syndromes. Other causes of fatigue should always be excluded, e.g. hypothyroidism, hypoadrenalism, primary Sjögren's syndrome and anaemia (Box 22.1).
- Both CWP and FM are associated with alterations in peripheral and central pain processing. Painful stimuli are detected at lower levels in affected patients. Allodynia (pain in response to non-painful stimuli) found in these conditions is thought to be due to central sensitization and an 'amplification' phenomenon.

*Diagnosis of FM*

There are two classification criteria for FM (ACR 1990 and ACR 2010 criteria). The 1990 criteria require diffuse tenderness at discrete anatomical sites. The 2010 criteria are based on mood, pain, and sleep disturbance. The 2010 criteria are designed to provide an alternative method of classification to allow long-term follow-up of FM patients and a method of evaluating the symptom severity of FM.

- Many FM tender points (Box 22.2) are over entheses which are scored for pain in enthesitis indices when assessing SpA conditions. It is of exceptional importance that SpA is distinguished from FM. Of course, both may coexist. An enthesitis predominant form of psoriatic arthritis is not uncommon (see CASPAR criteria for diagnosis of PsA in ➋ Chapter 8).
- FM is also found in up to 25% of patients with RA (see ➋ Chapter 5), and SLE (see ➋ Chapter 10). It is also commonly found in association with hypermobility spectrum disorders and hypermobility-EDS (➋ Chapter 19).
- Care must be taken to avoid misdiagnosing CWP/FM as the only cause for pain when there is an AICTD, axSpA, or PsA present.
- FM cases tend to aggregate within families but no genetic contribution has been defined as yet. It is implausible that genetic influences will not eventually be defined; thus common environmental triggers should be considered.
- The 2010 criteria for classification of FM are shown in Box 22.3.

### Box 22.2 ACR 1990 criteria for diagnosis of fibromyalgia

#### 1. History of widespread chronic pain

Pain is considered widespread and chronic when all of the following are present:

- Pain in the left and right side of the body
- Pain above and below the waist
- Axial skeletal pain
- Pain present for 3 months

*and*

#### 2. Pain in at least 11/18 tender point sites on digital palpation with 4 kg pressure*. One point is given for each side of the body at the following 9 sites:

| | |
|---|---|
| 1. | Occiput: at the suboccipital muscle insertions |
| 2. | Low cervical: at the anterior aspects of the inter-transverse spaces at C5–C7 |
| 3. | Trapezius: at the midpoint of the upper border |
| 4. | Supraspinatus: at origins above scapula spine near medial border |
| 5. | 2nd rib: at 2nd costochondral junction |
| 6. | Lateral humeral epicondyles: 2 cm distal from epicondyles |
| 7. | Gluteal: in upper outer quadrants |
| 8. | Greater trochanter: posterior to trochanter |
| 9. | Knees: at medial fat pad proximal to joint line |

* Positive tender point when subject says palpation was painful, ('tender' is not considered painful).

FM is said to be present when both criteria (CWP and tender point count) are satisfied. FM is not excluded by the presence of another disorder.

Criteria taken from Wolfe F et al. The American College of Rheumatology 1990 Criteria for the Classification of Fibromyalgia. *Arthritis and Rheumatism* 1990;33(2):160–72.

## Management of CWP and fibromyalgia

The ultimate goal of pain rehabilitation is to improve quality of life and sense of well-being rather than focus on pain reduction. With improvement in factors such as sleep or anxiety and improvements in physical activity and general participation, distraction from pain is improved and the overall sense of threat reduced. This will in turn reduce the volume of pain signal.

### Management issue 1: explanation and reassurance

It is of paramount importance to consider carefully the way in which an explanation is given as to the nature of the condition. This may take some time and may be best approached in the context of a multidisciplinary team (psychologists, physiotherapists, OTs, doctors).

### Box 22.3 ACR (revised) 2010 fibromyalgia criteria

A patient satisfies criteria for FM if the following three criteria are met:

1. Widespread pain index (WPI) ≥7 and a symptom severity (SS) scale score of ≥5 or WPI 3–6 and SS scale score ≥9.

2. Symptoms have been present at a similar level for ≥3 months.

3. The patient does not have a disorder that would otherwise explain the symptoms.

*WPI = the number of areas in the last week where there has been pain (score 0–19): left and right—shoulder girdle, upper arm, lower arm, 'hip' (buttock/ trochanter), upper leg, lower leg, jaw. Also: upper back, lower back, chest, abdomen, neck.*

*SS scale score (0–12) is calculated by:*
*Scoring each of these 3 symptoms: waking unrefreshed, fatigue, and cognitive symptoms, on a scale of 0–3 where:*

*0= no problem*
*1= slight or mild problems, generally mild or intermittent*
*2= moderate, considerable problems, often present and/or at a moderate level*
*3= severe: pervasive, continuous, life-disturbing problems.*

*And adding a score for the extent (severity) of somatic symptoms\* where:*

*0= no symptoms*
*1= few symptoms*
*2= a moderate number of symptoms*
*3= a great deal of symptoms.*

\* Somatic symptoms that might be considered: muscle pain, IBS, fatigue/tiredness, thinking or remembering problem, muscle weakness, headache, pain/cramps in the abdomen, numbness/tingling, dizziness, insomnia, depression, constipation, pain in the upper abdomen, nausea nervousness, chest pain, blurred vision, fever, diarrhoea, dry mouth, itching, wheezing, Raynaud's, hives, welts, ringing in ears, vomiting, heartburn, oral ulcers, loss of/change in taste, seizures, dry eyes, short of breath, loss of appetite, rash, sun sensitivity, hearing difficulties, easy bruising, hair loss, frequent urination, painful urination, bladder spasms.

New criteria summarized from Wolfe F et al. The American College of Rheumatology Preliminary Diagnostic Criteria for Fibromyalgia and Measurement of Symptom Severity. *Arthritis Care & Research* 2010;62:600–10.

- It is important to assess the effect of symptoms on the patient's life, and develop a good rapport so psychosocial issues can be discussed.
- The emphasis in the explanation should be reassurance that there is no serious underlying inflammatory or systemic condition, that nothing has been missed, and there is no damage to the joints and muscles. This fear blocks engagement with explanations and undermines rehabilitation strategies.

- Effective explanation uses appropriate language and stories to help the patient understand:
  - more about the complexity of pain processing and why it goes wrong.
  - why there isn't a quick switch to turn it off.
  - why a return to activities and routines including normalization of sleep helps.
  - why there needs to be a change in coping strategies.
- Explanations also challenge the value of ongoing litigation and it may be necessary to wait for this to be resolved before beginning a pain management programme
- Education of family and partners is invariably helpful and often essential.
- Both CWP/FM are conditions with relapses and remissions. Most patients will have ongoing symptoms. Patients with appropriate coping strategies, improvements in psychosocial stressors, and good social support networks are more likely to have a better outcome.

*Management issue 2: symptom management*
Often people with CWP limit activity due to a fear of provoking more pain. In addition to addressing physical symptoms such as pain and fatigue, psychological input (e.g. cognitive behavioural therapy) is helpful in providing tools to manage pain and activity levels.

- Although exercise may cause a short-term increase in pain, a graded exercise programme has been shown to be beneficial.
- Low-impact exercise, such as Pilates may be helpful. Pilates is helpful because it:
  - requires control avoiding jarring and unpredictable movements.
  - works all individual muscle groups including those that have become weak from previous unhelpful patterns of muscle use.
  - is tiring and releases endorphins.
  - encourages effective stretching.
  - builds confidence and resilience.
- A physiotherapist should help support and guide engagement with Pilates, yoga, and gym classes and may indicate what specific activity might be avoided in the first instance.
- Pacing of activities is important, avoiding 'boom and bust' patterns of over-activity when feeling well, followed by periods of inactivity due to subsequent pain and fatigue.
- Cognitive behavioural therapies (CBTs) provide a small incremental benefit over control interventions in reducing pain, negative mood and disability at the end of treatment and at long-term follow-up in FM.[2]
- Lack of adequate forms of sleep reduces resilience and promotes pain amplification. Poor sleep is one of the major barriers to improvement and is tackled at the outset of most pain programmes.
- Sleep disturbance needs to be addressed through sleep hygiene measures (e.g. have a quiet bedroom, reduce light and noise where possible, avoid eating late, reducing caffeine intake in the evening).
- Sleep health information is available at: ℠ https://www.sleepassociation.org/patients-general-public/insomnia/sleep-hygiene-tips/

*Management issue 3: pharmacological therapy*

The role of medication is to help establish and reinforce good sleep routines, reduce anxiety and fear of pain, and where possible allow improvements in pain severity to allow engagement with pain programme recommendations. Many of the techniques learnt in psychological-based treatment strategies help with this, reducing the reliance on often unhelpful pain medications.

- NSAIDs and GCs are not effective and may cause morbidity due to side effects.
- Narcotics should be avoided.
- Many patients will have tried analgesics with little effect. This in itself can fuel anxiety as to the cause and severity of their underlying condition, and frustration and lack of confidence in their doctor.
- Tricyclic antidepressants such as amitriptyline (10–50 mg 2 hours before bedtime) are often helpful in embedding changes to sleep routines and improving quality of sleep, decreasing morning stiffness, and alleviating pain.
- Patients should be warned of side effects of tricyclics such as dry mouth, self-limiting morning somnolence and weariness, and that they may take 3–4 weeks to take effect.
- Patients are often also wary of being given an 'antidepressant'. An explanation that a tricyclic is being used as a modifier of the impact of pain is important to improve adherence. Amitriptyline is one of a group of drugs that increase 5-hydroxytryptamine.
- Amitriptyline can be used with tramadol and this combination may be helpful in those with severe exacerbations or waves of pain.
- The efficacy of selective serotonin reuptake inhibitors (SSRIs) is debated given variable evidence of efficacy. The use of fluoxetine, duloxetine sertraline, or citalopram improves mood and anxiety, but SSRIs may be less effective than tricyclics in treating pain, fatigue, and sleep disturbance.
- Venlafaxine (a serotonin and noradrenaline reuptake inhibitor) in high doses is effective in treating multiple symptoms in FM. Low-dose treatment is ineffective.
- Pregabalin has shown efficacy on pain in some studies and can be combined effectively with duloxetine.[3]
- Sedative hypnotics have been reported to improve sleep in severe circumstances.
- A recent meta-analysis of RCTs[4] showed that duloxetine 60 mg, pregabalin 300 mg, milnacipran 100 mg, and 200 mg were more efficacious than placebo. However, there was no significant difference in the efficacy and tolerability between the medications at the recommended doses.
- Overall however, when treatments are judged against quite strict criteria for improvement there is not strong evidence for efficacy.[4]
- The conclusion from the meta-analysis report[4] was: 'The available data regarding efficacy . . . (treating pain, sleep, physical function, fatigue, anxiety, depression, and cognition) . . . were insufficient to draw definite conclusions . . . (regarding response of FM patients to reported

treatment modalities). . . . Indirect evidence indicates that efficacy may be expected with the use of serotonin noradrenaline reuptake inhibitors (SNRIs), noradrenaline reuptake inhibitors (NRIs), and multidisciplinary treatment. . . .'
- A number of meta-analyses of drug therapies are available in the Cochrane Library ( http://onlinelibrary.wiley.com/cochranelibrary).

## References

1. Okifuji A, Gao J, Bokat C, et al. Management of fibromyalgia syndrome in 2016. *Pain Manag* 2016;6:383–400.
2. Bernardy K, Klose P, Busch AJ, et al. Cognitive behavioural therapies for fibromyalgia. *Cochrane Database Syst Rev* 2013;9:CD009796.
3. Gilron I, Chaparro LE, Tu D, et al. Combination of pregabalin with duloxetine for fibromyalgia: a randomized controlled trial. *Pain* 2016;157:1532.
4. Papadopoulou D, Fassoulaki A, Tsoulas C, et al. A meta-analysis to determine the effect of pharmacological and non-pharmacological treatments on fibromyalgia symptoms comprising OMERACT-10 response criteria. *Clin Rheumatol* 2016;35:573–86.

# Localized pain syndromes

Localized pain syndromes are chronic pain conditions in a defined area. The diagnosis of a localized pain syndrome is a diagnosis of exclusion given conditions that can present with similar features. Often there is underlying neuropathic pain and abnormal neural activity.

## Chronic regional pain syndrome (CRPS)

### General considerations

CRPS is characterized by variable dysfunction of the MSK, skin, neurological, and vascular systems. CRPS may occur in a variety of situations with a number of clinical manifestations varying around central core features.

- Several terms have evolved, describing aspects of the same condition: reflex sympathetic dystrophy, Sudeck's atrophy, shoulder–hand syndrome, and transient osteoporosis.
- These terms have been superseded by the term CRPS, which is recognized by the International Association for the Study of Pain.
- There are two subtypes of CRPS: type 1 describes symptoms in the absence of peripheral nerve injury, and type 2 ('causalgia') in the presence of injury to a specific peripheral nerve.

### Epidemiology and aetiology

CRPS is a common disorder. It affects both sexes equally, and occurs at any age in all races and geographical regions. Although the exact aetiology is unclear, there is likely to be a combination of peripheral and central neurological factors involved.

- Trauma (e.g. fracture, burn, surgery, etc.) is the most common triggering event. The event may be trivial. Often no cause is identified.
- CRPS is reported in up to a third of series of distal forearm fracture.
- Several neurological conditions may act as triggers, including, for example, hemiplegia and meningitis. Peripheral nerve root injury may also lead to the syndrome.
- Pregnancy, tumours, and prolonged immobilization have also been linked as possible triggering factors. However, 25% of cases have no clear trigger.
- It is important to try and identify psychosocial stresses as these may have an effect on the persistence of symptoms.

### Clinical features

Typically, the syndrome involves the distal part of a limb, e.g. forearm or foot. Early clinical features of the condition include pain, soft tissue swelling (e.g. may be synovitis if over a joint), reticular/livedo rash, warmth over affected part. Occasionally there may be localized, sweating and piloerection.

- The pain has several particular characteristics and is often described as 'burning'. The features include:
  - *allodynia*—an otherwise innocuous stimulus produces pain.
  - *hyperalgesia*—increased pain perception to a given stimulus.
  - *hyperpathia*—delayed over-reaction, often after repetitive cutaneous stimulus.

- The affected limb is often guarded to avoid any contact as allodynia is usually extreme.
- Novel clinical signs described in recent years support involvement of the CNS and MRI studies show evidence of cortical reorganization. These clinical signs include digit misperception, astereognosis, altered hand laterality, and abnormal body schema.
- Patients become 'depersonalized' from their affected limb with a feeling that it no longer belongs to them and a desire to remove that limb.

*Investigation, staging, and diagnosis*

Clinical suspicion and knowledge, and a good history and examination will make the diagnosis of CRPS in all cases, but it is important to recognize changes that may occur in some radiological and functional imaging. These tests may be misinterpreted in other settings and may help with explanations with patients.

- Laboratory tests need to be interpreted cautiously. ESR, CRP, and FBC abnormalities may be present if there is underlying inflammatory rheumatic MSK disease.
- However, there may be evidence of bone demineralization (osteopenia on radiographs, CT or low bone density estimated using regional DXA) if the lesion is severe.
- High bone resorption can be indicated biochemically by hypercalciuria (hypercalcaemia would be very unlikely), and raised plasma/serum collagen crosslinks (e.g. CTX).
- Thermography can demonstrate changes in cutaneous temperature.
- Perhaps of most value, and high specificity, is the triple-phase bone scintigraphy ($^{99m}$Tc-MDP scintigraphy).
- An experienced nuclear medicine physician can specify CRPS based on characteristic patterns of bone scintigraphy abnormality in the early regional blood flow distribution, blood pool appearances, and late skeletal radionuclide uptake.
- CRPS stage I is essentially regional pain and swelling. In most cases, the symptoms fluctuate, then gradually resolve.
- Stage II CRPS is a period of dystrophic change (see ➲ Plate 10). This tends to occur several months after onset of the disorder. The affected region becomes cool, pale, and often cyanosed in colour with abnormal sensation (dysesthesia).
- Stage III CRPS is manifest by a decrease in hair and nail growth, osteopenia, and eventually atrophy of skin and subcutaneous tissue. Stage III CRPS is difficult to treat and reverse.
- Most cases of CRPS tend not to progress beyond stage I, or at most early stage II.
- The Budapest criteria for diagnosis of CRPS are shown in Table 22.1.

*Management of CRPS*

Success treating CRPS relies on an early and accurate diagnosis and early treatment in order to prevent chronicity.

- Once CRPS persists beyond 6–8 months, it is difficult to reverse.
- Early and ongoing treatment should focus on the whole individual and not simply the regional symptoms.

**Table 22.1.** The Budapest criteria for diagnosis of CRPS. *For a diagnosis of CRPS, all four criteria (A–D) must be met*

| Criteria | A: continuing pain disproportionate to the inciting event and |
|---|---|
| | B: ≥1 symptom in ≥3 categories (below) |
| | *and* |
| | C: ≥1 sign in ≥2 categories (below) |
| | *and* |
| | D: no other diagnosis better explains the symptoms and signs |
| Categories | *Sensory:* allodynia (to light touch and/or temperature sensation and/or deep somatic pressure and/or joint movement) and/or hyperalgesia (to pinprick) |
| | *Vasomotor:* temperature asymmetry (>1°C) and/or skin colour asymmetry between limbs |
| | *Sudomotor/oedema:* oedema and/or sweating changes and/or sweating asymmetry |
| | *Motor/trophic:* decreased range of motion and/or motor dysfunction (weakness, tremor, dystonia) and/or trophic tissue changes (hair, nail, skin) |

- Treatment is based around the broad categories of physical therapies (physiotherapy and desensitization therapy), psychological therapies (cognitive behavioural techniques), and pharmacotherapy.
- Attention to anxiety, psychosocial stressors, pain behaviour, and sleep disturbance is important.
- Patients often require repeated reassurance and counselling.
- The aim should be to resume premorbid levels of activity so early physical therapy (/hydrotherapy) input should be considered.
- Desensitization therapy of the affected region can help to normalize the sensations of hyperalgesia and allodynia.
- Desensitization is achieved by applying different textures to the affected area, concentrating particularly on the interface between normal and abnormal sensations.
- Mirror therapy to reflect the unaffected limb while performing synchronized movements can also help in regaining function and range of movement and relieving pain.
- In early acute disease, IV pamidronate may be helpful in relieving pain, especially if there are bony changes on imaging. Short courses of glucocorticoids (GCs) may also be helpful in the acute stages.
- Tricyclic antidepressants can help correct sleep disturbance and increase the pain threshold.
- Gabapentin or pregabalin may also be of value.
- Transcutaneous electrical nerve stimulation (TENS) may help pain control and allow entry into a physical activity programme.

- In some severe cases, regional sympathetic or ganglion blocks have been reported to control pain sufficiently to facilitate engagement with pain management programmes.
- Patients may request limb amputation as a result of their depersonalization from that limb. However, this should be discouraged as it does not guarantee improvement in pain and such patients may suffer with intractable phantom limb pain.

## Other adult regional pain syndromes

### Post-herpetic neuralgia

This neuropathic pain condition develops in a dermatomal distribution following an episode of herpes zoster. It is defined as pain that continues for 3 months following an attack of herpes zoster. Typically, the neuralgia begins as the vesicles start to heal and crust over.

- Pain can be variable in severity and is neuropathic in nature.
- Antivirals such as aciclovir are often used at the beginning of an attack of herpes zoster to limit the duration of the attack and reduce the chances of developing post-herpetic neuralgia. However, these are not useful in established disease.
- Treatment includes anticonvulsants such as carbamazepine and gabapentin as well as tricyclic antidepressants such as amitriptyline.
- Ganglion regional nerve blocks can be considered for severe cases.
- Analgesics such as paracetamol, anti-inflammatories, and opioids may all be helpful in managing pain.
- Short courses of GCs are often used to reduce the duration of pain.
- Conservative measures that may be helpful are TENS, acupuncture, relaxation techniques, and heat/cold therapy.

### Trigeminal neuralgia

This is a type of neuropathic pain affecting the trigeminal nerve and causing intense facial pain along the trigeminal nerve divisions. There are two main types: *typical* and *atypical* trigeminal neuralgia.

- The typical form causes attacks of severe sudden pain on one side of the face which can last for seconds to minutes while the atypical form causes constant burning pain.
- The exact aetiology is unknown but is thought to be due to loss of the myelin nerve sheath.
- Treatment is with anticonvulsants such as carbamazepine and tricyclics such as amitriptyline. Opioids are usually not effective.
- Surgery may be an option if conservative measures fail.

### Temporomandibular joint (TMJ) dysfunction

The most important feature of TMJ dysfunction is pain and restricted mandibular opening.

- There is often clicking associated with movement of the joint.
- About 20–30% of the general population have some degree of TMJ dysfunction.
- There is a link to the habit of teeth grinding so often prosthetic mouth guards are fashioned to wear particularly at night.
- The TMJ can be affected in all inflammatory arthritides such as RA and PsA and such causes should always be considered as an underlying cause of TMJ pain.

# Chronic pain in children and adolescents

## Introduction

In childhood and adolescence, pain is a ubiquitous experience affecting over 80% of individuals in any given preceding 3–6-month period. As in adults, this threat, or danger, sensation is associated with neuroendocrine, MSK, and inflammatory responses, and provokes threat appraisal and behavioural adaptation that may be attentive or avoidant.

- Prevalence rates of chronic (recurrent or persistent) pain in children and adolescents are high (11–38%) with 5% experiencing significant pain-related dysfunction.
- Chronic pain affects most body sites with a prevalence that increases with age (see Table 22.2)
- Over 10% of all GP contacts with adolescents are attributable to MSK pain and of those seeking medical intervention the direct cost to the USA is $19 billion.
- Although the international criteria for chronicity is 3 months' duration (constant or intermittent), taken from the definition in adults, a diagnosis can often be made sooner.
- On careful enquiry the site, character, and severity of pain, and any loss of function, are often incongruous with the mechanism of any injury or background disease state (JIA, sickle, IBD, etc.) and this frequently overrides the relevance of duration.

### Associations of chronic pain in children and adolescents

Most chronic MSK pain might reasonably be attributed to biomechanical imbalances and stresses that typically result from tissue tightness and changes in patterns of muscle use with normal growth and development.

- Inappropriate patterns of muscle use may also derive from previous injury, repetitive sport or dance activities, or commonly from deconditioning when sedentary behaviour predominates.
- Other common associations with chronic pain and pain amplification include obesity, poor sleep health, lower socioeconomic status, parental catastrophizing, risk aversion, thought and attention problems, anxiety, low mood, rule breaking, aggressive behaviour and hypermobile joints, but the extent to which these factors are contributory in childhood vary.
- Pain in multiple sites, including chest, abdomen, and head, is strongly associated with obesity in girls and a high number of psychosocial and mechanical factors.
- Multiple MSK pains in adolescence have a high tendency to persist (>2 years) with both psychosocial factors and lifestyle factors contributing to this vulnerability.

**Table 22.2** Prevalence of chronic pain in children and adolescents

| Pain type | Prevalence range from various studies (%) |
| --- | --- |
| Headache | 8–83 |
| Abdominal pain | 4–53 |
| Back pain | 14–24 |
| MSK pain | 4–40 |
| Multiple pains | 4–49 |
| Other/general pains | 5–88 |

## Chronic widespread pain in children and adolescents

The diagnosis term *chronic widespread pain (CWP)* is preferred to *juvenile FM* or *joint hypermobility syndrome/hypermobility spectrum disorder* or other labels which intimate poorly established aetiologies, have overlapping diagnostic criteria, marked heterogeneity, and may unnecessarily inculcate (or trap) patients into an expectation of lifelong disability.

- Due to variation in diagnostic labels and criteria, the epidemiology of CWP is poorly understood.
- The prevalence of juvenile fibromyalgia (JFM), defined by ACR criteria for adults (chronic MSK pain, multiple discrete tender points, fatigue, and sleep disturbance), is up to 6%.
- JFM accounts for 8% of diagnoses made by paediatric rheumatologists. The prevalence of joint hypermobility syndrome in children diagnosed with JFM is probably the same as in the general paediatric population.
- Enigmatic symptoms of dizziness, fatigue, blurring of vision, 'black outs', and tachycardia occur in 50% of children and adolescents with CWP and might reasonably be attributable to variations in 'threat signalling' and may be exacerbated by anxiety.
- Labels of 'postural orthostatic tachycardia syndrome' PoTS, 'autonomic dysfunction,' or 'chronic Lyme disease' are usually unhelpful and most of the clinical symptoms resolve with effective explanation and engagement in a rehabilitative programme.
- CWP may be triggered by or coexist in 5–20% of cases with an underlying disorder such as sickle cell disease, heart disease, or cancer. CWP in the presence of a SpA condition requires careful disentangling as enthesitis linked to SpA may be present (see ➲ Chapter 8).

### Management of CWP: general principles

- Irrespective of the medical setting there is always a potential to positively intervene, beginning with recognition of a primary pain disorder and making time for the patient to explain their history, the impact, and their understanding.
- The therapeutic consult acknowledges the pain and explains the role of pain as a threat signal.

- Further explanations about pain processing, in appropriate language, should assist an understanding to promote engagement in the treatment strategies described in the next subsection and reduce a sense of helplessness.
- Effective explanations of pain are therapeutic and can be enormously motivational.
- In particular, there should be an understanding of disruptions to the '4Ss' (sleep, sports/physical activity, social life, and school).
- A focus on returning to normal 4S routines should improve resilience and improve quality of life, with consequent reductions in the psychological impact of pain and enhanced biofeedback to counteract pain signals.

*Programmes of care for CWP*

- Effective programmes of care target an appropriate amount of resource to the level of need.
- Integration across a network of services is often required with community and secondary care services working with a tertiary hub.
- The focus of care is to return to normal function with an incident decrease in pain.
- Core features of a programme of care include:
  - adequate explanation about pain and rehabilitation.
  - an interdisciplinary and goal-orientated approach with a specific focus on self-management.
  - medication used to enhance engagement with advice and other self-management strategies.
- Pain workshops inform and educate in an engaging way, dispel myths, and create a narrative that helps to increase participation and improvements in quality of life despite minimal changes levels of pain. Workshops also provide the benefit of peer support.
- Physical therapies such as physiotherapy and occupational therapy treatment strategies are most effective when goal oriented.
  - Physiotherapists help to reduce the fear of movement and guide the patient through a programme of exercise and increase participation in general physical activity.
  - Physiotherapy promotes resilience, as well as reducing muscle tightness and building strength, stamina, balance, and normal patterns of muscle use.
  - Occupational therapists support upper limb physical activity, a graded return to school, sleep advice, management of bullying and a return to an active social life.
  - Physiotherapists often support such re-engagement with regaining normal 4S function too.

*Psychological therapies for CWP*

- Psychological intervention now draws from an array of treatment strategies in addition to CBT.
- Effective psychology programmes include a focus on resilience and promotion of patient strengths in addition to reducing barriers to engagement and coping modification.
- A Cochrane review in 2014 showed psychological treatments are effective in reducing pain intensity and disability in various forms of CWP and the benefits appear to be maintained.
- Evidence for the effects of psychological therapies on mood is limited as it is for effects on disability in children with headache.

### Active mind–body techniques

- Techniques are useful in promoting self-management.
- Techniques include breathing strategies (square breathing, diaphragmatic and slow exhale breathing), mindfulness, yoga, Pilates, and progressive muscle relaxation. This is not an exclusive list and the benefit varies between patients.

### Parent coaching

- A child or adolescent in pain exerts a considerable emotional, and often financial, toll on family life.
- Pain-related disability is more consistently related to poor family functioning than pain intensity.
- Parenting behaviours can act to maintain or even enhance their child's pain experience; e.g. if the child has to interpret ambiguous emotional parental expressions.
- There is a risk of increased anxiety and depression for a child of a parent with CWP. Familial dysfunction can follow.
- Normalizing parental protectiveness reduces guilt and defensiveness and refocuses parents' attention on healthy and adaptive behaviours.
- Parents are taught how to calm themselves and use skills to distract and avoid emotional escalation. A focus should be maintained on their child's function and participation.
- Parents' pain experiences should be addressed and discussed openly with the child present. It should be clearly pointed out that the child's pain is different from the parent's disability and pain, with an expectation that the child can become pain free.
- Parents are taught how to optimize the independence of teenagers and encourage self-management skills.

### Pharmacotherapy in CWP

- There is little evidence to support the sole use of medication but it may have a role in the integrated management plan described here.
- There are no RCTs which confirm the benefit of paracetamol in treating paediatric CWP but there is some limited evidence for ibuprofen although both are associated with potential long-term side effects including overuse headaches.
- Opiates should be avoided in primary pain disorders due to poor safety and side effect profiles associated with worse outcomes.
- Care should be taken with opiate use when IBD or sickle cell disease is associated with a primary pain disorder.
- Codeine has been withdrawn from the WHO pain ladder for children.
- Adjuvant therapies including low-dose tricyclic antidepressants, gabapentinoids, SSRIs, and melatonin may be helpful.
- There are no RCTs which support the use of gabapentin in treating paediatric CWP, and its use may result in cognitive impairment and reduced resilience.
- The anxiolytic effects of tricyclics and SSRIs may help to improve engagement with management strategies and resilience from improving sleep.
- Medication is associated with a strong placebo effect in CWP. For example, in various RCTs for migraine therapies, a placebo response is typically seen in 50–60% of study participants and can decrease headache frequency from six to three headaches/month.

# Complex regional pain syndrome in children and adolescents

CRPS is clinically distinct from adult CRPS in that the lower limb is more commonly involved than the upper limb, there is a marked female predominance, dystrophic changes and long-term disability are less common, and multiple limbs can typically become involved.

- The peak incidence is in early adolescence (median 13 years).
- MRI shows increased bone signal ('oedema') early in the condition.
- Thermography highlights abnormal regional blood flow changes, which can be compared to the other limbs.
- Later in the disease radiographs show osteopenia.
- Ultimately, limb deformity occurs in the most severe cases.

## Management of CRPS

- Effective management of CRPS requires a careful explanation of the condition to the child or adolescent and their family, a graded exercise programme supervised by a therapist experienced in chronic pain management, and frequent desensitization.
- Work on restoring normal 4S function improves resilience and most patients respond within 4–6 therapy sessions. Patients can expect to become pain free and return to all activities.
- 25–35% of children and adolescents with CRPS are resistant to routine management techniques and will benefit from more intense programmes of care as described for CWP (see ➐, 'Chronic widespread pain', pp. 639–41).

# Part III

# Medicine management and emergencies

# Drugs used in
# rheumatology practice

## Introduction

A variety of pharmacological agents are used across the breadth of rheumatic diseases. Therapeutic options are discussed in each of the disease-specific chapters in Part II of this book.

This chapter highlights common themes pertinent to prescribing for pain relief and control of autoimmune rheumatic disease. It is not the intention of this chapter to describe all of these in detail, although specific issues are discussed. Protocols for the use of certain agents such as pooled-immunoglobulin will also be described.

For a detailed description of a specific drug it is recommended the reader use a National Formulary and in the UK all medicine summary of product characteristics (SPCs) are available at ℘ http://www.medicines.org.uk

Table 23.1 lists the common classes of drug used in rheumatology and is the framework for the content of this chapter.

**Table 23.1** Pharmacotherapy of rheumatological diseases

| Drug type | Examples |
|---|---|
| Pain relief | Paracetamol and compound analgesics |
| | Opioid analgesics |
| | NSAIDs |
| | Antidepressants |
| | Gabapentin and pregabalin |
| | Hypnotics and muscle relaxants |
| | Topical agents |
| Glucocorticoids (GCs) | Prednisolone, triamcinolone, methylprednisolone |
| Conventional synthetic disease-modifying antirheumatic drugs (sDMARDs) | Azathioprine |
| | Ciclosporin |
| | Cyclophosphamide |
| | Gold (Myocrisin® IM or auranofin oral) |
| | Hydroxychloroquine (HCQ) |
| | Leflunomide |
| | Methotrexate (MTX) |
| | Mycophenolate mofetil (MMF) |
| | Penicillamine |
| | Sulfasalazine |
| Targeted sDMARDs | Tofacitinib |
| | Apremilast |
| Biological DMARDs | Anti-TNFα: etanercept, infliximab, adalimumab, certolizumab, golimumab |
| | Anti B-cell (CD 20): rituximab (RTX) |
| | Anti BLyS/BAFF: belimumab |
| | IL-1 receptor antagonists: anakinra |
| | IL-6 receptor antagonists: tocilizumab |
| | IL-12/23 antagonists: ustekinumab |
| | IL-17A antagonists: secukinumab |
| | CTLA4-Ig: abatacept |
| Other | Hyperuricaemia/gout: allopurinol, febuxostat |
| | *Osteoporosis:* bisphosphonates, denosumab, strontium, teriparatide |
| | Pulmonary hypertension and Raynaud's disease: iloprost, sildenafil, bosentan |
| | Intravenous immunoglobulin |

# Pain relief

### General considerations

The descriptors and assessment of the impact of pain are discussed in
➲ Chapters 1 and 22. Good pain management is associated with improvement in various physiological and psychological outcome measures.

- In general, pain management may be broadly divided into
  pharmacological and non-pharmacological methods. The individual
  description of each non-pharmacological method is beyond the scope
  of this chapter but may include the following:
  - Hot/cold/pressure compress.
  - Physical therapies—land based and hydrotherapy.
  - Transcutaneous electrical nerve stimulation (TENS).
  - Acupuncture.
  - Hypnosis.
  - Cognitive and behavioural therapy (CBT).
  - Pulsed radiofrequency and nerve ablation therapies.
  - Low-level laser therapy (LLLT).
  - Massage, relaxation therapy, and meditation.
  - Other complementary medicine methods.
- Effective pain management must begin with a thorough assessment of
  the patient's pain, treatment expectations, and concerns.
- Unrealistic expectations or misunderstanding of pain could mean that
  the management strategy may fail from the beginning.
- In chronic painful conditions please refer to Chapter 22. Patients
  should be aware that there might be a period of trial and error before
  the optimal combination of pain relief is found although in many
  circumstances medication may be unhelpful.
- In assessing efficacy of an oral analgesic, it is important to consider:
  - the analgesic effect.
  - the frequency and maximum dose tried.
  - any unwanted side effects.
- If there was temporary relief that then wore off, this may be due to
  either an insufficient dose, or the interval between doses is too long.
- Unpleasant side effects may also put patients off some medications.
- Patients may use the term 'addiction' to express concerns over the
  long-term use of analgesics, in particular, opioid-based pain relief. If such
  concerns are not addressed, patients may be reluctant to take opioids
  regularly which in turn leads to poor pain control.
- Rather than 'substance abuse', the patient is most likely reflecting on the
  possibility of 'tolerance,' when citing 'addiction', i.e. 'becoming used to'
  the analgesic so that a higher dose is required to sustain the effect over
  time. This often needs clarification during consultation.
- Abuse of opioids—addiction or recreational use and deliberate self-
  harm by overdosing—is a legitimate cause for concern.
- The safety and suitability of these agents are very much dependent on
  assessment of the individual patient.
- Follow-up appointments are important to allow both the patient and
  the clinician to evaluate the efficacy of a treatment regimen and to then
  make the necessary adjustments.
- There is very little high-quality evidence for the use of analgaesia in
  paediatric pain.

## Analgesic escalation: the 'analgesic ladder'

The WHO analgesic ladder (Fig. 23.1) is a useful framework to consider when commencing patients on pharmacological pain treatment. But see also more specific guides for managing and prescribing strong analgesics in chronic pain (e.g. SIGN-136: www.sign.ac.uk; and at CDC: www.cdc.gov/mmwr/volumes/65/rr/rr6501e1.htm).

- Escalation of pain relief modality follows a stepwise approach depending on the assessment of the severity of pain.
- Movement up the analgesic ladder is a balancing act between increasing analgesic potency versus increasing risk of side effects.
- At the bottom of the ladder (Step 1) are non-opioid compounds with relatively good safety profile such as paracetamol and non-steroidal anti-inflammatory drugs (NSAIDs). These are effective for mild to moderate pain severity.
- Step 2 involves adding in weak opioids such as tramadol or codeine phosphate for pain of moderate severity, although codeine is no longer included in the WHO ladder for pain relief in children. This is because children are variable metabolisers of codeine, leading to an unpredictable effect. Codeine should not be used in chronic pain in long term paediatric conditions.
- If long term opioid use is to be maintained consider converting to sustained-release form as a basal analgesia. This is supplemented with instant-release opioid for breakthrough pain. Caution should be taken when using opioids in long term paediatric conditions and alternative strategies to pain management should be sought.
- Opioids used for an extended period lead to tolerance, create physical dependency, and should not be withdrawn abruptly.

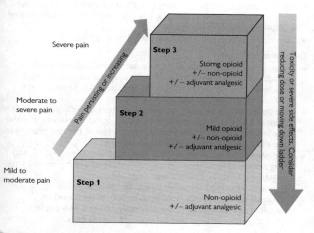

**Fig. 23.1** WHO analgesic ladder. Reprinted from WHO's cancer pain ladder for adults, Copyright (2014) http://www.who.int/cancer/palliative/painladder/en/. Accessed May 2017.

- If an episode of acute pain is superimposed upon chronic pain requiring regular strong opioids, any analgesia prescribed should be in addition to the regular opioid regimen.
- Some analgesics, when taken together, have a synergistic effect that is greater than the sum of its individual effects. It makes sense therefore to have a compound form (e.g. co-codamol which contains codeine and paracetamol).
- A compound agent may be easier for the patient to manage by reducing the number of separate pills to ingest. However, the ability to alter the dose of one of the component agents without altering the other is lost. There is also the additional risk of patients double dosing on a medication from failure to recognize the active components of the drug (e.g. taking co-codamol and paracetamol together).
- Clear advice on the options for increasing dose according to tolerability and efficacy should be given, including the principle of starting at the lowest dose whenever possible (particularly in the elderly). Clear guidance puts the patient in control of their pain relief.

## Simple and compound analgesics

### Paracetamol (acetaminophen)
Paracetamol is thought to reduce pain by inhibiting prostaglandin synthesis within the central nervous system. It has both analgesic and antipyretic activity without anti-inflammatory activity.

- It is available over the counter in many countries and is effective in managing soft tissue injury, joint pain, dental pain, and headache.
- It is usually given orally at 4 g/day (children 30–60mg/kg/day; max 4g) given in 4 divided doses. It is also available in suppository and IV formulations.
- It is reasonable to try paracetamol first. Most GPs will and it is important to assure the patient of its efficacy. The specialist may hear patients say 'my GP just gave me paracetamol'.
- Common concerns and interactions are shown in Table 23.2.

### Paracetamol compounds
- Paracetamol 500 mg is also available in compound analgesics, such as co-codamol (paracetamol and codeine), co-dydramol (paracetamol and dihydrocodeine), and paracetamol and tramadol. These are not recommended in chronic paediatric conditions.
- Care should always be taken, as with 'over-the-counter' aspirin products and other NSAIDs, that patients ensure they do not take more than the maximum daily dose of paracetamol, irrespective of the combination of single and compound medications used together.
- The codeine content varies in these formulations between 10, 15, and 30 mg per tablet to a maximum total daily dose of 240 mg divided into 8 tablets and taken as 2 tablets four times a day.
- Codeine is discussed later under opioid analgesics.
- Because of safety concerns (related to toxicity in overdose) co-proxamol (paracetamol and dextropropoxyphene) is only available in the UK by special arrangement on a named-patient basis.

**Table 23.2** Cautions and side effects with paracetamol

| Caution | Comment |
| --- | --- |
| Hepatic toxicity | Avoid in known significant liver disease and alcohol abuse |
| Renal toxicity | Note that the effervescent formulations contain sodium—avoid in moderate–severe renal impairment |
| Blood dyscrasia | E.g. thrombocytopenia and leucopenia can be induced or worsened |
| Pregnancy and breastfeeding | *Not* known to be harmful |
| **Common interactions** | |
| Coumarin (warfarin) | Paracetamol may enhance the anticoagulant effect |
| Absorption and metabolism | Metoclopramide increases absorption; carbamazepine accelerates metabolism of paracetamol |

## Opioid analgesics

Opioid drugs act as agonists at opioid receptors which are found mainly in the brain and spinal cord and also peripherally.

- For all opioid drugs, there are numerous cautions (See ➔ Table 23.3) and care should be taken in all chronic conditions, especially in children.

*Commonly used weak opioids: codeine and dihydrocodeine*

- Codeine and dihydrocodeine (also available as modified release) can be used as a single agent to maximum daily adult dosage of 240 mg (usually 2 × 30 mg tablets four times a day). It is available in 15 mg or 30 mg tablets.
- It is also available in compound agents with paracetamol as described earlier and with ibuprofen or aspirin.
- Codeine is marketed in various salt compounds including phosphate and sulfate (typical in the USA, Canada, and UK), hydrochloride (continental Europe), hydro-iodide, and citrate.
- Low-dose codeine is available 'over the counter' in some countries and is also found in cough suppressants. In the majority of countries however, it remains prescription only due to concerns over dependency and misuse. Its use is still classed as illegal in a few places. Travellers with legitimate prescriptions are advised to carry documentation of their condition from their physician.
- Cimetidine, acting as a P450 enzyme inhibitor, increases plasma concentration of codeine and dihydrocodeine.
- Metoclopramide and domperidone are antagonized by codeine and dihydrocodeine.

Table 23.3 Cautions and side effects of opioid analgesics

| Caution | Comment |
|---|---|
| Hypotension | Particular care when also taking antihypertensives, antipsychotics, or antidepressants |
| Sedation and respiratory suppression | Avoid in chronic obstructive pulmonary disease, head injury, any situation of reduced level of consciousness; take particular care when also taking antipsychotics, antidepressants, or antihistamines. Counsel caution over driving and use of machinery |
| Hepatic toxicity | Avoid in known significant liver disease, reduce dose in mild disease |
| Renal toxicity | Avoid in known significant renal disease, reduce dose in mild disease |
| Blood dyscrasia | E.g. thrombocytopenia; leucopenia can be induced or worsened |
| Porphyria | Avoid |
| Pregnancy | Avoid |
| Breastfeeding | Preferably avoid. Note codeine is not known to be harmful as concentration are very small; however, individuals vary in rate of metabolism and close observation should be made for signs of infant morphine overdose |
| Gastrointestinal | Opioids induce nausea, vomiting, constipation, pancreatitis, obstruction |
| Neuropsychiatric | Opioids induce headache, confusion, dys/euphoria, hallucinations, mood change, seizures |
| Genitourinary | Sexual dysfunction, urinary retention, avoid in significant obstructive prostatic hypertrophy |
| Age | Reduce dosage in the elderly, avoid in childhood |

*Tramadol and meptazinol*
Tramadol is a weak opioid agonist. It inhibits the reuptake of both serotonin and norepinephrine (noradrenaline) at the dorsal horn.
- The maximum recommended adult dose is 400 mg/day in divided doses. It is available in modified-release 12-hourly preparations (200 mg twice daily) and in combination with paracetamol.
- Meptazinol is a partial opioid receptor antagonist and is given at 800 mg/day in divided doses. Its mixed effect reduces the risk of dependence and is less likely to be used as a substance of abuse.
- These agents are often tried after or instead of codeine compounds given the difference in mechanisms of action.
- They have a more favourable gastrointestinal (GI) side effect profile than codeine and may be one of the reasons for trying them before codeine in those prone to constipation. However, this is offset by a greater risk of intolerance from neuropsychiatric effects.

*Commonly used strong opioids*

These include morphine sulfate and oxycodone hydrochloride 5–10 mg, both 4–6-hourly (can be titrated up to 400 mg per day in severe cases); the latter also has a compound of oxycodone/naloxone, which may be beneficial in those with severe constipation from opioids despite trials of different classes of laxative. Thereafter, escalation might move to morphine salts, but before any of these are utilized it is common to try patch formulations.

*Opioids delivered through transdermal patches*

These are applied to the skin and, therefore, in addition to the above-mentioned cautions, be aware of allergic reaction with localized sensitivity.

- *Buprenorphine* (also available in the UK as Temgesic® 200 micrograms sublingual) is produced as BuTrans® and Transtec®. Both have formulations that allow a wide variety of dosing, e.g. BuTrans 5 micrograms/hour 7-day patch, gradually building dose, perhaps every 2 weeks depending on tolerance and response of symptoms.

# Non-steroidal anti-inflammatory drugs

NSAIDs are commonly used. Most have a licensed indication for OA (see ◆ Chapter 6) and RA (see ◆ Chapter 5); some have a licence for ankylosing spondylitis (see ◆ Chapter 8).

- In reality, most NSAIDs are prescribed in effect 'off licence' for a number of rheumatic conditions outside these diagnoses, but based on being effective analgesics with the capacity to reduce inflammation such as occurs in soft tissues, tendonitis, and synovitis.
- NSAIDs are classified by their inhibitory action on cyclooxygenase 1 (COX-1), e.g. ibuprofen, naproxen, and diclofenac, or COX-2, e.g. celecoxib and etoricoxib. Some agents (e.g. oxicams) demonstrate inhibitory action against both enzyme pathways.
- It is reasonable to try a NSAID from a different class when another has failed.
- *Ibuprofen* and *aspirin* compounds are available over the counter in many countries. *Naproxen* (250–500 mg twice daily) and *diclofenac* (150 mg daily in divided doses) probably represent the two most commonly prescribed NSAIDs worldwide.
- *COX-2 inhibitors* are discussed later in this section.
- Oral preparations are most often used. Some are available as slow-release formulations, e.g. diclofenac.
- Although per rectum agents are also available in some, these do not appear to reduce side effect (specifically gastric) enough to warrant their preference over oral agents in the majority of cases.
- Topical agents have variable efficacy, often with limited evidence of benefit. That said, they are popular with patients as part of their management.
- Paediatric dosing includes: Ibuprofen 10mg/kg 4–6 times daily; naproxen 10–20mg/kg/day in 2–3 divided doses; diclofenac 3–5mg/kg/day in 2–3 divided doses.

*Adverse effects of NSAIDs*

A number of adverse reactions are recognized. Caution applies to all NSAIDs, particularly avoiding their use in hepatic and renal impairment, pregnancy, and GI ulceration (Table 23.4).

- Using the lowest possible dose for the shortest period of time lessens the adverse effects risk of NSAIDs. It is inevitable, however, that those with long-term conditions for which remission is less than optimal will require long-term therapy.
- While cardiovascular complications occur, many patients with cardiovascular disease and risk factors use NSAIDs, particularly if the benefit is considered to outweigh the risk (e.g. improved function/ exercise tolerance encourages a healthier lifestyle).
- It is imperative that blood pressure and renal function are monitored regularly (preferably every 3 months).
- The highest risk of cardiovascular complications is with diclofenac, COX-2 NSAIDs, and high-dose ibuprofen (2.4 g daily). The lowest risk is with naproxen (1 g daily) and ibuprofen (1.2 g or less daily).
- It is not uncommon for individuals to also be on aspirin for its platelet inhibitory function.
- All NSAIDs are contraindicated in severe heart failure.
- GI risks are documented in Table 23.4.

**Table 23.4** Adverse effects of NSAIDs

| Organ/complication | Occurrence | Comments |
|---|---|---|
| GI tract | Common | Gastritis, bleeding, and perforation. High risk in the elderly and those with a history of ulcers |
| Renal | Common | Fluid retention, papillary necrosis |
| Hypertension | Common | Interference with drugs such as thiazide diuretics |
| Cardiac/myocardial infarction | Increased risk in those with cardiovascular risk factors | COX-1 and COX-2 drugs |
| Lung | Not uncommon | Exacerbation of asthma, pneumonitis (naproxen) |
| Skin | Not uncommon | Hypersensitivity, erythema multiforme |
| Central nervous system (CNS) | Not uncommon | Tinnitus, fatigue, cognitive disturbance |
| | Rare | Aseptic meningitis |
| Liver | Uncommon | Drug-induced hepatitis |
| Haematological | Rare | Bone marrow dyscrasias |

- The highest GI risk is seen with *piroxicam* and *ketoprofen*; intermediate risk with *diclofenac*, *etodolac*, *indometacin*, *naproxen*, and *oxicams*; and the lowest risk with *ibuprofen*.
- In renal disease, NSAIDs should be used with caution and avoided if possible.
- NSAIDs can induce acute kidney injury, as well as exacerbate chronic impairment. The 'rule of thumb' of lowest possible dose for shortest possible period of time applies.
- NSAIDs can exacerbate asthma; however, it should not be an absolute contraindication to prescribing.
- Many patients may well have inadvertently tried aspirin and ibuprofen over-the-counter compounds without complication. The clinician may therefore gain some sense of tolerability. The decision to prescribe should always be based on the severity and responsiveness/stability of asthma in each individual.

### NSAID cautions: sDMARD co-prescribing

- Concern is often expressed over the co-administration of sDMARDs and NSAIDs. Toxicity monitoring is a fundamental responsibility when managing sDMARDs.
- sDMARD monitoring applies irrespective of NSAID use.
- In principle, as disease comes under control on sDMARDs it is appropriate to reduce the frequency of NSAID use if possible.

### NSAID cautions: pregnancy and breastfeeding

It is generally advised that NSAIDs should be avoided in pregnancy unless the benefits to well-being significantly outweigh the risk.

- NSAIDs can be used with caution in the first and second trimester but should be avoided in the third trimester due to the added risk including closure of the fetal ductus arteriosus *in utero*, delay in onset, and an increase in the duration of labour. In addition, pulmonary hypertension may affect the newborn infant.
- In some cases, studies show concentrations of certain NSAIDs to be too low in breast milk to warrant concern. In general, manufacturers advise avoiding NSAIDs for the duration of breastfeeding.
- Low-dose aspirin may be continued throughout pregnancy but high-dose aspirin should be avoided.
- There are limited data for COX-2 inhibitors, which have been shown to be teratogenic in animal studies and hence these should be avoided in pregnancy and breastfeeding.

### Aspirin

- As the prototype NSAID, aspirin is available in single and compound formulations over the counter. While it is rarely prescribed as an NSAID, it is important to acknowledge its availability, as well as its common use in lower dosage (75–150 mg daily) as a cardio-protective agent, when prescribing other NSAIDs, and advising on side effects and drug interactions.
- For analgesic effect, aspirin is dosed at 300–900 mg four times a day (maximum adult dose 4 g/day). It is available in oral and suppository formulations.

- Low-dose aspirin may be continued throughout pregnancy but high-dose aspirin should be avoided.
- Aspirin is avoided in children under the age of 16 years (except for cardiac conditions such as Kawasaki Disease) due to the risk of Reye syndrome.

*Oxicams*

- This group of NSAIDs was developed for their longer half-life.
- *Meloxicam* (7.5–15 mg daily) and *piroxicam* (20 mg daily) are the two most commonly used agents.
- *Piroxicam has a relatively high relative toxicity:efficacy ratio for GI adverse effects compared with other NSAIDs.*

*Coxibs/COX-2 inhibitors*

- These agents were introduced because of their efficacy and selective COX-2 inhibition, recognizing the value of preserving COX-1 'protective' enzyme activity, particularly in relation to GI tolerability.
- However, large-scale phase III control trials, an integral part of modern pharmacological practice and essential in seeking approval for a licence, demonstrated an appreciable cardiovascular risk. As a consequence, several COX-2 drugs (e.g. rofecoxib) have been withdrawn.
- *Celecoxib* (100–200 mg twice daily) and *etoricoxib* (30–120 mg once daily) are available in Europe. *Celecoxib* is available in the USA. In 2007, the Food and Drug Administration (FDA) voted not to approve etoricoxib.
- Regular blood pressure monitoring is required.

## Antidepressants

Several antidepressants are used in the management of pain, usually as a single agent given at bedtime, sometimes in combination with other drugs using different mechanisms of action, and often at lower doses than typically used for controlling depression. There is no compelling evidence for their use in chronic paediatric pain.

- There is often a need to explain to patients that these drugs are being used for pain control and not for depression, even if there is a degree of reactive-depression present as a consequence of chronic pain.
- Educating the patient and explaining the mechanisms of action (blocking pain messages from travelling up the spinal cord and modifying the response to pain in the midbrain), one can gain greater compliance and enhance the clinician–patient relationship.
- A detailed exploration of the mechanisms is beyond the scope of this book, but most agents are thought to have a dual effect by modifying responsiveness of spinal opioid receptors, and changing mood and perception centrally.
- These agents are perhaps most logically used when pain disturbs sleep. A mild sedative and relaxant effect may also be beneficial.

## Serotonin and norepinephrine reuptake inhibitors

### Tricyclics

Tricyclics are predominantly serotonin and/or norepinephrine re-uptake inhibitors. The 'typical' agents in this group include amitriptyline, clomipramine, imipramine, and dosulepin.

* *Amitriptyline* is the agent most frequently used (although sometimes nortriptyline is better tolerated). Given at doses up to 75 mg/day taken before bedtime, it is often titrated from a baseline of 10–25 mg in 10 mg steps gradually until a balance between maximum efficacy and tolerability is reached.
* Common side effects and interactions are shown in Table 23.5.

### Selective serotonin reuptake inhibitors (SSRIs)

* This group includes *fluoxetine* (20–40 mg once daily), *sertraline* (50 mg once daily), and *paroxetine* (20 mg once daily).
* Randomized control trials in fibromyalgia (FM; see ➋ Chapter 22) demonstrate SSRI efficacy similar to 25 mg amitriptyline; however, the average impact on pain reduction and quality of life is only about 15–20% and, as such, these agents are probably not suitable candidates as analgesics when used in isolation. The side effect profile in Table 23.5 applies.

**Table 23.5** Cautions and side effects of serotonin/norepinephrine reuptake inhibitors

| Caution | Comment |
| --- | --- |
| Sedative | Care needed when used with other potentially sedating agent. Note: CNS toxic effects of tramadol can be enhanced (serotonin syndrome). Also note caution with driving or using machinery |
| Antimuscarinic action | Caution in those with ocular (closed-angle glaucoma), genitourinary (retention, prostatic hypertrophy), dry eyes/mouth, constipation |
| Cardiovascular | Risk of dysrhythmias especially ventricular (e.g. increased with concomitant use of sotalol and amiodarone) |
| Hypotension | Increased risk in patients on diuretics |
| Thyroid disease | Amitriptyline enhances effects of thyroid drugs |
| Epilepsy | Amitriptyline antagonizes antiepileptics reducing the threshold for seizures |
| Sexual dysfunction | Sexual dysfunction may occur. |
| Hyponatraemia | Usually in the elderly and possibly due to inappropriate secretion of antidiuretic hormones. |
| Hepatic impairment | Try to avoid in severe liver disease—risk of sedation |
| Pregnancy and breastfeeding | Avoid unless being used for psychiatric reasons and in the best interests of well-being |
| Neuropsychiatric | Induction of hallucinations, delusions, (hypo)mania, neuroleptic malignant syndrome, and suicidal behaviour |
| Motor function | Tremor/extrapyramidal signs |
| Endocrine | Breast enlargement, galactorrhoea |

*Mixed serotonin-norepinephrine reuptake inhibitors (SNRIs)*

- Increasing interest in the complexities of central pain pathways and the action of SNRIs has led to several studies demonstrating SNRI efficacy in FM (see ➲ Chapter 22).
- The FDA (USA) approved *duloxetine* (2008) and *milnacipran* (2009) for treatment of FM in adults. Neither is approved for use in children.
- Duloxetine is given as 60–120 mg daily and milnacipran at 100 mg twice daily. Side effects include nausea, headache, insomnia, dizziness, constipation, hepatic dysfunction, hyponatraemia, and orthostatic hypotension (duloxetine) and hypertension (milnacipran).
- Like all antidepressants duloxetine carries a warning highlighting an increased risk of suicide, especially in children and young adults.
- Tramadol should not be co-administered with duloxetine; there is a risk of developing serotonin syndrome. Through cytochrome P450 enzyme system interactions, duloxetine may prolong opioid effects.

### Other adjuvant analgesics

*Gabapentin* and its analogue *pregabalin* (both structural analogues of γ-aminobutyric acid (GABA)), has been shown to have efficacy, particularly in studies of FM (see ➲ Chapter 22), although the NNT is 9 and there is a high incidence of side effects. There is no compelling evidence for their use in chronic pain in children and adolescents.

*Gabapentin*

- Dose: oral, titrated from 300 mg daily to maximum 3600 mg daily in divided doses, e.g. 300 mg once daily on day 1, then 300 mg twice daily on day 2, then 300 mg 3 times daily on day 3, then increased according to response and tolerability in increment of 300 mg daily every 2–3 days to maximum dose of 3600 mg daily.
- Dose needs to be reduced in renal impairment according to GFR.
- Side effects: dizziness/light-headedness, oedema, weight gain, and sedation/mental impairment. Other concerns include leucopenia, ataxia, Stevens–Johnson syndrome, hepatitis, and pancreatitis.
- Avoid during pregnancy and breastfeeding.
- Discontinuation has to be done gradually over minimum of 1 week.

*Pregabalin*

- Dose: oral, titrated after 3–7 days from 150 mg to maximum 600 mg daily in 2–3 divided doses.
- Dose needs to be reduced in renal impairment according to GFR.
- Side effects: dizziness/light-headedness, oedema, weight gain, and sedation/mental impairment. Other concerns include visual disturbance, neutropenia, ataxia, arrhythmia, Stevens–Johnson syndrome, and pancreatitis.
- Avoid during pregnancy and breastfeeding.
- Discontinuation has to be done gradually over minimum of 1 week.

*Muscle relaxants*

The most likely agent to consider is *diazepam*, a benzodiazepine.

- Given at doses of 2–5 mg three times a day for up to 14 days diazepam can be helpful in alleviating acute severe pain associated with spasm, particularly across the neck and shoulder girdle, and the lumbar spine.
- Diazepam should be avoided in hepatic and renal impairment, pregnancy, and breastfeeding.
- As with opioids, care should be taken to counsel the patient over perceived risk of dependency of benzodiazepines, and prescription should be avoided if there are any concerns over potential abuse.
- Drugs such as baclofen, dantrolene, methocarbamol, and tizanidine usually sit within the realm of the neurologist and may be valuable in controlling muscle spasm and pain in conditions such as stroke and multiple sclerosis. Where indicated, the rheumatologist should seek advice from a neurologist if spasm pain is considered to be the consequence of a neurological condition.
- *Quinine sulfate* is often used in doses of 200–300 mg to control cramps. It should be prescribed with caution in patients with arrhythmia and avoided or dose halved in hepatic and renal impairment.
- *Quinine sulfate* is contraindicated in haemoglobinuria, myasthenia gravis, optic neuritis, and tinnitus; and it may be teratogenic (certainly in higher dosage) in the first trimester of pregnancy, but safe during breastfeeding.

*Topical agents*

- The most common classes to be used (excluding opioid transcutaneous delivery by patch) include a variety of 'over-the-counter' preparations (rubefacients), NSAIDs, and capsaicin.
- *Capsaicin* is an active component of chili peppers. It is licensed to treat post-herpetic neuralgia and diabetic neuropathy. It can be considered an adjunct to treating OA. One risk is a severe burning and irritation if contact is made with mucous membranes, including the lips and conjunctiva. Hand-washing after use should be meticulous.
- Capsaicin is prescribed as a 45 g tube of 0.025% or 0.075% concentration, to be applied twice daily in the smallest of volume; literally a tiny amount squeezed onto the tip of the little finger and then rubbed in over the site of pain.

# Glucocorticoids

Glucocorticoids (GCs; 'steroids') are powerful anti-inflammatories and range in use from short duration of low and high dosage to gain control of a condition (including intra-articular; see ➲ Chapter 24), through to prolonged and even lifelong therapy.

Commonly used GCs are prednisolone, methylprednisolone, and triamcinolone. Disease-specific indications and dosing regimens are stated in each relevant chapter of this book.

Table 23.6 highlights the major and common cautions and concerns that should be monitored and discussed with the patient. Patients on long-term GC treatment should be encouraged to hold a steroid treatment card or some form of alert bracelet, etc.

## Glucocorticoid interactions

- Because of the tendency for GCs to increase blood pressure, the effect of antihypertensives may be blunted. Monitoring is key.
- *Barbiturates and antiepileptics* increase the metabolism of GCs.
- *Diuretics* may be antagonized by GCs.
- *Erythromycin and azoles* may inhibit the metabolism of GCs thus increasing their effect.
- *GCs may amplify the severity of NSAIDs* peptic ulceration risk.
- *GCs may increase the* risk of bone marrow suppression with methotrexate (MTX).
- *GCs in combination with theophylline* increases hypokalaemia risk.
- *GCs may increase or decrease the anticoagulant effect of warfarin.*

**Table 23.6** Cautions and complications of glucocorticoid use

| Caution | Comment |
|---------|---------|
| Adrenal insufficiency | Long-term use can lead to adrenal atrophyAbrupt withdrawal should be avoided |
| | Replacement (even higher dosing) should be given during surgery, inter-current illness (especially associated vomiting) |
| Diabetes | Induction and exacerbation of hyperglycaemia |
| Hypokalaemia | Can cause hypokalaemia |
| Infection | GCs are immunosuppressive—there is an increased susceptibility to infections and severity of infections especially after prolonged use |
| | Live viral immunization should be avoided |
| | Exposure to chickenpox or measles leading to concern over significant infection should be managed with passive immunoglobulin |
| | May expose latent TB |
| Neuropsychiatric | Can induce mania, confusion, delirium, and suicidal thoughts—can occur early after starting corticosteroid (3–5 days on average) and take several weeks to resolve having discontinued therapy |
| Weight gain | This may be either as a consequence of peripheral oedema or increased appetite—patients should be warned to be careful of this and to use tricks like drinks of water to reduce sense of hunger |
| Skin | Long-term use leads to atrophy and bruising |
| Eyes | Increased risk of cataracts and glaucoma |
| Cardiovascular | Induction and exacerbation of hypertension and congestive cardiac failure |
| Peptic ulceration | |
| Bone and muscle | Induction and exacerbation of osteoporosis |
| | Growth retardation |
| | Myopathy |
| | Osteonecrosis |
| Pregnancy | GCs can be used or continued if indicated—preferably lowest dose possible. No evidence of teratogenic effects; occasional neonatal adrenal suppression which usually resolves spontaneously |
| Breastfeeding | Doses of prednisolone up to 40 mg daily are unlikely to result in systemic effect in infants |

# Disease-modifying antirheumatic drugs

Disease-modifying antirheumatic drugs (DMARDS) are the cornerstone of disease management aimed at the slowing or arrest and remission of chronic inflammatory rheumatic disease. For additional detail see also ➲ Chapter 5 (RA) and ➲ Chapter 8 (SpAs). Terminology can be confusing since the introduction of 'biologics', which are also 'disease-modifying'. A new nomenclature of DMARD terminology has been proposed by Smolen et al.[1]:

- Firstly: 'synthetic DMARDs', which are subdivided into conventional synthetic DMARDs (csDMARDs), i.e. traditional DMARDs, and targeted synthetic DMARDs (tsDMARDs), which are oral synthetic drugs designed to target a particular molecular structure.
- Secondly: 'biologic DMARDs' (bDMARDs), which are subdivided into biologic original DMARDs (boDMARDs) and biosimilar DMARDs (bsDMARDs).
- At the time of writing it is unknown whether this proposed nomenclature will be generally accepted. In this book we have mainly used the terminology sDMARDs and bDMARDs, and have avoided introducing the other terms extensively, with the exception being this chapter with the distinction being made clear in the following subsections.

## Conventional synthetic DMARDs

### General considerations

Conventional synthetic DMARDs (csDMARDs) are slow-acting drugs that take 8–12 weeks to begin to demonstrate benefit, and even then, possibly longer to achieve maximum benefit as the dose is escalated (typically >6 months). Patients should always be informed of this, clarifying expectations and improving compliance.

- It is not uncommon for combinations of csDMARDs to be used either by sequential 'step up' (adding one after the other over time) or 'step down' (starting with two or three, and reducing to one over time).
- In the UK, it is unlikely that more than three csDMARDs would be used since the introduction of bDMARDs: UK guidance allows use of bDMARDs after failure of at least two csDMARDs (see later).
- The most common drugs used are: hydroxychloroquine (HCQ), leflunomide (LEF), MTX, and sulfasalazine (SSZ).
- Of these drugs, MTX is probably the drug of first choice for most conditions (e.g. RA, PsA, JIA) at doses of 7.5–30 mg weekly.
- csDMARDs are not without their toxicity and the protean complications and monitoring requirements can seem daunting.
- Tables 23.7–23.10 describe principles applicable to all csDMARDs.
- Advice on immunization and risk assessment of viral infection is shown in Box 23.1.
- General monitoring of csDMARDs—see Table 23.7 (please refer to Box 23.2 for common side effects to assess for, at every blood test check and clinical review).
- Common csDMARD side effects and advice on initial action to be taken—see Box 23.2.

## Box 23.1 Immunization and assessment of infection risk before commencing csDMARDs

*Disclaimer:* all readers should refer to their own local practice guidelines. Information here is incomplete and brief and a skeleton guide only.

- In some circumstances it may be appropriate to give live vaccines to patients on DMARDs. Refer to local guidelines. (e.g. oral polio, BCG, MMR, yellow fever).
- Patients should receive the pneumococcal vaccine.
- Annual flu vaccination is recommended.
- Patients exposed to chickenpox (who have no clear history of chicken pox in the past) or to shingles, should receive passive immunization using varicella zoster immunoglobulin.
- Patients should be screened for hepatitis B and C risk by history, and, if required, serum antibodies.
- Patients should be assessed for risk of HIV and tested if applicable.
- Patients should be assessed for risk of active/latent TB.

---

- Use in pregnancy and breastfeeding—see Table 23.10.
- All csDMARDs should be used with caution in hepatic and renal impairment, blood dyscrasias (including suspected or known G6PD deficiency and porphyria), recurrent infection, and in the elderly.

*csDMARD management for surgery and during infective illness*

- csDMARDs do not need to be discontinued before surgery though some surgeons/surgical specialties request csDMARDs are discontinued. There is a lack overall of robust data as few randomized trials have been undertaken.
- If the surgeon wishes csDMARDs to be stopped then, as a 'rule of thumb', it is reasonable to discontinue for 2 weeks before and up to 2 weeks after surgery.
- It is not possible to predict the risk of a flare of inflammation during this period, although many patients report a level of tolerance for up to 4 weeks.
- csDMARDs are discontinued during severe infective illness if there is concern their immunosuppressant effect outweighs the risk of a disease flare.

*Family planning, pregnancy and breastfeeding, while taking csDMARDs*

- Some csDMARDs can be taken reasonably safely while pregnant and breastfeeding; see guidelines (e.g. BSR guideline on prescribing for pregnancy and breastfeeding can be found at: ℘ http://www. rheumatology.org.uk/resources/guidelines/default.aspx).
- Table 23.8 shows specific regimens advised before trying to conceive, and which drugs to avoid during pregnancy and breastfeeding.
- LEF should be stopped 2 years before trying to conceive, or 'washed' out as described later in this section (see ➔ 'Leflunomide', p. 670).
- Advice on use of analgesics and GCs in pregnancy and breastfeeding is given in the previous sections.

**Table 23.7** Principles of monitoring of csDMARDs.
*Disclaimer:* all readers should refer to their own local practice guidelines. Information here is incomplete and brief and a skeleton guide only.

| Time line | Action |
|---|---|
| Pre-treatment assessment | FBC, creatinine, U&E, LFTs, CRP and ESR, urinalysis (protein), CXR (pre-MTX), blood pressure, exclude current infection, exclude unexplained rash/skin lesion, complete applicable disease activity assessment tools, request visual acuity measurement before starting HCQ |
| Monitoring for the first 6–8 weeks | FBC and LFT every 2 weeks (4 weekly in children for MTX and Aza and 2 weekly MMF and LFD) for 6–8 weeks (except for AZA and MMF (weekly), HCQ (not required), gold (FBC and urinalysis before every dose), SSZ (every 4 weeks)). Also, creatinine, U&E for ciclosporin |
| 6–8-week clinical assessment | FBC, creatinine, U&E, LFTs, CRP, ESR, urinalysis, blood pressure, exclude infection and skin lesions, complete applicable disease activity assessment tools |
| Monitoring between 2 and 6 months if drug dose stable | FBC and LFT every 4 weeks (except for HCQ (not required), gold (before every dose), SSZ (3-monthly if stable in first 3 months)). Some drugs require close monitoring of creatinine and urinalysis—see ciclosporin |
| 6-month clinical assessment | FBC, creatinine, U&E, LFTs, CRP and/or ESR (as part of assessment criteria), urinalysis (protein and blood), blood pressure, exclude current infection and rash/skin lesions, complete applicable disease activity assessment tools |
| Monitoring after 6 months if stable drug dose | FBC and LFT every 8–12 weeks. Some drugs require close monitoring of creatinine, U&E, and urinalysis—see ciclosporin |
| Yearly clinical assessment | FBC, creatinine, U&E, LFTs, CRP, and ESR |
| Assessment every 6 months if dose stable | Urinalysis (protein), blood pressure, exclude current infection, exclude unexplained rash/skin lesion, complete applicable disease activity assessment tools |

*General principles*
Return to the early monitoring protocol whenever increasing drug dose after a period of stable dosage, or when introducing another csDMARD or an NSAID or other potentially toxic drug (by interaction) for the first time.

See published guidelines, e.g. at British Society of Rheumatology: ℔ http://www.rheumatology. org.uk/resources/guidelines/default.aspx

*Malignancy risk with csDMARDs*
- Establishing the risk of malignancy from csDMARDs is challenging owing to the excess incidence of malignancy in some of the conditions being treated and a lack of 'real-world' data of csDMARD use.
- MMF, CYC, and AZA are associated with increased incidence of malignancy but SSZ, HCQ, MTX, and LEF are probably not.

**Table 23.8** Disease-modifying antirheumatic drugs in pregnancy and breastfeeding

| Drug | Effects |
|------|---------|
| Azathioprine | *Pregnancy*: compatible throughout pregnancy with dose ≤2 mg/kg/day<br>*Breastfeeding*: compatible with breastfeeding |
| Ciclosporin | *Pregnancy*: compatible throughout pregnancy with lowest possible dose. Suggested monitoring of blood pressure, renal function, blood glucose and drug levels<br>*Breastfeeding*: compatible—though from limited data |
| HCQ | *Pregnancy*: compatible throughout pregnancy<br>*Breastfeeding*: compatible with breastfeeding |
| Leflunomide (LEF) | *Pregnancy*: potential teratogenic—avoid<br>*Note*: LEF has a long half-life. Rapid removal of the active metabolite can be achieved using washout with colestyramine 8 g three times a day or activated charcoal 50 g four times a day for 11 days. Blood concentrations should be checked twice, 14 days apart prior to conceiving (levels should be <0.02 mg/L)<br>*Breastfeeding*: avoid LEF |
| Methotrexate (MTX) | *Pregnancy*: teratogenic and abortifacient. Termination not mandatory. Stop MTX 3 months before starting to try to conceive<br>*Breastfeeding*: avoid drug |
| Mycophenolate mofetil (MMF) | *Pregnancy*: teratogenic and abortifacient avoid MMF. Stop MMF >6 weeks before starting to try to conceive. Recommend use of two forms of contraception otherwise.<br>*Breastfeeding*: avoid MMF |
| Sulfasalazine | *Pregnancy*: compatible throughout pregnancy with folate supplement of 5 mg/day<br>*Breastfeeding*: compatible with full-term, healthy infants |
| CYC, gold, penicillamine | Avoid in pregnancy and breastfeeding |

*Shared care information on csDMARDs and their use*

- It is essential that the patient receives information and advice on csDMARDs and their primary care physician has access to correspondence from the prescribing clinician and results of monitoring.
- It is essential that there is clarity over the roles and responsibilities of the prescribing and primary/community clinicians and the patient.
- Various guidelines on csDMARD monitoring exist (e.g. see UK BSR guidelines 2017 at: ℘ http://www.rheumatology.org.uk/resources/guidelines/default.aspx).
- Box 23.2 broadly outlines management of csDMARD side effects.

## Box 23.2 csDMARD monitoring and side effects management

*Disclaimer:* all readers should refer to their own local practice guidelines. Information here is incomplete and brief and a skeleton guide only.

- *Abnormal AST or ALT.* Stop csDMARD if enzyme level > twice upper limit of normal. As with all blood indices listed below, repeat weekly until normalized.
- *Abnormal leucocyte count.* Stop csDMARD if neutrophils <1.5 × 10$^9$/L, or if steep downward trend in count, and assess for infection. With eosinophilia >0.5 × 10$^9$/L, increased vigilance required but may be unassociated atopy.
- *Low platelets.* Stop csDMARD if platelet count <100 × 10$^9$/L or serial results show significant trend downwards.
- *Abnormal bruising.* Check clotting screen and platelets urgently. If abnormal withhold csDMARD immediately. Bruises are common in children.
- *Abnormal MCV.* If MCV >110 fL, check folate, vitamin B12, TSH, and for excess alcohol intake. MCV+ may be an effect of AZA, MTX, SSZ, or allopurinol
- *Proteinuria.* Send urine for microscopy/culture + treat infection. Quantify proteinuria, check creatinine, U&E, exclude haematuria + urinary casts and obtaining 'KUB' ultrasound. Consider withdrawing csDMARD.
  - Note: proteinuria may indicate worsening disease so stopping the csDMARD may be inappropriate.
- *Rash.* If mild in adults, drop csDMARD dose. If moderate/severe, then stop csDMARD. Rashes are common in children but advice may be sought.
- *Mucosal ulceration.* Consider cause of ulceration and add folate (for MTX) and adjust dose if persistent. If severe consider trial off csDMARD.
- *Hair loss.* Consider cause of alopecia and adjust dose if persistent. A trial off treatment may be appropriate but hair growth may not recover for ≥1 hair cycle, i.e. several months.
- *Hypertension.* If mild rise, may respond to small drop in csDMARD dose or leave alone and monitor. If moderate to severe, treat hypertension first (see advice for ciclosporin on dose reduction).
- *Weight loss.* Consider the cause of weight loss and reduce the dose or stop for a trial period depending on the severity.
- *Dyspnoea.* Chest exam + CXR. Treat infection and cardiac failure. If pulmonary fibrosis suspected stop csDMARD and arrange further investigation.
- *Advisable actions if stopping a csDMARD.* Repeat blood test after 1 or 2 weeks. Assess for any recent change in medication, alcohol consumption, illness, csDMARD dosing error. Treat disease 'flare' with GCs. If trend downwards in laboratory indices, then csDMARD should be reviewed irrespective of laboratory value. Once abnormalities return to normal, start csDMARD at a lower dose, or switch to a new csDMARD, and in both cases return to the early monitoring phase.

*Azathioprine*

Azathioprine (AZA) is prescribed for a number of autoinflammatory and autoimmune conditions. AZA inhibits purine synthesis by generating thioguanine nucleotides from its metabolite: 6-mercaptopurine (6-MP).

- The typical dose of AZA is 0.5–1 mg/kg/day orally in twice-daily divided doses, increasing after 4–6 weeks to 2–3 mg/kg/day with an anticipated response within 6–12 weeks.
- Thiopurine methyl transferase (TPMT) activity status can be checked before AZA is started:
  - 99% of people will have high or intermediate TPMT levels and be at low risk of AZA toxicity (from slow AZA clearance).
  - In a TPMT deficiency homozygous state (0.3% of population (1:300)) it may be fatal—toxicity occurring in the first 6 weeks.
  - In the heterozygous state (10% of population), there may be delayed (up to 6 months), but usually reversible, bone marrow toxicity.
  - Although measurement of TPMT is advised in guidelines, it may be impractical so close FBC monitoring in the first 6–12 weeks of treatment is imperative.
- AZA can cause a photosensitivity reaction—patients should be advised to wear sunscreens and protective covering.
- AZA has some specific drug interactions:
  - *Allopurinol:* AZA dose should be reduced to 0.25–0.5 mg/kg/day.
  - *Angiotensin-converting enzyme (ACE) inhibitors:* co-prescription may exacerbate anaemia.
  - *Anticonvulsants:* AZA may reduce absorption.
  - *Aminosalicylates: (mesalazine (ME)/SSZ):* increase risk of bone marrow toxicity.
  - *Ciclosporin:* AZA can decrease ciclosporin levels.
  - *Co-trimoxazole/trimethoprim:* bone marrow toxicity.
  - *Warfarin:* AZA inhibits anticoagulant effects.

*Ciclosporin*

Ciclosporin is considered in PsA, RA, AICTDs, uveitis, and MAS. It is a calcineurin inhibitor and has a fairly selective action on lymphocytes: blocking mitosis and inhibiting lymphokine release.

- Ciclosporin dose is typically 2.5 mg/kg/day orally in twice-daily doses for 6 weeks, then may be increased at 4-weekly intervals in 25 mg increments up to a maximum of 4 mg/kg/day. Response in <12 weeks.
- Pre-monitoring (Table 23.8) should include fasting lipids, repeated 6-monthly and the drug discontinued if an uncontrollable significant rise in lipids occurs.
- Monitoring includes checking creatinine clearance/GFR. A rise in creatinine >30% above baseline on two consecutive readings 7 days apart warrants stopping the drug and reassessing.
- It is essential that blood pressure monitoring be commenced at baseline. If uncontrollable hypertension occurs, the drug should be stopped.
- Electrolyte balance should be checked every 2 weeks until stable dose achieved and then every 3 months with other routine monitoring (Table 23.8). If the potassium rises above the laboratory threshold the drug should be stopped and re-assessed (having ensured it is not a result of other medication changes).

- Grapefruit (including juice) increases the bioavailability of ciclosporin. Grapefruit should be avoided for an hour before and after taking the drug.
- Ciclosporin has some specific drug interactions. Ciclosporin is an inhibitor of CYP3A4, which metabolizes some drugs:
  - *Calcium channel blockers:* reduce dose of ciclosporin to 50%.
  - *Statins:* use in low dose as ciclosporin can elevate concentration of all these drugs.
  - *Colchicine:* should be avoided.
  - *Diclofenac:* reduce the maximum dose of diclofenac to 75 mg daily.
  - *Digoxin:* measure levels and reduce dose accordingly as ciclosporin can increase serum levels.
  - *Diuretics:* caution with electrolyte imbalance.
  - *Hydroxychloroquine (HCQ):* may increase plasma concentrations of ciclosporin.
  - *PUVA:* avoid ciclosporin given significant increase risk of invasive squamous cell carcinoma.
  - *Concomitant use of potentially nephrotoxic drugs requires special concern and monitoring.*
  - *Simvastatin:* avoid dosing above 10 mg/day.
  - *St. John's wort:* decreases ciclosporin activity.

*Cyclophosphamide*

The main use of the cytotoxic drug cyclophosphamide (CYC) is for organ- or life-threatening manifestations of autoimmune connective tissue diseases (AICTDs) and for remission induction of vasculitis.

- CYC can be administered either orally at a dose of 1.5–2 mg/kg/day or IV given as a pulsed regimen.
- IV CYC dose is typically calculated based on weight or body surface area and adjusted for renal function and age; given once every 2–4 weeks for up to 3–6 months.
- For ANCA-associated vasculitis (AAV), the CYCLOPS regimen is used: IV CYC at dose of 15 mg/kg (reduced for age and renal function) each 2 weeks for 6 weeks then each 3 weeks for 3 months.
- Pulsed IV CYC regimens are associated with lower total lifetime doses and reduced toxicity.
- CYC-induced suppression of gametogenesis is often irreversible. Prior to the decision to use CYC, patients should be counselled about infertility and offered the use of GNRH analogue and/or harvesting and storage of sperm/ova.
- Urothelial toxicity from the active CYC metabolite acrolein can cause haemorrhagic cystitis. Patients should be well hydrated before receiving CYC and for 24–48 hours after IV administration.
- Mesna is given to reduce risk of CYC-induced urothelial toxicity. The usual dose is 2 g before and repeated 2 and 6 hours after IV therapy.
- Common side effects include nausea, vomiting, diarrhoea, arthralgia, fatigue, headache, tachycardia, and hypotension.
- Prophylactic antiemesis treatment should be offered to patients who are receiving IV CYC.
- Co-trimoxazole 960 mg three times a week should be prescribed for prophylaxis against *Pneumocystis* during treatment with CYC.

- Leucopenia/neutropenia is a significant risk and CYC dose should be reduced if this happens. FBC may be checked on days 0, 7, 10, and 14 after the first infusion and with any subsequent infusions where the dose is changed. An FBC is often checked on day 12 (the usual nadir in neutrophil count) in anticipation of the next infusion.
- After induction of disease remission, the usual practice is to switch from CYC to alternative maintenance therapy such as AZA or MTX) to maintain remission.
- There are a few CYC drug interactions:
  - *Avoid clozapine:* increased risk of agranulocytosis.
  - *Digoxin:* CYC reduces absorption.
  - *Phenytoin:* CYC reduces absorption.

## Gold (auranofin and sodium aurothiomalate)

Gold was used extensively in the management of RA and JIA but its use has become infrequent since the widespread adoption of relatively high-dose MTX and the availability of bDMARDs.

- The precise mode of action of gold is unknown though numerous *in vitro* actions which may be relevant have been observed.
- Gold is given as 3 mg 2–3 times daily (oral; auranofin) or as a 50 mg IM injection (sodium aurothiomalate), usually monthly.
- A test dose of 10 mg IM sodium aurothiomalate should be given on the first treatment; thereafter 50 mg is given weekly until disease response achieved. Thereafter, the injection is given every 4 weeks.
- In children, IM gold is given at 1 mg/kg up to a maximum of 50 mg.
- If no response is seen after a cumulative dose of 1 g (about 20 weekly doses) of sodium aurothiomalate, it should be discontinued.
- Both formulations of gold are contraindicated in severe renal or hepatic disease, ulcerative colitis, history of marrow dysplasia, porphyria, exfoliative dermatitis, SLE, pulmonary fibrosis, and bronchiolitis.

## Hydroxychloroquine (HCQ) and chloroquine phosphate

HCQ and chloroquine phosphate are (old) antimalarials. Their use is common in the management of RA, and in all the AICTDs. HCQ is especially popular for its use as maintenance treatment in SLE (see ➲ Chapter 10).

- Antimalarial drugs have a number of anti-inflammatory and immunomodulatory actions.
- HCQ is produced as a sulphate. Some side effects to HCQ may be a consequence of the sulphate component of the drug (e.g. rash) thus a phosphate form of HCQ can be used instead.
- The therapeutic dose of HCQ is 200 mg once or twice daily. The dose of chloroquine phosphate is 250 mg once daily.
- The daily dose of chloroquine should not exceed 6.5 mg/kg. Alternate daily regimes may be used in small children.
- Enquire about visual impairment and measure acuity. Near-vision testing should demonstrate the capacity to read small print N8 or N6 on an acuity chart.

- A thorough baseline visual assessment, including a view of the retina, may be requested of an optometrist, optician or ophthalmologist prior to drug onset.
- Once on an antimalarial, patients should report any changes in visual acuity/blurring; this would trigger re-assessment at any time and immediate withdrawal of the drug until the nature of the problem is found. Otherwise, accurate visual acuity assessment should take place annually.
- Antimalarials can exacerbate psoriasis.
- Antimalarials can cause skin rash, nausea, diarrhoea and can in rare cases cause cardiac conduction abnormalities.
- There are a few drug interactions:
  - Antimalarials can increase the plasma concentration of digoxin, MTX, and ciclosporin.
  - Avoid antimalarial use with amiodarone, quinine, mefloquine, and quinolones for risk of hypersensitivity reaction.

*Leflunomide*

LEF is used in RA, PsA, and JIA and can be used in csDMARD combination regimens. LEF is an 'antiproliferative' drug inhibiting the enzyme dihydro-orodate dehydrogenase.

- A loading dose of 100 mg daily for 3 days is suggested (see SPC) but often this causes GI upset and most rheumatologists avoid it, starting at the long-term maintenance dose of 20 mg daily.
- A dose of 10 mg daily may be sufficient if there are side effects on 20 mg.
- The dose in children over 3 years of age is 5mg daily if <10kg; 10mg daily is 10–40kg; 20mg daily if >40kg.
- LEF has a long half-life and requires a washout when severe toxicity is suspected. A washout is achieved using colestyramine 8 g three times a day or activated charcoal 50 g four times a day for 11 days. Blood concentrations should be checked twice, 14 days apart prior to conceiving (levels should be <0.02 mg/L).
- Caution is recommended when using LEF with MTX, since this combination has been associated with liver dysfunction and failure. Cytopenia has also been observed.
- Blood pressure is monitored with blood monitoring since LEF may cause an increase in BP and destabilize controlled hypertension.
- Rarely, LEF can cause pneumonitis, acute allergic reaction and neuropathies.
- Women planning a family should have stopped LEF for 2 years (teratogenic) (and men 3 months) before trying to conceive.
- There are a few drug interactions with LEF:
  - LEF can increase the anticoagulant effect of warfarin.
  - LEF enhances the hypoglycaemic effects of tolbutamide.
  - LEF may lead to increased concentrations of anticonvulsants.

*Methotrexate*

MTX is the most commonly used csDMARD. It is used as a first-line csD-MARD in RA, JIA and PsA, and in managing some AICTDs and vasculitides.

- The action of MTX as an immunomodulator is not clear, although it is known to be an inhibitor of dihydrofolate reductase in high doses. This is associated with an inhibition of DNA, RNA, and protein synthesis and may effect cell division.
- The typical maintenance dose of MTX is 15–25 mg once a week.
- The use of MTX varies across centres, but typically begins at 10–15 mg per week and increase by 2.5–5 mg every 2 weeks for a period of 6–8 weeks.
- In children and adolescents the subcutaneous route is commonly used at initiation at a dose of 10–15mg/m$^2$. Higher doses of up to 20–25mg/m$^2$ may be used but are associated with more side effects and a lower rate of additional benefit.
- A lower dose and slower escalation is recommended in the elderly and frail and where there is reduced renal clearance.
- The subcutaneous route is associated with reduced risk of GI side effects and higher bioavailability, compared to oral.
- MTX tablets should be taken whole, not crushed or chewed.
- MTX tablets come in 2.5 mg and 10 mg formulations. It is recommended that only 2.5 mg tablets are prescribed and dispensed to avoid confusion and risk of overdose.
- *Folic acid* (5mg once per week) is often given to reduce the risk of side effects. It may be increased up to 6 days of the week avoiding the same day as MTX.
- Folic acid may be increased when there is: raised MCV, mildly deranged LFTs, anaemia, mucositis symptoms, nausea, mucosal ulceration; hair loss.
- Emergency *folinic acid* 'rescue' (15–25 mg four times a day IV or oral) should be given if any concern over severe toxicity (primarily pneumonitis and marrow suppression) and in overdose usually above a cumulative of 100 mg MTX. If serum MTX levels can be measured it is advisable to continue rescue until MTX levels fall below <0.1 μmol/L. In most cases, the response is judged by the daily improvement in haematological indices.
- The role of liver biopsy and serum pro-collagen III (PIIINP) testing remains unclear. Some centres consider obtaining a liver biopsy when there has been three consecutive elevations in PIIINP over a 12 month period. The decision to stop therapy would be based on a risk/benefit assessment in each individual.

- History should be taken at each monitoring visit for new dyspnoea as a screening assessment for pneumonitis or pulmonary fibrosis. Further investigation may require high-resolution CT and lung function tests detailing lung volume and gas transfer coefficients.
- The antifolate effect of some drugs, particularly co-trimoxazole and trimethoprim, may increase the toxicity of MTX.
- MTX concentration can be increased slightly by regular NSAIDs.

*Mycophenolate mofetil*

MMF has been routinely used in organ transplantation. MMF has also been used in the control of lupus nephritis, myositis, and vasculitis, often in 'remission maintaining' or in 'steroid-sparing' roles.

- MMF is the 2-morpholinoethyl ester of mycophenolic acid (MPA). MPA is a potent, selective, uncompetitive and reversible inhibitor of inosine monophosphate dehydrogenase, and therefore inhibits the *de novo* pathway of guanosine nucleotide synthesis without incorporation into DNA.
- Because T and B lymphocytes are critically dependent for their proliferation on *de novo* synthesis of purines whereas other cell types can utilize salvage pathways, MPA has more potent cytostatic effects on lymphocytes than on other cells.
- MMF dose is 1–3 g/day (300–600mg/m$^2$ in children and adolescents) orally in divided doses, starting at 500 mg daily for the 7 days, then 500 mg twice daily for 7 days, building sequentially by an additional 500 mg daily every 7 days over the ensuing weeks to an optimal/tolerable dose.
- MMF is monitored using FBC, LFTs, and urinalysis (screening for nephrotoxicity).
- Main drug interactions of MMF:
  - Decreased absorption of MMF can occur with antacids (magnesium and aluminium hydroxide) and colestyramine.
  - Increased concentration may arise with the use of aciclovir.
  - Concomitant NSAIDs may add to nephrotoxic risk.

*Sulfasalazine*

Sulfasalazine (SSZ) is a useful csDMARD in treating peripheral and entero-pathic SpA and RA. There is weak to moderate evidence for efficacy in PsA.

- A SSZ is an active substance although most is converted by bacteria in the colon into the active metabolites colon where bacteria split the drug into sulfapyridine (SP) and mesalazine (ME). Most SP is absorbed, hydroxylated, or glucuronidated and a mix of unchanged and metabolized SP appears in the urine. Some ME is taken up and acetylated in the colon wall. SSZ is also excreted unchanged in the bile and urine.
- Overall SSZ and its metabolites exert immunomodulatory effects, antibacterial effects, effects on the arachidonic acid cascade, and alteration of activity of certain enzymes.
- SSZ therapeutic dose range is from 1.5 g to 3 g daily in divided doses. The dose in children and adolescents is 30-50mg/kg/day (maximum 3g daily) in two divided doses.

- A dose increment regimen is typically advised starting at 500 mg/day (approximately 10mg/kg in children) for 7 days and increasing by an additional 500 mg daily every 7 days over the ensuing weeks to the planned therapeutic dose.
- Patients should be warned that bodily fluids may turn a darker yellow/orange and not to be alarmed.
- SSZ may lead to staining of contact lenses.
- The enteric-coated formulation is well tolerated. SSZ also can be prescribed in liquid form.
- Slow acetylators of SSZ may develop a drug-induced lupus-like syndrome. It is not necessary to check acetylator phenotype since the drug will have been stopped when suspicion occurs.
- The majority of patients who develop SSZ side effects do so in the first 3 months of taking the drug. Correspondingly, laboratory test monitoring can be relaxed and in most guidelines, in long-term use, is only advised once every 3–6 months.
- A history of hypersensitivity to sulfonamides/co-trimoxazole should deter use of the drug.
- SSZ contains in part salicylic acid thus it can produce aspirin and NSAID-like side effects (e.g. peptic lesions, interstitial nephritis, tinnitus).
- SSZ can reduce sperm count and viability directly and can affect fertility by reducing gonadotrophin production.
- SSZ in combination with AZA may potentiate the risk of bone marrow toxicity from either drug.

## Targeted synthetic DMARDs (tsDMARDs)

### Tofacitinib

Tofacitinib is a JAK (Janus kinase) inhibitor that impairs the JAK-STAT signalling pathway and affects immune cell function.

- Tofacitinib has been shown to be effective in RA as monotherapy or co-therapy with MTX. Trials have also taken place in psoriasis and colitis.
- It has been approved in the USA for treatment of RA and it is being reviewed by NICE in the UK.
- It is given orally 5 mg twice daily for the immediate-release tablet or 11 mg once daily for the extended-release tablet.
- The dose needs to be adjusted in moderate renal and hepatic impairment to 5 mg once daily and avoided in severe impairment.
- It is not recommended to co-prescribe tofacitinib with strong CYP3A4 inducers such as rifampicin and the dose should be reduced with concomitant use of CYP3A4 inhibitors.
- Test and treatment for latent TB is recommended prior to commencement of tofacitinib.
- Lymphoma and other malignancies including skin cancers have been reported.
- EBV-associated post-transplant lymphoproliferative disorders have been reported in renal transplant patients treated with tofacitinib and concomitant immunosuppressants.

- Bone marrow suppression, lipid abnormalities, and hepatotoxicity can occur and hence monitoring should include FBC, lipid profile, and liver function tests.
- GI perforation has been reported in clinical trials so use with caution in patients at increased risk such as diverticulitis.

### Apremilast

Apremilast is a phosphodiesterase 4 (PDE4) inhibitor, which results in increased intracellular cAMP levels and consequently affects the regulation of numerous inflammatory mediators including decreasing the expression of TNFα:

- Apremilast is licensed for the use of PsA.
- It is approved in the USA and Europe but it is yet to be approved by NICE as 'cost-effective' in the UK.
- Apremilast is given orally initially at 10 mg in the morning on day 1, titrate upward by additional 10 mg per day on days 2 to 5 and maintenance dose of 30 mg twice daily from day 6.
- Dose needs to be adjusted when creatinine clearance is <30 mL/min.
- Apremilast may cause weight loss and discontinuation should be considered with significant weight loss.
- Neuropsychiatric effects such as depression and mood changes have been reported.

## Biological DMARDs

### Anti-TNFα therapy

TNFα is a potent pro-inflammatory cytokine and the levels are elevated in autoinflammatory/autoimmune inflammatory conditions.

- At present, there are five main anti-TNFα bDMARDs available: adalimumab, etanercept, certolizumab pegol, infliximab, and golimumab.
- Infliximab is a chimeric human–murine anti-TNFα monoclonal antibody, etanercept a recombinant human TNFα receptor fusion protein, certolizumab pegol a pegylated Fab fragment of a fully humanized anti-TNF monoclonal antibody, adalimumab and golimumab are both fully humanized anti-TNFα monoclonal antibodies.
- Infliximab is administered by slow IV infusion at 0, 2, 4, and every 4–8 weeks, thereafter depending on response.
- Etanercept is administered by SC injection and can be given once (50 mg) instead of twice (25 mg) weekly.
- Certolizumab pegol is given by SC injection at a dose of 400 mg in weeks 0, 2, and 4, followed by a dose of 200 mg every 2 weeks.
- Adalimumab is given by SC injection: 40 mg (20mg if the child weighs <30kg) every 2 weeks.
- Golimumab is given by SC injection at a dose of 50 mg every 4 weeks. An increase in dose to 100 mg every 4 weeks can be given in patients who weigh >100 kg.
- With all anti-TNFα agents, co-administration with MTX is recommended for treating RA and JIA when MTX is tolerated as this has been shown to increase efficacy. In addition, MTX use with infliximab and adalimumab reduces the risk of antibodies to the anti-TNF agent.

- For efficacy alone there appears to be no additional effect of adding MTX to anti-TNFα therapy for PsA or AS/axSpA.
- For RA patients who cannot take MTX, adalimumab, etanercept and certolizumab pegol can be used as monotherapy.
- Notably, and particularly in PsA and axSpA/AS, there is evidence that patients may respond to a second anti-TNFα if there is an inadequate response to a first therapy.
- In the UK, anti-TNFα is restricted by criteria for use (NICE has published guidelines for NHS use based on cost-effectiveness assessments; Table 23.9).
- Infliximab has been used to treat conditions ('off-licence') such as Behçet's disease (see ➲ Chapter 18).

*Anti-TNFα: cautions and monitoring*

All the assessment and monitoring principles set out in Table 23.7, Table 23.8, and Box 23.2 apply to bDMARDs as much as they do to csD-MARDs, particularly the assessment of infection and malignancy risk.

- Active bacterial or severe viral infection and current/recent malignancy are exclusion criteria for treatment with anti-TNFα. Paediatric judgment is required in children.
- Anti-TNFα should not be given to patients with a history of multiple sclerosis or severe heart failure (NYHA grade 3 or 4).
- Guidelines for using anti-TNFα therapy in pregnancy have recently been published (Table 23.10).
- Common reactions include headache, nausea, and injection-site reactions.

---

**Table 23.9** Summary of UK (NICE) guidelines for the use of the anti-TNFα therapy in RA in NHS practice

| | |
|---|---|
| 1 | Patients with clinical diagnosis of RA: 'recent onset' (disease duration of up to 2 years and established (>2 years) |
| 2 | A Disease Activity Score (DAS 28) of >5.1 |
| 3 | Adequate trial of at least 2 conventional DMARDs, one of which should be methotrexate. An adequate trial is defined as: |
| | Treatment for at least 6 months, with at least 2 months at standard target dose (unless toxicity) |
| | Treatment for <6 months where treatment was withdrawn due to intolerance or toxicity, normally after at least 2 months of therapeutic doses |
| 4 | *Exclusion criteria:* active infection or high risk of infection. Malignant or pre-malignant states |
| 5 | *Criteria for withdrawal of therapy:* adverse events or inefficacy |
| 6 | An alternative anti-TNFα therapy may be considered for patients in whom treatment is withdrawn due to an adverse event before the initial 6-month assessment of efficacy |

Information taken from ℐ⅁ https://www.nice.org.uk/guidance/TA375 and ℐ⅁ https://www.nice.org.uk/guidance/CG79.

**Table 23.10** Biologics in pregnancy and breastfeeding
*Disclaimer:* all readers should refer to their own local practice guidelines. Information here is incomplete and brief and a skeleton guide only.

| Drugs | Effects |
|---|---|
| Infliximab | Pregnancy: compatible peri-conception and with first trimester, stop at 16 weeks<br>Breastfeeding: compatible |
| Etanercept<br>Adalimumab | Pregnancy: compatible peri-conception and with first and second trimester, stop at third trimester<br>Breastfeeding: compatible |
| Certolizumab | Pregnancy: compatible peri-conception and throughout pregnancy<br>Breastfeeding: compatible |
| Golimumab | Pregnancy: no data to recommend<br>Breastfeeding: no data to recommend |
| Rituximab | Pregnancy: stop 6 months before conception<br>Breastfeeding: no data to recommend |
| Tocilizumab | Pregnancy: stop 3 months before conception<br>Breastfeeding: no data to recommend |
| Anakinra<br>Abatacept<br>Belimumab | Pregnancy: no data to recommend<br>Breastfeeding: no data to recommend |

- Serious bacterial infections have been reported, and patients with active infection should have their treatment stopped.
- For patients at risk of recurrent infection (e.g. in-dwelling urinary catheter, immunodeficiency states) it is usually recommended to avoid anti-TNFa therapy.
- Other reported side effects include demyelination, worsening of heart failure, lupus-like syndromes, and blood dyscrasias.
- Reactivation of TB has been reported mainly with infliximab and adalimumab use (3–4× increased risk compared with etanercept) and most commonly within 3 months of beginning of treatment. Patients should be assessed for TB risk.
- There are guidelines for assessing risk and managing TB infection in patients due to start anti-TNFα therapy (e.g. British Thoracic Society available at: http://www.brit-thoracic.org.uk). Use of anti-TNFα therapy is not contraindicated but patients may require up to 3–6 months' treatment for latent TB.
- The long-term safety of anti-TNFα especially with regard to malignancy is not known. It is well known that RA patients have a 2× risk of developing lymphoma compared with the general population. Debate continues as to whether reports of lymphoma in RA patients on anti-TNFα therapy reflect a real drug effect or the known increased incidence of lymphoma in RA patients.

- There is no increased risk of developing solid tumours. However, there appears to be an increased risk of some skin cancers especially melanoma and hence patient should be advised on preventive skin care and close monitoring of skin.

## B-cell depletion therapy

B cells play an important role in the pathogenesis of RA and other autoimmune conditions generating antibodies and, through their surface receptors, in processing and presenting antigen to T cells.

### Rituximab

RTX is a chimeric monoclonal antibody against human CD20 that is present on developing B cells prior to the plasma cell stage. Administration of RTX leads to rapid CD20 positive B-cell depletion in the peripheral blood. Normal B-cell repopulation (measured by monitoring the CD19 count) occurs variably but typically over the next 6–9 months.

- RT. RCTs have shown that in RF-positive RA patients who have failed several csDMARDs, a course of RTX (two infusions, 1 g 2 weeks apart with methylprednisolone infusions) achieves a significant improvement in RA disease activity at 6 months compared to MTX alone.
- In RA, the time to next infusion regimen can range from 6 to 18 months, but has a mean of 9 months.
- There is concern about persistent hypogammaglobulinaemia after repeated courses of RTX. The possibility of increased risk of infection with hypogammaglobulinaemia should be discussed with patients before re-treatment.
- In the UK, NICE allows RTX to be used with MTX in the treatment of severe RA for NHS patients, where there has been an inadequate response to other DMARDs and one or more other anti-TNFα therapy.
- Open-label studies in SLE initially suggested efficacy of RTX, with benefits extending to 6 months; however, a RCT failed to show that RTX was beneficial to patients with moderate-to-severe SLE.
- Repeated RTX infusions in SLE appear to increase BAFF/BLyS (see later), which is associated with increasing severity of post-treatment flares in some patients.
- Rituximab is as effective as CYC in the treatment of AAV as induction or maintenance therapy and is used if avoidance of CYC is preferable or there is an inadequate response to CYC.
- There is a growing literature suggesting benefit of RTX in other conditions, e.g. polymyositis and dermatomyositis.
- The serious condition progressive multifocal leucoencephalopathy (PML) has been reported with RTX in a small number of patients. Patients should be counselled appropriately before treatment.
- The assessment and monitoring recommended for RTX is similar to that recommended for anti-TNFα therapy.
- A lymphocyte CD19 count can be checked before and 6 weeks after administering RTX. The observation of it falling with treatment and then rising as the disease 'flares' is evidence in favour of drug efficacy and a means of predicting need for retreatment.

*Belimumab*

- Belimumab is monoclonal antibody that depletes B cell by blocking the binding of soluble BAFF/BLyS to receptors on B lymphocytes, reducing the activity of B-cell-mediated immunity. BAFF/BLyS is a TNF superfamily member (TNFSF13B) best known for its role in the survival and maturation of B cells.
- Belimumab may be used in SLE resistant to other agents.
- Belimumab is given as an infusion initially at 10 mg/kg every 2 weeks for 3 doses and maintenance of 10 mg/kg every 4 weeks.

## Interleukin-1 receptor antagonists

Interleukin-1 (IL-1) is a pro-inflammatory cytokine. Anakinra is an IL-1 receptor antagonist that competes with Il-1 for binding.

- Anakinra is given by 100 mg (in children 1–4mg/kg) SC injection daily.
- RCTs have shown that anakinra is more effective than placebo in RA but smaller disease responses are evident compared to anti-TNFα.
- Anakinra is used in treating MAS, systemic onset JIA and autoinflammatory conditions, e.g. TNF receptor-1 associated periodic syndrome (TRAPS), SAPHO syndrome, and adult-onset Still's disease (see ➲ Chapter 18).
- Side effects include injection-site reactions, blood dyscrasias, and infection.
- Anakinra should not be used together with anti-TNFα therapies.
- Clearance is reduced in renal impairment.

## Interleukin-6 inhibition

Interleukin-6 (IL-6) is a potent pro-inflammatory cytokine and mediator of the acute-phase response. High levels of Il-6 have been found in serum and synovial fluid of RA patients.

- Recent work has shown that both upstream and downstream signalling pathways for IL-6 differ between myocytes and macrophages.
- It appears that unlike IL-6 signalling in macrophages, which is dependent on activation of the NFκB signalling pathway, intramuscular IL-6 expression is regulated by a network of signalling cascades, including the $Ca^{2+}$/NFAT and glycogen/p38 MAPK pathways.
- IL-6 signalling in monocytes or macrophages, creates a pro-inflammatory response, whereas IL-6 signalling in muscle (independent of a preceding TNFα response or NFκB activation) is anti-inflammatory.

*Tocilizumab*

Tocilizumab is a humanized monoclonal antibody specific for the Il-6 receptor. It is licensed for use in treating RA, systemic JIA, and Castleman's disease.

- Tocilizumab is given by monthly IV infusion at a dose of 8 mg/kg. It is also available as SC injection at 162 mg every other week if weight is <100 kg or 162 mg every week if weight >100 kg. In children >2y with systemic JIA the dose is: weight <30kg–12mg/kg every two weeks by infusion; weight >30kg–8mg/kg every two weeks. In children with polyarticular JIA the dose is 8–10mg/kg every 4 weeks by infusion.
- Tocilizumab is effective in controlling disease and limiting radiographic progression in RA patients in whom MTX and anti-TNFα therapy have been ineffective or not tolerated.

- Tocilizumab can be used as monotherapy if MTX is not tolerated or contraindicated.
- Tocilizumab is currently under trial for use in large vessel vasculitis and uveitis.
- Lipids should be monitored 6-monthly given the association with drug-induced hyperlipidaemia.
- Bone marrow side effects are more frequent in the first few months of treatment. FBC and liver function tests should be monitored monthly.

## Biologic DMARDs targeting Th17 cell activation

Common to a number of conditions, Th17 cell activation is driven by Il-12 and Il-23, which triggers the activated T-cell to produce Il-17 and elaborate other cytokines, which have downstream pro-inflammatory effects in various tissues then having tissue-specific effects. Diseases where Th17 cell activation is pertinent include psoriasis and the SpAs (see ➲ Chapter 8).

### Ustekinumab

Ustekinumab is a human monoclonal antibody directed against the pro-inflammatory cytokines IL-12 and IL-23. Ustekinumab binds to the (common sequence) p40 subunit of both cytokines so that they cannot activate their receptors on Th17 cells.

- In PsA, ustekinumab has shown superior efficacy in treating synovitis, dactylitis and enthesitis compared to MTX alone. Responses are positive in both anti-TNFα naïve and anti-TNFα treated patients.
- Ustekinumab is given by SC injection: dose 45 mg (weight <100 kg) or 90 mg (weight >100 kg) at week 0, 4, and 12-weekly thereafter.
- In the UK, NICE has approved use for NHS patients with PsA when disease is still active despite treatment with DMARDs and if anti-TNFα has failed or is contraindicated.
- Common side effects include infection, fatigue, and headache.
- Uncommon side effects include exfoliative dermatitis, encephalopathy, and facial palsy.

### Secukinumab

Secukinumab is a recombinant fully human monoclonal IgG1k antibody which binds Il-17A inhibiting its receptor binding. It is licensed for use in treating plaque psoriasis and has shown efficacy in treating AS.[2]

- For AS, the recommended dose is 150 mg once weekly subcutaneously at weeks 0, 1, 2, and 3; followed by a maintenance dose monthly from week 4.
- Secukinumab may be effective in some adults with PsA whose response to csDMARDs has been inadequate. Case reports suggest effectivity in patients defined as having axSpA.
- It should be used with caution in patients with Crohn's disease as it can cause exacerbation of inflammatory disease.

## Other biologic DMARDs

### Abatacept (CTLA4-Ig)

Abatacept disrupts the CD80/86 co-stimulatory signal required for T-cell activation by competing with CD28 for binding.

- Abatacept is effective in patients with RA whose disease is not controlled with one or more csDMARDs including MTX or anti-TNFα.
- Abatacept is administered IV at a dose according to body weight; 500 mg (<60 kg), 750 mg (60–100 kg), and 1000 mg (>100 kg) at weeks 0, 2, and 4 and then monthly thereafter. In children <75kg the dose is 10mg/kg by infusion in the same frequency as adults.
- Abatacept can also been given SC at a dose of 125 mg once weekly. In children 25–50kg the dose is 87.5mg and if >50kg an adult equivalent dose is used.
- A recent systematic review has shown that the incidence of serious infections was low, and compared with placebo was equal.

### The use of bDMARDs in pregnancy and breastfeeding

There is a paucity of data on the effect of bDMARDs in pregnancy and in women breastfeeding but consensus opinion is summarized in a number of guidelines (e.g. UK BSR guidelines available at: ℜ http://www.rheumatology.org.uk/resources/guidelines/default.aspx).

### References

1. Smolen JS, van der Heijde D, Machold KP, et al. Proposal for a new nomenclature of disease-modifying antirheumatic drugs. *Ann Rheum Dis* 2014;73:3–5.
2. Baeten D, Sieper J, Braun J, et al. Secukinumab, an interleukin-17A inhibitor, in ankylosing spondylitis. *N Engl J Med* 2015;373:2534–48.

# Other medications

### Drugs used in treating osteoporosis

The treatment of osteoporosis is described in ➲ Chapter 6. A summary of currently licensed osteoporosis drugs is shown in Table 23.11.

Table 23.11 Drugs used in the treatment of osteoporosis

| Drugs | Dose | Comments |
|---|---|---|
| Alendronic acid | 70 mg orally once weekly | Fracture reduction broadly 20–40% for oral bisphosphonates over 3–5 yrs and 70% for vertebral fracture reduction for zoledronate at 3 yrs. Initial treatment course is 3–5 yrs |
| Risedronate | 35 mg orally once weekly | Optimum response occurs if not calcium and vitamin D deficient |
| Ibandronic acid | 150 mg oral monthly or 3 mg IV every 3 months | Avoid all bisphosphonates in renal impairment (estimated GFR <30 mL/min) |
| | | Oral bisphosphonates can cause dyspepsia, oesophagitis, and oesophageal ulcers |
| Zoledronic acid | 5 mg IV once yearly | Oral bisphosphonates must be taken with water, fasting and at least 1 hr before food or liquid (other than water) |
| | | Regular review for adherence is advisable |
| | | Atypical femoral fractures have been reported—but rarely and chiefly with long-term treatment |
| | | Osteonecrosis of the jaw is very rare |
| Denosumab | 60 mg SC injection once every 6 months | Fracture reduction risk about 70% over 3 yrs for vertebral fractures |
| | | Side effects include cellulitis, urinary tract infection, and upper respiratory tract infection |
| | | Hypocalcaemia can occur and the risk is increased if estimated GFR <30 mL/min—give calcium supplements and monitor serum calcium |
| | | Atypical femoral fractures and osteonecrosis of jaw (advise dental check-up) are rare but can occur |
| Strontium ranelate | 2 g oral daily; avoid food for 2 hrs before and 2 hrs after | RCTs showed fracture prevention after 3 yrs of continuous use. Continued use to 8 yrs suggested maintained fracture prevention |
| | | Side effects: GI; now used sparingly because of increased risk of cardiovascular disease and venous thrombosis. Use banned in some countries |
| Teriparatide | 20 micrograms SC injection daily for 2 years | Side effects include GI disorders, palpitation, hypercalcaemia, myalgia |
| | | Contraindicated in hypercalcaemia, skeletal malignancies or bone metastases, Paget's, and previous radiation to the skeleton |
| | | Avoid in severe renal impairment |

## Drugs used in the treatment of Raynaud's disease and pulmonary artery hypertension

The treatment of Raynaud's disease (RD) and pulmonary artery hypertension (PAH) associated with SScl is described in ➲ Chapter 13. Table 23.12 provides a summary of the drugs used.

**Table 23.12** Drugs used in the treatment of Raynaud's disease (RD) and pulmonary artery hypertension (PAH)

| Drugs | Adverse effects |
|---|---|
| *Nifedipine:* 5–20 mg three times a day for RD. Start dose low with dose adjustments following response<br><br>*Amlodipine* 5–10 mg daily for RD | Oedema, hypotension, headache, nausea |
| *Losartan:* 25–50 mg oral daily for RD | Hypotension, hyperkalaemia |
| *Fluoxetine:* 20–40 mg oral daily for RD | See SNRI cautions, ➲ p. 658 and Table 23.5, p. 657 |
| *Topical GTN:* available in 5 mg/24 hrs. For RD. Apply to affected area for up till 12 hrs | Hypotension, headache, application site reactions |
| *Sildenafil:* 25–50 mg orally three times a day for RD, or<br>*Tadalafil:* 40 mg orally daily.<br>Reduce doses in renal and hepatic impairment | Hypotension, priapism, headache, flushing, diarrhoea, visual defects |
| *Iloprost (prostacyclin analogue)*<br>Nebulized form for PAH. First inhaled dose should be 2.5 micrograms increased to 5.0 micrograms if tolerated and given 3–4-hourly. Typically, 6–9 doses/day but no more than 45 micrograms/day advisable.<br>IV infusion for PAH initially 0.5 ng/kg/min for 30 mins then increased at intervals of 30 mins in steps of 0.5 ng/kg/min up to 2 ng/kg/min. Exact infusion rate should be calculated on body weight to effect infusion rate range of 0.5–2 ng/kg/min. Final dose given over 6 hrs daily (e.g. over 5 days). | Hypotension, headache, jaw or limb pain. Monitor pulse, blood pressure, and oxygen saturation. If effects severe consider reducing dose or stopping infusion temporarily and restarting at lower dose |
| *Bosentan:* for PAH. Initially 62.5 mg twice daily orally increased after 4 weeks to 125 mg twice daily. *Macitentan:* for PAH only: 10 mg oral daily.<br>*Ambrisentan:* for PAH only: 5 mg oral daily, increased if necessary to 10 mg daily | Low haemoglobin (Hb) so monitor Hb before and during treatment. Also check LFTs at start and at monthly intervals on treatment |
| *Riociguat:* for PAH only; initially 1 mg three times a day daily for 2 weeks, increased by 0.5 mg each dose every 2 weeks up to maximum 2.5 mg three times a day | Hypotension—reduce dose if systolic BP falls <95 mmHg |

## Drugs used in treating gout and hyperuricaemia

The management of gout is described in ➜ Chapter 7. The treatment of acute gout is with NSAIDs, colchicine, and GCs. Urate lowering drugs are used if gout is severe (e.g. chronic/tophaceous) and/or recurrent. See also Cochrane review CD010069 (⅋ http://www.cochranelibrary.com).

### Colchicine

- Colchicine is anti-inflammatory and used in gout and CPPD disease for both acute attacks and chronic disease.
- Colchicine can also be used long term in the treatment of Behçet's disease and familial Mediterranean fever.
- It is given initially at a dose of 0.5 mg twice daily in acute gout and CPPD. The dose in children is 0.3 – 2.4mg in one to two divided doses increasing in 0.3mg/day increments as tolerated.
- Dose should be adjusted with renal impairment and avoided completely in severe renal impairment (estimated GFR <10 mL/min).
- Dose is increased to three or four times daily but is limited by dose-related diarrhoea.
- Colchicine frequently causes nausea, vomiting, and abdominal pain. Larger doses may cause profuse diarrhoea, GI haemorrhage, skin rashes, and renal and hepatic damage.
- The rare side effects are myopathy, rhabdomyolysis, alopecia, with prolonged treatment, bone marrow suppression can occur.

### Allopurinol

- Allopurinol is a xanthine oxidase inhibitor which is usually the first-line urate-lowering drug.
- Initiate at 100 mg orally daily then adjust according to plasma uric acid concentration each month by 100 mg to maximum 900 mg daily.
- The dose should be adjusted down in renal impairment, and in severe renal impairment, reduce daily dose below 100 mg.
- The dose should be changed inversely (e.g. each 4–6 weeks) titrated against urate level to a target <360 nmol/L or in severe disease <300.
- About 2% of patients develop a rash which is typically pruritic and maculopapular. If mild, withdraw therapy and re-challenge can be undertaken with caution but discontinue promptly if recurrence.
- Life threatening hypersensitivity reactions such as Stevens–Johnson syndrome, toxic epidermal necrolysis, or drug rash with eosinophilia and systemic symptoms (DRESS) can occur rarely and re-challenge should not be undertaken.
- GI disorders, e.g. nausea and diarrhoea, are uncommon and bone marrow suppression is rare even in high doses.
- Allopurinol can interfere with the metabolism of AZA and 6-MP, potentiating side effects. The dose of AZA or 6-MP should be ~25% of the usual dose if they are given concurrently with allopurinol.
- Other interactions include warfarin (monitor INR), theophylline (monitor drug level), and ACE inhibitors (haematological reactions).

*Febuxostat*

Febuxostat is a non-purine xanthine oxidase inhibitor used to treat hyperuricaemia. It is appropriate for patients who are allergic to allopurinol, do not reach the target uric acid level with maximal allopurinol doses, or have severe renal insufficiency.

- Febuxostat is initiated at 80 mg orally daily then increase to 120 mg daily after 2–4 weeks if serum uric acid >6 mg/dL.
- The most common side effects are diarrhoea, nausea, headache, liver function test abnormalities, and rash.
- Severe hypersensitivity reactions such as Stevens–Johnson syndrome, toxic epidermal necrolysis, or DRESS occur but are rare.
- Mild liver function abnormalities were observed in 5% in clinical studies, hence checking LFTs is recommended before starting febuxostat and periodically thereafter. In known mild hepatic impairment, the dose is reduced to 40–80 mg daily.
- Febuxostat is not advised for people with ischaemic heart disease or heart failure because initial trials showed a higher incidence of cardiovascular side effects from febuxostat compared with allopurinol; however, the observation has not been substantiated in further trials.
- Febuxostat can interfere with metabolism of AZA and 6-MP and hence concomitant use is not recommended.

*Probenecid*

Probenecid is a uricosuric agent, which is effective by altering renal handling of urate and increasing urine excretion. It has been used to increase the concentration of some antibiotics.

- The recommended dose is 250 mg oral twice daily for 1 week and 500 mg twice daily thereafter.
- Probenecid should not be started until after an acute attack of gout.
- In some countries, including the UK, probenecid is only available from 'special-order' manufacturers or distributors.
- It is important to ensure adequate fluid intake.
- Probenecid is contraindicated in patients with a history of blood disorders, renal stones, and renal impairment where estimated GFR is <30 mL/min.

*Sulfinpyrazone (sulphinpyrazone)*

Sulfinpyrazone is a uricosuric agent. It should not be started during an acute gout attack.

- Sulfinpyrazone is initiated at 100–200 mg orally daily with food increasing over 2–3 weeks to 600 mg daily until target serum uric acid concentration is reached and then reduced to maintenance dose which may be as low as 200 mg daily.
- Dose should be reduced in renal impairment. It should be avoided in severe renal impairment and is ineffective if GFR is <30 mL/min.
- It is contraindicated in patients with history of blood disorders.
- Regular FBC/CBC monitoring is advisable as sulfinpyrazone can cause blood disorders.
- Caution is advised in prescribing where there is cardiac, cerebrovascular, or hypertension disease as the drug may cause salt and water retention.

- Other side effects include GI disturbances and ulceration, allergic skin reactions, acute kidney injury, and hepatitis.
- See also: ℘ http://www.medicines.org.uk/emc/medicine/26935.

### Benzbromarone

Benzbromarone is a uricosuric agent and non-competitive inhibitor of xanthine oxidase, available in Europe. Benzbromarone also inhibits cytochrome CYP2C9, which is responsible for metabolizing a number of drugs including drugs with a narrow therapeutic index such as warfarin and phenytoin and other drugs such as tolbutamide, losartan, and some NSAIDs.

- Benzbromarone offers advantages over some uricosuric drugs as it may be safer and better tolerated in patients with renal insufficiency.
- Liver function must be monitored for drug-induced hepatitis; fulminant liver failure has been described.
- Given its effects on CYP2C9 caution with co-prescribing, any medication is mandatory.

### Rasburicase

Rasburicase is a recombinant uricase/urate-oxidase enzyme produced by genetically modified *Saccharomyces cerevisiae* strain. Urate oxidase exists in many mammals but does not occur in humans.

- Rasburicase catalyses enzymatic oxidation of uric acid into a metabolite, allantoin, which is 5–10× more soluble than uric acid, with $CO_2$ and hydrogen peroxide as by-products in the chemical reaction.
- Rasburicase is licensed in the USA and Europe for treatment of acute hyperuricaemia associated with tumour lysis syndrome in patients receiving lymphoma or leukaemia chemotherapy.
- The recommended dose is 0.2 mg/kg/day given as a once-daily 30-minute IV infusion in 50 mL of 0.9% saline.
- The duration of treatment may be up to 7 days, the exact duration should be based upon adequate monitoring of uric acid levels in plasma and clinical judgement.
- Long-term use for hyperuricaemia associated with gout at doses of 0.15–0.2 mg/kg is being investigated.

### Pegloticase

Pegloticase is a recombinant porcine-like uricase and like rasburicase it metabolizes uric acid to allantoin.

- Pegloticase is pegylated to increase its elimination half-life from about 8 hours to 10–12 days and to decrease the immunogenicity of the foreign uricase protein. So pegloticase is given every 2–4 weeks.
- Pegloticase might be considered* for patients with severe gout in whom other urate-lowering agents have been ineffective.
- Pegloticase produces rapid reduction in signs and symptoms of gout.
- Pegloticase is given as an IV infusion, 8 mg every 2 weeks, infused over >2 hours with premedication to decrease infusion reactions including oral paracetamol, hydrocortisone, and antihistamine.
- All patients should be given prophylaxis for prevention of acute gout during the first 6 months of treatment.
- Trials have shown that the urate-lowering effect can be attenuated or lost in some patients due to high titre anti-pegloticase antibodies.

- In the UK, pegloticase has not been sanctioned for use in gout by NICE for NHS-treated patients, citing poor cost-effectivity but also noting reported severe anaphylaxis reactions have occurred with it.
- * In 2016, the European Commission withdrew the marketing authorization for pegloticase in the EU.

## Pooled intravenous immunoglobulin (IVIg)

Pooled IVIg is primarily used as replacement therapy in primary immunodeficiency conditions. However, IVIg can have an immunosuppressive effect though the mechanism of effect is not precisely known. A number of theories exist.

- Apart from immunodeficiency, the main indications for IVIg are in Guillain–Barré syndrome, myasthenia gravis, immune thrombocytopenic purpura, SLE (see ➔ Chapter 10), dermatomyositis (see ➔ Chapter 14), and Kawasaki disease (see ➔ Chapter 15).
- The typical dosing regimen is 400 mg/kg/day as a single infusion over 2–4 hours as tolerated and for 5 days; or 1 g/kg/day for 2 days. This is repeated every 4–8 weeks for up to 6 months in the first instance according to efficacy.
- Side effects occur in <5% of patients and most often within 24 hours of an infusion.
- However, the FDA (USA) requires IVIg products to carry a black box warning, cautioning that IVIg has been associated with renal dysfunction, acute kidney injury, osmotic nephrosis, and death, especially in the elderly or with simultaneous use of other nephrotoxic drugs or other pre-existing issues that affect the kidneys.
- Side effects at the time of infusion include headache, flushing, chills, myalgia, wheezing, tachycardia, lower back pain, nausea, and hypotension. If these occur, the infusion should be slowed or stopped. Most cases will respond to antihistamines and IV hydrocortisone if symptoms persist.
- Other significant, but rare complications include acute kidney injury, arteriovenous thrombosis, disseminated intravascular coagulation, transient serum sickness, transient neutropenia, aseptic meningitis, post-infusion hyperproteinaemia with pseudohyponatraemia, eczematous dermatitis, and alopecia.

## Resources

All UK-licensed drug SPCs are available at EMC: ✍ http://www.medicines.org.uk
Patient drug information available at: ✍ http://www.arthritisresearchuk.org
Selective therapy meta-analyses at: ✍ http://www.cochranelibrary.com

# Glucocorticoid injection therapy

Relevant anatomical drawings for each region of the body are found in ➔ Chapter 3

# Introduction

Local anaesthetic and glucocorticoid (GC; 'steroid') injection into joints, tendons, bursae, and soft tissues is a very effective treatment for localized pain and inflammation.

- Injection offers a local maximal anti-inflammatory effect with minimal systemic absorption.
- As a general rule, it is recommended that any one joint should not be injected more than four times in 12 months and there are at least 6 weeks between injections.
- The indications for local steroid injection include:
  - reduction of inflammation.
  - relief of pain from inflammatory lesions.
  - relief of inflammation at sites of nerve compression.
  - reduce the size of nodules and ganglia.
- The contraindications are:
  - *absolute*: septic arthritis/sepsis, a febrile patient with cause unknown, serious allergy to previous injection, sickle cell disease.
  - *relative*: unknown cause of lesion, neutropenia, thrombocytopenia, anticoagulation, or bleeding disorder.
- Common steroid preparations used include:
  - hydrocortisone acetate—a short-acting, weak steroid useful for superficial lesions such as tendons and bursae: 25mg is typical.
  - methylprednisolone acetate 40 mg/mL.
  - prednisolone acetate 25 mg/mL.
  - triamcinolone acetonide 10 and 40 mg/mL.
- The latter three agents are long-acting synthetic glucocorticoids.
- Choice of strength of steroid remains empiric.
- Volume of steroid/anaesthetic 'accepted' by joints varies:
  - Small joints accept only a small volume; thus, for IPJs, MCPJs, MTPJs, and temporomandibular joints, 0.5 mL only is appropriate.
  - All other joints should accept at least 1 mL.
  - There may be merit in diluting the steroid in sterile saline, to increase volume for better distribution in larger joints.
  - alternatively, larger volume levobupivacaine (10 mL) is of value.
- Potential, though uncommon, side effects (see also → Chapter 23) are:
  - exacerbation of pain for 24–48 hours.
  - septic arthritis and reactivation of TB.
  - tissue atrophy (less likely with hydrocortisone than others).
  - depigmentation of skin.
  - anaphylaxis.
  - nerve damage.
  - tendon rupture.
  - osteonecrosis.
  - cartilage damage.
  - soft tissue calcification.
  - temporary exacerbation of hyperglycaemia in diabetes.

# Principles of injection techniques

The procedure need not necessarily be done in a sterile environment. However, there is a need to maintain an aseptic technique. Efficacy may be greater using US-guided injection but will be more accurate. US should only be done by appropriately qualified clinicians.

• Mark the exact spot of needle insertion.
• Wash hands. Use sterile gloves for the procedure.
• Clean the skin with povidone-iodine and allow it to dry.
• Anaesthetize the skin (either with local anaesthetic or refrigerant alcohol spray). Children and some adolescents may require a light general anaesthetic given the procedure can be traumatic. An alternative is to use local anaesthetic gel pads (e.g. EMLA® patch).
• Insert a clean needle with empty syringe and aspirate back.
• Leave the needle in place, detach the syringe, and place the syringe containing steroid/local anaesthetic onto the end of a new needle.
• Insert needle into site to be injected.
• Pull back the syringe plunger again before injecting to confirm placement, ensuring the needle is not in a blood vessel.
• Introduction of steroid should be effortless. Resistance implies the end of the needle is in the wrong space. Stop if it causes more pain.
• On completion of the procedure, remove the syringe and needle and throw away the 'sharps'.
• Cover the injection site with clean gauze or a bandage.
• Rest the joint for 24 hours (consider up to 48 hours for a weight-bearing joint), including using a non-rigid splint (e.g. Velcro® attached semi-rigid splint for wrist, or modified Robert-Jones bandaging for the knee).
• Advise that icing the area/joint may reduce post-injection discomfort, and re-emphasize possible side effects and benefits.

# The shoulder

## The glenohumeral joint (for glenohumeral joint synovitis or adhesive capsulitis)

### US-guided injection technique

It is difficult to be confident a needle is placed in the glenohumeral joint space without confirmation imaging with US. The default technique for injecting the glenohumeral joint should be with US.

- US-guided injection is the gold standard for comparing therapy options in research studies (e.g. steroid injection vs hydrodilation for adhesive capsulitis).
- US is probably not required, however, when an injection is done as the second part of a linked procedure when the first part is aspirating a large effusion (e.g. in CPPD-pseudogout).

### Non-US-guided injection technique

Sometimes it is not possible to obtain US and a 'blind' injection may need to be done. It is essential that anyone undertaking the injections has been appropriately trained or is supervised and is knowledgeable about anatomy and functional anatomy.

- The approach may be anterior or posterior.
- The anterior approach is favoured for adhesive capsulitis given the predominant pathology involves the anterior part of the joint complex including coracoacromial ligament and subscapularis bursa.
- The anterior route is undertaken thus:
  - Palpate the coracoid process anteriorly and acromion posteriorly.
  - The injection is made just lateral to the coracoid with the needle pointing towards the acromion (see ➲ Plate 4).
- The posterior route is done thus:
  - The clinician palpates the spine of the scapula with the thumb to its lateral end where it bends forward as the acromion.
  - With the forefinger, palpate the coracoid anteriorly. The line between finger and thumb then marks the position of the joint line.
  - The needle is advanced from behind, 1 cm below the acromion, and towards the coracoid. There should be no resistance.
- By either approach, the joint can be injected with relatively large volumes such as 1 mL (40 mg) methylprednisolone acetate mixed with 5 mL 1% lidocaine.
- A long needle is needed.
- Withdrawing the needle slightly and redirecting 30° upward will allow one to reach the rotator cuff with the same procedure.

## Subacromial space (for subacromial impingement disorders)

*US-guided injection technique*

It is difficult to be confident a needle is placed in the subacromial space without confirmation with US. The default technique for injecting the subacromial space should be with US.

- US may be used diagnostically and, with appropriate sonographer experience and skill, calcific supraspinatus lesions and tears can be identified.
- Radiological expertise varies from department to department and local advice on choosing MRI or US for specific lesion identification would be appropriate.

*Non-US-guided injection technique*

Sometimes it is not possible to obtain US and a 'blind' injection may need to be done. It is essential that anyone undertaking such an injection has been appropriately trained or is supervised and is knowledgeable about anatomy and functional anatomy.

- The subacromial space is injected most effectively from the lateral aspect of the shoulder.
- The arm is placed in a neutral position, hanging to the side, and the gap between the acromion and the humeral head is palpated.
- A long, narrow-gauge (e.g. 23) needle is directed medially and slightly posterior (but on a horizontal plane) for about 2–3 cm (see ➜ Plate 5).
- Usually a volume of 3–4 mL can be accepted (e.g. 40 mg methylprednisolone acetate in 1 mL with up to 5 mL 1% lidocaine).
- Advise avoidance of overarm activity or heavy lifting for a few days and consider arranging physiotherapy to start 2 weeks after the injection to work on restoring rotator cuff function.

## Acromioclavicular joint (ACJ)

The ACJ is sometimes very difficult to locate so US to help mark the joint is desirable. US is somewhat limited in its utility however, given the amount of bone present—usually an ACJ which needs injecting is somewhat arthritic with osteophytes and periarticular sclerosis—thus interfering with US imaging data.

- The ACJ is located by following the clavicle laterally to a ridge in the bone. The joint is often tender to palpate.
- Marking the bony edge/landmarks with a pen will be helpful.
- With the patient either sitting or lying supine, a small-gauge needle with 20 mg methylprednisolone (or equivalent) in 0.5 mL mixed with 0.5 mL of 1% lidocaine is directed in to the joint.

# The elbow

### Lateral epicondylitis/'tennis elbow'/common extensor tendon origin enthesitis

Please see ➜ Chapter 3 for advice on clinical assessment and making a diagnosis. This lesion may be secondary to trauma or associated with a SpA condition or PsA.

- US imaging is not required. The injection is best placed at the point of maximum tenderness. The target is usually very superficial.
- The lateral humeral epicondyle and surrounding tissue is injected with the elbow resting on a pillow—or similar—on the examination table and flexed at 90°.
- Use hydrocortisone initially 25 mg because other steroid preparations may cause local fat atrophy and depigmentation (as this is necessarily often a very superficial injection just under the skin).
- Use 0.5–1 mL 1% lidocaine mixed with the hydrocortisone.
- The injection is aimed at 45° to the end of the tendon origin.
- A fair amount of pressure is required for this injection. Efficacy of the injection may rely partly on disruption of the periosteum of the epicondylar bone. It is often painful (see ➜ Plate 6).
- Advise rest and icing post procedure.
- Autologous blood injection has been reported anecdotally as effective, though the technique is controversial, convincing data on efficacy is lacking and in the UK NHS, the technique is not recommended. Guidance on this procedure may be found at: ✍ https://www.nice.org.uk/guidance/ipg438/.

### Medial epicondylitis/'golfer's elbow'/common flexor tendon origin enthesitis

Please see ➜ Chapter 3 for advice on clinical assessment and making a diagnosis. This lesion may be secondary to trauma or associated with a SpA condition or PsA.

- US imaging is not required. The injection is best placed at the point of maximum tenderness. The target is usually very superficial.
- The medial humeral epicondyle and surrounding tissue is injected with the elbow extended and resting on a pillow—or similar—on the examination table.
- Use hydrocortisone initially 25 mg because other steroid preparations may cause local fat atrophy and depigmentation (as this is necessarily often a very superficial injection just under the skin).
- Use 0.5–1 mL 1% lidocaine mixed with the hydrocortisone.
- The injection is aimed at 45° to the end of the tendon origin.
- The needle is directed to the flexor tendon origin. However, care should be taken to avoid the groove just behind the medial epicondyle—the site of the ulnar nerve.
- Advise rest and ice post procedure.

## Olecranon bursitis

An olecranon bursa can be aspirated and injected without US guidance. Needle position is confirmed by the aspiration of fluid.

- The usual causes of bursitis are gout, infection, and RA.
- Fluid aspirated may reasonably be sent initially for microscopy and culture and infection ruled out before steroid is injected.
- Always send fluid for polarized light microscopy.
- Use triamcinolone acetonide or methylprednisolone at a dose of 20–40 mg and advise icing and rest for 48 hours.
- Arrange appropriate follow-up as the olecranon bursa is prone to develop infection and may need prompt reassessment—advise the patient accordingly.

## Elbow joint (e.g. RA synovitis)

US guidance may help though often, when there is an effusion, needle placement is relatively straightforward and can be confirmed by fluid aspiration.

- The elbow joint is most easily reached by a posterior approach.
- Use 40 mg methylprednisolone or equivalent, with 2–3 mL 1% lidocaine.
- Injection into a swollen elbow joint after fluid aspiration, when there is a distended capsule is relatively straightforward; however, an effusion may be present and not readily clinically identified—so landmark identification is necessary.
- Place the thumb on the lateral epicondyle and the third finger on the olecranon. The groove between the two fingers identifies the joint line.
- Inject at 90° to the skin, just above and lateral to the olecranon.
- Alternatively, the radial head can be palpated (by feeling for it during forearm pronation/supination) and the needle sited tangentially just under the capsule (an anterolateral approach).
- Advise rest and icing post procedure and advise to avoid lifting or gripping with the arm for a few days.
- Consider arranging physiotherapy to encourage/exercise the elbow back to full range. There is a high chance, with persistent inflammatory disease in the elbow, of progression to permanent loss of elbow extension.

# The wrist and hand

### Lesions of the wrist

#### Radiocarpal joint

(Please see also ➋ Chapter 3.)

- The radiocarpal joint is best identified for injection with the patient's forearm supported and their hand—also supported—palm down with the wrist then in slight flexion. A triangular gap is felt between the radius scaphoid and lunate.
- The needle (small gauge) is pointed directly down into the space.
- For most causes of wrist joint inflammation and synovitis, 40 mg methylprednisolone acetate with 2 mL 1% lidocaine is appropriate.
- Image-guided injection technique is not usually needed for this injection as the wrist space is easily gained.

#### Carpal tunnel syndrome

For anatomy and clinical assessment see ➋ 'Upper limb peripheral nerve lesions', pp. 124–7.

- The carpal tunnel is injected on the palmar surface of the wrist in the first crease, midline. Position the patient's supported arm, volar side up and with gentle extension at the wrist; hand supported also.
- US guidance for this injection is not needed.
- Sit opposite the patient so their arm and hand is pointing towards your own position.
- Advance the needle at 30–45° to the skin towards the hand for about 2 cm (i.e. towards you).
- Improvement of neurogenic symptoms can be gained with hydrocortisone 25 mg but most rheumatologists will use triamcinolone 20 mg or methylprednisolone acetate 20 mg.
- Do not use lidocaine.
- If the palmaris tendon is present, the injection should be sited just medial (i.e. closer to the 'little finger') to the midline, by about 1cm.
- There should be no resistance on injection or nerve pain (see ➋ Plate 12).

### Extensor pollicis brevis/abductor pollicis longus

De Quervain's tenosynovitis should be injected at the point of maximal tenderness, advancing the needle through the tendon sheath at a very shallow angle to the skin, along the line of the tendon rather than at 90° to the tendon.

- For functional anatomy and clinical assessment please, see ➋ 'Wrist pain in adults', pp. 106–10.
- Inject 25mg hydrocortisone initially. If a second injection is required, consider either using methylprednisolone or asking for a US-guided injection.
- A US can also rule out other lesions of the wrist and tendon area (e.g. ganglia, carpal bone disruption, lateral wrist compartment synovitis, 1st CMCJ synovial cyst, etc.).

### The small hand joints

The small joints of the hand are frequently affected by synovitis in patients with chronic inflammatory arthritis. Excess joint fluid and capsule extension and thickening can be confirmed by US. Effusions are usually under high pressure, though cannot easily be aspirated without a large-gauge needle. Use of the latter, however, is somewhat brutal and is best not attempted except under anaesthetic.

- US to confirm joint synovitis is often very useful and there are specific diagnostic signs potentially available with it (e.g. double contour sign in detecting MSU crystals in gout and calcium pyrophosphate deposits in CPPD arthritis).
- The MCPJs and PIPJs will normally 'accept' 0.5–1 mL of injected fluid (e.g. 0.5 mL triamcinolone acetonide or methylprednisolone (20 mg) and 0.5 mL 1% lidocaine).
- For MCPJ injection, ensure the patient's forearm and hand are supported. Sit opposite the patient.
- Use a small 23- or 25-gauge needle and 'run' the needle under the skin parallel to the finger just to the side of the metacarpal head (Fig. 24.1), away from you but aiming very slightly towards the metacarpal head—envisage entering the needle under the distended joint capsule and in this way, avoid contacting the bone (which will be painful). Look for a subcutaneous bleb appearing (a sign of not getting the injection into the joint).

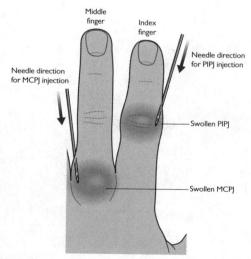

**Fig. 24.1** Direction of needle access to a swollen metacarpophalangeal joint (MCPJ) or proximal interphalangeal joint (PIPJ). Synovitis swells the joint capsule which can be accessed by running the needle virtually parallel with the digit but slightly angled.

- Using the same needle access point but angling the needle appropriately, two MCPJs can be accessed in the one procedure (but plan this and fill the syringe with appropriate amount of steroid/lidocaine).
- The approach to a PIPJ is probably best undertaken from the ulnar side of the digit but the technique is similar to MCPJ injection.
- The small joint injections can cause discomfort and so advise icing and NSAID use in the post-injection period for 2–3 days.
- As always with joint injections, advise against mobilizing the joint too much in the first few days after injection.

# The hip and periarticular lesions

## Hip joint

Hip injection is not a routine outpatient procedure. Aspiration and injection of the joint either under US or fluororadiographic guidance is recommended.

## Greater trochanter pain syndrome

Pain at and around the greater trochanter may be due to referred lumbosacral pain, gluteus medius (or other tendon) tear or insertional tendonitis/enthesitis, or a local bursitis. Lesions can coexist.

- Imaging to confirm the lesion and to rule out a tendon tear—when an injection would be contraindicated—is advisable.
- Trochanteric bursitis or enthesitis at this site, however, often responds well to local steroid injection.
- US-guided injection is preferable as the inflamed tissue is deep and 'blind' injection placement may be quite inaccurate.
- However, occasionally 'blind' injection is appropriate.
- The patient should lie on their side with knees drawn up and the most tender area located with markers—e.g. with pen on the skin.
- The usual point of maximum tenderness in gluteus medius enthesitis is just posterior and high to the greater trochanter apex.
- The site of injection is at the point of maximal tenderness.
- The injection target is deep and therefore a pragmatic approach using a large volume is sensible (e.g. 5–10 mL).
- Use 20–40 mg triamcinolone or methylprednisolone (thus 1–2 mL) and then diluted with sterile saline or 1% lidocaine.
- Injection failure should raise the possibility of poor needle position thus US-guidance on a second injection attempt is advisable.

## Other lesions around the pelvis and hip

- Meralgia paraesthetica occurs as a consequence of lateral cutaneous nerve entrapment (see ➲ Chapter 3) as it traverses the fascia 10 cm below and medial to the anterior superior iliac spine. If this spot can be clearly demarcated because of localized tenderness, steroid injection has a greater chance of success.
- The ischial tuberosities are located deep in the medial side of the buttocks. The hamstring entheses or overlying bursae can become inflamed, causing pain on sitting. These tender points can be injected. The differential diagnosis is coccidynia.
- The coccyx can be palpated with the patient prone or lying on their side) and is amenable to local anaesthetic and steroid injection.
- Adductor enthesitis/insertional tendonitis is amenable to steroid injection but is technically difficult. Imaging initially is essential as there is a differential diagnosis—which includes symphysitis, osteitis pubis, ischiopubis fracture, inguinal hernia, and medial hip joint lesions. An inflamed symphysis pubis is best injected under US guidance.

# The knee and periarticular lesions

### The knee joint

Knee joints are, with appropriate training and experience, straightforward to access with a needle without imaging guidance.

- Access to the joint is perhaps simplest by the lateral approach so the procedure does not have to take place 'over' the patient's other leg/ knee, and the person undertaking the procedure can sit comfortably without having to reach over the patient.
- The patient should be supine and comfortable with support under the knee (which may not, when there is an effusion, be able to extend fully and rest on the couch).
- Mark a point about a third of the way down the patella but midway between the upper and lower parts of the leg—this should be where an effusion will 'balloon' out because of pressure distribution within the joint, and thus be most easily accessed.
- A wide-gauge needle is most appropriate given aspiration of synovial fluid is often also required for symptom relief and diagnostics.
- If the procedure may be long because of anticipation that a large volume of fluid will need to be aspirated, then consider anesthetizing the skin and subcutaneous tissues first.
- The needle is advanced at 90° to the skin surface (see ➔ Plate 19).
- A joint effusion should be reached, in all but the most obese patients, within 2 cm. A common mistake that inexperienced operators can make is to insert the needle too far and cause pain by hitting the femur or patella bone with the needle.
- If sepsis or crystal arthritis is suspected, send a sample of fluid for microscopy and culture, and polarized light microscopy, respectively.
- If a sample is needed to assess for infection, take great care to harvest the sample in a sterile way—with the aid of an assistant to help collect the sample in a sterile pot.
- Aspirate the joint to dryness or until aspiration becomes difficult. Try not to reposition the needle too many times as this will cause trauma and bleeding—effusions with PsA and infection can be large (e.g. author's personal record is 300 mL from a TB effusion!).
- Access to the joint space may be improved, and greater fluid removal facilitated, by pressing on the medial side of the knee and pressing on, and tilting, the patella with your other hand.
- Disengage the needle from the syringe and re-attach the syringe containing steroid: 40 mg triamcinolone or methylprednisolone is appropriate for most size joints and conditions—but add perhaps 5 mL of either sterile saline or 1% lidocaine because the joint space is potentially quite large.
- The efficacy of a steroid injection may relate to the amount of rest following the procedure—avoidance of weight-bearing on a flexed knee for example. Advise 48 hours rest ideally.
- Icing and NSAID use for 24 hours after the procedure may ease discomfort associated with the procedure.
- Consider follow-up physiotherapy if there is poor extension range and/o quadriceps wasting associated with chronicity of the knee synovitis.

### Knee periarticular injections

- Prepatellar bursitis, patellar ligament enthesitis, pes anserinus enthesitis or bursitis, and trigger points around the knee may all respond to local steroid and anaesthetic.
- US scanning to confirm diagnosis may reasonably be combined with a US-guided procedure but the details of this need to be agreed with an appropriate radiologist in advance.
- Popliteal cysts can be directly aspirated and injected but due to the risk of damaging superficial neurovascular structures, should be done under US guidance.

# The ankle and foot

## Ankle and subtalar joints and tarsal tunnel

The ankle joint can sometimes be accessed without US guidance though the technique is difficult when affected by the common occurrence of subcutaneous oedema.

- The ankle joint is located most easily with the patient supine on a couch and whole leg rested and supported.
- The joint line can be palpated just lateral to the extensor digitorum tendon as it crosses the ankle crease.
- The needle is initially advanced downwards over the dome of the talus and parallel to the sole of the foot for about 1–2 cm in most cases— when there is an effusion, the swelling will balloon out/forward towards this point.
- It is quite frequent to hit bone with the needle so caution in needle placement is advised (see ➲ Plate 20a).
- It is unusual to be able to aspirate fluid from an ankle joint though a small volume is accessible with a larger-gauge needle. The ankle is a common joint to be affected by gout and CPPD arthritis so sending any sample for PLM is appropriate.
- For an inflammatory ankle arthritis, 40 mg of triamcinolone or methylprednisolone acetate with 2–3 mL of 1% lidocaine is typical.
- Advise elevation, rest, and icing post procedure and avoiding all but necessary weight-bearing for 48 hours.
- Subtalar joint can be affected by synovitis and infection but accessing the joint without US guidance is very difficult.
- The tarsal tunnel (see ➲ Plate 20b) is injected under the flexor retinaculum between the calcaneum and the medial malleolus.

## Plantar fasciitis

The origin of the plantar fascia at the medial calcaneal tubercle of the os calcis is frequently affected by recurrent trauma and inflammation. The latter occurs commonly in axSpA, PsA, reactive (SpA-associated) arthritis, and IBD-related arthritis.

- The plantar fascia origin is injected from the medial side after carefully localizing the position of maximal pain (see ➲ Plate 20c).
- Never inject through the sole of the foot (i.e. at 90° to the skin) but a point of needle entry at the medial edge of the foot, angled towards the point of maximal tenderness may be optimal.
- Some clinicians will numb the area with local anaesthetic injection of the posterior tibial nerve, in the tarsal tunnel (see ➲ Plate 20b).
- Use 40 mg triamcinolone acetonide or methylprednisolone mixed with 1–2 mL of 1% lidocaine.
- Advise post-procedure foot elevation, restricting of weight-bearing, and icing if the heel is sore.
- Many rheumatologists will consider it appropriate to offer a second injection if the first is only partly helpful. Allow 4–6 weeks to tell if the first injection has been satisfactorily effective or not.

## Small joints of the feet

- The MTPJs are injected most easily via the dorsal approach (20 mg triamcinolone or methylprednisolone) through the toe web.
- The needle is directed towards the appropriate metatarsal head.
- The same technique is used to inject around an interdigital neuroma (Morton's neuroma).
- Care should be taken with sterilizing the skin prior to the procedure as there is a particular risk of infection after the procedure.

# Rheumatological emergencies

# Septic arthritis

Infection in a joint can progress rapidly, causing tissue destruction, permanent deformity, and disability. When septic arthritis is suspected, investigation and antibiotic initiation should be prompt, and where feasible, infected tissue resected. The epidemiology and aetiopathogenesis of septic arthritis is reported in ➔ Chapter 17.

## Septic arthritis: in adults

- Patients may not appear systemically unwell, so a high index of clinical suspicion is required.
- Septic arthritis is more common in patients with established joint disease, prosthetic joints, and where there are comorbidities such as diabetes, chronic renal disease, immunosuppression, and IV drug abuse.
- *Staphylococcus* and *Streptococcus* are the most common pathogens. Septic arthritis from *Haemophilus influenzae* type b is becoming rare due to vaccination programmes.
- Crystal arthropathy and cellulitis are differential diagnoses.
- Consider primary or secondary infective endocarditis in high-risk cases, (e.g. IV drug users and prosthetic/diseased cardiac valves).
- Gonococcal arthritis is the most common cause of monoarthritis in a young, sexually active adult; women during menstruation may be at particular risk. Disseminated gonococcal infection may present as a clinical triad of pustular skin lesions, tenosynovitis, or migratory arthralgias. The cutaneous manifestations are fleeting and are not required to make this diagnosis.

## Septic arthritis: in children

- Diagnosis is considered if there is high or spiking fever, loss of weight bearing or limp, or joint swelling. There may be focal bony tenderness if there is associated osteomyelitis (especially in infants).
- Most cases occur in young children (50% of cases aged <2 years).
- The lower limb is involved in 75% of cases (knee > hip > ankle). The shoulder is a commonly affected site.
- Presentation depends on organism and host immunity. Infants may have few signs and not appear unwell or pyrexial.
- Although >2 joints may be affected, this is rare, and alterative diagnoses should be considered, e.g. JIA.
- The yield from joint/bone aspirate and biopsy is poor.
- *Staphylococcus aureus* is the most common cause in children, but community-acquired methicillin-resistant *Staphylococcus aureus* (MRSA-CA) is increasingly common. Consider other pathogens by age:
  - Neonates: *Escherichia coli* and group B streptococci.
  - 2 months to 5y group A Strep, and *Strep. pneumoniae*.
  - Adolescents: *Neisseria gonorrhoeae*.
- *Mycobacterium tuberculosis* is an increasingly recognized, albeit rare cause of chronic pyogenic arthritis. Mantoux and an IFNγ release assay (IGRA) should be done in high-risk cases.
- Consider *Haemophilus influenzae* type B in non-vaccinated children.

- Viral-induced transient synovitis of the hip is an important differential diagnosis. It is a benign condition, far more common than septic arthritis of the hip, presenting with hip pain, impaired mobility, apyrexia, and without systemic upset.

## Immediate management of septic arthritis in adults

- Joint immobilization, analgesia, and fluid resuscitation if septic.
- Laboratory testing (FBC, U&E, creatinine, LFT, ESR, and CRP) and blood cultures.
- Complete joint drainage synovial fluid analysis with Gram stain, culture, and polarized light microscopy.
- Joint fluid with a white blood cell count >50,000/mm³ (mainly neutrophils) and a glucose <400 mg/L is highly suggestive of infection (see ➲ Chapter 17).
- If crystals are evident, and cultures are negative after 48 hours, a diagnosis of a crystal arthropathy should be considered (see ➲ Chapter 7).
- Antibiotic therapy initiation immediately after joint samples have been obtained. Culture and sensitivity results may change antibiotic therapy as they become available, but broad-spectrum IV therapy should be given initially.
- Joints with implants or prostheses should not be aspirated without prior discussion with an orthopaedic specialist, and should only be aspirated in sterile theatre environments; ideally prior to antibiotic administration.
- For a non-gonococcal septic arthritis, seek orthopaedic input for joint washout, and microbiology input to arrange a Gram stain of joint fluid and set up cultures/special tests for atypical organisms (especially for a septic arthritis resistant to empiric antibiotics).
- Empiric antibiotic treatment in the absence of a positive Gram stain in adults in a straightforward clinical scenario should be guided by local policies; some examples regimens are detailed as follows:
  - Common regimens include flucloxacillin 2 g IV four times a day ± gentamicin IV or a third-generation cephalosporin.
  - In cases of suspected MRSA infection, discussion with microbiology and consideration of vancomycin is advised.
  - *Pseudomonas* spp. should be suspected in IV drug users (Table 25.1) and treated with cephalosporin IV with an aminoglycoside (e.g. gentamicin 3–5 mg/kg IV).
  - For further information see ➲ Chapter 17.

## Management of septic arthritis in children

Follows a similar line to adults and includes a hip ultrasound in children if the cause of the limp is not obvious. IV antibiotics and analgesia will depend on local policies, but as a guide according to age (see Table 25.1 and Table 25.2) the following are recommended

- <3 months old: IV cefotaxime and amoxicillin.
- 3 months: 5 years old: IV cefuroxime.
- >5 years old: IV flucloxacillin

Table 25.1 Post-immediate management of septic arthritis in children

| Diagnostic status | Management |
| --- | --- |
| Diagnosis not confirmed Clinically improved | Splint and continue IV antibiotic 1–2 weeks Then switch to oral co-amoxiclav for a total treatment of 4–6 weeks according to clinical condition |
| Confirmed diagnosis (pus ± 50,000 leucocytes ± pathogen isolated in blood or synovial fluid) | Splint and continue IV antibiotic 1–2 weeks and adjust based on culture/susceptibility Then switch to oral co-amoxiclav for a total treatment of 4–6 weeks according to clinical condition and pathogen Weekly clinical and laboratory follow-up |
| Diagnosis not confirmed Clinically not improved | Review antibiotics Obtain paediatric infectious disease specialist advice Further evaluation to consider other types of non-infectious arthritis |

Table 25.2 Summary of antibiotics by age group

| | |
| --- | --- |
| Neonate (<3 months) | Benzylpenicillin and gentamicin Or cefotaxime Add amoxicillin if listeria suspected Oral switch to co-amoxiclav |
| 3 months–5 years | Cefuroxime Oral switch to cefalexin or co-amoxiclav |
| >5 years | Flucloxacillin or clindamycin Consider ceftazidime or ciprofloxacin if pseudomonas suspected Oral switch to co-amoxiclav suspension or flucloxacillin or clindamycin tablets |

Reproduced from Watts et al. (2013) *Oxford Textbook of Rheumatology* with permission from Oxford University Press.

## Post-immediate management of septic arthritis in adults

- Regular analgesia review.
- Assess for multiple foci of infection.
- Discontinue any immunosuppressants, but consider stress-dose glucocorticoids (GCs) if the patient is systemically unwell and has been on long-term GCs.
- Adjust antibiotics according to culture sensitivities and in discussion with an infectious disease specialist.

- For affected weight-bearing joints, keep non-weight-bearing until there is obvious improvement in pain and swelling, and you are confident the patient is on appropriate antimicrobials.
- Physical therapists should be involved early to help passive mobilization of joint before patient weight-bears.
- The evidence for routine duration of antibiotic course is not strong and the regimen should be tailored to the individual. A common protocol is IV antibiotics for 1–2 weeks, followed by oral antibiotics for 2–4 weeks.
- Reasons for limited/no response to treatment can include:
  - Alternative diagnosis. Consider crystal-induced MSK disease (see ⧓ Chapter 7), RA (see ➔ Chapter 5), and spondyloarthritis (see ⧓ Chapter 8).
  - Concomitant crystal-induced MSK disease, reactive arthritis, foreign body, or flare of underlying arthritis, e.g. RA.
  - Inappropriate antimicrobial choice for an atypical organism (e.g. *Mycobacterium marinum, Borrelia,* fungus) or multiple infecting organisms (see ➔ Chapter 17).
  - Secondary osteomyelitis—especially if treatment had been delayed (see ➔ Chapter 17).
  - Surgical lavage may need to be repeated, and surgical synovectomy considered. Recalcitrant cases may require joint excision ± subsequent arthroplasty.

## Gonococcal septic arthritis

- Synovial fluid and blood cultures can be negative. If gonococcal infection suspected, re-culture blood but also urethra, cervix (80–90% positive), rectum, pharynx, any skin pustules, and joint fluid.
- Urine can be tested for gonococcal nucleic acid by PCR.
- Treatment should be guided by local policies but a common regimen is ceftriaxone 1 g IM or IV every 24 hours. An oral switch can be considered after 24–48 hours when clinical improvement is seen. Treatment should continue for 7 days.
- Due to increasing organism microbial resistance, treatment with ciprofloxacin is no longer advisable.
- Consider empiric therapy for *Chlamydia* with doxycycline 100 mg for 7 days or one dose of azithromycin 1 g, and concurrent testing for HIV and syphilis.
- All sexual partners should receive one dose of ceftriaxone 125 mg IM and empiric treatment for *Chlamydia*.

# Infections in patients on biologics

- Over the last 10 years, immunosuppressants that specifically inhibit the actions of TNFα, Il-6, and T cells, and deplete B cells have become widely used to treat multiple rheumatic diseases (see → Chapter 23).
- The risk of infections is increased with use of these 'biologic' drugs, although is probably greater with anti-TNFα agents than other classes. Patients with a history of serious infections should be treated with this class of drug with extreme caution and vigilance.
- The risk and severity of infections may be increased in those also taking other immunosuppressants, typically MTX or GCs.

## Common pathogens

- Patients are at particular risk for tuberculosis (TB).
- Disseminated fungal and viral infections can occur (Table 25.3).
- Reactivation of latent infections may be a particular problem.

Table 25.3 Organisms and infections reported with biologics

| Organisms | | Nature of infection |
|---|---|---|
| Bacteria | Mycobacterium tuberculosis | Disseminated Pulmonary |
| | Atypical mycobacteria | |
| | Listeria | Septicaemia Septic arthritis Meningitis |
| | Staphylococcus | Septicaemia Cavitating pneumonia |
| | Salmonella | Septicaemia Septic arthritis |
| | Moraxella | Septic arthritis |
| | Actinobacillus | Septic arthritis |
| | Nocardia | Respiratory tract |
| Viruses | Varicella | Disseminated |
| | Herpes simplex | Severe |
| | Hepatitis B/C | Reactivation |
| | CMV | Disseminated |
| Fungi/yeasts | Candida | Septicaemia |
| | Cryptococcus | Pneumonia |
| | Aspergillus | Disseminated |
| | Sporothrix | Skin |
| | Pneumocystis | Pneumonia |
| | Histoplasmosis | Disseminated |
| Parasites | Leishmania | Visceral |

- Latent histoplasmosis should be considered in patients from endemic regions or with a history of potential exposure (e.g. caving/potholing, construction).
- Listeriosis should be considered in the context of unpasteurized dairy consumption.

## Tuberculosis and its risk

Reports of TB occurring with biologics advocate taking precautions:
- Screen for latent TB prior to initiation of therapy.
- Screen people who travel to endemic areas and healthcare workers.
- Screen using intradermal injection of PPD and CXR given the possibility of anergy.
- With PPD injection, induration of ≥5 mm should be considered a positive response for most patients with rheumatic disease.
- If active TB is found, patients should be treated as per the British Thoracic Society Guideline and treatment should be postponed until ≥2 months of anti-TB therapy has been received.
- Reactivation of TB should be considered in biologic-treated febrile patients and those not screened for TB before biologic treatment.
- Patients may need a longer than normal course of antibiotics and need careful reassessment before restarting therapy.

## Varicella infections

- If a patient on a biologic, or a household contact, develops primary varicella (chickenpox), then varicella immunity should be checked.
- People not immune and at significant risk of infection should be given varicella zoster immunoglobulin within 72 hours. This will provide temporary immunity.
- If a patient develops shingles, standard treatment should be given and the biologic withheld.

# Acute systemic lupus erythematosus

Acute systemic lupus erythematosus (SLE) will manifest either as a flare in patients with an established diagnosis or as the first presentation of the disease. Declining C3 and increasing dsDNA titres may predict acute disease flares in some patients. The reader is referred to ➔ Chapter 13 for SLE and to ➔ Chapter 11 for antiphospholipid syndrome (APS) and catastrophic APS.

## Diagnosing SLE in an acute medical context

- Consider SLE as a diagnosis in all young and middle-aged women who present with a history of joint pain, photosensitive rash, or pleuritic chest pain.
- Raynaud's disease (RD) and recurrent mouth ulcers are non-specific, but may also appear in association with SLE.
- ANA serology and complement levels may not be available at initial assessment.
- Inflammatory markers such as the ESR or CRP are not reliable indicators of SLE activity.
- Although pericardial effusions are common with SLE, they are generally trivial. Cardiac tamponade is found in <1% of patients. Since the effusion tends to reflect the overall disease state, generally treatment of the underlying disease is adequate to resolve the effusion. Rarely, therapeutic pericardiocentesis is required.

## Acute renal SLE (adults)

- Check the BP, send blood for creatinine, U&E, send urine for culture, a spot urine protein/creatinine ratio (as an estimate of proteinuria) and organize a renal tract US to rule out post-renal obstruction.
- Quantification of urinary protein and creatinine grades severity of the renal lesion and guides management approach (Fig. 25.1).
- Control BP aggressively. Use an ACE inhibitor or ARB for those with proteinuria.
- Biopsy can inform treatment decisions. Induction treatment is usually given with GCs and oral mycophenolate mofetil (titrate to 1–1.5 g twice daily) or IV cyclophosphamide.
- GC-induced osteoporosis and cardiovascular risk should be managed from the outset. Consider getting the following done early: DXA scan, ECG, and fasting lipid panel.
- Daily calcium (1000–1500 mg) and vitamin D (800 IU) should be administered to all patients receiving GCs.
- With cyclophosphamide, there is a need to counsel patients about the risks of infertility, malignancy, and haemorrhagic cystitis, the dosing schedules (e.g. using mesna), monitoring (FBC at day 10 after and prior to IV pulse), and *Pneumocystis* prophylaxis chemotherapy (e.g. trimethoprim-sulfamethoxazole; Fig. 25.1).

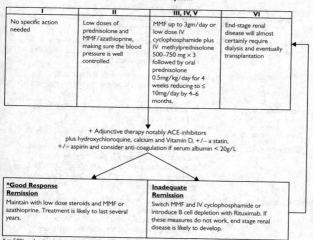

Fig 25.1 Flow diagram of the management of renal systemic lupus erythematosus based on our own practice. Reproduced from Watts et al. (2013) *Oxford Textbook of Rheumatology* with permission from Oxford University Press.

## Acute cardiorespiratory SLE (adults)

- Cardiac and isolated pulmonary manifestations of SLE are rare and in many patients with SLE, acute cardiac and pulmonary features may be due to other common conditions (Table 25.4).
- CRP elevation may reflect infection or significant pleuropericardial SLE. Lupus pericarditis alone without evidence of cardiac compromise can be treated with NSAIDs and prednisone 20–40 mg daily for 2–4 weeks with subsequent GC dose taper.
- If not due to cardiac failure, acute dyspnoea in SLE may be due to intercurrent infection, pneumonitis, pulmonary vasculitis, pulmonary embolism, pulmonary hypertension, or dyspnoea from the pain of pleural serositis.
- Cyclophosphamide should be considered for severe or life-threatening manifestations of SLE.

**Table 25.4** Important aspects in management of acute cardio-respiratory SLE (adults)

| | |
|---|---|
| Initial clinical cardiac assessment | ECG, blood for CK, troponin T, echo |
| Initial lung assessments | ABGs, CXR, spirometry, HRCT chest, VQ scan |
| Consider pulmonary embolus | Consider empirical anticoagulation early and check for lupus anticoagulant, APL antibodies, and complete thrombophilia screen |
| Pulmonary vasculitis (very rare) | Features: severe dyspnoea, CXR abnormal. Requires ICU and respiratory physician support and consider plasma exchange |
| Interstitial lung disease | Requires high-dose steroids and either cyclophosphamide, azathioprine, or mycophenolate mofetil |
| Antiphospholipid syndrome | PE-associated with APL syndrome in SLE requires lifelong anticoagulation |
| **Specific therapies** | |
| Glucocorticoids | Assuming non-viral infections excluded or treated most cardiopulmonary SLE features respond to oral prednisone 0.5–1 mg/kg/day. Consider methylprednisolone 1 g IV × 3 days if clinical situation extreme |
| Mycophenolate | Mycophenolate mofetil (0.5 mg twice daily initially increasing after 1–2 weeks to 1–1.5 g twice daily) can be considered if AZA or cyclophosphamide contraindicated or patient intolerant. It is increasingly being used instead of cyclophosphamide for inducing remission in lupus nephritis |
| Anti-CD20 | Though evidence minimal, rituximab (anti-CD20) 1 g infusion repeated after 2 weeks may be considered if other immunosuppressants are contraindicated or cause side effects |
| Fragility fracture/ osteoporosis prevention | All patients treated with GCs require daily calcium (1 g) and vitamin D (800 IU). For all >50 yrs a bisphosphonate should be offered initially (and withdrawn if DXA scan and overall fracture risk assessment (e.g. FRAX) suggests fracture risk is low. Local guidelines may exist |

## Acute haematological SLE (adults)

- Many patients with SLE are Coombs (direct antiglobulin) test positive without having haemolysis (and do not need treating as such).
- Features of haemolysis include fever, shivers, pyrexia, anaemia, elevated bilirubin in serum and urine, low serum haptoglobins, and reticulocytosis.

- Acute thrombocytopenia is a relatively frequent presentation.
- If severe, both haemolytic anaemia (Hb <70 mg/L) and thrombocytopenia (platelets <25,000) require high-dose prednisone 60–80 mg/day and AZA or CYC (pulsed IV or oral).

## Acute renal SLE (paediatrics)

- The most common lesion is Class IV diffuse proliferative glomerulonephritis (30–45% of cases), and carries the worst prognosis.
- One-third of children with acute renal SLE have hypertension which often needs aggressive management.
- All have microscopic haematuria and proteinuria >3 mg/kg/day. Most have >25 mg/kg/day proteinuria. Up to 33% have serum albumin >35 g/L. About 50% maintain GFR >100 mL/min/1.73 m².
- Prognosis and therapy of nephritis is guided by the histopathology active ISN-grade pathological lesion and chronicity index, thus obtaining a biopsy is important.
- Management should be in a specialist unit, and includes high-dose GCs and MMF 600mg/m² BD. In some cases IV CYC uitilising the low- or high- dose Eurolupus protocol is used for induction or flare of lupus nephritis.
- The value of plasma exchange and IVIg in crescenteric or fulminant renal disease is unclear but its often considered, and dialysis may ultimately be necessary.

## Acute haematological SLE (paediatrics)

- Overt haemolysis occurs in <10%, thrombocytopenia in 15–45%.
- Bleeding is uncommon.
- Autoimmune haemolytic anaemia is treated with oral GCs, but, when there is rapidly progressing anaemia, IV methylprednisolone and IVIg may be needed.
- Most patients with thrombocytopenia respond to oral GCs. If there is active haemorrhage or no response to oral GCs, then IV methylprednisolone and IVIg may be needed.
- Splenectomy should be avoided.
- A high index of suspicion is needed to diagnose catastrophic APS. It is characterized by multiple organ thromboses and microangiopathy.
- Leucopenia usually resolves as disease activity improves.
- If there is neutropenia with infection, granulocyte colony stimulating factor can be used to increase the neutrophil count. If neutropenia is due to drug toxicity and infection is absent, this usually improves with stopping or decreasing the dose of the offending medication.
- Close working with haematologists will assist interpretation of coagulation studies and advise on anticoagulant use including factor 10a inhibitors.

# Systemic vasculitis

A vasculitis flare should be treated aggressively because permanent damage from tissue ischaemia may occur rapidly. Patients diagnosed with pulmonary capillaritis or glomerulonephritis will typically benefit from treatment with pulse GCs. The specific management of each type of vasculitis is outlined in ➜ Chapter 15. See ➜ Table 4.2 p. 212 for precipitants and associations of leucocytoclastic small vessel vasculitis and ➜ Table 4.3 p. 214 for the range of laboratory tests needed in patients with suspected vasculitis.

## Giant cell (temporal) arteritis

- Since giant cell arteritis (GCA) can lead to cranial ischaemic events including blindness and stroke, treat empirically if suspected.
- The prevalence of GCA increases with age. Visual changes, jaw claudication, and diplopia in the setting of B-type symptoms all support the diagnosis of GCA.
- Empiric therapy is with prednisone 40–60 mg daily for 1 month but if there are visual symptoms, urgent ophthalmology examination is essential.
- Ischaemic GCA-related ocular pathology is treated with methylprednisolone 1 g IV for 3 days.
- Daily low-dose aspirin decreases the risk of cranial ischaemic events, and should be used as part of standard therapy unless there is a clear contraindication.
- Treatment should not be delayed. Biopsy is diagnostically useful for up to some weeks after GC therapy is initiated.
- To optimize yield, temporal artery biopsy should be bilateral, with samples >1.5 cm in length.

## 'Severe' vasculitis

- Patients with active vasculitis can quickly develop manifestations that threaten life or the function of a vital organ.
- Patients with a potential flare of vasculitis, already on immunosuppression, need thorough assessment to rule out infection initially—see ➜ Tables 4.2 and 4.3 (p. 212 and p. 214).
- Severe manifestations of the small vessel vasculitides include pulmonary haemorrhage (or capillaritis) and glomerulonephritis. Severe manifestations of medium vessel vasculitis include mononeuritis multiplex (e.g. foot drop/wrist drop) and mesenteric angina/ischaemia.
- When glomerulonephritis is suspected, renal biopsy should always be considered.
- Severe vasculitis is generally treated with pulse methylprednisolone 1 g IV for 3 days, followed by prednisone 1 mg/kg/day.
- Most patients with severe vasculitis will also be treated with cyclophosphamide 1.5–2.0 mg/kg/day. Lower doses should be used in the elderly or in patients with renal insufficiency.

- Plasmapheresis can be life-saving for AAV-related pulmonary vasculitis; not all centres have a facility to give plasmapheresis though.
- Cyclophosphamide places patients at risk for *Pneumocystis* infection, and appropriate chemoprophylaxis should be instituted.
- In patients who decline on clinical grounds, despite immunosuppression, then infections mimicking vasculitis should be considered.

# Systemic sclerosis 'crises'

## Renal crisis

- This may manifest as an acute or subacute hypertensive crisis, usually within the first 4 years after diagnosis of diffuse systemic sclerosis (dcSScl). It can be the presenting feature of SScl (see ➔ Chapter 13). It rarely occurs in limited cutaneous SScl (lcSScl).
- An abrupt increase in BP >150/85 and new renal insufficiency are consistent with this diagnosis. Very occasionally patients are normotensive, and paradoxically subject to a poorer prognosis.
- Other manifestations include those of a hypertensive emergency: microangiopathic haemolytic anaemia, encephalopathy, and hypertensive retinopathy.
- Urinalysis is usually normal.

### Management

- ACE inhibitors are the cornerstone of renal crisis management.
- The patient should be treated with escalating doses of captopril until BP is brought under control. Calcium channel blockers can be added sequentially if captopril is inadequate.
- Fast drops in BP should be avoided, as low perfusion pressures in abnormal renal vessels may worsen renal failure.
- Early consulting with a nephrologist about the potential need for haemodialysis is prudent.
- Prompt initial treatment can lead to return of good renal function.

## Pulmonary hypertension crisis

(See also ➔ Chapter 13.)

- Primary pulmonary arterial hypertension (PAH) occurs as a complication of lcSScl, although it can also occur in dcSScl (both as a primary feature and secondary to pulmonary fibrosis).
- Echocardiography can be used to screen for PAH. A RVSP estimate of >40 mmHg is suggestive, but the diagnosis must be confirmed by right heart catheterization.
- Decompensated PAH presents with dyspnoea, syncope, raised JVP, loud P2 heart sound, and ankle oedema.

### Management

- Intensive coronary care unit monitoring is essential.
- Patients with rapidly decompensating heart failure secondary to PAH should be treated with supplemental oxygen, diuresis.
- Continuous IV epoprostenol can be considered but decreasing cardiac preload too much can reduce overall pulmonary perfusion if the PA is not responsive.
- Diuretics decrease right ventricular preload, and can lead to significant symptomatic relief.
- A large pulmonary embolism can also result in rapidly worsening of PAH, and should be considered contributory if the PAH was known to be high previously, if there is APS and in the appropriate setting.

# Methotrexate-induced pneumonitis

This is rare but can occur in any patient taking methotrexate (MTX).

## Epidemiology and risk factors

- Incidence 5–70 per 1000 patients per year taking MTX. It is probably much rarer in children/adolescents compared with adults.
- Life-threatening pneumonitis requiring hospital admission occurs in <1% patients taking MTX.
- Mild pneumonitis likely resolves on drug withdrawal alone.
- Most patients suffering from pneumonitis do so within the first few months of starting MTX or after a significant dose change.
- In patients on stable-dose MTX, blood levels may change in the setting of progressive renal insufficiency or low levels of folate.
- Consider the diagnosis in all patients on MTX with acute onset of dry cough, dyspnoea, headache, and fever.
- The differential diagnosis lies between chest infection, acute pulmonary oedema, or acute interstitial lung disease associated with the underlying condition.

## Management of severe toxicity

- Stop MTX.
- Intensive respiratory care is not often needed but should be considered. Severe cases need supplemental oxygen and blood transfusion.
- Assess for infection. Consider bronchoalveolar lavage for samples and high-resolution lung CT. It may be necessary to treat empirically for the most likely pathogens, while awaiting results.
- Optimal therapy for MTX-induced pneumonitis has not been well defined. Folinic acid (15–25 mg orally four times a day) may reverse MTX toxicity.
- Anecdotally, GCs accelerate recovery. In cases of severe respiratory decompensation, treat with methylprednisolone 1 g IV for 3 days, followed by prednisone 1 mg/kg/day. Prednisone can be tapered over the subsequent 1–6 months, depending on disease severity.
- Most patients with MTX-induced lung injury will recover, but may have chronic lung damage as a result.

# Macrophage activation syndrome

Macrophage activation syndrome (MAS) is rare but is life-threatening (mortality is 8–22%). MAS can complicate other diseases. MAS is also termed secondary haemophagocytic lymphohistiocytosis (HLH). For a summary, see ℘ http://www.the-rheumatologist.org/article/macrophage-activation-syndrome/6/

## Pathology

- Activated macrophages engulf other haematopoietic cells in the bone marrow, liver, and spleen.
- Polyclonal T- and NK-cell activation is associated with a cytokine 'storm' with consequent extensive immunological abnormalities.

## Presentation and clinical features

- A high level of suspicion remains key to MAS diagnosis as it may present insidiously in an already unwell child.
- Unremitting fever and high levels of persistent inflammation despite broad-spectrum antibiotics or an unexpected fall in ESR associated with new-onset cytopenia and hyperferritinaemia should raise suspicion of MAS.
- MAS can be the initial presentation or a complication of oncologic, infectious, and rheumatic disorders, including systemic-onset JIA, SLE, and Kawasaki disease and less commonly juvenile DM, PAN, polyarticular JIA, MCTD, and other autoimmune and autoinflammatory conditions.
- Sepsis should be considered as a cause.
- Infective triggers of MAS include EBV, VZV, CMV, coxsackievirus, parvovirus B19, hepatitis A, *Salmonella*, and enterococcus.
- If MAS is the initial presentation of an inflammatory illness, assessment should be made for malignancy.
- By contrast to MAS/secondary HLH, *primary* HLH is usually seen in children <2 years old, with consanguineous parents. There may be a history of death of young family member with unexplained fever, and a primary central nervous system presentation.

## Diagnosis

Clinical features are not specific for diagnosis. Combinations of typical features are often present and high suspicion for the diagnosis remains important; see Table 25.5.

- New diagnostic criteria for MAS in the context of active SoJIA[1] include:
  - Ferritin >684 ng/mL.
  - Plus ≥2 of the following: platelet count <181 × 10$^9$/L, AST >48 U/L, triglycerides >156 mg/dL, fibrinogen <360 mg/dL.
- The value of testing for CD25 and CD163 positive circulating lymphocytes, low NK-cell activity, haemophagocytosis in bone marrow, liver, spleen, or lymph nodes, high D-dimer, and abnormal perforin expression, is debatable.

**Table 25.5** Clinical and laboratory features of macrophage activation syndrome

| Clinical signs | Laboratory findings |
| --- | --- |
| • High, persistent, unremitting fever or change in pattern of fever | • Low/falling ESR in context of active inflammatory disease or high CRP |
| • New-onset hepatosplenomegaly | • Low/rapidly falling white blood cells, Hb, or platelet count |
| • Neurological manifestations including irritability | • Low/falling or unexpectedly normal platelet count |
| • Lymphadenopathy | • Low/falling or unexpected normal fibrinogen |
| • New-onset heart, lung, or kidney failure | • Rising AST, ALT, GGT, bilirubin, triglycerides and LDH |
| • Petechiae or haemorrhages | • Ferritin higher than would be expected for patient's diagnosis |

*Haemophagocytosis in the bone marrow aspirate is present in 60% of MAS cases, and tends to be a relatively late sign. Absence of haemophagocytosis does not rule out MAS.*

## Treatment

- Treatment should be started promptly as delayed treatment is associated with poor prognosis.
- Broad-spectrum antibiotic treatment is usually started in cases other than those with active autoimmune conditions.
- First-line treatment of IV then oral GCs is effective in >50% of cases. For example: methylprednisolone 30 mg/kg/day (maximum 1 g) for 3 consecutive days, followed by oral prednisolone 1 mg/kg/day and then dose tapering.
- If there is a poor response to steroids, IVIg 1–2g/kg is recommended.
- IL-1 inhibition (e.g. anakinra) is dramatically effective in MAS associated with SoJIA (and increases survival rate vs placebo in *adult* sepsis + MAS features). Anakinra is given SC or IV 2–8 mg/Kg/day (max 100mg/ dose) in 1–4 divided doses.
- In refractory disease other options include anti-IL-6r (tocilizumab), anti-TNFα, etoposide, rituximab (anti-CD20+ B-cell therapy) for EBV-driven MAS, and cyclophosphamide in SLE-associated MAS.

## Reference

1. Ravelli A, Minoia F, Davì S, et al. 2016 Classification Criteria for Macrophage Activation Syndrome Complicating Systemic Juvenile Idiopathic Arthritis: A European League Against Rheumatism/ American College of Rheumatology/Paediatric Rheumatology International Trials Organisation Collaborative Initiative. *Ann Rheum Dis* 2016;75:481–9.

# Paediatric osteomyelitis

In children, osteomyelitis is most common in infants; 50% of cases occur before 5 years of age.

- There is usually a history of trauma, typically involving the metaphysis of long bones.
- Osteomyelitis can arise from haematogenous spread of pathogens from a primary site (e.g. lung, skin ear, nose, or throat) or by direct inoculation from open fractures or penetrating wounds.
- There are acute, subacute (2–3 weeks' delay), chronic (rare in children), and non-bacterial (e.g. CRMO or SAPHO) forms of osteomyelitis (see also ➔ Chapter 17).

# Malignancies presenting with musculoskeletal symptoms in children

## Causes

The annual incidence of primary malignant tumours of bone, synovium, or muscle is 6 per 1 million children. The main causes are osteosarcoma (about 50% of cases) and Ewing sarcoma (40–45% of cases).

- Widespread MSK symptoms may of course be from bone metastases from osteosarcoma or Ewing sarcoma.
- Bone marrow infiltration by different lymphoproliferative disorders can present with MSK symptoms.

## Presentation and clinical features

- Malignancy should be suspected, particularly in an adolescent if there is persistent pain of long bones or vertebrae of >2 weeks with associated:
  - point tenderness.
  - night awakening.
  - pain out of proportion for clinical findings.
- Other features can include bony swelling or enlargement, weight loss, malaise, pathological fracture (5–10%), and rarely, lung involvement.
- A mass increasing in size, extending deep into soft tissues, or a presumed exostosis >5 cm, should raise the possibility of malignancy.
- The associated arthritis usually involves large joints, is mild, migratory, and often without morning joint stiffness.

## Investigation and management

- Early referral to a paediatric oncologist is essential.
- Making a diagnosis prior to metastasis greatly enhances the prognosis. Mortality rate following metastasis is 40%.
- Blood tests may show increased inflammatory markers and LDH. FBC is often normal initially, but there may be a reduction trend in platelet count and haemoglobin. A low leucocyte count is a late sign.
- A blood film showing blast cells is pathognomonic for leukaemia.
- A bone marrow aspirate or tissue biopsy provides a histological diagnosis and can facilitate tumour grading.
- Tumour staging is dependent on the diagnosis, histological grade, and both size and location of the tumour.

### Imaging

- Plain radiographs characterize the primary bone tumour.
- US is important to screen for hepatosplenomegaly, lymphadenopathy, and further define soft tissue masses such as lipoma or vascular malformation.
- MRI provides specific information regarding the tumour nature and size and the surrounding soft tissue involvement.
- MRI images facilitate the planning of a biopsy.

- CT helps define tumour anatomy prior to surgery and to evaluate for metastases locally, though bone scintigraphy or whole-body MRI are useful investigations to get an overview of any skeletal metastases.

*Treatment*

- Therapy measures are beyond the scope of the text here. However, for overviews see references 2 and 3 for osteosarcoma and Ewing sarcoma management respectively.

## Other malignancies

Many childhood malignancies have MSK features at presentation, in particular acute lymphoblastic leukaemia (ALL), lymphoma, and neuroblastoma.

- Isolated hip or back involvement in a young child raises the suspicion of leukaemia in the absence of sepsis. Risk factors for leukaemia include conditions such as Down's syndrome.
- Back pain can be a presenting feature of neuroblastoma in young children and toddlers and is attributable to metastases which occur in 75% of patients at diagnosis.
- Limb pain in leukaemia and lymphoma is due to marrow invasion. Pain is usually intense and continuous and associated with night awakening. Local signs, such as arthritis or erythema, may be absent.
- All malignancies can be associated with systemic features such as pallor, petechiae, bruising, weight loss, and fever.
- In lymphoma, there may be hypertrophic osteoarthropathy associated with painful periostitis and lymphadenopathy.
- Investigations should include checking FBC, LDH, LFTs, a blood film, measuring urinary catecholamines/metadrenalines, CXR, and abdominal US.
- Bone marrow aspirate and whole-body MRI are then more definitive investigations.

## References

2. Lindsey BA, Markel JE, Kleinerman ES. Osteosarcoma overview. *Rheumatol Ther* 2017;4:25–43.
3. Kridis WB, Toumi N, Chaari H, et al. A review of Ewing sarcoma treatment: is it still a subject of debate? *Rev Recent Clin Trials* 2017;12:19–23.

# Index

Note: Tables, figures, and boxes are indicated by an italic *t*, *f*, and *b* following the page number.